AGE-RELATED
MACULAR DEGENERATION

AGE-RELATED MACULAR DEGENERATION

EDITORS

D. VIRGIL ALFARO III, MD
Attending Surgeon
Retina Consultants of Charleston
Faculty Advisor
The Citadel
Charleston, South Carolina

ERIC P. JABLON, MD
Partner
Retina Consultants of Charleston
Charleston, South Carolina

JOHN BARNWELL KERRISON, MD
Partner
Retina Consultants of Charleston
Assistant Clinical Professor
Department of Ophthalmology
Medical University of South Carolina
Charleston, South Carolina

KENNETH A. SHARPE, MD
Partner
Retina Consultants of Charleston
Charleston, South Carolina

MONICA RODRIGUEZ FONTAL, MD
Clinical Trial Director
Retina Consultants of Charleston
Charleston, South Carolina

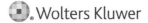
. Wolters Kluwer

Philadelphia • Baltimore • New York • London
Buenos Aires • Hong Kong • Sydney • Tokyo

Acquisitions Editor: Ryan Shaw
Product Development Editor: Kate Marshall
Production Project Manager: Bridgett Dougherty
Senior Manufacturing Coordinator: Beth Welsh
Marketing Manager: Stephanie Manzo
Design Coordinator: Holly McLaughlin
Production Service: SPi Global

Second Edition

Copyright © 2015 by Wolters Kluwer
Two Commerce Square
2001 Market Street
Philadelphia, PA 19103 USA
LWW.com

First Edition © 2006, Lippincott Williams & Wilkins

Printed in China

Library of Congress Cataloging-in-Publication Data
Age-related macular degeneration (Alfaro)
Age-related macular degeneration / editors, D. Virgil Alfaro, III, Eric P. Jablon, John B. Kerrison, Kenneth A. Sharpe, Monica Rodriguez-Fontal. — Second edition.
     p. ; cm.
Includes bibliographical references and index.
ISBN 978-1-4511-5169-5
 I. Alfaro, D. Virgil, III, editor of compilation. II. Jablon, Eric P., editor of compilation. III. Kerrison, John B., editor of compilation. IV. Sharpe, Kenneth A., editor of compilation. V. Rodriguez-Fontal, Monica, editor of compilation. VI. Title.
  [DNLM: 1. Macular Degeneration. 2. Choroidal Neovascularization.   WW 270]
  RE661.D3
  618.97'7735—dc23
                                                        2014000607

To purchase additional copies of this book, call our customer service department at (800) 638-3030 or fax orders to (301) 223-2320. International customers should call (301) 223-2300.

Visit Lippincott Williams & Wilkins on the Internet: at LWW.com. Lippincott Williams & Wilkins customer service representatives are available from 8:30 am to 6 pm, EST.

10 9 8 7 6 5 4 3 2 1

RRS1407

DEDICATION

This textbook is dedicated to Stephen J. Ryan, MD. Steve succumbed to cancer this year, reminding us all of life's fragility and fleeting nature.

Steve's introduction to ophthalmology and retina began at the Wilmer Eye Institute at Johns Hopkins University in the early 1970s. Dr. Edward Maumenee influenced many young ophthalmologists during his tenure as professor and chairman. Dr. Morton F. Goldberg, who was Steve's chief resident and became chairman of the Wilmer Eye Institute, recalls that Steve was a glutton for work and highly motivated to do research. Steve had a severe allergy to cats, rabbits, and other animals; however, this did not impair his research or home life where his landlady had pets. In fact, he wore a surgeon's mask at work in the lab and at home. This illustrates how energetic he was, allowing nothing to get in his way.

Steve served as chief resident at Wilmer and went on to become chairman of ophthalmology at the Los Angeles County Hospital and the University of Southern California School of Medicine.

For nearly 40 years, Steve dedicated his professional life to the University of Southern California and the Doheny Eye Institute. Under his leadership and guidance, the reputation of the institute soared, and it has been listed as one of the top 10 eye centers in the country for two decades.

Steve had many passions in the academic world of ophthalmology, but his name will always be remembered as one considers management of the severely injured eye. Using animal models, he defined the importance of the vitreous as it relates to proliferative vitreoretinopathy after penetrating eye injury. He and his international fellow from Ireland, Paul Cleary, published numerous papers that became widely known as the Ryan-Cleary model of ocular trauma.

As an editor of this textbook, it would be an oversight not to mention the great personal impact that Steve had on my professional life. His compelling personality and ability to affect those whom he trained has had a life-long influence. I have no doubt that there are many, many ophthalmologists around the world who have also been blessed by his mentorship.

D. Virgil Alfaro III, MD

CONTRIBUTORS

D. Virgil Alfaro III, MD
Attending Surgeon
Retina Consultants of Charleston
Faculty Advisor
The Citadel
Charleston, South Carolina

Madhu Amara, MD
University Retina
Oak Forest, Illinois

Gisela Barcat Angelelli, MD
Ophthalmologist
Department of Retina
Santa Lucia Ophthalmologic Hospital
Buenos Aires, Argentina

Richard J. Antcliff, MD, FRCOphth
Consultant Ophthalmic Surgeon
Department of Ophthalmology
Royal United Hospital
Bath, Somerset, England

J. Fernando Arévalo, MD, FACS
Professor
Wilmer Eye Institute
Johns Hopkins University
Baltimore, Maryland
Chief
Vitreoretinal Division
The King Khaled Eye Specialist
   Hospital
Riyadh, Kingdom of Saudi Arabia

Irene A. Barbazetto, MD
Clinical Assistant Professor
Department of Ophthalmology
School of Medicine
New York University
Attending Physician
Department of Ophthalmology
Manhattan Eye and Ear Hospital, NSLIJ
New York, New York

Harit K. Bhatt, MD
Clinical Assistant Professor
Illinois Eye and Ear Infirmary
University of Illinois at Chicago
Chicago, Illinois
Attending Physician/Partner
University Retina and Macula Associates
Bedford Park, Illinois

Antonio López Bolaños, MD
Associate Professor
Department of Retina
Instituto de Oftalmologia
Hospital Conde de Valenciana
Ciudad de México, Mexico

Jamel L. F. Brown, BS, MA
Retina Consultants of Charleston
Ladson, South Carolina

Wissam Charafeddin, MD
Retina Fellow
Retina Department
Centro de Oftalmologia Barraquer
Barcelona, Spain

Yan Chen, PhD
Postdoctoral Fellow
The Vanderbilt Eye Institute
Vanderbilt University
Nashville, Tennessee

Lucienne C. Collet, MD
Admiravisión
Department of Ophthalmology
Barcelona, Spain

Borja F. Corcóstegui, MD
Professor
Department of Ophthalmology
Universitat Autonomous Barcelona
Barcelona, Spain

Michelle L. Crouse, MA
Clinical Trial Coordinator
Retina/Vitreous
Retina Consultants of Charleston
Charleston, South Carolina

Matías E. Czerwonko, MD
Advisor
Department of Quality and Patient Safety
Hospital Universitario Austral
Buenos Aires, Spain

Mary Alexander Deas-Hamrick
Clinical Trial Coordinator
Retina Consultants of Charleston
Charleston, South Carolina

Francis Char DeCroos, MD
Retina Fellow
Department of Ophthalmology
Wills Eye Institute/Mid Atlantic Retina
Philadelphia, Pennsylvania

Diana V. Do, MD
Associate Professor of Ophthalmology
Wilmer Eye Institute
School of Medicine
Johns Hopkins University
Baltimore, Maryland

Jay S. Duker, MD
Professor
Department of Ophthalmology
School of Medicine
Tufts University
Chairman
Department of Ophthalmology
Tufts Medical Center
Boston, Massachusetts

Carlos F. Fernández, MD
Chief
Department of Ophthalmology
Clinica Oftalmolaser
Lima, Peru

Monica Rodriguez Fontal, MD
Clinical Trial Director
Retina Consultants of Charleston
Charleston, South Carolina

Reinaldo A. Garcia, MD
Associate Professor
Retina and Vitreous Disease
Clinica Oftalmologica El Vinedo
Valencia, Edo. Carabobo, Venezuela

Gerardo Garcia-Aguirre, MD
Attending Physician
Retina Department
Asociacion para Evitar la Ceguera en
   Mexico
Clinical Professor of Ophthalmology
Escuela de Medicina
Instituto Tecnológico y de Estudios
   Superiores de Monterrey
Mexico City, Mexico

Jose M. Garcia-Gonzalez, MD
Retina Fellow
Section of Ophthalmology
University of Chicago
Chicago, Illinois

Peter L. Gehlbach, MD, PhD
Associate Professor
Department of Ophthalmology
School of Medicine
Johns Hopkins University
Associate Professor
Biomedical Engineering
School of Medicine
Johns Hopkins University
Baltimore, Maryland

Isobel V.L. Goldsmith
Clinical Trial Coordinator
Retina Consultants of Charleston
Charleston, South Carolina

JoAnna L. Goulah, PhD
Clinical Trial Research Coordinator
Retina Department
Charleston Neuroscience Institute
Charleston, South Carolina

Sundeep Grandhe, MD
University Retina
Oak Forest, Illinois

Gabriela E. Granella, MD
Director and Retina Specialist
Oftalmológico Santa Lucía
Buenos Aires, Argentina

Craig M. Greven, MD
Professor and Chairman
Department of Ophthalmology
School of Medicine
Wake Forest University
Winston-Salem, North Carolina

Mariana Ingolotti, MD
Assistant Professor
Department of Pathophysiology
Austral University
Buenos Aires, Argentina

Eric P. Jablon, MD
Partner
Retina Consultants of Charleston
Charleston, South Carolina

Timothy L. Jackson, PhD,
FRCOphth
HEFCE Senior Clinical Lecturer
School of Medicine
King's College London
Consultant Ophthalmic Surgeon
Department of Ophthalmology
King's College Hospital
London, United Kingdom

Rama D. Jager, MD
Attending Physician/Partner
University Retina and Macula Associates
Bedford Park, Illinois

John Barnwell Kerrison, MD
Partner
Retina Consultants of Charleston
Assistant Clinical Professor
Department of Ophthalmology
Medical University of South Carolina
Charleston, South Carolina

Claudia M. Krispel, MD, PhD
Vitreoretinal Fellow
Department of Ophthalmology
Wilmer Eye Institute
Johns Hopkins Hospital
Baltimore, Maryland

Nancy Kunjukunju, MD
Assistant Professor
School of Medicine
University of Missouri–Kansas City
Assistant Program Director
Department of Ophthalmology
University of Missouri–Kansas City
Kansas City, Missouri

Henry Alexander Leder, MD
Assistant of Ophthalmology
Department of Ophthalmology
School of Medicine
Johns Hopkins University
Baltimore, Maryland

Maria Lozano-Vazquez, MD
Ophthalmology Attending
Department of Surgery
University of Santiago de Compostela
Santiago de Compostela, Spain
Ophthalmology Attending
Department of Surgery
Hospital Naval
Ferral, Spain

Ana Machín Mahave, MD
Attending Physician
Department of Ophthalmology
Sierrallana Hospital
Torrelavega, Cantabria, Spain

Mariana Mata-Plathy, MD
Glaucoma Specialist
Glaucoma Service
Clinica Oftalmologica El Viñedo
Valencia, Carabobo State, Venezuela

Pablo Carnota Méndez, MD
Attending Physician
Department of Retina and Vitreous
  Surgery
Centro de Ojos de La Coruña
La Coruña, Spain

Keisuke Mori, MD, PhD
Professor
Department of Ophthalmology
Saitama Medical University
Iruma, Saitama, Japan

Amelia Nelson
Student
Retina Consultants of Charleston
Charleston, South Carolina

Quan Dong Nguyen, MD, MSc
Associate Professor of Ophthalmology
Diseases of the Retina and Vitreous, and
  Uveitis
Wilmer Eye Institute
School of Medicine
Johns Hopkins University
Baltimore, Maryland

Maximiliano Olivera, MD
Assistant Lecturer
Molecular and Cell Medicine
Facultad de Ciencias Biomédicas
Universidad Austral
Pilar, Buenos Aires, Argentina

Veronica Oria, MD
Retina and Vitreous Service
Clínica Oftalmológica El Vinedo
Valencia, Carabobo State,
  Venezuela

Carlos E. Ortiz, BS
Retina Consultants of Charleston
Charleston, South Carolina

Gabriela Papa-Oliva, MD
Associate Professor
Department of Ophthalmology
Hospital Miguel Pérez Carreño. IVSS
Caracas, Venezuela

Samir Patel, MD
Co-founder and President
Ophthotech Corporation
New York, New York

Robert Petrarca, MBBS, BSc (Hons), MCOptom
Ophthalmologist
Department of Ophthalmology
King's College Hospital NHS Foundation Trust
Honorary Research Fellow
King's College London
London, United Kingdom

Hugo Quiroz-Mercado, MD
Director of Ophthalmology
Vitreo-Retina Specialist
Denver Health Medical Center
Professor of Ophthalmology
School of Medicine
University of Colorado
Denver, Colorado

Ernesto Romera Redondo, MD
Ophthalmologist
Department of Ophthalmology
Hospital Sierrallana
Torrelavega, Cantabria, Spain

Caio V. Regatieri, MD, PhD
Assistant Professor
Department of Ophthalmology
Tufts University
Boston, Massachusetts
Adjunct Professor
Department of Ophthalmology
Federal University of São Paulo
São Paulo, Brazil

Carl D. Regillo, MD, FACS
Director of Retina Research
Wills Eye Institute
Professor of Ophthalmology
Thomas Jefferson University
Philadelphia, Pennsylvania

Richard B. Rosen, MD, FACS, FASRS
Professor and Vice Chair
Director of Research
Surgeon Director and Chief
Retinal Services
Department of Ophthalmology
New York Eye and Ear Infirmary
New York, New York

Scott D. Schoenberger, MD
Instructor
Department of Ophthalmology
Vanderbilt University Medical Center
Nashville, Tennessee

Kenneth A. Sharpe, MD
Partner
Retina Consultants of Charleston
Charleston, South Carolina

Veeral Sheth, MD
Clinical Assistant Professor
Department of Ophthalmology
University of Illinois at Chicago
Chicago, Illinois
Director
Scientific Affairs
University Retina and Macula Associates
Lemont, Illinois

Jason S. Slakter, MD
Clinical Professor
Department of Ophthalmology
School of Medicine
New York University
Partner
Vitreous–Retina–Macula Consultants of New York
New York, New York

Paul Sternberg Jr., MD
G.W. Hale Professor and Chairman
Department of Ophthalmology
Vanderbilt University Medical Center
Nashville, Tennessee

Luis M. Suárez Tata, MD
Chief
Retina-Vitreo
Clínica oftalmológica El Viñedo
Valencia, Carabobo State, Venezuela

Carlos Méndez Vázquez, MD
Director
Department of Retina and Vitreous Surgery
Centro de Ojos de La Coruña
La Coruña, Spain

Robin A. Vora, MD
Fellow, Medical Retina
Department of Ophthalmology
New England Eye Center
Boston, Massachusetts
Attending Physician
Department of Ophthalmology
Kaiser Permanente
Oakland, California

Andre J. Witkin, MD
Retina Fellow
Retina Department
Wills Eye Institute
Philadelphia, Pennsylvania

Lawrence Yannuzzi, MD
Professor of Clinical Ophthalmology
Columbia University Medical School
Founder and Chairman
Vitreous–Retina–Macula Consultants of New York
New York, New York

FOREWORD

It is an honor for me to write the foreword to the second edition of *Age-Related Macular Degeneration*, by Dr. Virgil Alfaro and his colleagues at Retina Consultants of Charleston.

Our colleagues at Retina Consultants of Charleston represent the ideal model to emulate, as they are academic physicians in private practice. Collectively, they have published eight textbooks. Two of these books, *The Essentials of Neuroophthalmology* and *Vitreoretinal Surgery of the Injured Eye*, are regarded as true classics in their field. On Index Medicus, I find many peer-reviewed articles that they have authored in the most selective ophthalmology journals.

The publication of this textbook comes at a poignant time, as we see historic and significant advances in the diagnosis and treatment of age-related macular degeneration (AMD). The book has excellent chapters written on intravenous fluorescein angiography, indocyanine green angiography, and optical coherence tomography. These narratives provide classic teaching and instruction for residents and fellows to obtain a solid foundation in their use to diagnose and treat AMD.

Certainly, one of the most significant changes that we have noted in our field is the classification system of choroidal neovascular membranes in AMD. *Age-Related Macular Degeneration*, second edition, provides a concise and understandable discussion of this classification system.

The advent of anti-VEGF therapy has revolutionized the treatment of wet AMD. Newer treatments and newer treatment regimens have contributed to improvement of vision in these patients and in prevention of visual loss. Macugen, Avastin, and Lucentis remain potent and reliable sources of anti-VEGF therapy, and newer drugs such as Eylea appear to provide patients with more sustained efficacy necessitating fewer injections.

Lastly, their "Frontiers of Therapy" section provides up-to-date information for treating AMD secondary to geographic atrophy through cell transplantation and pharmacologic therapies.

Francisco Gomez-Ulla, MD
Dean of Ophthalmology
Universidad de Santiago de
    Compostela
Santiago de Compostela, Spain

PREFACE

We should not forget our mentors, those who went before us and influenced us to our own personal successes. Just as we are busy and our schedules are saturated with patients, surgeries, meetings, and the like, so, too, our teachers lived and flourished. Somehow, they managed to find time to guide and teach us. Those who influenced me were and are personally involved with the current status of the diagnosis and treatment of age-related macular degeneration.

In 1984, Drs. Stanley Chang, Harvey Lincoff, and D. Jackson Coleman walked the eighth floor of Cornell University Medical School and the New York Hospital and took me under their wing. These iconic figures in the world of vitreoretinal diseases taught me and countless other students, residents, and fellows the great balance of clinical practice and significant research.

Stephen J. Ryan served as chairman of the Los Angeles County Hospital department of ophthalmology and president of the Doheny Eye Institute. During my residency, he had put together a world class group of retina and macula specialists, including Peter E. Liggett, John Lean, Edgar Thomas, and others. They all served as investigators in the Macular Photocoagulation Studies that were to provide important clinical guidelines for years to follow. Coresidents Baruch Kuppermann, Pravin Dugel, Victor Gonzales, Keith Pince, Vinh Tran, Colin Ma, David Wagner, James Tsai, and others immersed themselves in this great clinical pearl, called the L.A. County Hospital.

Marvin Sears and Peter Liggett provided the leadership and mentorship during my fellowship at the Yale Eye Center. Marvin was proudest of his great teaching skills and his publication in *Science* that showed for the first time the presence of prostaglandins in the eye.

Age-Related Macular Degeneration represents 2 years of hard work by my fellow editors and authors. Our plan was to author, edit, and publish a body of work that would be a source of salient information for our students and colleagues. Each book chapter has been written to stand alone as a significant and inclusive text that the reader can use to learn and understand the topic at hand. It is our hope that patients around the world will benefit from our labor, as their doctors read and study this book.

D. Virgil Alfaro III, MD
Charleston, South Carolina

ACKNOWLEDGMENTS

The editors are indebted to the hard work and dedication of Sarah M. Granlund, who served as our project manager during all phases of this textbook. Indeed, her great diplomacy and administrative skills provided the editorial team with someone to turn to for help to bring this project to completion.

CONTENTS

NORMAL ANATOMY OF THE MACULA

J. FERNANDO ARÉVALO • CARLOS F. FERNÁNDEZ

◼ INTRODUCTION

Francisco Buzzi in Milan, Italy, was the first to anatomically define the macula at the end of the 18th century (1782–1784). He described it as the yellow portion of the posterior retina, lateral to the optic nerve, with a depression in its center. Also in the 18th century (1797), Fragonard, a French ophthalmologist, made a very detailed description of the foveal zone, but he failed to mention the central foveola. In addition, Soemmering (1795–1798) described the macula lutea; however, he thought that the foveola was a hole or foramen (foraminulum centrale retinae) and correlated it to the blind spot of the visual field. Finally, Michaelis in 1838 established the role of the macula, and it was confirmed by Müller in 1856. At the end of the 19th century, Tratuferi in Italy showed the first schematic drawings with the topographic localization of the retinal layers. The relationship between the retinal axonal layer, cones, and rods was established by Ramon y Cajal in 1894 (1).

The macula is recognized as the specialized region of the retina in charge of high-resolution visual acuity. Anatomically, it can be defined as the central part of the posterior retina that contains xanthophyll pigment and two or more layers of ganglion cells. In this chapter, we focus primarily on the aspects of the normal anatomy of the macula as an introduction to the understanding and management of age-related macular degeneration.

◼ EMBRYOLOGY

The neural components of the eye are an extension of the forebrain, and thus part of the central nervous system (Table 1.1).

The Neuroretina

The embryogenesis of the neuroretina occurs during the first month of life. The forebrain consists of a single layer of neuroectodermal cells. The optic vesicle extends laterally from the forebrain and then invaginates to form the optic cup. There is a double layer of neuroectodermal cells in the optic cup; the apices are together and basal aspects apart. The macular area appears at the end of the 4th week.

The inner layer of neuroectoderm becomes the sensory retina posteriorly. Part of the inner limiting membrane is the basement membrane of the sensory retina, next to the vitreous. The foveal pit forms late in embryonic life, and morphologic maturity does not occur until the age when it is possible to obtain 20/20 visual acuity in small children (2). The induction of the foveal pit requires a normal pigment epithelium (3). The inner layer of neuroectoderm is divided into the inner neuroblastic layer (Müller, amacrine, and ganglion cells) and the outer neuroblastic layer (cone and rod, horizontal, and bipolar cells). Between the inner neuroblastic layer and the outer neuroblastic layer is the transient fiber layer of Chievitz; this layer will progressively disappear.

Table 1.1	DEVELOPMENT OF THE SENSORY RETINA[a]		
4th–5th Week	6th Week–3rd Month	3rd–7th Month	Adult
Surface of the marginal layer	Superficial portion of the marginal layer	Nerve fiber layer	Internal limiting membrane Nerve fiber layer
	Inner neuroblastic layer	Ganglion cells Amacrine cells	Ganglion cells
Primitive neuroepithelium	Outer neuroblastic layer	Müllerian fiber nuclei Bipolar cells Horizontal cells Nuclei of rods and cones	Inner nuclear layer Outer nuclear layer
Cilia		Primitive rods and cones	Rods and cones

[a]The marginal layer free from nuclei (not included) appears between the 4th and 5th wk, after which it disappears. In addition, the transient layer of Chievitz (not included) appears between the 6th wk and 3rd mo and disappears after the 3rd mo.

The central and peripheral retinae start to differentiate between the first and third months. The ganglion cell layer becomes thicker, as do the inner plexiform layer and the amacrine cell layer. The cones appear in the 5th month. They are a protoplasmic extension of the outer neuroblastic layer (4–6). The rods appear in the 6th month (5). The macula becomes thinner in the 7th month because the cells of the different layers move laterally, and the foveal pit appears more evident (Fig. 1.1) (7,8).

The Retinal Pigment Epithelium

The outer layer of neuroectoderm (toward the sclera) becomes the retinal pigment epithelium (RPE), the pigmented ciliary epithelium, and the iris dilator muscle. The basement membrane of the RPE forms the innermost part of the Bruch's membrane (9).

Pigmentation of the neuroectodermal cells occurs early and is completed during embryonic life (10), whereas pigmentation of the uveal stroma, which is derived from the neural crest, starts much later and is not complete until several weeks after birth (9). The melanin granules of the neuroectoderm are larger and chemically different from those of the uveal stroma (11). Moreover, melanin content of the RPE is similar in all persons, regardless of race, in contrast to the amount of uveal stromal pigmentation, which corresponds to the racial pigmentation of the skin and hair (10).

Vascularization

Vascularization of the retina begins during the 16th week of gestation at the optic nerve head (12) and normally reaches the ora serrata nasally by term. It is not quite complete temporally at term because the distance from the optic nerve head to the ora is greater.

There are differing theories as to how vascularization of the macula occurs. Some have proposed that the capillary-free zone (CFZ) develops by regression of previously formed capillaries, because the retina is thin enough in this area that sufficient oxygen can diffuse inward from the choroidal circulation (12). Others believe that the CFZ forms primarily, with the embryonic vessels gradually encircling the center of the fovea and with no evidence of regression (13).

The Choroid

In the first phase, at 4 weeks, the choroid begins to take form in the undifferentiated mesenchyma surrounding the optic cup. At 5 to 6 weeks, endothelial tubes near the pigment epithelium differentiate into capillaries. Simultaneously, the Bruch's membrane and the vortex veins appear. With the appearance of the posterior ciliary arteries at 8 weeks, the choriocapillaris is fully established as a discrete layer.

During the growth phase in the 3rd month, the anterior capillaries arrange themselves in a linear and radial pattern. The anterior supply of the choriocapillaris is complete by 3 months, even though the ciliary body and iris are not yet formed. The capillaries drain into the supra- and infraorbital venous plexi.

The second phase of choroidal growth includes the formation of large vessels (Haller's layer) at 4 months. The third phase begins around the 5th month and is characterized by the formation of medium-sized vessels posterior to the equator. Anterior to the equator, there are only two layers of vessels, the choriocapillaris and medium-sized vessels.

Pigmentation of the choroidal melanocytes commences in the 5th month and continues until after birth, beginning outward near the sclera and progressing inward toward the Bruch's membrane. The peripapillary, intrascleral vascular circle of Haller and Zinn develops between 3 and 6 months. Between the 6th and 10th month, the major arterial circle of the iris forms recurrent arterial branches that supply the anterior choroid during its rapid growth phase (14).

■ TOPOGRAPHIC ANATOMY

The terms *macula* and *fovea* are used in different ways by the anatomist and the clinician. Anatomically, the macula (macula lutea or central retina) is defined as the portion of

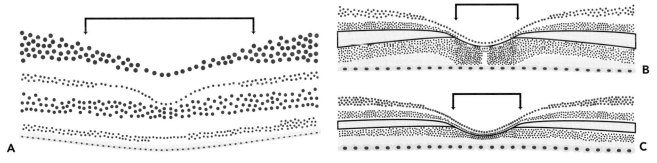

Figure 1.1 ■ Diagram showing the development of the human fovea. **A.** Human fovea at birth. **B.** Human fovea at 45 months. **C.** Human fovea at 72 years of age. *Black lines* mark the width of the rod-free foveola; at birth, the foveola is wider (A) than at 45 months (B). Full foveal development is not complete until sometime between 15 and 45 months of age.

the posterior retina that contains xanthophyll and two or more layers of ganglion cells. This region is about 5.5 mm in diameter and is centered approximately 4 mm temporal and 0.8 mm inferior to the center of the optic disk (15). It corresponds clinically to the posterior pole and is approximately bounded by the superior and inferior temporal vascular arcades. On the basis of microscopic anatomy, the macular area can be further subdivided into several zones (Fig. 1.2).

What is clinically referred to as the macula corresponds to the anatomic fovea. The fovea (fovea centralis) is a depression in the inner retinal surface in the center of the macula. It measures approximately 1.5 mm, or one disk diameter in size, and it is more heavily pigmented than the surrounding retinal tissue. The central floor of the fovea is called the foveola. The anatomic foveola, often referred to clinically as the fovea, measures approximately 0.35 mm in diameter. It lies within the CFZ, which measures approximately 0.5 mm in diameter in most patients. A small depression in the center of the foveola is called the umbo, where the retina is only 0.13 mm thick. A 0.5-mm-wide ring zone where the ganglion cell layer, inner nuclear layer, and outer

plexiform layer of Henle are the thickest is called the parafoveal area. This zone is in turn surrounded by a 1.5-mm zone referred to as the perifoveal area (16).

CLINICAL APPEARANCE

The anatomic subdivisions of the macula are ill-defined ophthalmoscopically. The margins of either the 0.35-mm diameter foveola or the 1.5-mm diameter fovea are difficult to define. A poorly defined zone of greater pigmentation (one-fourth to one disk diameter in size) corresponds to the center of the macula, which is maximum in the foveolar area. The foveal reflex is present in most normal eyes, and it lies just in front of the center of the foveola (Fig. 1.3). We can see the foveal depression with the narrow slit lamp beam.

The central retinal artery supplies the inner half of the retina. It usually divides into a superior and inferior trunk within the optic nerve head. These trunks divide into a nasal branch and a temporal branch. The corresponding retinal venous branches have much the same distribution as the

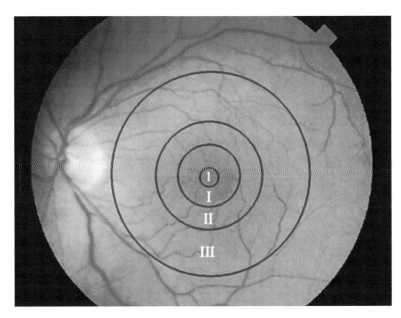

Figure 1.2 ■ Topographic anatomy of the normal macula. On the basis of microscopic anatomy, the macular area can be further subdivided into several zones. *I.* Fovea containing the foveola (*1*). *II.* Parafovea. *III.* Perifovea.

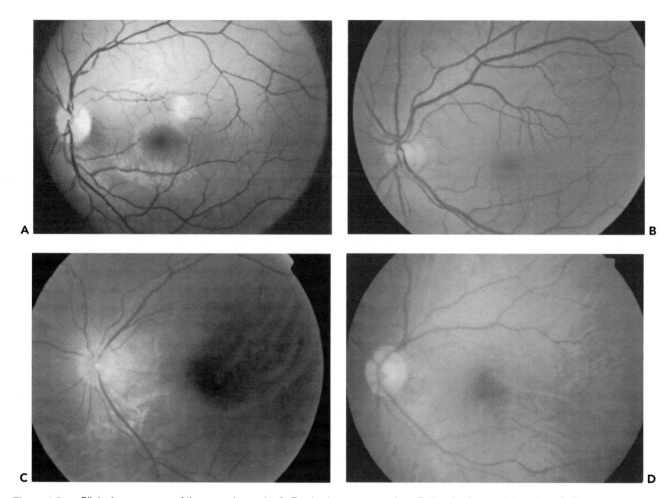

Figure 1.3 ■ Clinical appearance of the normal macula. **A.** Fundus in a young patient. **B.** Fundus in an adult patient. **C.** Fundus in a moderately myopic patient. **D.** Tessellated fundus in an older patient. Large choroidal vessels are visible in the macular area in (D) because of relative hypopigmentation of the RPE. (B and D courtesy of Dario Fuenmayor-Rivera and Enrique Murcia.)

arteries. They give off arteriolar and venular branches that posteriorly occur primarily at right angles to the parent vessel. They divide in a dichotomous way as they course peripherally. The right-angle branches are referred to as first-order arterioles and venules. One or more cilioretinal arteries derived from the ciliary circulation supply the papillomacular area in approximately 20% of patients (17), and occasionally the entire macula (Fig. 1.4). The blood vessel walls are normally transparent (16,18).

GROSS ANATOMY

The retina loses its normal transparency within hours after death. Xanthophyll is a yellow pigment made up of two carotenoids (zeaxanthin and lutein) (19,20). It is apparent in the center of the macula and is highly concentrated in the foveolar area. The maximal concentration of xanthophyll pigment is in the outer nuclear and outer plexiform layers. However, we can find xanthophyll within the inner plexiform layer inside the foveal area (19,21–23). The greatest concentration of pigment is in the cones' central axons (23).

The entrance site for the short and long posterior ciliary arteries can be visualized after removal of the choroid. There is no retinal circulation at the foveola. The short posterior ciliary arteries are concentrated in the macular area along the temporal margin of the fovea and the peripapillary area. The temporal long posterior ciliary artery and ciliary nerve enter about one and one-half disk diameters temporal to the center of the fovea (16).

HISTOLOGY

In the macula, we find the thickest portion of the retina surrounding the thinnest portion, the foveolar area. At the umbo, the neural retina consists only of the inner limiting membrane, the Henle's fiber layer, the outer nuclear layer, the external limiting membrane, and the photoreceptors' outer and inner segments (Fig. 1.5). The typical neural–retinal histology is established out of the foveola (Fig. 1.6). The neural retina consists of the inner limiting membrane, the nerve fiber layer (NFL), the ganglion cell layer, the inner plexiform layer (synaptic processes between bipolar

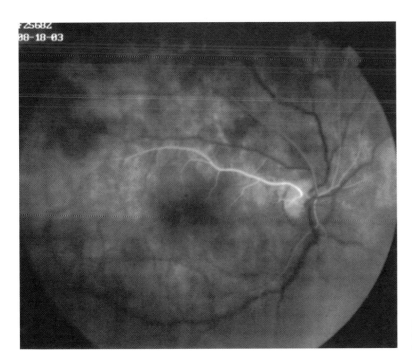

Figure 1.4 ■ FA shows a cilioretinal artery. (Courtesy of Dario Fuenmayor-Rivera and Enrique Murcia.)

cells and ganglion cells), the inner nuclear layer (nuclei of bipolar, horizontal, amacrine, and Müller cells), the outer plexiform layer (synaptic processes between bipolar cells and photoreceptors), the outer nuclear layer (nuclei of the rods and cones), the external limiting membrane (formed by cell junctions between photoreceptors and the terminal optical processes of Müller cells), and the photoreceptor layer (rod and cone cells). The bipolar cells, ganglion cells, fibers of the outer plexiform layer (Henle's fiber layer), and Müller cells are displaced circumferentially and show an oblique orientation in the macula that causes thickening of

the marginal zone and a central thinning of the retina, forming the fovea.

Müller cells are modified glial cells. They span the region from the internal limiting membrane to the external limiting membrane, and they give support to the neural elements of the retina. The internal limiting membrane consists of a basement membrane, which is a surface modification of the vitreous body, and the expanded vitreal processes of Müller cells. This membrane is relatively thick in the macular region except in the area of the foveola. The internal limiting membrane serves as

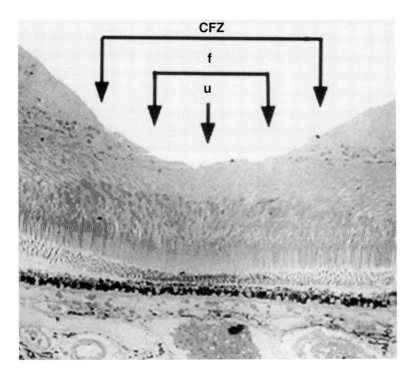

Figure 1.5 ■ Histology of the normal macula. CFZ, capillary-free zone; f, foveola; u, umbo. (Microphotograph courtesy of Dario Savino-Zari.)

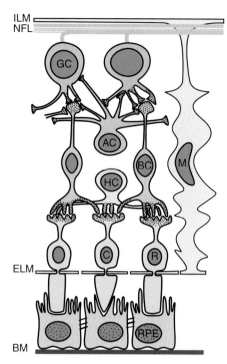

Figure 1.6 ■ Schematic representation of the human retina illustrating its organization into discrete layers. AC, amacrine cell; BC, bipolar cell; BM, Bruch's membrane; C, cone photoreceptor; ELM, external limiting membrane; GC, ganglion cell; HC, horizontal cell; ILM, internal limiting membrane; M, Müller cell; NFL, nerve fiber layer; R, rod photoreceptor; RPE, retinal pigment epithelium.

an anchoring structure for the collagen framework of the vitreous. The outer limiting membrane is formed by junctional complexes between cell membranes of the Müller cells and inner segments of photoreceptors. Müller cells are connected to the visual cells by a system of terminal bars (24,25). These junctional complexes probably provide at least a partial barrier to the passage of large molecules in either direction.

The retinal blood vessels supply the inner half of the retina. The major branches of the retinal arterial system have the structure of small arteries, persisting even beyond the equator (15). Retinal arteries do not have an internal elastic lamina; however, they have a well-developed muscularis (five to seven layers of smooth muscle cells posteriorly; one or two layers peripherally). Near the optic disk, the retinal veins have three to four layers of smooth muscle cells, and after a short distance, the muscle cells are replaced by fibroblasts. There is controversy concerning the pattern of distribution of the capillary network in the retina (diffuse arrangement or a two- or three-tier arrangement) (15,26,27). The superficial network is predominantly postarteriolar and the deep network prevenular. There is a distinct radial peripapillary

capillary network; this network richly interconnects with the inner retinal capillary layer (27). The large arterioles and venules of the retinal circulation travel in the NFL and ganglion cell layer. Close to the CFZ (0.4–0.5 mm in diameter), the capillaries form a single layer, but elsewhere, the capillaries are present in two or more layers and extend into the inner nuclear layer. The CFZ is normally vascularized during prenatal development of the retina. This vascularization undergoes spontaneous capillary obliteration just before or shortly after birth, forming the CFZ (28).

The foveola is composed entirely of cones; the central 100 μm of the foveola contains only red and green cones (29). The peak foveal cone density averages nearly 200,000 per mm² and falls rapidly with increasing eccentricity, such that cone density decreases nearly 10-fold within 1 mm of the umbo. Blue cone density is highest in a zone between 100 and 300 μm from the center of the fovea. The foveal cones take on a more rodlike shape; blue cones in the macula tend to have inner segments 10% taller and a more cylindrical shape than their red and green counterparts (29). Rod cells differ from cones, with their outer segments consisting of stacks of flattened membrane disks that are separate from the plasma membrane.

The RPE is a monolayer of hexagonal cells densely adherent to one another by a system of tight cellular junctions or terminal bars that make up the outer blood-retinal barrier, which maintains the subretinal space in a state of deturgescence. In the fovea, there are 30 cones per RPE cell, while in the periphery, there are 22 rods per RPE cell. Interdigitation of the RPE cells with the rod and cone outer segments provides only a tenuous adhesion of the RPE to the sensory retina. The RPE cells in the macular region are taller and contain increased amounts of melanin pigment than elsewhere (30,31). There is an inverse relationship between melanin and lipofuscin pigment concentration in the RPE. Lipofuscin concentration increases initially during the first two decades of life, and then again in the sixth decade. The concentration of lipofuscin in the RPE is significantly greater in light- than dark-skinned persons, whereas the concentration of melanin in the pigment epithelium is similar in light- and dark-skinned persons. The melanin content of the pigment epithelium and choroidal melanocytes decline with age (Fig. 1.3).

In young and middle-aged individuals, the RPE is tightly adherent to the underlying Bruch's membrane by means of its own basement membrane. This adherence decreases with advancing age. The Bruch's membrane consists of the basement membrane of the RPE, the inner collagenous layer, an elastic layer, an outer collagenous layer, and the basement membrane of the choriocapillaris. Because of its porous structure, it probably plays a minimal role in regulating movement of substances across it.

The choroid is the posterior aspect of the uveal tract; it is supplied by the short ciliary arteries, and they are concentrated in the macula and peripapillary region. These

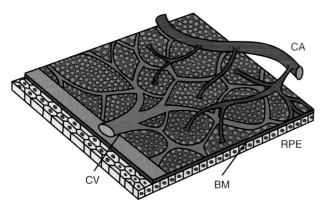

Figure 1.7 ■ Schematic representation of the lobular pattern of the choriocapillaris. Each lobule is supplied by an arteriole. BM, Bruch's membrane; CA, choroidal artery; CV, choroidal vein; RPE, retinal pigment epithelium.

arteries form a rich anastomotic network that quickly empties large quantities of blood into the choriocapillaris (sinusoidal network). The choriocapillaris is fenestrated and arranged in a lobular pattern, with a feeding arteriole in the center of each lobule and several venules peripherally (Fig. 1.7) (32–40).

The prelaminar part of the optic nerve is supplied by the peripapillary branches of the short posterior ciliary arteries. The choriocapillaris does not communicate directly with the optic disk capillaries. The prelaminar capillaries freely anastomose at the disk margin with those of the retina. Both capillary systems drain into the venules leading to the central retinal vein (33,40).

The RPE is an integral part of the visual cycle. It is an important component of photoreceptor renewal; new outer segment disks are continually added proximal to the base, and the oldest disks at the distal end of the outer segments are phagocytized by the RPE cells. The RPE also transports metabolic wastes from the retina into the choriocapillaris. The melanin within the RPE cells absorbs light that has not been captured by the photoreceptors, thus preventing excessive light scattering within the eye. Melanin absorption may also confer protection from photo-oxidative stress (41). The RPE cells are also thought to secrete growth factors essential for proper differentiation of photoreceptors during development (42).

The macula has the highest rate of blood flow of any tissue in the body. It probably functions to stabilize the temperature environment of the retina (43) because blood flow is greatly in excess of that needed to meet the nutritional demands of the retina. The choriocapillaris supplies the RPE and outer retinal layers. The choriocapillaris has an endothelium with a pore size sufficient to allow some larger molecules, including proteins, to escape into the extravascular space. There are no lymphatic channels in the eye; the perivascular and perineural spaces in the sclera probably function as lymphatic channels. Thus, the choriocapillaris endothelium controls the amount of extracellular fluid normally present in the choroid.

BLOOD–RETINAL BARRIERS

Retinal perfusion is accomplished by a nonoverlapping, dual system of blood circulation. For each system, there is a blood–retinal barrier analogous to the blood–brain barrier. Both barriers confine even relatively small molecules, because of a nonleaky tight junction between cells (44).

The outer blood–retinal barrier is constituted by the RPE; it blocks the inward migration of small molecules from the choriocapillaris into the subretinal space. Anatomically, these junctions include a zonula adherens and adjacent zonula occludens of the RPE, both situated near the apex of the cell and encircling it (45). The inner blood–retinal barrier is the retinal vascular endothelium, including the capillary endothelium. The site of the barrier is the specialized tight junctions (zonulae occludentes) between individual endothelial cells (44,46).

NORMAL FLUORESCEIN ANGIOGRAPHIC FINDINGS

Fluorescein angiography (FA) was developed in the 1950s as a means of studying vascular flow. FA is still used for this purpose, but it provides much additional information. Sodium fluorescein is excited by a blue light (465–490 nm), and it emits a fluorescent yellow-green light (peak wavelength of 520–530 nm). Because of its molecular weight (376 kDa), it diffuses freely out of all the body capillaries except the retina. Approximately 80% of the dye is bound to plasma proteins (albumin), and it is the unbound fluorescein that is detected angiographically (16).

FA is performed using a fundus camera. Filters are used to produce the exciting wavelength. The FA is photographed digitally or with black and white film because of its superior resolution and speed. On the positive images, fluorescein appears white and nonfluorescent areas appear black (46). The normal FA shows the dual nature of the retinal circulation. The larger choroidal vessels fill first, with almost immediate filling of the choriocapillaris. Rapid perfusion of the choroid and leakage of the dye from the choriocapillaris give the fairly uniform background fluorescence.

The tight junctions of the retinal pigment epithelial cells (the outer blood–retinal barrier) block the fluorescein that leaks from the choriocapillaris and diffuses through the Bruch's membrane. Normally, the fluorescein does not gain access to the subsensory retinal space. The retinal vessels, including the capillaries (the inner blood–retinal barrier), normally do not leak fluorescein. Thus, the angiogram evaluates both of the blood–retinal barriers (44).

The normal macular region is hypofluorescent or has a barely visible fluorescence because of the greater density of the RPE in this area and the presence of xanthophyll in the outer retinal layers. In darkly pigmented individuals, the increased density of choroidal melanocytes in the macula helps obscure the background choroidal fluorescence. In addition, the capillaries appear particularly distinct, because there is only one capillary layer surrounding the foveal avascular zone (47). Only in the extramacular area, before the arteriovenous phase, can details of perfusion of the larger choroidal vessels be detected.

The FA consists of five phases (Fig. 1.8):

1. Prearterial phase: The choroid and choriocapillaris fill with dye. A cilioretinal vessel, if present, usually fills at the same time as the choroidal circulation, before fluorescein is detectable in the other retinal vessels, approximately 1 second before that of the proximal branches of the central retinal artery (Fig. 1.4).

2. Arterial phase: Lasts until the arteries are completely filled.
3. Arteriovenous phase: Characterized by complete filling of the arteries and capillaries and the first evidence of laminar flow in the veins.
4. Venous phase: Begins as the arteries are emptying and persists until the veins are filled with dye.
5. Recirculation phase: Follows the venous phase and represents the first return of blood to the eye after fluorescein has passed through the kidneys. During the recirculation phase, the outer edges of the major retinal vessels appear relatively hyperfluorescent because of the greater amount of fluorescein in the tangential section of the plasma cuff near the edge of the blood vessels.

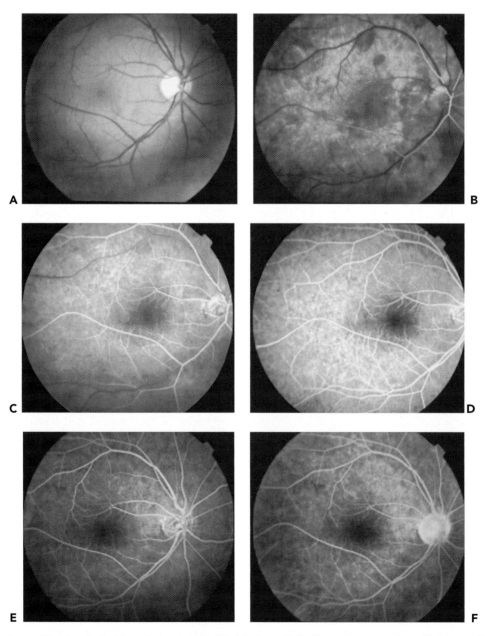

Figure 1.8 ■ FA of normal fundus. **A.** Red-free photograph. **B.** Arterial phase. **C.** Early arteriovenous phase. **D.** Intermediate arteriovenous phase. **E.** Venous phase. **F.** Recirculation phase. (Courtesy of Dario Fuenmayor-Rivera and Enrique Murcia.)

All abnormalities in the FA can be understood as the presence of either too much fluorescein (hyperfluorescence) or too little (hypofluorescence) in a specific location (48).

In evaluating diseases of the macula, FA can be of value in detecting alterations in blood flow, in permeability of the retinal blood vessels, in the retinal vascular pattern, in the density of the pigment epithelium, and other changes affecting the normal angiographic pattern in this area (16).

NORMAL INDOCYANINE GREEN ANGIOGRAPHY FINDINGS

Indocyanine green (ICG) is a dye that was originally used in the photographic industry. It was first used in ophthalmology by Flower and Hochheimer (49) in the early 1970s to image the choroidal circulation. Although both experimental and clinical investigations with ICG continued, it was not until the early 1990s that it became an established method of investigation. This was because of the increasing interest in the contribution of the choroid to retinal diseases and improvements in technology. ICG, a tricarbocyanine dye, is injected intravenously and is imaged as it passes through ocular vessels. An excitation filter with a peak at 805 nm and a barrier filter with a transmission peak of 835 nm, corresponding to the maximum fluorescence emitted by the dye in whole blood, are required. The standard technique is to inject 25 mg of ICG in 5 mL of water slowly and to begin photographs 7 to 10 minutes after injection with late photographs at 20 and 40 minutes. The circulating dye is rapidly excreted by the biliary system. A preinjection infrared fundus photograph showing pseudofluorescence or autofluorescence may help to avoid misinterpretation of the angiograms (50).

Adverse reactions to ICG are more rare than those with intravenous fluorescein. Mild reactions such as nausea, vomiting, sneezing, and transient itching occur in 0.15% of cases (51). More severe reactions such as urticaria, syncope, fainting, and pyrexia may also occur. Severe reactions such as hypotensive shock (52), anaphylactic shock (53), and death have been reported. Crossover allergy to iodine can occur in patients with seafood allergies, making iodine and seafood allergy a contraindication to ICG angiography. Because the liver primarily metabolizes ICG, it should be avoided in patients with hepatic disease. Those undergoing hemodialysis are also at increased risk of complications.

Photographic film with a conventional camera is not sensitive enough to acquire ICG images—more sensitive digital systems are required (54–57). Low-contrast individual images are digitally enhanced to allow better interpretation of choroidal structures (58,59). ICG and FA can each be performed and the images superimposed (60,61). New technologic developments now permit dynamic, simultaneous FA and ICG using the confocal scanning laser ophthalmoscope (62,63). The use of a wide-angle contact lens to visualize 160 degrees of the fundus may help in the evaluation of flow characteristics and simultaneous assessment of the periphery and posterior pole (64).

Interpretation of ICG angiography is difficult because multiple vascular layers are displayed at one time. After choroidal arteries fill, the capillary phase is characterized by a rather diffuse hyperfluorescence resulting from the additive fluorescence effects of multiple crossing arterioles and venules. This fluorescence is brighter in the foveolar area. However, because xanthophyll does not efficiently absorb infrared light, the foveola cannot be located exactly during ICG angiography (Fig. 1.9). The choriocapillaris layer itself can only be sensed as a faint haze that becomes visible in the early venous phase. The images do not change

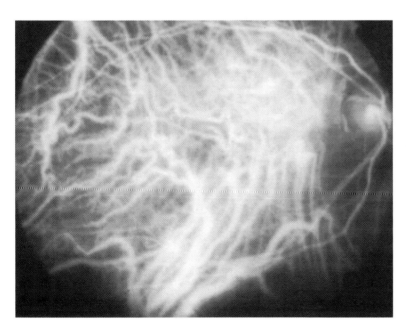

Figure 1.9 ■ Indocyanine green video angiography (ICG-V) of the normal fundus. (Courtesy of Dario Fuenmayor-Rivera.)

significantly during the next several minutes. With reduction in dye fluorescence after about 5 minutes, discernibility of single choroidal vessels decreases and there is a fairly uniform background fluorescence on which larger retinal vessels are visible as brighter structures; after 10 to 15 minutes, however, these vessels appear as darker structures. This rapid decrease in retinal vessel fluorescence reflects the fast hepatic extraction of the dye from the blood. In contrast, fluorescence in the choroid lasts much longer and could be interpreted as exudation of the dye. However, a comparative examination of ICG fluorescence demonstrates that plasma fluorescence of the dye is much brighter than that of whole blood and lasts much longer (65,66). In fact, it decreases at the same rate as background ICG fluorescence in the fundus. We therefore believe that plasma gaps in choroidal capillaries must be sufficiently large to become the main source of late choroidal fluorescence. As with fluorescein, ICG hyperfluorescence cannot always be attributed to extravasation of the dye. Focal, short-term hyperfluorescence is a common finding in the early venous phase and probably is caused by a plasma vortex in venous loops or additive fluorescence of crossing vessels. Though the pigment epithelium blocks only 10% of infrared light, that is still enough to create a window-like hyperfluorescence at the site of pigment epithelial atrophic defects (67).

NORMAL OPTICAL COHERENCE TOMOGRAPHY FINDINGS

Time-domain optical coherence tomography (TD-OCT, Zeiss-Humphrey Instruments, Dublin, CA) uses a continuously emitting, optically coherent laser diode centered at 850 nm and focused at the retina. The superluminescence low-coherence diode emits light with a 20 to 25 nm bandwidth. For thickness measurements, the time delay of reflected or backscattered light is determined using coherence interferometry. Reflectivity and distance information is contained in the interference signal between a probe beam, reflected from different structures within the investigated tissue, and light returning from a variable-reference optical delay path. The length of one scan is adjustable for 43 nm working distance up to 3 mm in air (in vivo approximately 6 mm), and one line can be measured within 1 second. The displayed image has a resolution of 500 × 500 pixels. The axial resolution of OCT is reported by the manufacturer to be 10 to 20 μm (68).

The recent introduction of spectral-domain OCT (SD-OCT) allows imaging of the macula with a much faster scan rate and at a higher scan resolution. Compared with the commercially available time-domain OCT (Stratus OCT, Carl Zeiss Meditec, Dublin, CA), the scan rate of SD-OCT is capable of obtaining at least 18,000 axial measurements per second with an axial resolution of 5 μm. The basic working principle of SD-OCT is similar to that of TD-OCT. Both systems measure the echo time delay of backscattered light

signals via an interferometer. The light spectrum from the interferometer is detected by a spectrometer. The interference spectrum data are then Fourier transformed to generate axial measurements of the retina. SD-OCT has been shown to improve visualization of the intraretinal structures, and the measurement repeatability is even better despite the fact that three-dimensional SD-OCT generally has greater macular thickness measurements compared with Stratus OCT (69).

The difference in foveal thickness measured by the two OCT instruments would lie between 3.9 and 37.8 μm in 95% of pairs of observation. The normal foveal thickness with SD-OCT is 216.4 ± 18 on the central fovea. The poor agreement between three-dimensional SD-OCT and Stratus OCT may be attributable to the different definitions of the posterior retinal boundary. In Stratus OCT, the inner segment–outer segment (IS/OS) interface of the photoreceptor layer is set as the posterior retinal boundary. Having a higher axial resolution, delineation of the IS/OS photoreceptor interface and the RPE is possible in three-dimensional SD-OCT, and the RPE is set as the posterior retinal boundary (Fig. 1.10). The more posteriorly located reference line results in greater values of macular measurement obtained by three-dimensional SD-OCT. Measurement obtained from one system may not be used interchangeably with the other.

Wakitani et al. (70) reported a study of macular thickness measurements in 203 healthy subjects with different axial lengths using TD-OCT. The thickness values of three circular areas centered on the central fovea with diameters 350 μm, 1,850 μm, and 2,850 μm were 167 ± 21 μm, 212 ± 17 μm, and 231 ± 15 μm, respectively. There was no significant difference in retinal thickness with age or with increasing axial length of the eye. However, the average thickness of the macula in females was significantly thinner than in males.

The contrast between different retinal layers is delineated by a narrow-field-of-view image of a normal fovea. The anterior and posterior margins of the retina are defined by highly reflective layers (the NFL and retinal pigment epithelium/choriocapillaris). In the area of the fovea, the retinal pigment epithelium/choriocapillaris appears distinct from

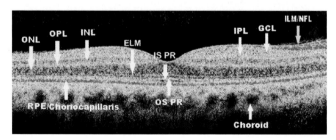

Figure 1.10 ■ Spectral-domain optical coherence tomography (SD-OCT) of the normal macula. ELM, external limiting membrane; GCL, ganglion cell layer; ILM/NFL, internal limiting membrane/nerve fiber layer; INL, inner nuclear layer; IPL, inner plexiform layer; ONL, outer nuclear layer; OPL, outer plexiform layer of Henle; IS/OS PR, photoreceptor's inner and outer segments (ellipsoid zone); RPE, retinal pigment epithelium.

the external segments of the photoreceptors. The stratified structure of the retina is composed of alternating layers of moderate and low reflectivity, and the photoreceptors appear minimally reflective. Moderate backscattering is observed from the inner and outer plexiform layers, which, like the NFL, consist of fibrous structures running perpendicular to the incident beam. In contrast, the nuclear layers show minimal backscattering because the cell bodies of the nuclear layers, like the photoreceptors, are oriented parallel to the incident light. The increased backscatter and the shadowing of the reflections from the RPE and choriocapillaris identify the retinal blood vessels. The larger choroidal vessels may also appear in the image and have minimally reflective dark lumens (71).

We can obtain information on three-dimensional structure, thanks to the ability of OCT to acquire images of consecutive slices through the retina (Fig. 1.11). Characteristic features of the retina appear consistently in the serial sections. The anterior and posterior surfaces of the neural retina are defined by backscattering at the NFL and vitreoretinal interface, while the highly backscattering red layer represents the RPE and choriocapillaris. The development and resolution of the foveal depression, which reaches its maximum depth at the fovea centralis, are revealed by the sequence of tomograms. Retinal blood vessels derived from the superior and inferior branches of the central retinal artery are evident in the tomograms from the partial shadowing of the deep retinal structure beneath the vessels (71).

NORMAL FUNDUS AUTOFLUORESCENCE IMAGING

Autofluorescent imaging of the ocular fundus relies on the stimulated emission of light from molecules, chiefly lipofuscin, in the RPE, in the photoreceptor outer segments, and in the space between the photoreceptor outer segments and the RPE (72). Currently, there are two ways to acquire fundus autofluorescence imaging: one is using a fundus camera-based system (73) and the other is by confocal scanning laser ophthalmoscopy (74).

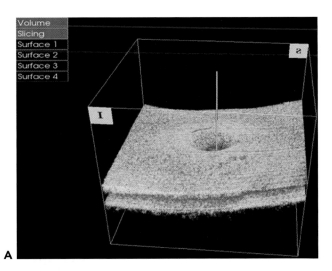

A

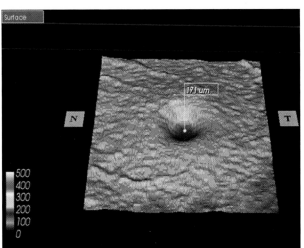

B

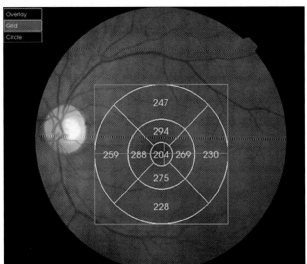

C

Figure 1.11 ■ Spectral-domain optical coherence tomography of normal macula. **A.** Three-dimensional image of the macula. **B.** Retinal thickness map. **C.** Normal fundus retinography.

Confocal Scanning Laser Ophthalmoscopy for Fundus Autofluorescence Imaging

Confocal scanning laser ophthalmoscopy (SLO, Heidelberg Retina Angiograph II, HRA II, Heidelberg Engineering, Heidelberg, Germany) has an argon laser source that is able to emit a 488-nm excitation wavelength and a barrier filter to detect emission from lipofuscin fluorophores over 500 nm. The illumination beam is 3 mm in diameter and the full aperture of the dilated or undilated pupil is used to collect the emitted fluorescence light from the posterior pole. The confocal detection unit employs a 400-µm pinhole aperture to suppress light from below or above the confocal plane. The size of the scanning field used is 30° × 30°. The frame grabber of the HRA can digitize image frames at a programmable rate of up to 5 frames per second. Each frame contains 1,536 pixels vertically and 1,536 pixels horizontally in the high-resolution mode (digital resolution 5 µm/pixel). All frames must be aligned and averaged to create a final image. One of the difficulties encountered during fundus autofluorescence imaging besides careful and standardized image acquisition is the influence of media opacities, with cataract being the most prominent adverse factor (74).

Fundus Camera–Based System

Ordinary fundus cameras can image autofluorescence of the fundus using the same wavelengths. However, autofluorescence of the crystalline lens would also be imaged, particularly in patients with nuclear sclerosis, creating fogging of the image. To avoid this problem, a new filter set is used with a fundus camera to image autofluorescence. A barrier filter of 695 nm (bandwidth 675–715 nm) is selected (Spectrotech, Saugus, MA) to avoid imaging the autofluorescence of the lens, which lies chiefly from 510 to 670 nm. SLOs use wavelengths to stimulate fluorescence that are preferentially attenuated by increasing nuclear sclerotic changes. Therefore, a bandpass filter for the excitation light of 580 nm (bandwidth 500–610 nm) is selected to help reduce any variation in stimulating light reaching the fundus caused by absorptive changes in the crystalline lens. The gain for the digital camera is set at the maximum level through the IMAGEnet software (Topcon, IMAGEnet, Oakland, NJ). The wavelengths selected are well outside of that used for both fluorescein and ICG angiography. The light exposure to the fundus is calculated to be orders of magnitude less than that used for a typical fluorescein angiographic evaluation. The autofluorescence photographs with confocal SLO imaging are noisier than the autofluorescence photographs with the fundus camera–based system (73).

Interpretation of Fundus Autofluorescence

All autofluorescence values are adjusted using a histogram distribution for the pixels in the image. A gaussian curve of values from 0 to 255 is obtained; 0 corresponds to black and 255 corresponds to pure white. A cumulative frequency distribution is calculated, and the determination of the pixel value at the 1 percentile value is performed. Then, subtraction of this pixel value from the values greater than 1 percentile is done. This process converts all values at or lower than 1 percentile to black and shifts all other corresponding values in an objective manner not influenced by operator interaction. Finally, these final pixel values are evaluated to calculate the mean and standard deviation of the brightness values. Fundus autofluorescence images usually are evaluated for the presence of areas of decreased (hypoautofluorescence) or increased (hyperautofluorescence) fundus autofluorescence. So, we consider that the RPE cells are normal if the autofluorescence imaging shows some autofluorescence. However, when autofluorescence imaging shows large autofluorescence, we consider that the RPE is sick or stressed RPE cells, and the absence of autofluorescence reflects the death of the RPE cells (73).

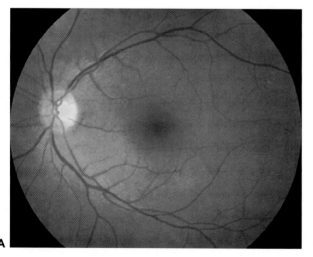 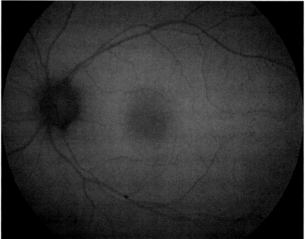

Figure 1.12 ■ **A.** Normal fundus retinography. **B.** Autofluorescence image of normal macula.

Normal Fundus Autofluorescence

A normal pattern of fundus autofluorescence is characterized by decreased intensity at the fovea, under the retinal blood vessels, and in the peripapillary region and further decrease over the optic nerve head, which appears dark (Fig. 1.12). The autofluorescence in the fovea is decreased because there is less accumulation of lipofuscin in the fovea than nasally or temporally to the macula (73). However, the autofluorescence in the fovea is minimally affected by the absorption of the macula luteal pigments at a 580 nm excitation wavelength. In addition, it has some effect of absorbance at a 488 nm excitation wavelength, and it is not significantly affected by ocular pigmentation depending on the choice of the wavelength excitation and barrier filters, because the higher the wavelength, the less the absorption by melanin. There is a topographic distribution of RPE lipofuscin content throughout the fundus, being higher at the posterior pole, with a localized dip at the fovea, lower toward the peripheral retina. This is consistent with histologic findings demonstrating a decay of lipofuscin correlating to the density of photoreceptors toward the periphery. The distribution by quadrants is highest temporally, then nasally, superiorly, and lowest inferiorly. There are some facts that we must have in mind to understand the normal autofluorescent pattern; one fact to be considered is the spatial distribution of the photoreceptors. It is difficult to perform a correlation between lipofuscin and cone photoreceptors because they decrease their density rapidly between the fovea. At 3 or 3.5 degrees, the maximal density of the cones is found at the fovea, and at 3 degrees from the fovea, we can find only 10% of their maximal density. In the case of the rod photoreceptors, the distribution is different: the rods' highest density is in a ring between 10 and 15 degrees, and the highest loss of rods happens between 5 and 12 degrees (inside the highest density ring of rods); after 15 degrees, the density of the rods starts to decrease toward the periphery (73). It is important to address that the zone of minimal fluorescence in the fovea overlaps the rod-free zone, and this fact can suggest that the rate of lipofuscin formation in the cones may be slower than in the rods; it would be confirmed if studies in humans correlated the study in rhesus monkeys where the number of phagosomas in the RPE of the fovea (derived from cones) is only one-third of the number of extrafoveal phagosomes in the RPE (derived mainly from rods). Despite the fact that the greatest lipofuscin accumulation overlaps the regions in which the rod loss is greatest, the prediction of rod loss cannot be done by lipofuscin accumulation, because the inferior retina had greater rod loss and lower fluorescence than the superior retina.

In the case of the Bruch's membrane, the fluorescence is only significant if the excited wavelength used is in the blue light spectrum: the higher the wavelength excitation, the lower the fluorescence of the Bruch's membrane. In the red edge of the spectrum, the Bruch's membrane has little contribution to autofluorescence.

ACKNOWLEDGMENTS

Supported in part by the Arevalo-Coutinho Foundation for Research in Ophthalmology, Caracas, Venezuela.

REFERENCES

1. Amalric P. The macula: 50 years of study: from clinical aspects to genetics. Points de Vue. 1998;39:4–20.

2. Hendrickson AE, Yuodelis C. The morphological development of the human fovea. Ophthalmology. 1984;91:603–612.

3. Fulton AB, Albert DM, Craft JL. Human albinism. Light and electron microscopy study. Arch Ophthalmol. 1978;96:305–310.

4. Leuenberger P. Stereo-ultrastructure of the retina. Comparative transmission and scanning electron microscope study. Arch Ophthalmol Rev Gen Ophthalmol. 1971;31:813–822.

5. Mann I. Development of the Human Eye. New York: Grune & Stratton; 1964.

6. Duke-Elder S, Cook C. Normal and abnormal development. In: System of ophthalmology, vol 3, part 1. St. Louis, MO: Mosby; 1963.

7. Streeten BW. Development of the human retinal pigment epithelium and the posterior segment. Arch Ophthalmol. 1969;81:383–394.

8. Provis JM, Van Driel D, Billson FA, et al. Development of the human retina: patterns of cell distribution and redistribution in the ganglion cell layer. J Comp Neurol. 1985;22:429–451.

9. Moore KL. The developing human: clinically oriented embryology. 3rd Ed. Philadelphia, PA: WB Saunders; 1982:413–416.

10. Weiter JJ, Delori FC, Wing GL, et al. Retinal pigment epithelial lipofuscin and melanin and choroidal melanin in human eyes. Invest Ophthalmol Vis Sci. 1986;27:145–152.

11. Duvall J. Structure, function, and pathologic responses of pigment epithelium: a review. Semin Ophthalmol. 1987;2:130–140.

12. Garner A. Retinal angiogenesis: mechanism in health and disease. Semin Ophthalmol. 1987;2:71–80.

13. Engerman RL. Development of the macular circulation. Invest Ophthalmol. 1976;15:835–840.

14. Federman JL, Gouras P, Schubert H, et al. Retina and vitreous. In: Podos SM, Yanoff M, eds. Textbook of ophthalmology, vol 9. London, UK: Gower Medical; 1994.

15. Hogan MJ, Alvarado JA, Weddell JE. Histology of the human eye: an atlas and textbook. Philadelphia, PA: WB Saunders; 1971:508–519.

16. Gass JD. Stereoscopic atlas of macular diseases: diagnosis and treatment, 4th Ed, vol 1. St. Louis, MO: Mosby-Year Book Inc.; 1997:1–17.

17. Justice J Jr, Lehmann RP. Cilioretinal arteries: a study based on review of stereo fundus photographs and fluorescein angiographic findings. Arch Ophthalmol. 1976;94:1355–1358.

18. Michaelson IC. Retinal circulation in man and animals. Springfield, IL: Charles C. Thomas; 1954.

19. Wald G. Human vision and the spectrum. Science. 1945;101:653–658.

20. Bone RA, Landrum JT, Hime GW, et al. Stereochemistry of the human macular carotenoids. Invest Ophthalmol Vis Sci. 1993;34:2033–2040.

21. Nussbaum JJ, Pruett RC, Delori FC. Historic perspectives: macular yellow pigment; the first 200 years. Retina. 1981;1:296–310.

22. Snodderly DM, Auran J, Delori FC. Localization of the macular pigment. Invest Ophthalmol Vis Sci. 1979;18:80.

23. Snodderly DM, Auran J, Delori FC. The macular pigment. II. Spatial distribution in primate retinas. Invest Ophthalmol Vis Sci. 1984;25:674–685.

24. Fine BS. Limiting membranes of the sensory retina and pigment epithelium: an electron microscopic study. Arch Ophthalmol. 1961;66:847–860.

25. Blanks JC. Morphology and topography of the retina. In: Ryan SJ. Retina, vol 1, 3rd Ed. St Louis, MO: Mosby; 2001:32–53.

26. Marquardt R. Ein Beitrag zur Topographie and Anatomie der Netzhautgefasse des menschlichen Auges. Klin Monatsbl Augenheilkd. 1966;148:50–64.

27. Shimizu K, Ujiie K. Structure of ocular vessels. Tokyo, Japan: Igaku Shoin; 1978.

28. Henkind P, Bellhorn RW, Murphy ME, et al. Development of macular vessels in monkey and cat. Br J Ophthalmol. 1975;59:703–709.

29. Curcio CA, Allen KA, Sloan KR, et al. Distribution and morphology of human photoreceptors stained with anti-blue opsin. J Comp Neurol. 1991;312:610–624.

30. Tso MOM, Friedman E. The retinal pigment epithelium I. Comparative histology. Arch Ophthalmol. 1967;78:641–649.

31. Green WR. Retina. In: Spencer WH, Ophthalmic pathology: an atlas and textbook, vol 2, 4th Ed. Philadelphia, PA: W.B. Saunders Company; 1996:667–681.

32. Amalric PM. Choroidal vessel occlusive syndromes—clinical aspects. Trans Am Acad Ophthalmol Otolaryngol. 1973;77:OP291–OP299.

33. Hayreh SS. The choriocapillaris. Albrecht von Graefes Arch Klin Exp Ophthalmol. 1974;192:165–179.

34. Hayreh SS. Segmental nature of the choroidal vasculature. Br J Ophthalmol. 1975;59:631–648.

35. Hayreh SS. Submacular choroidal vasculature pattern: experimental fluorescein fundus angiographic studies. Albrecht von Graefes Arch Klin Exp Ophthalmol. 1974;192:181–196.

36. Krey HF. Segmental vascular patterns of the choriocapillaris. Am J Ophthalmol. 1975;80:198–206.

37. Dollery CT, Henkind P, Kohner EM, et al. Effect of raised intraocular pressure on the retinal and choroidal circulation. Invest Ophthalmol. 1968;7:191–198.

38. Hayreh SS. Recent advances in fluorescein fundus angiography. Br J Ophthalmol. 1974;58:391–412.

39. Perry HD, Hatfield RV, Tso MOM. Fluorescein pattern of the choriocapillaris in the neonatal rhesus monkey. Am J Ophthalmol. 1977;84:197–204.

40. Ernest JT, Stern WH, Archer DB. Submacular choroidal circulation. Am J Ophthalmol. 1976;81:574–582.

41. Sarna T. Properties and functions of the ocular melanin: a photobiophysical view. J Photochem Photobiol B. 1992;12:215–258.

42. Tombran-Tink J, Shivaram SM, Chader GJ, et al. Expression, secretion, and age related down regulation of pigment epithelium-derived factor, a serpin with neurotrophic activity. J Neurosci. 1995;15:4992–5003.

43. Parver LM, Auker CR, Carpenter DO. The stabilizing effect of the choroidal circulation on the temperature environment of the macula. Retina. 1982;2:117–120.

44. Cunha-Vaz J. The blood-ocular barriers. Surv Ophthalmol. 1979;23: 279–296.

45. Dubai J. Structure function, and pathologic responses of pigment epithelium: a review. Semin Ophthalmol. 1987;2:130–140.

46. Kincaid MC. Topographic anatomy, histology and fluorescein angiography. In: Grossniklaus HE, Kincaid MC. Ophthalmology clinics of North America: macular diseases, vol 6. Philadelphia, PA: WB Saunders Company; 1993:181–189.

47. Iwasaki M, Inomata H. Relation between superficial capillaries and foveal structures in the human retina. Invest Ophthalmol Vis Sci. 1986;27: 1698–1705.

48. Rabb MF, Burton TC, Schatz H, et al. Fluorescein angiography of the fundus: a schematic approach to interpretation. Surv Ophthalmol. 1978;22: 387–403.

49. Flower RW, Hochheimer BF. Clinical infrared absorption angiography of the choroid (letter). Am J Ophthalmol. 1972;73:458.

50. Piccolino FC, Borgia L, Zinicola E, et al. Pre-injection fluorescence in indocyanine green angiography. Ophthalmology. 1996;103:1837–1845.

51. Hope-Ross M, Yannuzzi LA, Gragoudas ED, et al. Adverse reactions due to indocyanine green. Ophthalmology. 1994;101:529–533.

52. Bonte CA, Ceuppens J, Leys AM. Hypotensive shock as a complication of indocyanine green injection. Retina. 1998;18:476–477.

53. Olsen TW, Lim JI, Capone A Jr, et al. Anaphylactic shock following indocyanine green angiography. Arch Ophthalmol. 1996;114:97.

54. Hyvärinen L, Flower RW. Indocyanine green fluorescence angiography. Acta Ophthalmol (Copen) 1980;58:528–538.

55. Bischoff PM, Flower RW. Ten years experience with choroidal angiography using indocyanine green dye: a new routine examination or an epilogue? Doc Ophthalmol. 1985;60:235–291.

56. Slakter JS, Yanuzzi LA, Guyer DR, et al. Indocyanine green angiography. Curr Opin Ophthalmol. 1995;6:25–32.

57. Bartsch DU, Weinreb RN, Zinser G, et al. Confocal scanning infrared laser ophthalmoscopy for indocyanine green angiography. Am J Ophthalmol. 1995;120:642–651.

58. Klein GJ, Baumgartner RH, Flower RW. An image processing approach to characterizing choroidal blood flow. Invest Ophthalmol Vis Sci. 1990;31: 629–637.

59. Maberly DAL, Cruess AF. Indocyanine green angiography: an evaluation of image enhancement for the identification of occult choroidal neovascular membranes. Retina. 1999;19:37–44.

60. Flower RW, Hochheimer BF. Indocyanine green dye fluorescence and infrared absorption choroidal angiography performed simultaneously with fluorescein angiography. Johns Hopkins Med J. 1976;138:33–42.

61. Bischoff PM, Niederberger HJ, Torok B, et al. Simultaneous indocyanine green and fluorescein angiography. Retina. 1995;15:91–99.

62. Scheider A, Schroedel C. High resolution indocyanine green angiography with a scanning laser ophthalmoscope (letter). Am J Ophthalmol. 1989;108:458–459.

63. Holz FG, Bellmann C, Rohrschneider K, et al. Simultaneous confocal scanning laser fluorescein and indocyanine green angiography. Am J Ophthalmol. 1998;125:227–236.

64. Spaide RF, Orlock DA, Herrmann-Delemazure B, et al. Wide angle indocyanine green angiography. Retina. 1998;18:44–49.

65. Scheider A, Voeth A, Kaboth A, et al. Fluorescence characteristics of indocyanine green in the normal choroid and in subretinal neovascular membranes. Ger J Ophthalmol. 1992;1:7–11.

66. Scheider A, Neuhauser L. Fluorescence characteristics of drusen during indocyanine green angiography and their possible correlation with choroidal perfusion. Ger J Ophthalmol. 1992;1:328–334.

67. Yannuzzi LA, Flower RW, Slakter JS, eds. Indocyanine green angiography. St. Louis, MO: Mosby; 1997.

68. Neubauer AS, Priglinger S, Ullrich S, et al. Comparison of foveal thickness measured with the retinal thickness analyzer and optical coherence tomography. Retina. 2001;21:596–601.

69. Jo YJ, Heo DW, Shin YI, et al. Diurnal variation of retina thickness measured with time domain and spectral domain optical coherence tomography in healthy subjects. Invest Ophthalmol Vis Sci. 2011;52(9):497–500.

70. Wakitani Y, Sasoh M, Sugimoto M, et al. Macular thickness measurements in healthy subjects with different axial lengths using optical coherence tomography. Retina. 2003;23:177–182.

71. Puliafito CA, Hee MR, Schuman JS, et al. Optical coherence tomography of ocular diseases. Thorofare, NJ: SLACK Inc.; 1996.

72. Delori FC, Dorey K, Staurenghi G, et al. In vivo autofluorescence of the ocular fundus exhibits retinal pigment epithelial lipofuscin characteristics. Invest Ophthalmol Vis Sci. 1995;36:718–729.

73. Schmitz-Valckenberg S, Holz FG, Bird AC, et al. Fundus autofluorescence imaging: review and perspectives. Retina. 2008;28:385–409.

74. Holz FG. Autofluorescence imaging of the macula. Ophthalmologe. 2001; 98:10–18.

2

ANIMAL MODELS FOR AGE-RELATED MACULAR DEGENERATION

MATÍAS E. CZERWONKO • MARIANA INGOLOTTI • AMELIA NELSON
JAMEL L. F. BROWN • D. VIRGIL ALFARO III

INTRODUCTION

Age-related macular degeneration (AMD) is a late-onset, multifactorial, neurodegenerative disease of the retina and the leading cause of irreversible vision loss in the elderly in the Western world (1). It affects 30 to 50 million individuals, and clinical hallmarks of AMD are observed in at least one-third of persons over the age of 75 in industrialized countries (2). Animal models, in particular, have contributed greatly to current knowledge regarding the etiology, molecular mechanisms, and histologic features of this extremely prevalent condition.

As we consider animal models of AMD, with the potential for preclinical investigation, various pathologic and nonpathologic histologic elements must be considered. In the particular case of AMD, we can roughly divide its typical features into two types: histologic and functional alterations.

Among the *histologic features* that have been reported from the eyes of patients with AMD are the following:

- Thickening of the Bruch's membrane (BM)
- Subretinal pigmented epithelium (RPE) basal laminar deposits and basal linear deposits (i.e., drusen)
- Hyperplasia
- Changes in the RPE including loss of the basal infoldings

- Accumulation of immune cells (i.e., macrophages and microglia)
- Atrophy
- Photoreceptor atrophy
- Deposition of activated complement proteins
- Retinal or choroidal neovascularization (CNV)
- Fibrosis
- Accumulation of lipofuscin in RPE cells with increased levels of A2E and corresponding increases in autofluorescence

Functional changes refer to decreased signals on electroretinograms (ERGs) secondary to photoreceptor atrophy (3–7). Although AMD disease mechanisms are still poorly understood, several pathogenic pathways have been proposed, each associated with manifestations of AMD, including oxidative damage, metabolic deregulation, and chronic inflammatory processes. These pathways have been tested and confirmed in studies based on animal models, most of which are explained in this chapter.

Mice have been widely used for generating models that simulate human AMD features for investigating the pathogenesis, treatment, and prevention of the disease. Focal atrophy of photoreceptors and RPE, lipofuscin accumulation, and increased A2E can be present in aged mouse eyes, even though the mouse does not have a macula.

15

Unfortunately, drusen are rarely seen in mice because of their simpler BM and different process of lipofuscin extrusion compared with humans. Analyzing basal deposits at the ultrastructural level and understanding the ultrastructural pathologic differences between various mouse AMD models are therefore critical to comprehend the significance of research findings. More recently, some other animal models have entered the world of AMD research. While nonhuman primate models have gained popularity over the past few years because of their resemblance to the ocular anatomic features of humans, rabbits and pigs are less often used.

The purpose of this chapter is to provide a framework for better understanding some of the existing animal models and the knowledge that has been derived from their study regarding both dry and wet types of AMD. Some of these models have encouraged the development of some promising lines of investigation concerning novel therapeutic approaches. Nevertheless, it is important to understand that most of these models are not necessarily etiologic representations of human disease.

ETHICS OF ANIMAL USE

The use of animals in biomedical research dates back to the fifth century BCE. Our ancient ancestors realized the homogenous relationship between humans and other animals and the subsequent medical discoveries that come from experimentation. Since then, nonhuman animals have proved themselves to be appropriate models for scientific inquiries, contributing to medical science. However, with the use of animals in research must come a regard for the ethical treatment and general welfare of the animals used.

The first mention of animal usage in the medical field occurred around 500 BCE. Pythagoras, an ancient philosopher and mathematician, recognized a common soul between animals and humans—a connection that could be used to make certain comparisons. Hippocrates was the first to directly compare specific organs. Vivisection was even practiced among certain scientists, including Alcmaeon, Herophilus, and Erasistratus, at this time in history. Years later, the use of vivisection was exercised even more so by one of the fathers of medical experimentation, Galenus. The first true published experiment involving animals did not occur until 1638 CE by English physician William Harvey. However, the issue of ethics in these experiments was not mentioned until the 18th century. British philosopher Jeremy Bentham published his ideas on the welfare of animals, which led to the start of regulations and protection of animals. Bentham is responsible for projecting the idea of utilitarianism, the ethical doctrine stating if an action provides benefit to society, it is indeed morally right. He was the first to question the actual suffering of animals in experiments, and laws regarding such would be the result.

Britain was the first country to pass laws concerning animal welfare. The first association to establish themselves as protectors of animals in medical research was the Society for the Prevention of Cruelty to Animals, begun in the year 1824 in England. The first law to pass was the British Cruelty to Animals Act in 1876. The issue of animal rights did not die in England during the 1900s; in 1969, FRAME (Fund for the Replacement of Animals in Medical Experiments) was established.

In 1909, Americans started publishing on behalf of animal rights. The first federal law passed in America regarding animal cruelty was created in 1966 and called the U.S. Animal Welfare Act, serving to protect the welfare of laboratory animals. Animal rights organizations such as PETA (People for the Ethical Treatment of Animals) and the Johns Hopkins Center for Alternatives to Animal Testing began forming in the 1980s. The three R's, replace, reduce, and refine, became a sentiment for animal activists across the globe. Laws and regulations on the ethics of animals in the laboratory are still fighting to be passed, and the conflict lingers with a conclusion still remaining to be determined.

The first topic to be addressed when discussing animal research is the obvious question: What is the purpose? Or, in other words, is there indeed a need for animal experimentation? Some claim that animals and humans are simply too different to make valid comparisons and that ultimately society does not benefit from animal research. Of course, this is true if one was to compare completely dissimilar organisms, such as two animals in entirely different animal kingdoms. Nonetheless, properly executed animal experiments have led to many historical medical breakthroughs, including the discovery and refinement of insulin in dogs.

Another concern when evaluating the ethics of using animals in the laboratory is the actual success rate of the research itself. How often does an experiment involving animals actually lead to something valuable and how often does it simply fail to achieve useful results? To answer this question, one must determine what constitutes a low success rate, a term whose meaning is relative to the person who is using it. Since a "low success rate" is not attached to a tangible number, there is no way of knowing if animal experimentation would qualify as such. The rebuttal to this argument points out that trial and error is one of the characteristics of scientific research and explains that upon comprehension of the scientific method should come a realization of the inevitable chance of failure.

While there is still disagreement among people on opposing sides of the issue, there is common ground being reached. Scientists have resorted to alternative methods of experimentation. In many instances, in vitro techniques can replace animal testing. Scientists take stem cells from humans to mimic real human responses to testing. They can also use brain imaging, such as MRI or CT scans, to study human brains instead of animal brains and even imitate real human responses through computer simulation. Although the two different sides of the issue conflict, alternative methods to animal testing serve as a satisfying compromise.

Another point to be addressed is the inclusion of policies on ethical standards in lab experiments and reports. One study shows that 40.7% of published work involving animal testing was performed with a respect for ethical standards. A different study, using articles from PubMed, shows that 53% of the research had ethical policies. Both of these studies show that there is much improvement to be done in this field. Inclusion of ethical standards in animal research should hopefully reach 100%, proving that all research involving animals displays ethical treatment to the laboratory animals. Not only does reporting ethical standards in studies show that the science has taken a moral standpoint, but it also implies scientific integrity and respect in the medical field (8–12).

ANIMAL MODELS OF DRY MACULAR DEGENERATION

Rodent Models for Dry AMD

The active role of oxidative stress, inflammation, and metabolic deregulation in AMD pathogenesis has been well established (13). Pathologic hallmarks of the dry type of AMD include drusen accumulation, BM thickening, RPE, and photoreception degeneration followed by atrophy. Mice have been the most commonly used models for retinal disease because their retina resembles the human nasal and peripheral retina. The described murine models for dry AMD have drusen-like lesions and RPE atrophy on funduscopy, ERG abnormalities, lipofuscin accumulation, sub-RPE basal deposits, and BM thickening. Undoubtedly, one of the most seductive advantages of murine models is the ease to manipulate them genetically, surgically, and pharmacologically.

The aforementioned dry AMD murine models can be conveniently classified into three categories:

- Genetically engineered mice
- Immunologically manipulated mice
- Naturally occurring mouse strains

Most murine models are genetically engineered to manipulate genes that are suspected to cause macular degeneration-like disorders in humans or might be somehow associated to AMD pathogenesis. Inflammatory genes (Cfh, Ccl2, Ccr2, and Cx3cr1), oxidative stress–associated genes (Sod1 and Sod2), and metabolic pathway genes (mcd, Cp, Hepb, ApoE, and ApoB100) have been manipulated to create models with features that are typical of dry AMD. The immunologically manipulated mouse model is immunized against carboxyethylpyrrole (CEP), an endogenous biomarker of oxidative stress. Finally, the naturally occurring mouse models include retinal degeneration models with mice exposed to nocive and AMD-related conditions and the senescence-accelerated mouse (SAM) models with systemic and retinal age-related pathology, including BM thickening, basal deposits, and CNV.

In the following paragraphs, we explain the most important models of each of the groups mentioned above. Overall, these models contrast with the murine models of wet AMD that are mostly induced mechanically and are explained later in this chapter.

LIPID AND GLUCOSE METABOLISM MODELS

A growing body of the literature indicates the involvement of lipids, lipoproteins, and glucose in the formation of extracellular lesions in aging BM, basal deposits and drusen, and other AMD hallmarks. Observational studies have indicated that maintaining adequate levels of fatty acids or a low glycemic index (GI) diet may be particularly beneficial for early stages of the disease. From a pathophysiologic perspective, lipids and cholesterol that concentrate within the BM with aging are believed to restrict the metabolite transference between the RPE and the choriocapillaris (14–18). From a structural point of view, lipids and cholesterol deposits may promote the formation of both basal laminar and basal linear deposits. We could fairly claim that there are three major metabolism-related risk factors that have been associated to AMD pathogenesis:

- *Diet*: High intakes of cholesterol and monounsaturated, polyunsaturated, and saturated fats have been associated with the onset and progression of AMD (19).
- *Cardiovascular diseases*: An apparent correlation between the deposition of cholesterol and lipids in atherosclerotic plaques and the material accumulated in the BM was described. Nevertheless, numerous studies have shown opposing results so that controversy still exists as to how tight this association really is, if there is any (20–22).
- *Genetics*: Polymorphisms in genes that code for lipid transport mediators (apolipoproteins) showed a significant association with the risk of AMD (23,24).

The following sections are dedicated to mention and describe the most important animal models that have been designed to assess the potential connection between lipid and glucose metabolism and AMD pathogenesis.

Aging and a High-Fat Diet

To examine the histologic, histochemical, and ultrastructural changes in the BM in C57BL/6 mice on a high-fat (HF) diet, Dithmar et al. compared 2-month-old models on a normal diet and 8-month-old mice on a normal or HF diet. Confirming the importance of aging, thickening of the BM was found in 8-month-old mice on both normal and HF dietary regimens. However, 8-month-old mice exposed to HF diets showed greater thickness compared to that of nonexposed counterparts. Since the plasma cholesterol level was significantly higher in mice on HF diets than the controls, the results were consistent with the suspected role of lipids in the pathogenesis of AMD. A year later to

Dithmar's studies, Cousins et al. (25) compared 2-month-old and 16-month-old C57BL/6 mice fed normal and HF diets. In this case, basal laminar deposits were observed in the 16-month group exclusively.

Aging and High Glycemic Index Diet

The GI indicates how fast blood glucose is raised after consuming a carbohydrate-containing food. Human metabolic studies indicate that GI is related to abnormal responses after meals. Recent epidemiologic evidence indicates positive association between GI and risk for AMD in people without diabetes. Therefore, it is reasonable to suspect low GI diets as protective factors for the development of AMD (26–30).

Based on these assumptions, Uchiki et al. (31) compared mice that consumed low and high GI diets, showing that the latter promote the apparition of AMD-like lesions. Mice that consumed the lower GI diet displayed a significantly reduced frequency and severity of age-related retinal lesions such as basal deposits. Glycation-altered proteolysis is accounted for linking dietary GI, aging, and age-related diseases like AMD. Not surprisingly, consuming higher GI diets was associated with over threefold higher accumulation of advanced glycation end products (AGEs) in the retina in the age-matched mice. Both incidence and severity of retinal changes aggravated with age, as older mice exhibited more thickening of the BM, more basal laminar deposits, disorganization of RPE basal infolding, and increased photoreceptor atrophy compared to 17-month-old counterparts (32).

Apolipoproteins

Cholesterol and its transporter, apolipoprotein E (ApoE), are major constituents of sub-RPE deposits in AMD eyes. Based on these findings, the following murine models were designed and studied:

■ *ApoE knockout mice*: ApoE is a constituent of very-low-density lipoprotein (VLDL) synthesized by the liver and of a subclass of high-density lipoprotein (HDL) involved in cholesterol transporting among cells. ApoE mediates high-affinity binding of ApoE-containing lipoprotein particles to the low-density lipoprotein (LDL) receptor and is thus responsible for the cellular uptake of these particles. Mice with inactivated endogenous ApoE gene exhibited very high levels of circulating cholesterol (33,34) and revealed thickening of the BM combined with electrolucent particles and membrane-bounded material at 8 months of age (35).

■ *ApoEe2/ApoEe4 transgenic mice*: With the purpose of studying the multiple ApoE alleles seen in humans, transgenic mice were created replacing native ApoE with human ApoE equivalents (36–38). Eyes of aged mice expressing human ApoE2, ApoE3, or ApoE4 and maintained on a high fat and cholesterol (HF-C) diet showed ApoE isoform–dependent pathologies of diverse severity. They develop a constellation of changes that mimic the pathology associated with human AMD such as

■ Diffuse subretinal pigment epithelial deposits
■ Drusenoid deposits
■ Thickened BM
■ Atrophy, hypopigmentation, and hyperpigmentation of the RPE

Interestingly, ApoE4 mice were the most severely affected, to the point of having sometimes developed CNV. Transgenic ApoE4 mice fed HF-C diets have also shown to accumulate amyloid b (Ab), a well-known constituent of human drusen (39). What is more, systemic anti-Aβ immunotherapy was shown to protect against loss of visual function and retinal damage, suggesting a role for Ab in the AMD pathogenesis and functional manifestations (40). Ironically, while the ApoEe4 allele is correlated with relative protection for AMD in humans, in the mice, the opposite appears to be true (23,41–43). The reason for this discrepancy between species still remains unclear.

■ *ApoE3-Leiden transgenic mice*: ApoE3-Leiden is a dysfunctional form of ApoE3 that is associated with a dominantly inherited form of familial dysbetalipoproteinemia and early onset of atherosclerosis (44). With the intention of investigating the ApoE3-Leiden mouse as an animal model for retinal extracellular deposits, transgenic mice carrying the ApoE3-Leiden gene were created. Eyes were obtained from ApoE3-Leiden transgenic mice on a HF-C diet or on a normal mouse chow diet for 9 months. As controls, eyes were collected from ApoE knockout mice on the same dietary regimens. All eyes of the ApoE3-Leiden mice on a HF-C diet exhibited basal laminar deposit, whereas ApoE3-Leiden mice on normal chow displayed basal laminar deposits only occasionally. In both cases, however, the ultrastructural features of these deposits were comparable with those seen in human eyes, and they all showed immunoreaction with antihuman ApoE antibodies. Importantly, no deposits were found in any of the control mice. These results indicate that ApoE3-Leiden mice can be used as an animal model for the pathogenesis of basal laminar deposits and that a HF-C diet enhances the accumulation process. Furthermore, this study supports the previously suggested involvement of dysfunctional ApoE in the accumulation of extracellular deposits in the human disease (45,46).

■ *ApoB100 transgenic mice*: ApoB100 is the major apolipoprotein in LDL cholesterol. Lipoprotein particles in the BM have been shown to contain ApoB100. To study how ApoB100 might contribute to the formation of lipoproteinaceous deposits in AMD, several groups have examined mice that express human ApoB100. Young ApoB100 mice developed basal laminar deposits when fed with a HF diet and exposed to oxidative blue-green light (47). At older ages, ApoB100 mice exposed to normal diets exhibited BM thickening, loss of the basal infoldings of the RPE, and basal laminar deposits (48,49). When these animals were additionally fed HF diets, more basal linear deposits were observed.

Lipoprotein Receptors

LDL receptor (LDLR) knockout mice are incapable of importing cholesterol, leading to increased plasma cholesterol levels and development of atheromatosis. Since atherosclerosis is a well-established risk factor for developing AMD, a murine knockout model with LDLR deficiency was used to evaluate changes in the BM. As it was expected, mice lacking LDLR exhibited a degeneration of the BM with accumulation of lipid particles, which was further increased after fat intake due to elevated blood lipid levels.

Alternatively, alterations in the gene that codes for VLDL receptor (VLDLR) have also shown some impact on the onset and progression of retinopathies. Mice with both alleles mutated do not show signs of dyslipidemia but still develop retinal neovascularization as early as 2 weeks of age (50–52). These vessels grow toward the subretinal space, and can form choroidal anastomosis or cause retinal hemorrhages between 30 and 60 days. Deeper analysis of this model revealed the development of CNV, elevated levels of vascular endothelial growth factor (VEGF), and dysregulation of the Wnt pathway all of which suggested VLDLR as a negative regulator of CNV (53). Therefore, modulation of the VLDLR may have a great potential from a therapeutic perspective.

More recently, polymorphisms in CD36 have also been shown to be protective factors in AMD (54). CD36 is a scavenger receptor that binds oxidized LDL (OxLDL) and is mostly expressed in the apical and basolateral membrane of the RPE (55–57). Mice deficient for CD36 accumulate subretinal OxLDL even when fed a regular diet (58). Even though lipids in the RPE come mostly from photoreceptor outer segments and are exocytosed through the base of the RPE to be eliminated via the choroid, RPE cells can also take up oxidized lipids from their cell base, suggesting they may be involved in clearing the subretinal space from such deposits. Laminar deposits in the BM have been found to contain OxLDL among other compounds. Consistently, CD36 deficiency in mice resulted in both age-associated accumulation of oxidized lipids and BM thickening. Coherently, treatment of HF-C-fed ApoE null mice with a CD36 agonist was shown to diminish thickening of the BM notably as well as to partially lessen photoreceptor atrophy and preserve function (58).

Cathepsin D

Cathepsin D is an aspartic protease that is highly expressed in the RPE and plays a decisive role in processing photoreceptor outer segments (59,60). Cathepsin D is secreted as a proenzyme, which accumulation has been linked to RPE dysfunction (61). To study the mechanism, transgenic mice

with a mutant form of cathepsin have been developed (62). Mice homozygous for the transgene demonstrated areas of RPE atrophy as early as 9 months of age (63). Between 10 and 18 months old, these mice exhibited areas of RPE hypertrophy, photoreceptor atrophy, and reduced ERGs. Remarkably, they also displayed small yellowish spots in the fundus that were similar to basal laminar and basal linear spots.

OXIDATIVE DAMAGE MODELS

Clinical and experimental evidence supports that chronic oxidative stress is a primary contributing factor to numerous retinal degenerative diseases, specially AMD (64–66). Oxidative damage is normally minimized by the presence of a wide range of antioxidant and efficient repair systems. Unfortunately, aging intensifies oxidative damage while decreasing antioxidant capacity, thereby perturbing the oxidative homeostasis. Postmortem eye examinations from AMD patients have shown signs in line with extensive free radical damage (67). Consistently, antioxidant-enriched diets have been shown to reduce the progression from dry to wet AMD (68).

Several mouse models of chronic oxidative stress displayed many of the most characteristic hallmarks of AMD. These models can be classified into two groups: those that lack intrinsic antioxidant mechanisms and those where additional oxidative stress is applied. However, whether oxidative stress is an etiologic component or if it is just involved in disease progression is still controversial.

Carboxyethylpyrrole-Adducted Products

Recent evidence has implicated AMD as an immunologically mediated disease (69). The protein adduct CEP is present in AMD eye tissue and in the blood of AMD patients at higher levels than found in age-matched non-AMD tissues. Autoantibodies to CEP are also higher in AMD blood samples than in controls. It has been suggested that a signal from the outer retina initiates an immune response in AMD. CEP acts as a reliable biomarker of oxidative stress and is currently suspected to be one of those signals (70,71).

To test such hypothesis, Hollyfield et al. (72,73) created a mouse model by immunizing animals with CEP-adducted mouse serum albumin. Essentially, two groups were compared: a short-term group that received a strong immunologic challenge over 3 months and a long-term group that was inoculated with a weaker challenge but over a year. Both groups successfully developed antibodies to CEP-adducted albumin. At 3 months, the short-term group showed deposition of complement component C3d in BM, RPE swelling and lysis, sub-RPE deposits, pyknosis of overlying photoreceptors, and invasion of macrophages. Long-term counterparts, on the other hand, exhibited a three- to fivefold thickening of BM. There existed a solid correlation between the levels of CEP-specific antibodies and the severity of pathologic alterations. Importantly, although CEP is also proangiogenic via a VEGF-independent pathway (74), neither the short-term nor long-term group exhibited signs of CNV, confirming that the utility of this model is limited for dry AMD only.

SOD Models

Superoxide dismutases (SODs) are one of the major antioxidant defense systems, which consist of three isoforms in mammals: the cytoplasmic SOD (SOD1), the mitochondrial SOD (SOD2), and the extracellular SOD (SOD3). All of these isoforms require catalytic metal (Cu or Mn) for their activation (75). To investigate the role of oxidative stress in AMD pathogenesis, transgenic mice targeting the SOD oxidative stress recovery pathways have been created and examined. With some significant variances, knockout mice for different SOD genes showed typical features of AMD.

SOD1 levels are particularly high in the retina, and its protective role against oxidative damage is unquestionable. Imamura et al. showed that SOD1 knockout mice display age-related pathologic changes in the retina reminiscent of AMD as early as 7 months of age. Among the most frequent findings were the presence of drusen, the thickening of BM, and the development of CNV (being thereby suitable for simulating wet forms of AMD as well) (76). However, prior to the 7-month period, retinas from these animals were absolutely indistinguishable from age-matched wild-type animals (76). As with many other models, lesions increased in number and severity with age: At 10 months of age, 86% of mice had drusen, compared to very few drusen in age-matched wild-type mice (76), and at a year of age, RPE vacuolization and degenerative changes were noted. Remarkably, yellowish drusen-like deposits between the RPE and BM stained for some of the most typical drusen biomarkers such as vitronectin, carboxymethyl lysine, and tissue inhibitor metalloproteinase 3 (TIMP3) (76,77). Senescent SOD1 knockout mice demonstrated evidence of necrotic death of cells in the inner nuclear layer (INL) and reduced ERGs (78).

SOD2 knockout mice have been used as models for dry AMD as well, but not without some difficulties. Contrary to SOD1, the antioxidant enzyme manganese superoxide dismutase (MnSOD), encoded by SOD2, is in the mitochondrial matrix, and polymorphisms in its encoded gene have been strongly associated with the development of AMD (79). Unfortunately, most SOD2 knockout mice died of dilated cardiomyopathy by the early age of 10 days, limiting their use as a model for maculopathies (80). Nevertheless, retinal histology from some of the few that survived over 3 weeks demonstrated significant central thinning of all retinal layers (81). Justilien et al. (82) managed to overcome the limitations of this model by transfecting mouse retina and RPE with an adenovirus that expresses a ribozyme that degrades SOD2, thereby reducing its levels only locally and

diminishing major systemic consequences. Thickening of BM, degeneration of the RPE, increased autofluorescence, elevation of A2E levels, and atrophy of the photoreceptors were among the most remarkable histologic findings.

Ceruloplasmin and Hephaestin

Iron is an essential cofactor for many enzymes, but ferrous iron (Fe^{2+}) can cause oxidative damage via the Fenton reaction. Such oxidative stress increases in the body with aging and may contribute to AMD pathogenesis when affecting the retina (83). Indeed, compared to normal eyes, AMD eyes show a statistically significant increase in total iron in the RPE and BM (84). Since ceruloplasmin is believed to facilitate iron export from cells, it is reasonable to expect humans without functional ceruloplasmin to develop drusen and retinal pigmentary changes later in life (85–87). Nevertheless, mice lacking functional ceruloplasmin only showed a trivial iron overload (88) with mild retinal alterations. The most satisfactory explanation for such discrepancies lies in the presence of a second ferroxidase named hephaestin (Heph), which may compensate, at least partially, the impact caused by the ceruloplasmin loss (88–90). As a result, it was necessary to create mice with combined deficiencies in Cp and Heph so as to assess the potential influence of iron overload in AMD (91). By 5 months of age, these double knockout models had fruitfully increased iron levels and displayed subsequent iron-laden electron-dense vesicles inside the RPE cells. Focal areas of RPE hypertrophy and hypopigmentation in the midperipheral retina, subretinal deposits, photoreceptor atrophy, and subretinal neovascularization start appearing at the age of 6 to 9 months, and after a year, these models showed infiltration of macrophages, focal areas of hyperautofluorescence, and complement disposition (92). It is of interest to note that the RPE hypertrophy in this model was greater than what had been observed in AMD retinas (91,92). Unfortunately, most double knockout mice die from a movement disorder at a very young age, thus hindering possibility to study long-term effects.

Exogenous Oxidative Conditions: Cigarette Smoke, Hydroquinone, High-Fat Diet, and Blue Light

It is unanimously accepted that smoking constitutes the major preventable risk factor for AMD (93–97). Cigarette smoke contains over 4,000 potentially damaging toxins, many of which are pro-oxidants including carbon monoxide, nitric oxide, and hydroquinone (98). The association between AMD pathogenesis and oxidative harm caused by environmental factors has been studied in multiple animal models. Espinosa-Heidmann et al. described the histologic alterations of mice exposed to combinations of HF diets, blue light, and whole cigarette smoke versus oral hydroquinone. Animal exposed to these conditions exhibited changes to the BM and had increased basal laminar deposits (25,99). Plus, several mice exhibit invasion of the choriocapillaris into the BM suggestive of early AMD. Wild-type mice treated with hydroquinone in their drinking water develop decreased expression of Ccl-2 in the RPE and choroid and demonstrated altered ratios of proangiogenic VEGF versus antiangiogenic pigment epithelium-derived factor (PEDF) (100). Therefore, it was hypothesized that hydroquinone may raise the risk of CNV by disturbing the normal balance between angiogenic factors. Nevertheless, some studies have reached different results regarding hydroquinone activity so that it remains a matter of debate.

OXY Rat

The term OXY rats refer to an inbred strain of Wistar rats that were chosen for susceptibility or resistance to the early development of cataracts when fed with diets rich in galactose (101). The susceptible line (OXYS) displays high levels of hydroxyl radical formation and lipid peroxidation causing mitochondrial oxidative damage and a senescence-accelerated model. As a result, these rodents show premature aging and suffer age-related conditions such as cataracts, emphysema, scoliosis, tumors, and myocardiopathy relatively early in life (101–104). As for the retina, funduscopic analysis on these rats revealed choriocapillaris and atrophic areas in the RPE at the age of 45 days (105). Eventually, rats also exhibited thickening of BM, drusen and RPE detachments, and, by the age of a year, photoreceptor atrophy, decreased ERGs, destruction of the choriocapillaris with signs of fibrosis, and even hemorrhagic detachment of the retina secondary to neovascularization (101,105,106).

COMPLEMENT PATHWAY AND INFLAMMATION MEDIATORS

Chronic inflammation contributes to the onset and progression of multiple age-related degenerative diseases including AMD (107,108). The pathology of AMD lesions reveals signs of chronic persistent inflammatory damage such as macrophage infiltration and microglial accumulation. Plus, several acute-phase reactant proteins, in particular elements of the complement cascade, have been identified as molecular components of drusen shaft (69,109–112).

Interestingly, underneath the AMD-related inflammatory processes, there is a strong genetic connotation. Polymorphisms in many of the genes that have been accounted for AMD encourage a proinflammatory state in the eye denoted by increased C-reactive protein and decreased inhibitory complement factors (113,114). Such polymorphisms include genes that code for factor H (CFH), complement component 2 (C2), complement component 3 (C3), complement factor B (FB), and complement

factor I (FI) (115–119). Suffice to mention the particular case of the Y402H polymorphism in CFH to understand the great role, these genetic variations may have within AMD pathogenesis. Not only does such polymorphism increase the risk of AMD five- up to sevenfold, but it has also been found in half of AMD cases. Additional polymorphisms related to toll-like receptor (TLR) (e.g., TLR-3 and TLR-4) and chemokines (e.g., CX3CR1 and CCR3) have been also linked to the development and progression of AMD (120–124). In fact, the association between chronic inflammation and AMD is strong, and murine models that target specific aspects of the inflammatory process have been created to further elucidate this connection. These models are as varied as interesting and are discussed in detail in the following sections.

COMPLEMENT CASCADE

CFH Models

CFH negatively regulates the complement system by inhibiting the alternative pathway either by promoting factor I–mediated inactivation of C3b or by displacing factor Bb from the C3bBb complex and blocking the formation of C3 convertase (125,126). CFH dysfunction may lead to excessive inflammation and tissue damage, which may contribute to the pathogenesis of AMD in the retina (127). Patients and mice lacking functional CFH develop macular drusen similar to those seen in AMD (128–131). At the age of 2 years, these genetically engineered mice suffered decreased visual acuity, reduction in rod-driven ERG a- and b-wave responses, increased subretinal autofluorescence, complement deposition in the retina, and disorganization of photoreceptor outer segments. However, though there is an association between CFH and AMD, the CFH knockout mice do not display many of the hallmark AMD features. Contrary to other models of AMD, almost 30% of these animals showed a substantial thinning of their BM. Plus, since CFH itself is a main component of drusen, the loss of this protein may reduce the volume of sub-RPE deposits.

Transgenic CFH Y402H Mice

Recent studies have shown an increase risk of AMD in individuals with the Y402H polymorphism in the complement factor H gene (132). This polymorphism has been located to a region of CFH that binds heparin and C-reactive protein (124). In order to understand the role that such particular CFH mutation have in AMD pathogenesis, Ufret-Vincenty et al. (133) created transgenic mouse lines expressing the Y402H polymorphism under control of the human ApoE.

At the age of 1 year, transfected mice showed larger amounts of drusen-like deposits than those observed in either wild-type mice or even CFH knockout mice. While immunohistochemistry has revealed an increased amount of both microglial and macrophages in the subretinal space, the electron microscopy showed thickening of the BM and deposits of C3d in the basement membrane. Contrary to the CFH knockout mice, transgenic CFH Y402H models did not show signals of photoreceptor atrophy. This occurrence might be explained either by the younger age at which these animals were examined (1 year vs. 2 years) or by the existence of some functional activity of CFH protein that disallowed a more severe dysregulation of the alternative pathway.

Transgenic Mice Overexpressing C3

C3 plays a major role in the complement activation and generation of immune responses by integrating signals from every complement-activating pathway. Since C3 can activate complement system and the complement system is a major risk factor for developing AMD, it is reasonable to expect that overexpression of this protein might lead to accelerated development of retinal pathology. To put this theory in practice, Cashman et al. (134) injected mice in the subretinal space with a recombinant adenovirus-expressing murine C3. Such delivery of C3 induced significant functional and anatomic changes that reproduce not only many of the features of AMD but also those of other retinal diseases. Examination of transfected eyes revealed more retinal changes (significantly increased vascular permeability, endothelial cell proliferation and migration, RPE atrophy, loss of photoreceptor outer segments, reactive gliosis, retinal detachment, and reduced retinal function) relative to those injected with a control adenovirus. Deposition of the membrane attack complex was observed on endothelial cells and photoreceptor outer segments.

This novel model may be useful in assessing the role of complement in retinal pathology and in developing anti-complement therapies for retinal diseases associated with complement activation. However, as for its accuracy to emulate AMD, there are some limitations that could not be ignored. In particular, the fact that C3-overexpressing animals demonstrated an unexpectedly high incidence of retinal detachments (a feature not shared with AMD) raises question about its similarity to the actual disease. Plus, it is unknown whether or not the mere activity of the transfected adenovirus could contribute to the pathologic features, thereby biasing the results.

C3a and C5a Receptor

Both C3 and C5 have been found in drusen (39,135). Although these proteins are best known for their role in opsonization and formation the membrane attack complex, their activity is multifaceted. In fact, mice lacking the receptors for these components showed smaller lesions in the laser-induced CNV model, decreased levels of VEGF expression, and impaired leukocyte recruitment (136). Such data support the hypothesis that activation of the C3a and C5a receptors contributes in the appearance of CNV in AMD.

Chemokines and Chemokine Receptors

Chemotactic cytokines, also named chemokines, are a family of small cytokines, which name is derived from their ability to induce directed chemotaxis in nearby responsive cells (137). Some chemokines are considered proinflammatory and can be induced during an immune response to recruit cells of the immune system to a site of infection, while others are considered homeostatic and are involved in controlling the migration of cells during normal processes of tissue maintenance or development. From a structural perspective, however, chemokines are frequently divided into four families: CXC, CX3C, CC, and C (138,139).

As for AMD, chemokines appear to be crucial in the subretinal microglia/macrophage accumulation observed and may also participate directly in the genesis of several abnormal processes such as retinal degeneration and CNV (108,140,141). The CCL2/CCR2 and CX3CL1/CX3CR1 ligand/receptor pairs excel among all the chemokines studied (142). Particularly, the T280 M allele of CX3CR1 gene has been shown to be associated with AMD in diverse patient populations (143–146). There are several reports using knockout mice for these ligand/receptor pairs in an attempt to decipher the inflammatory mechanisms of AMD. These models have successfully displayed many of the most distinctive AMD characteristics.

Ccl2 and Ccr2 Single Knockout Mice

Ccl2, also known as monocyte chemoattractant protein 1 (MCP-1), enables the binding of monocytes to the endothelium for subsequent tissue extravasation (147,148). RPE cells under oxidative stress can upregulate Ccl2 (149), so that increased intraocular levels have been reported both in exudative AMD (150) and in mouse models of CNV (151). Macrophages extracted from eyes undergoing the laser-induced CNV model, which are primarily responsible for the angiogenic reaction (152), managed to get in the eye by moving toward this higher concentration of the chemical in question. Bearing this in mind, it is easy to understand why the recruitment of macrophages/microglia to the injury site and the subsequent CNV happened to be diminished in both Ccr2 and Ccl2 knockout mice (153). Nevertheless, Ambati et al. (154) reported the spontaneous appearance of yellowish drusen-like subretinal deposits in these mice after 9 months of age, combined with other AMD features including thickening of BM, an increase in autofluorescence and lipofuscin granules, photoreceptor malfunction, and the occurrence of CNV. It had been hypothesized that the deficiency in macrophages/microglia recruitment through a CCL2-/CCR2-dependent pathway could have prevented the clearance of accumulating debris in BM, which would have eventually taken to drusen formation. Nevertheless, further studies from Ccl2 knockout mice have rebutted such initial interpretation (153), since drusen-like subretinal deposits initially happened to be accumulations of swollen macrophages. Finally, Luhmann et al. found no difference between thickening of BM, RPE and photoreceptor atrophy, and ERG amplitudes compared to age-matched wild-type animals. Consequently, the actual influence of the Ccl2/Ccr2 pathway to AMD pathogenesis still remains unclear.

CX3CR1 Single Knockout Mice

CX3CR1 is a chemokine receptor that has been found in microglial cells in the retina (144,155,156). T280M allele of the CX3CR1 gene leads to a dysfunctional monocyte migration associated with AMD. Studies of two independently generated CX3CR1-deficient mice (157,158) have exposed alterations in line with AMD (144). By the year of age, these animals displayed drusen-like deposits that were not apparent in age-matched wild-type counterparts. However, these lesions were lipid-bloated subretinal microglia and not sub-RPE extracellular deposits. By the 18 months of age, CX3CR1 knockout mice also experienced significant retinal thinning. It is generally believed that deficiency of functional CX3CL1 on retinal microglia may reduce egress of these cells from the retina, causing in term the formation of subretinal deposits.

Ccl2/Cx3cr1 Double Knockout Mice

Ccl2 and CX3CR single knockout mice only exhibit signs of maculopathy at older ages (16 and 18 months, respectively), and the phenotype was not fully penetrant. In an attempt to accelerate the development of AMD-like features, Tuo et al. (145) created double knockout (DKO) mice. The model was a success: DKO mice displayed retinal alterations early in life (with the earliest occurrence at 6 weeks) making a seductive alternative to single knockout animals. By 9 weeks of age, all DKO mice had developed subretinal drusen, which worsen with aging. Immunostaining revealed increased complement in BM, RPE, and choroidal capillaries (159). DKO mice had focal thickening of BM, increased levels of A2E, infiltration of microglial, and photoreceptor atrophy. In older animals, areas of atrophy and chorioretinal scars were observed. Up to 15% of eyes displayed CNV as early as at 3 months. These data support DKO mice as convenient models for both dry and wet AMD.

Nonetheless, the validity of this model has been recently rebutted by Raoul et al. (142), whose independently developed lines of DKO mice did not display well-defined features and were not phenotypically different from single knockout counterparts. According to the authors, differences in the results exist because of a bias in the previous selection regarding the breeding of animals, since those worst drusen may have been unintentionally chosen for AMD factors independent of CCL2 or CXCR1. Besides, it has been also reported that such lines may have been adulterated with concomitant unrelated mutations, which may had an impact in the ultimate phenotypes as well (160,161). Therefore, the conclusions concerning this murine model should be taken with caution.

Nonhuman Primates for Dry AMD

Macular degeneration occurs in rhesus and cynomolgus macaques. In both, retinal lesions are characterized by drusen accumulation in the central retina. However, onset of fundus changes and inheritance patterns differ in these two primate species. Macular degeneration in the cynomolgus macaque appears to be a model for early-onset maculopathies rather than AMD. In contrast, adult-onset macular degeneration in rhesus macaques resembles human AMD. Genetic studies in rhesus macaques may resolve, which of two closely linked adjacent genes on human (HTRA1 and LOC387715/ARMS2) are responsible for the disease.

Early-Onset Macular Degeneration in Cynomolgus Monkeys (*Macaca fascicularis*)

At the Tsukuba Primate Center, an early-onset macular degeneration with autosomal dominant inheritance occurred in a large pedigree of cynomolgus macaques (*Macaca fascicularis*) (162–165). A similar syndrome has been identified in the Japanese macaque (*Macaca fuscata*) (161). Symptoms appeared as early as 2 years of age and exacerbate gradually with aging. While funduscopy revealed fine, yellowish white dots within the macula of affected animals, drusen from these animals have been confirmed by histopathology to closely resemble human equivalents and have been shown by immunohistochemistry and proteomic analysis to contain many human hallmarks, such as:

- Apolipoprotein E
- Amyloid P component
- Various-sized complement component C5
- The terminal C5b-9 complement complex
- Vitronectin, membrane cofactor protein
- Annexins
- Crystallins
- Immunoglobulins

Young age of onset and inheritance pattern in this model are reminiscent of a number of early-onset maculopathies in humans, rather than AMD. Umeda et al. assessed the contribution of early-onset human maculopathy susceptibility genes in this cynomolgus colony. They found no association between the monkey phenotype and 13 genes that are known to underlie early macular degeneration syndromes in humans (162). The dominant inheritance and early onset of this disease could facilitate production of animals for preclinical therapy development.

Adult-Onset Macular Degeneration in Rhesus Monkeys (*Macaca mulatta*)

Even though natural developments of both dry and wet forms of advanced AMD are only occasionally found in monkeys, many groups have been capable of documenting the signs of early to intermediate AMD in older rhesus macaques (*Macaca mulatta*) (164,166–175). Funduscopic examination of a closed colony of rhesus macaques found in Cayo Santiago revealed macular drusen in approximately half of animals older than 9 years and all specimens older than 25 years (168,176–178). Both histologic and ultrastructural examination set the presence of small and large drusen within the BM as well as beneath the RPE. In some cases, RPE cells overlying drusen were atrophic. Among the composites found in the drusen of cynomolgus macaques, we can remark the following:

- The apolipoprotein E
- Amyloid P component
- Complement component C5
- The terminal C5b-9 complement complex
- Vitronectin, membrane cofactor protein
- Annexins
- Crystallins
- Immunoglobulins

For further studying, a breeding colony derived from these macaques was established at the University of Florida in 1994, and equivalent features were displayed (179). In spite of the much higher occurrence of macular drusen in young adult to middle-age macaques compared to that observed in humans, the disease seems to progress more slowly and only occasionally lead to geographic atrophy or CNV (167,176,178). Contrary to early-onset macular degeneration in cynomolgus macaques, rhesus macaques appear to have a nonmendelian inheritance pattern. Francis et al. (169) genotyped a population of rhesus macaques and found that a susceptibility locus in the rhesus homologue of human 10q26 was associated with macular phenotype. These genes contain sequence variants significantly associated with affected status in humans and macaques. As expected, the LOC387715/ARMS2 gene is present in simians only, thus corresponding with development of the macula. In contrast to human studies, this study indicated that only the promoter polymorphism in HTRA1 appears to be significantly associated with the disease phenotype.

ANIMAL MODELS OF WET MACULAR DEGENERATION

Only about 10% of patients suffering from AMD have the wet type. This form, known also as exudative or neovascular, is characterized by the formation of a pathologic CNV responsible for most cases of severe blindness (180).

Bleeding, leaking, and scarring from these abnormal blood vessels eventually cause irreversible damage to the photoreceptors and rapid vision loss if left untreated. Yet, studies based on animal models have opened the door toward a new era as far as treatment, prognosis, and morbidity in wet AMD are concerned. In fact, it was the better

understanding of the molecular basis for this condition that allowed the replacement of aggressive ablative therapies with more sophisticated and seductive alternatives (181). Agents that delay neovascular growth and moderate subretinal hemorrhages are one of the most hopeful breakthroughs in the field of therapeutics for advance AMD and are currently under evaluation.

The majority of present models for wet AMD rely on either laser or direct mechanical injury to the RPE/BM complex or alteration of the RPE and surrounding environment by external interventions (such as exogenous compounds injected in the subretinal space). Nonetheless, genetically altered mice have been gaining popularity among experts, who use these "internal" interventions to explore angiogenic homeostasis within the RPE–choroidal interface, specially the equilibrium between proangiogenic VEGF and antiangiogenic PEDF. The interface of these two approaches has brought several antiangiogenic agents into clinical use. Even though these studies currently focus on inhibiting VEGF (182), additional use of PEDF via gene therapy constitutes a realistic idea and may occur in the future (183).

Even though these exudative AMD models recapitulate many of the clinical and histologic manifestations of CNV in humans, the time to develop, course of progression, size, and appearance of the lesion vary significantly among them (184). These models and the differences between them are going to be discussed in detail in the following sections.

LASER-INDUCED MODELS OF CNV

Laser Injury in Rodents

Laser-induced neovascularization can be achieved in both mice (136,185,186) and rats (187,188). Although this laser trauma model was first tried in nonhuman primates (189), rodent adaptations are nowadays more popular mainly because they offer attractive advantages in terms of cost, number of CNV lesions for statistical analysis, and time course. In fact, both mice and rats showed an early-phase CMV over the first week, displaying mature membranes after only 10 days (184,190). Laser trauma models basically consist of using high-powered, focused laser energy in order to induce several breaks in BM. The power employed to generate CNV must be fixed carefully, as burns without enough intensity to break the BM may not result in CNV and extremely intense burns may result in extensive choroidal hemorrhage followed by avascular scarring without CNV.

There is no ideal method to detect laser-induced neovascularization; each approach has their own strengths and weaknesses and often complements each other. Neovascular development can be monitored in anesthetized rodents with high-resolution angiography with fluorescein isothiocyanate–dextran to assess vessel leakage, although quantifying is sometimes challenging as mature CNV complexes may not leak at all (190). Plus, tissues can be scanned postmortem with paraffin histology. Since these studies have an important quantitative component, care must be taken during processing so that pathology of each laser site can be correlated with its in vivo angiographic progression. Histochemical visualization and immunochemical methods using antibodies may contribute in detecting endothelial cells and thereby neoformed vessels (187,191). However, histologic examinations are overall demanding and time-consuming processes, which may be also limited by the technical difficulty to achieve adequate sampling, as was previously mentioned. Finally, using image analysis software is an appealing alternative to investigate the histologic area of CNV in these models (192). Sclera–choroid–RPE flat mounts may be created and combined with fluorescein-ated high molecular weight dextran angiography to allow computer-assisted, quantitative imaging (184). However, there are two major problems regarding this method: First, there is no certainty that the vascular tissue imaged in this technique is choroidal in origin (187), and second, nonper-fused vessels sometimes are not detected (193). Recently, Campos et al. have proposed another method of assessment in which rat eye cups were fluorescently labeled with markers for nuclei, endothelial cells, microglia, and filamentous actin and then flat-mounted specimens were evaluated with confocal microscope. Computer software generated three-dimensional reconstructions for qualitative and quantitative analysis of confocal image stacks. This technique provides excellent morphologic detail and facilitates the study of critical early events in CNV, including the rupture of the BM and the formation of endothelial clusters before vessel formation.

Laser-induced CNV models have several differences with the actual wet AMD that must be taken into consideration. First, laser use may ominously harm the overlying neural retina to a larger extent than what is normally observed in eyes of AMD patients. Second, laser trauma models fail to emulate the complex sequence of events that leads ultimately to CNV in the actual maculopathy. Such functional disparity is a consequence inherent to the model fabrication process: Trauma-induced CNV occurs secondary to an acute injury and inflammation response and not to long-standing senescent degeneration and chronic inflammation as happens in the genuine disease.

Regardless of the drawbacks mentioned above, rodent laser trauma models have contributed greatly toward our present understanding of the pathogenesis of CNV, including

- The role of angiogenic cascade (80,194–202)
- The role of intracellular kinase signaling of growth factors (192,203)
- The participation of numerous cell types involved in CNV formation (194,204,205) and the role of RPE (206)
- The role of the complement cascade in experimental CNV (207)
- The proof of concept for pharmacotherapy of CNV and gene therapy (192,208–223)

Laser Injury in Nonhuman Primates

Just as in rodents, laser photocoagulation is used to break the BM and induce a subsequent fibrovascular proliferative response in the choroid. This response is the basis for modeling CNV in late-stage AMD regardless of the animal employed. The primate model of experimental CNV, created by Ryan et al. (224,225), was termed "subretinal neovascularization" at the time and was the first animal model of CNV more than 30 years ago. Although this procedure was originally tried in rhesus and cynomolgus macaques, the technique has been recently adapted for use in the squirrel monkey (226). Ryan (189) used an argon laser to induce small spots of photocoagulation in a reproducible grid pattern in the temporal retina, avoiding the capillary-free zone of the fovea. This method continues to be in use. Typical argon laser exposure parameters for the induction of CNV have included a 50-μm spot size, 100-ms duration, and powers ranging from 300 to 700 mW but in some studies as high as 1,500 mW. Spots are funduscopically visible as bubbles at the time of photocoagulation. Photocoagulation is sometimes repeated to produce a break in the BM and bubble formation.

Photocoagulation induced thrombosis of choroidal vessels followed by reendothelialization 48 hours later and growth of new vessels into the subretinal space by a week (227). As explained above, newly formed vessels are more permeable so that neovascular development can be monitored with fluorescein angiography to assess vessel leakage. As a matter of fact, outcome measures of efficacy include the extent of growth of laser-induced new vessels, the total area of blood vessel leakage, and the percentage of laser lesions resulting in clinically significant vessel leakage, as visualized by fluorescein angiography and in some cases confirmed by histopathology. By these criteria, CNV peaks at approximately 2 to 4 weeks after photocoagulation. Similar to the CNV that occurs in human ocular disease, laser-induced CNV follows predictable stages of development: early membrane formation, establishment of a mature fibrovascular network, and involution (228). Experimental agents are typically given at approximately 1 month after injury, before vessels begin to resolve (226,229). Spontaneous neovascular involution (indicated by decreased fluorescein leakage) commences at approximately 3 to 7 weeks and then gradually progresses (over a period of approximately 2 to 13 months) until leakage is no longer apparent at the site (230). The extent of new vessel growth compared to poorly vascularized scarring can be variable in all models and is influenced by species, location of injury in the retina, and intensity of the laser beam. In some cases, laser injury can result in anastomotic vessels between choroidal and retinal circulations (229). This lesion, known as retinal angiomatous proliferation, can be present as part of advanced AMD in humans, and it holds a poor prognosis.

Advantages of the primate model include the close approximation of the monkey retina and macula to the human, size of the primate eye for drug delivery studies, and utility of the model for development of human clinical trials. Disadvantages include the expense of the animals, animal care and husbandry, length of experiments, and ethical issues regarding use of primates when rodents (mice and rats) are a reliable model. The primary drawback of the model is that not all eyes respond with new vessel formation, with an incidence of CNV as low as 30% (225,231). Latest studies have managed to optimize laser parameters to produce advanced lesions more frequently (232). Still, group sizes of 10 monkeys are typically required to document significant effects, and in some studies, smaller group sizes have generated inconclusive results (233,234).

Laser Injury in Rabbits and Pigs

Rabbit

elDirini et al. (235) used rabbits in an attempt to find an intermediate laser-induced CNV model between rodents and primates, thereby avoiding the expense and ethical issues concerning the latter. Nonetheless, rabbits exhibit significant anatomical discrepancies, as they do not have a macula and their retina vascular supply is different. The model utilized subretinal endophotocoagulation to create histologically identified CNV.

Pig

Another intermediate laser-induced CNV model is the pig. Saishin et al. (219) used a laser to create defects in the BM in the pig eye and establish histologic evidence of CNV in 100% of lesions. Image analysis of histologic sections was used to evaluate drug delivery for the treatment of the CNV. Kiilgaard et al. studied xenon laser versus diode laser versus mechanical disruption of the BM in a pig model of CNV. The authors found histopathologic evidence of CNV in 54%, 83%, and 100% of the animals, respectively (236). The pig eye is approximately the same size as the human eye, and the retina vascularization is similar to the human. Like the rabbit, the pig circumvents the cost and ethical issues of the primate. The utility of the pig is for drug delivery experiments. However, the pig lacks the advantages of high-throughput, short-duration experiments as available in rat and mouse models of laser-induced CNV.

Surgically BM Rupture

Trauma to the BM can cause localized fundus areas of hemorrhage and infarction with subsequent neovascular connections between the retina and choroid (237). Pioneer studies undertaken by Kiilgaard et al. (236) compared eyes in pigs that underwent retinal photocoagulation with a xenon lamp and retinal laser photocoagulation with those exposed to mechanical ruptures of the BM following surgical debridement of the RPE without damage to the neuroretina. The results were conclusive: Not only did the surgical method show higher success rates of CNV induction (100% vs. 83% and 54%), but it has also produced CNV

membranes that were morphologically more similar to those present in human exudative AMD. Contrary to CNV obtained by using laser or xenon burns, morphology of surgically induced lesions was not dominated by retinal gliosis and retinal neovascularization, probably due to a preservation of the neuroretina.

Also, Lassota et al. (238) found that the original surgical technique could be optimized by avoiding RPE removal prior to the BM perforation. Compared to those obtained with the original surgical intervention, CNV membranes induced by using this method were significantly thicker and had a higher cellular content, were more richly vascularized, and also exhibited the highest propensity to leak in fluorescence angiograms. It is important to note that even when the surgical model offers benefits of reduced neuroretinal damage, the technique is limited by higher cost and the necessity of a three-port vitrectomy.

■ SUBRETINAL INJECTION MODELS

CNV has been immunologically and mechanically induced in animal models, primarily by injection of synthetic peptides, viral vectors containing VEGF, cells, and inert synthetic materials. The proximity to the choroidal vasculature along with the perturbation of the RPE caused by the injection itself, when combined with proper angiogenic signals, appears to be sufficient stimuli to encourage invasion of the subretinal space by CNV complexes (196).

Subretinal Matrigel Injection

Although the pathogenesis of CNV in AMD is not entirely clear, it has been strongly associated with the presence of abnormal extracellular deposits in the space between the RPE and BM (4,6,239,240). Supporting this notion, recent studies have shown that artificially created sub-RPE deposits are sufficient to induce the development of CNV in mice (241) and in rabbits (242). Subretinal/RPE injection of Matrigel, a basement membrane extract (243) that solidifies after implantation in tissue, was reported to induce CNV in both ccl2-deficient and wild-type rodents, possibly by encouraging the release of angiogenic factors and recruit host cells (242). As mentioned in previous sections, the normal functioning of CCL2/CCR2 pair confers protection against age-related maculopathies. Consistently, data revealed that CCL2 knockout mice developed more severe disease than wild-type counterparts. These findings support Matrigel subretinal injection as a useful generator of AMD-like pathologic changes while confirmed the importance of CCL2 in AMD pathogenesis. More recently, studies showed that rabbits exposed to subretinal injection of Matrigel alone or Matrigel with VEGF also responded positively, developing CNV in 100% of the lesions (242). Zhao et al. used Matrigel injection to assess the necessity of a proper relationship between the RPE and BM so as to prevent abnormal angiogenesis. Matrigel was injected to the subretinal space of rats to create an amorphous deposit, causing RPE cells to migrate toward photoreceptors and then form a new layer between the deposit and photoreceptors, resulting in RPE translocation. The BM devoid of RPE attachment becomes susceptible to invasion by new blood vessels from the choroid, thereby resulting in CNV (241).

Subretinal Lipid Injection

Lipid and oxidized lipid depositions are found in eyes of AMD patients as well as non-AMD aged BM (244). Rabbits and rats exposed to subretinal injections of an oxidized lipid (HpODE) have displayed CNV (245,246). Since animals in which subretinal injections caused breaks in the BM were excluded from the study, the authors were in position to blame the lipid injection for the histologic changes.

Subretinal Complement Compounds Injection

The role of the complement cascade in the formation of drusen and CNV is unquestionable and has been already discussed (122,136,247). Lyzogubov et al. (248) employed different doses of subretinal PEG-8 to create a new model of CNV. PEG-8 is an activator of both the classical and alternative pathways of the complement system. In this model, PEG-8 injection induced activation of the complement cascade and dose-dependent CNV production.

Macrophages

Macrophages are believed to have a pivotal role in the development of CNV (249,250). Subretinal injection of macrophages on wild-type or Ccl2 knockout mice (251) caused CNV with concomitant fibrosis. Nevertheless, since the protocol included rupture of the BM with a laser at the site of injection, the meaning of the findings is indefinite.

GENETICALLY ENGINEERED ANIMAL MODELS OF CNV

Subretinal VEGF Gene Therapy

VEGF is the quintessential promoter of vasculogenesis and angiogenesis processes in both CNV models and human wet AMD (252,253). In effect, CNV membranes removed from AMD patients showed VEGF remarkable immunoreactivity (254,255). It has been hypothesized, therefore, that overexpression of VEGF would result in concomitant angiogenesis within the eye.

Numerous groups have sought to put into practice this theory by giving subretinal injections of adenovirus vectors expressing VEGF to rodents. Transgenic expression of VEGF in RPE cells resulted in choroidal vascular permeability, leukocyte adhesion, and intrachoroidal neovascularization, as measured by angiography and histology. If the VEGF transgene is expressed in the photoreceptor layer, new vessels originate from the inner retinal vasculature within the retina and extend into the subretinal space, where they form clusters of vessels surrounded by RPE cells (256). Adeno-associated virus–mediated delivery of PEDF to the subretinal or vitreous space results in significant reduction of neovascularization resulting from laser injury in mice (223). Plus, pharmacologic blocking of its signaling has shown results as promising as consistent by successfully inhibiting laser-induced CNV in experimental animal models (219,257).

The advantage of these models is the ability to study various biologic components of CNV by comparison with controls and crossbreeding experiments. Disadvantages relate to the length of time for the CNV to develop, the relatively small percentages of eyes that develop CNV, and the small size of the CNV. These models have supported the concept that the best models of CNV are those that incorporate physical disruption of the BM into the model.

SOD1 Knockout Mice

Senescent Cu–Zn SOD–deficient mice displayed fundus and histologic evidence of CNV in 8.3% and 10%, respectively (76). A marker of oxidative damage to DNA (I-OHdG) was detected in the RPE of senescent Sod 1 knockout mice but not in controls. The CNV appeared to connect with retinal vessels in 16-month-old compared with year-old mice.

Ccr2-/Ccl2-Deficient Mice

The Ccr2-/Ccl2-deficient mouse model of AMD has received considerable attention (154). In this model, transgenic mice deficient in either Ccl2 or Ccr2 fail to recruit macrophages to the area of the RPE and BM. This allows for accumulation of C5a and IgG, both of which induce VEGF production. Thorough examination of these transgenic mice showed a CNV incidence of 25% (154). These findings have contributed to the understanding of the pathophysiology of CNV, specifically regarding to macrophage recruitment. Although the areas of CNV are very small, recent work has shown that CCR3 is specifically expressed in choroidal neovascular endothelial cells in either of these knockout mice (258).

Ccl2/Cx3cr1 DKO Mice

RPE changes and drusen-like lesions exhibited by these mice have been already mentioned. However, approximately 15% of these animals eventually exhibit histologic evidence of CNV. The fact that lesions in these mice take only 6 weeks to appear makes it a very appealing model for studying spontaneous development of neovascularization. However, further work is required to assess the molecular mechanisms underneath this neovascularization.

VLDLR-Targeted Mutant

Homozygous strains of mice with targeted mutations for VLDLR gene developed new blood vessels in the area of the outer plexiform layer of the retina and choroidal anastomoses by 3 months (51).

ApoE Overexpression

Eyes in hypercholesterolemic mice displayed AMD-like changes in the BM/RPE complex (35). ApoE4 overexpressing transgenic mice fed with HF-C diet developed CNV in addition to drusen-like and basal laminar deposits as early as 65 weeks of age (36). The CNV was observed in 19% of male and 18% of female mice and was demonstrated by several methods.

Cp Heph Knockout Mice

Iron overload, observed in these transgenic mice, causes AMD-like alterations. The mice developed funduscopically evident lesions at the level of the RPE, and 100% of the mice developed histologically identified subretinal neovascularization, although it is not apparent if the neovascularization arose from the retina or choroid (91). Furthermore, the mice do not appear to develop the drusen-like or basal laminar deposit-like lesions as seen in AMD.

Spontaneous Bst Chromosome 16 Mutant

An angiogenic phenotype has been described in Bst/+ mice that is age related and clinically evident and resembles human CNV. This represents a spontaneous, genetically determined model of CNV. Bst/+ mice offer the possibility of exploring the molecular mechanisms of CNV without the need for exogenous agents. The Bst mutation demonstrates a broad range of phenotypic expression that includes CNV, focal retinal detachment, retinal dysplasia, persistence of the hyaloid vascular system, patchy absence of retinal differentiation, and colobomas. Almost 90% of the mice exhibited subretinal neovascularization identified with histologic examinations. The CNV was associated with RPE abnormalities, retinal hamartoma-like lesions, and connections of the neovascularization with the retina and choroid through defects in BM. Although the CNV was age related, there were neither drusen-like nor basal laminar deposit-like lesions in this model.

ANIMAL MODELS FOR ANTI-VEGF THERAPY

Anti-VEGF therapies are widely used to treat wet AMD. Bevacizumab (BVZ), a full-length antibody originally developed to treat advanced colon adenocarcinoma, found its way through ophthalmology, and it is chosen for diseases as relevant as exudative AMD, diabetic retinopathy (DR),

retinal vein occlusions, and retinopathy of prematurity. Likewise, pegaptanib, an aptamer to VEGF165, and ranibizumab (RVZ), the Fab fragment of the VEGF, were developed exclusively for intravitreal usage (259). We must note that both in vitro and in vivo preclinical studies were performed in order to determine its efficacy and safety (260).

Animal models used to test these therapies were mostly rabbits, rats, mice, and nonhuman primates. Rabbits were used primarily to describe the pharmacokinetics of intravitreal RVZ and BVZ. These studies showed that BVZ had longer half-life but was detected in low concentrations in serum and humor vitreous of the fellow uninjected eye (261,262). Pharmacokinetics and serum bioavailability were studied in cynomolgus monkeys as well. Six to twenty-four hours after intravitreal injection, retina levels of the anti-VEGF drug were one-third that in the vitreous, and its half-life was 3 days with a parallel clearance from all ocular compartments. Consequently, it would be suitable for clinical use in wet AMD by an intravitreal injection once a month (263).

Rats were chosen to investigate the toxicity of all three anti-VEGF therapies using two different doses in both healthy and N-methyl-D-aspartate (NMDA)–induced retinal ganglion cell (RGC)–damaged animals. No toxic effects of BVZ and RVZ were found in either healthy or damage rat models (264).

Mouse models of subretinal neovascularization and exudative retinal detachment were employed in order to compare the effects of intravitreal injections of RBZ and BVZ. For this purpose, Miki et al. selected two models: transgenic mice, in which the *rhodopsin promoter* derived expression of human VEGF in photoreceptors (*rho/VEGF* mice), and double transgenic mice, which had doxycycline-inducible expression of VEGF in the retina (Tet/opsin/VEGF). This last one represented an aggressive model of proliferative retinopathy due to high VEGF expression. The gathered data suggest that BVZ is not only as useful as RBZ for treatment of subretinal neovascularization in mice but also superior in severe models (265).

New antiangiogenic approaches are being studied including small RNA (ribonucleic acid) interfering molecules and multikinase inhibitors. Two small interfering RNAs that selectively silence messenger RNA encoding for VEGF are under investigation:

- Bevasiranib (bevasiranib, OPKO Health, Miami, FL) targets against VEGF—an mRNA.
- SIRNA-027 (AGN211745 or SIRNA-027, Allergan, Irvine, CA) targets VEGF receptor 1.

Tyrosine kinase inhibitors, which block the phosphorylation of all known VEGF receptors such as Vatalanib® (formerly PTK-787, Novartis International AG, Basel, Switzerland), have shown efficacy in mice animal models of retinal and CNV. Maier et al. investigated the effect of this drug in a mouse model of ischemia-induced retinopathy.

Mice were exposed to 75% oxygen on postnatal day 7, and on day 12, they injected the drug intravitreally. The authors concluded that a single intravitreal injection was capable of significantly reducing angioproliferative retinopathy (266).

ANIMAL MODELS OF OTHER RETINAL DEGENERATIONS

Retinal degenerations reunite a group of entities characterized by the progressive loss of retinal function due to cell death. These conditions comprise different phenotypes that can be present at birth and develop during infancy or even during adulthood. Plus, the spectrum of vision impairment is also wide and can range from night blindness and loss of peripheral or central vision to total loss of vision.

Retinal degenerations are usually classified in heritable and nonheritable. In the heritable retinal degeneration group, we can include retinitis pigmentosa (RP), Leber congenital amaurosis (LCA), and Stargardt disease. On the other hand, AMD, glaucoma, and DR belong to the nonheritable group, which affect a larger number of people worldwide (267).

Retinitis Pigmentosa

RP is an inherited disorder that leads to blindness because of the loss of photoreceptor cells. It is caused by the mutation of multiple genes that encode for proteins responsible for the maintenance and function of cones and rods. Its prevalence is around 1 case per 3,000 to 5,000 individuals (268), and the inheritance can be sporadic, X-linked, and autosomal recessive or dominant, being the latest accounted for 25% to 30% of all cases of RP (269).

Since neither successful treatment nor cure has been discovered, exploiting animal experimentation to develop new strategies may be crucial. The greatest number of known mutations that cause RP occurs in 32 genes, specially in the rhodopsin (RHO), retinitis pigmentosa 1 (RP1), and retinitis pigmentosa GTPase regulator (RPGR) genes. However, no single mutation accounts for more than 10% in related patients (270).

RP pathogenesis and therapy have been studied in a wide range of animals including rodents, dogs, cats, and pigs. Of those, two animal models described in literature stand out for their utility, and they differ in their Mendelian inheritance. RPGR mutations are the most common cause of X-linked retinitis pigmentosa (XLRP). Most of these mutations are present in ORF15, the purine-rich terminal exon of the predominant splice variant expressed in retina. A naturally occurring mouse animal model of XLRP has been recently defined. The retinal degeneration 9 mice carry a 32-base-pair duplication at ORF15 that leads to a shift in the reading frame causing a nonsense mutation. Therefore, no protein is translated, and thus, mice exhibit pigment loss and thinning of the outer nuclear layer (271).

The second model corresponds to an autosomal dominant retinitis pigmentosa (adRP) miniature pig that carries the most common human mutation Pro23His (P23H) RHO. Miniature pigs were chosen instead of domestic pigs because its smaller size makes it easier to manipulate. Mini pigs with the Pro23His (P23H) RHO mutation successfully developed the clinical phenotype of human RP: a dramatic reduction in the scotopic b-wave amplitude in the full-field ERG, reflecting rod photoreceptor dysfunction, and a subsequent, albeit delayed, reduction in the photopic b-wave amplitude, reflecting cone photoreceptor dysfunction along with extensive degeneration of the outer nuclear and reduced thickness of the INLs. Authors supported this model over rodents on the grounds of convenient eye size, better access to the subretinal space improving surgical interventions, and a more appropriate biologic model (since approximately 14% of the photoreceptors in the pig are cones, compared to only 1% in mice (272)). Cat and dog models of inherited RP are currently used in research as well (273,274). However, its restricted genetic information, the presence of major and minor histocompatibility differences using cell-based therapies, the societal concern over experimentation in them, and the limited access to retinal progenitor and stem cells in these species constitute major limitations that frequently impede their use.

Diabetic Retinopathy

DR is a major microvascular complication of diabetes mellitus and the leading cause of preventable blindness among the working-aged population with a significant impact on the world's health systems. DR's most accepted classification includes a nonproliferative (NPDR) and a proliferative form (PDR) (275). NPDR, previously called background retinopathy, is determined by the presence of microaneurysms and dot and blot hemorrhages. According to these microscopic findings, NPDR can be further subdivided into three stages:

- *Mild*: microaneurysms only.
- *Moderate*: more than just microaneurysms but less than in the severe nonproliferative form.
- *Severe*: more than 20 intraretinal hemorrhages in each of four quadrants or definite venous beading in two quadrants or prominent intraretinal microvascular abnormalities (IRMAs) in one quadrant. No signs of proliferation must be found.

On the other hand, PDR is characterized by the presence of neovessels that conduct to vitreous/preretinal hemorrhages, fibrosis, and tractional retinal detachments.

Animal models have been extensively used in diabetes research. To date, species such as mice, rats, cats, dogs, pigs, and nonhuman primates are being used to understand the pathogenic mechanisms underneath DR. Models of DR are complex and can be achieved by genetic alteration, pharmacologic induction, feeding a galactose diet, and

Table 2.1	DIABETIC RETINOPATHY RODENTS ANIMAL MODELS

Rats

Type 1 diabetes
- Biobreeding rat (278)

Type 2 diabetes
- Zucker diabetic fatty rat (279)
- Wistar Bonn Kobori rats (280)
- Otsuka Long-Evans Tokushima fatty (281)
- Goto-Kakizaki rat (282)
- Spontaneously diabetic Torii rat (283)

Mice

Type 1 diabetes
- Nonobese diabetic mice (284)

Type 2 diabetes
- Db/db (*Leprdb*) mice (285)
- Ins2Akita mice (286)

spontaneous selection inbreeding. Recently, protein molecular biologic techniques have produced a large number of new animal models for the study of diabetes, including knockin, generalized knockout, and tissue-specific knockout mice.

Rodents, especially mice, are the most widely studied animal DR models due to their short generation time, easy manipulation, and the inherited hyperglycemia that affect certain strains. They are suitable for reproducing early stages of the disease but less useful in demonstrating all neural and vascular complications typical of the advanced phases, so they do not exactly mirror the human condition (276). Consequently, researchers have chosen nondiabetic animals to study proliferative retinopathy where VEGF and IGF-1 factors can be manipulated independently.

Rodent DR models can be either spontaneous or chemically induced. Currently, diabetes can be provoked by destroying the pancreatic β-cells with alloxan or streptozotocin, generating a type 1 diabetic model. These animals maintained a hyperglycemic state for up to 24 months with small amounts of insulin and develop early-stage DR findings. This method is frequently performed in rats because mice can be difficult to maintained alive once diabetic. Interestingly, variations in the retinal response to diabetes in between rat species have been reported (277). By contrast, spontaneously diabetic rodents, for both type 1 and type 2 diabetes, have been broadly described in literature (Table 2.1).

Larger animals, including dog, cats, and pigs, have been used in DR research with relative success, but not exempt from limitations. All of these models, although morphologically similar to human DR, tend to be expensive and complex because of the lack of specific antibodies and molecular biology reagents. To add more, techniques for manipulation and genetic characterization are somewhat experimental and therefore less precise than in small animal models. Indeed, nonhuman primates stand out among

other models discussed above because of the presence of a macula. Cynomolgus monkeys (*Macaca fascicularis*) that were pancreatectomized or treated with streptozotocin and obese rhesus monkeys (*Macaca mulatta*) that spontaneously develop diabetes at middle age have been used in DR studies. As in humans, DR develops fairly slowly in these models. Johnson et al. reported ophthalmoscopical changes in aged monkeys with spontaneous diabetes. Their findings showed intraretinal hemorrhages and large areas of retinal capillary nonperfusion along with macular edema (287). These models can almost perfectly mimic every aspect of the human condition. However, the longer gestational periods, the lack of reagents for experimentation, the high cost of maintenance, and the ethical issues involved represent disadvantages that cannot be ignored.

REFERENCES

1. Klein R, et al. Ten-year incidence and progression of age-related maculopathy: the Beaver Dam eye study. Ophthalmology. 2002;109(10):1767–1779.

2. Gehrs KM, et al. Age-related macular degeneration—emerging pathogenetic and therapeutic concepts. Ann Med. 2006;38(7):450–471.

3. Sparrow JR, et al. A2E, a fluorophore of RPE lipofuscin: can it cause RPE degeneration? Adv Exp Med Biol. 2003;533:205–211.

4. Green WR, Enger C. Age-related macular degeneration histopathologic studies. The 1992 Lorenz E. Zimmerman Lecture. Ophthalmology. 1993;100(10):1519–1535.

5. Green WR. Histopathology of age-related macular degeneration. Mol Vis. 1999;5:27.

6. Sarks SH. Ageing and degeneration in the macular region: a clinico-pathological study. Br J Ophthalmol. 1976;60(5):324–341.

7. Gerth C. The role of the ERG in the diagnosis and treatment of age-related macular degeneration. Doc Ophthalmol. 2009;118(1):63–68.

8. Gluck JP, Bell J. Ethical issues in the use of animals in biomedical and psychopharmacological research. Psychopharmacology (Berl). 2003;171(1):6–12.

9. Rands SA. Inclusion of policies on ethical standards in animal experiments in biomedical science journals. J Am Assoc Lab Anim Sci. 2011;50(6):901–903.

10. Miziara ID, et al. Research ethics in animal models. Braz J Otorhinolaryngol. 2012;78(2):128–131.

11. Pluhar EB. Experimentation on humans and nonhumans. Theor Med Bioeth. 2006;27(4):333–355.

12. Ringach DL. The use of nonhuman animals in biomedical research. Am J Med Sci. 2011;342(4):305–313.

13. Ding X, Patel M, Chan CC. Molecular pathology of age-related macular degeneration. Prog Retin Eye Res. 2009;28(1):1–18.

14. Curcio CA, et al. Accumulation of cholesterol with age in human Bruch's membrane. Invest Ophthalmol Vis Sci. 2001;42(1):265–274.

15. Pauleikhoff D, et al. Aging changes in Bruch's membrane. A histochemical and morphologic study. Ophthalmology. 1990;97(2):171–178.

16. Sheraidah G, et al. Correlation between lipids extracted from Bruch's membrane and age. Ophthalmology. 1993;100(1):47–51.

17. Sunness JS, et al. Peripheral retinal function in age-related macular degeneration. Arch Ophthalmol. 1985;103(6):811–816.

18. Sunness JS, et al. Retinal sensitivity over drusen and nondrusen areas. A study using fundus perimetry. Arch Ophthalmol. 1988;106(8):1081–1084.

19. Seddon JM, et al. Progression of age-related macular degeneration: association with body mass index, waist circumference, and waist-hip ratio. Arch Ophthalmol. 2003;121(6):785–792.

20. Klein R, et al. The association of cardiovascular disease with the long-term incidence of age-related maculopathy: the Beaver Dam Eye Study. Ophthalmology. 2003;110(6):1273–1280.

21. Tomany SC, et al. Risk factors for incident age-related macular degeneration: pooled findings from 3 continents. Ophthalmology. 2004;111(7):1280–1287.

22. Hyman L, et al. Hypertension, cardiovascular disease, and age-related macular degeneration. Age-Related Macular Degeneration Risk Factors Study Group. Arch Ophthalmol. 2000;118(3):351–358.

23. Klaver CC, et al. Genetic association of apolipoprotein E with age-related macular degeneration. Am J Hum Genet. 1998;63(1):200–206.

24. Simonelli F, et al. Apolipoprotein E polymorphisms in age-related macular degeneration in an Italian population. Ophthalmic Res. 2001;33(6):325–328.

25. Cousins SW, et al. The role of aging, high fat diet and blue light exposure in an experimental mouse model for basal laminar deposit formation. Exp Eye Res. 2002;75(5):543–553.

26. Chiu CJ, et al. Association between dietary glycemic index and age-related macular degeneration in nondiabetic participants in the Age-Related Eye Disease Study. Am J Clin Nutr. 2007;86(1):180–188.

27. Chiu CJ, et al. Dietary carbohydrate and the progression of age-related macular degeneration: a prospective study from the Age-Related Eye Disease Study. Am J Clin Nutr. 2007;86(4):1210–1218.

28. Chiu CJ, et al. Dietary glycemic index and carbohydrate in relation to early age-related macular degeneration. Am J Clin Nutr. 2006;83(4):880–886.

29. Chiu CJ, Taylor A. Dietary hyperglycemia, glycemic index and metabolic retinal diseases. Prog Retin Eye Res. 2011;30(1):18–53.

30. Chiu CJ, et al. Informing food choices and health outcomes by use of the dietary glycemic index. Nutr Rev. 2011;69(4):231–242.

31. Uchiki T, et al. Glycation-altered proteolysis as a pathobiologic mechanism that links dietary glycemic index, aging, and age-related disease (in nondiabetics). Aging Cell. 2012;11(1):1–13.

32. Weikel KA, et al. Natural history of age-related retinal lesions that precede AMD in mice fed high or low glycemic index diets. Invest Ophthalmol Vis Sci. 2012;53(2):622–632.

33. Plump AS, et al. Severe hypercholesterolemia and atherosclerosis in apolipoprotein E-deficient mice created by homologous recombination in ES cells. Cell. 1992;71(2):343–353.

34. Zhang SH, et al. Spontaneous hypercholesterolemia and arterial lesions in mice lacking apolipoprotein E. Science. 1992;258(5081):468–471.

35. Dithmar S, et al. Ultrastructural changes in Bruch's membrane of apolipoprotein E-deficient mice. Invest Ophthalmol Vis Sci. 2000;41(8):2035–2042.

36. Malek G, et al. Apolipoprotein E allele-dependent pathogenesis: a model for age-related retinal degeneration. Proc Natl Acad Sci U S A. 2005;102(33):11900–11905.

37. Malek G, et al. Initial observations of key features of age-related macular degeneration in APOE targeted replacement mice. Adv Exp Med Biol. 2006;572:109–117.

38. Sullivan PM, et al. Targeted replacement of the mouse apolipoprotein E gene with the common human APOE3 allele enhances diet-induced hypercholesterolemia and atherosclerosis. J Biol Chem. 1997;272(29):17972–17980.

39. Mullins RF, et al. Drusen associated with aging and age-related macular degeneration contain proteins common to extracellular deposits associated with atherosclerosis, elastosis, amyloidosis, and dense deposit disease. FASEB J. 2000;14(7):835–846.

40. Ding JD, et al. Anti-amyloid therapy protects against retinal pigmented epithelium damage and vision loss in a model of age-related macular degeneration. Proc Natl Acad Sci U S A. 2011;108(28):E279-E287.

41. Baird PN, et al. The epsilon2 and epsilon4 alleles of the apolipoprotein gene are associated with age-related macular degeneration. Invest Ophthalmol Vis Sci. 2004;45(5):1311–1315.

42. Schmidt S, et al. A pooled case–control study of the apolipoprotein E (APOE) gene in age-related maculopathy. Ophthalmic Genet. 2002;23(4):209–223.

43. Souied EH, et al. Macular dystrophy, diabetes, and deafness associated with a large mitochondrial DNA deletion. Am J Ophthalmol. 1998;125(1):100–103.

44. Havekes L, et al. Apolipoprotein E3-Leiden. A new variant of human apolipoprotein E associated with familial type III hyperlipoproteinemia. Hum Genet. 1986;73(2):157–163.

45. Kliffen M, et al. The APO(*)E3-Leiden mouse as an animal model for basal laminar deposit. Br J Ophthalmol. 2000;84(12):1415–1419.

46. van den Maagdenberg AM, et al. Transgenic mice carrying the apolipoprotein E3-Leiden gene exhibit hyperlipoproteinemia. J Biol Chem. 1993;268(14):10540–10545.

47. Espinosa-Heidmann DG, et al. Basal laminar deposit formation in APO B100 transgenic mice: complex interactions between dietary fat, blue light, and vitamin E. Invest Ophthalmol Vis Sci. 2004;45(1):260–266.

48. Fujihara M, et al. A human apoB100 transgenic mouse expresses human apoB100 in the RPE and develops features of early AMD. Exp Eye Res. 2009;88(6):1115–1123.

49. Sallo FB, et al. Bruch's membrane changes in transgenic mice overexpressing the human biglycan and apolipoprotein b-100 genes. Exp Eye Res. 2009;89(2):178–186.

50. Frykman PK, et al. Normal plasma lipoproteins and fertility in gene-targeted mice homozygous for a disruption in the gene encoding very low density lipoprotein receptor. Proc Natl Acad Sci U S A. 1995;92(18):8453–8457.

51. Heckenlively JR, et al. Mouse model of subretinal neovascularization with choroidal anastomosis. Retina. 2003;23(4):518–522.

52. Tiebel O, et al. Mouse very low-density lipoprotein receptor (VLDLR): gene structure, tissue-specific expression and dietary and developmental regulation. Atherosclerosis. 1999;145(2):239–251.

53. Chen Y, et al. Very low density lipoprotein receptor, a negative regulator of the wnt signaling pathway and choroidal neovascularization. J Biol Chem. 2007;282(47):34420–34428.

54. Kondo N, et al. Positive association of common variants in CD36 with neovascular age-related macular degeneration. Aging (Albany NY). 2009;1(2):266–274.

55. Gordiyenko N, et al. RPE cells internalize low-density lipoprotein (LDL) and oxidized LDL (oxLDL) in large quantities in vitro and in vivo. Invest Ophthalmol Vis Sci. 2004;45(8):2822–2829.

56. Hayes KC, et al. Retinal pigment epithelium possesses both LDL and scavenger receptor activity. Invest Ophthalmol Vis Sci. 1989;30(2):225–232.

57. Ryeom SW, et al. Binding of anionic phospholipids to retinal pigment epithelium may be mediated by the scavenger receptor CD36. J Biol Chem. 1996;271(34):20536–20539.

58. Picard E, et al. CD36 plays an important role in the clearance of oxLDL and associated age-dependent sub-retinal deposits. Aging (Albany NY). 2010;2(12):981–989.

59. Bosch E, Horwitz J, Bok D. Phagocytosis of outer segments by retinal pigment epithelium: phagosome–lysosome interaction. J Histochem Cytochem. 1993;41(2):253–263.

60. Regan CM, et al. Degradation of rhodopsin by a lysosomal fraction of retinal pigment epithelium: biochemical aspects of the visual process. XLI. Exp Eye Res. 1980;30(2):183–191.

61. Rakoczy PE, et al. Correlation between autofluorescent debris accumulation and the presence of partially processed forms of cathepsin D in cultured retinal pigment epithelial cells challenged with rod outer segments. Exp Eye Res. 1996;63(2):159–167.

62. Zhang D, et al. A model for a blinding eye disease of the aged. Biogerontology. 2002;3(1–2):61–66.

63. Rakoczy PE, et al. Progressive age-related changes similar to age-related macular degeneration in a transgenic mouse model. Am J Pathol. 2002;161(4):1515–1524.

64. Cruickshanks KJ, et al. The prevalence of age-related maculopathy by geographic region and ethnicity. The Colorado-Wisconsin Study of Age-Related Maculopathy. Arch Ophthalmol. 1997;115(2):242–250.

65. Vingerling JR, et al. Age-related macular degeneration and smoking. The Rotterdam Study. Arch Ophthalmol. 1996;114(10):1193–1196.

66. Wenzel A, et al. Molecular mechanisms of light-induced photoreceptor apoptosis and neuroprotection for retinal degeneration. Prog Retin Eye Res. 2005;24(2):275–306.

67. Nowak M, et al. Changes in blood antioxidants and several lipid peroxidation products in women with age-related macular degeneration. Eur J Ophthalmol. 2003;13(3):281–286.

68. Age-Related Eye Disease Study Research Group. A randomized, placebo-controlled, clinical trial of high-dose supplementation with vitamins C and E and beta carotene for age-related cataract and vision loss: AREDS report no. 9. Arch Ophthalmol. 2001;119(10):1439–1452.

69. Patel M, Chan CC. Immunopathological aspects of age-related macular degeneration. Semin Immunopathol. 2008;30(2):97–110.

70. Anderson RE. Lipids of ocular tissues. IV. A comparison of the phospholipids from the retina of six mammalian species. Exp Eye Res. 1970;10(2):339–344.

71. Gu X, et al. Carboxyethylpyrrole protein adducts and autoantibodies, biomarkers for age-related macular degeneration. J Biol Chem. 2003;278(43):42027–42035.

72. Hollyfield JG, et al. Oxidative damage-induced inflammation initiates age-related macular degeneration. Nat Med. 2008;14(2):194–198.

73. Hollyfield JG, Perez VL, Salomon RG. A hapten generated from an oxidation fragment of docosahexaenoic acid is sufficient to initiate age-related macular degeneration. Mol Neurobiol. 2010;41(2–3):290–298.

74. Ebrahem Q, et al. Carboxyethylpyrrole oxidative protein modifications stimulate neovascularization: implications for age-related macular degeneration. Proc Natl Acad Sci U S A. 2006;103(36):13480–13484.

75. Behndig A, et al. Superoxide dismutase isoenzymes in the human eye. Invest Ophthalmol Vis Sci. 1998;39(3):471–475.

76. Imamura Y, et al. Drusen, choroidal neovascularization, and retinal pigment epithelium dysfunction in SOD1-deficient mice: a model of age-related macular degeneration. Proc Natl Acad Sci U S A. 2006;103(30):11282–11287.

77. Crabb JW, et al. Drusen proteome analysis: an approach to the etiology of age-related macular degeneration. Proc Natl Acad Sci U S A. 2002;99(23):14682–14687.

78. Hashizume K, et al. Retinal dysfunction and progressive retinal cell death in SOD1-deficient mice. Am J Pathol. 2008;172(5):1325–1331.

79. Kimura K, et al. Genetic association of manganese superoxide dismutase with exudative age-related macular degeneration. Am J Ophthalmol. 2000;130(6):769–773.

80. Li Y, et al. Dilated cardiomyopathy and neonatal lethality in mutant mice lacking manganese superoxide dismutase. Nat Genet. 1995;11(4):376–381.

81. Sandbach JM, et al. Ocular pathology in mitochondrial superoxide dismutase (Sod2)-deficient mice. Invest Ophthalmol Vis Sci. 2001;42(10):2173–2178.

82. Justilien V, et al. SOD2 knockdown mouse model of early AMD. Invest Ophthalmol Vis Sci. 2007;48(10):4407–4420.

83. Dunaief JL. Iron induced oxidative damage as a potential factor in age-related macular degeneration: the Cogan Lecture. Invest Ophthalmol Vis Sci. 2006;47(11):4660–4664.

84. Hort GM, et al. Delayed type hypersensitivity-associated disruption of splenic periarteriolar lymphatic sheaths coincides with temporary loss of IFN-gamma production and impaired eradication of bacteria in Brucella abortus-infected mice. Microbes Infect. 2003;5(2):95–106.

85. Miyajima H, et al. Familial apoceruloplasmin deficiency associated with blepharospasm and retinal degeneration. Neurology. 1987;37(5):761–767.

86. Morita H, et al. Hereditary ceruloplasmin deficiency with hemosiderosis: a clinicopathological study of a Japanese family. Ann Neurol. 1995;37(5):646–656.

87. Yamaguchi K, et al. Retinal degeneration in hereditary ceruloplasmin deficiency. Ophthalmologica. 1998;212(1):11–14.

88. Patel BN, et al. Ceruloplasmin regulates iron levels in the CNS and prevents free radical injury. J Neurosci. 2002;22(15):6578–6586.

89. Harris ZL, et al. Targeted gene disruption reveals an essential role for ceruloplasmin in cellular iron efflux. Proc Natl Acad Sci U S A. 1999;96(19):10812–10817.

90. Vulpe CD, et al. Hephaestin, a ceruloplasmin homologue implicated in intestinal iron transport, is defective in the sla mouse. Nat Genet. 1999;21(2):195–199.

91. Hahn P, et al. Disruption of ceruloplasmin and hephaestin in mice causes retinal iron overload and retinal degeneration with features of age-related macular degeneration. Proc Natl Acad Sci U S A. 2004;101(38):13850–13855.

92. Hadziahmetovic M, et al. Ceruloplasmin/hephaestin knockout mice model morphologic and molecular features of AMD. Invest Ophthalmol Vis Sci. 2008;49(6):2728–2736.

93. Evans JR. Risk factors for age-related macular degeneration. Prog Retin Eye Res. 2001;20(2):227–253.

94. Klein R, et al. Further observations on the association between smoking and the long-term incidence and progression of age-related macular degeneration: the Beaver Dam Eye Study. Arch Ophthalmol. 2008;126(1):115–121.

95. Seddon JM, et al. A prospective study of cigarette smoking and age-related macular degeneration in women. JAMA. 1996;276(14):1141–1146.

96. Smith W, et al. Risk factors for age-related macular degeneration: pooled findings from three continents. Ophthalmology. 2001;108(4):697–704.

97. Thornton J, et al. Smoking and age-related macular degeneration: a review of association. Eye (Lond). 2005;19(9):935–944.

98. Smith CJ, Hansch C. The relative toxicity of compounds in mainstream cigarette smoke condensate. Food Chem Toxicol. 2000;38(7):637–646.

99. Espinosa-Heidmann DG, et al. Cigarette smoke-related oxidants and the development of sub-RPE deposits in an experimental animal model of dry AMD. Invest Ophthalmol Vis Sci. 2006;47(2):729–737.

100. Pons M, Marin-Castano ME. Cigarette smoke-related hydroquinone dysregulates MCP-1, VEGF and PEDF expression in retinal pigment epithelium in vitro and in vivo. PLoS One. 2011;6(2):e16722.

101. Salganik RI, et al. Inherited enhancement of hydroxyl radical generation and lipid peroxidation in the S strain rats results in DNA rearrangements, degenerative diseases, and premature aging. Biochem Biophys Res Commun. 1994;199(2):726–733.

102. Kolosova NG, et al. OXYS rats as a model of senile cataract. Bull Exp Biol Med. 2003;136(4):415–419.

103. Marsili S, et al. Cataract formation in a strain of rats selected for high oxidative stress. Exp Eye Res. 2004;79(5):595–612.

104. Salganik RI, et al. Impairment of respiratory functions in mitochondria of rats with an inherited hyperproduction of free radicals. Biochem Biophys Res Commun. 1994;205(1):180–185.

105. Markovets AM, et al. Alterations of retinal pigment epithelium cause AMD-like retinopathy in senescence-accelerated OXYS rats. Aging (Albany NY). 2011;3(1):44–54.

106. Neroev VV, et al. Mitochondria-targeted plastoquinone derivatives as tools to interrupt execution of the aging program. 4. Age-related eye disease. SkQ1 returns vision to blind animals. Biochemistry (Mosc). 2008;73(12):1317–1328.

107. Xu H, et al. Age-dependent accumulation of lipofuscin in perivascular and subretinal microglia in experimental mice. Aging Cell. 2008;7(1):58–68.

108. Xu H, Chen M, Forrester JV. Para-inflammation in the aging retina. Prog Retin Eye Res. 2009;28(5):348–368.

109. van der Schaft TL, et al. Histologic features of the early stages of age-related macular degeneration. A statistical analysis. Ophthalmology. 1992;99(2):278–286.

110. Spraul CW, Grossniklaus HE. Characteristics of Drusen and Bruch's membrane in postmortem eyes with age-related macular degeneration. Arch Ophthalmol. 1997;115(2):267–273.

111. Anderson DH, et al. A role for local inflammation in the formation of drusen in the aging eye. Am J Ophthalmol. 2002;134(3):411–431.

112. Chan CC, et al. Ccl2/Cx3cr1-deficient mice: an animal model for age-related macular degeneration. Ophthalmic Res. 2008;40(3–4):124–128.

113. Boekhoorn SS, et al. C-reactive protein level and risk of aging macula disorder: the Rotterdam Study. Arch Ophthalmol. 2007;125(10):1396–1401.

114. Seddon JM, et al. Association between C-reactive protein and age-related macular degeneration. JAMA. 2004;291(6):704–710.

115. Gold B, et al. Variation in factor B (BF) and complement component 2 (C2) genes is associated with age-related macular degeneration. Nat Genet. 2006;38(4):458–462.

116. Maller J, et al. Common variation in three genes, including a noncoding variant in CFH, strongly influences risk of age-related macular degeneration. Nat Genet. 2006;38(9):1055–1059.

117. Montes T, et al. Functional basis of protection against age-related macular degeneration conferred by a common polymorphism in complement factor B. Proc Natl Acad Sci U S A. 2009;106(11):4366–4371.

118. Reynolds R, et al. Plasma complement components and activation fragments: associations with age-related macular degeneration genotypes and phenotypes. Invest Ophthalmol Vis Sci. 2009;50(12):5818–5827.

119. Yates JR, et al. Complement C3 variant and the risk of age-related macular degeneration. N Engl J Med. 2007;357(6):553–561.

120. Edwards AO, et al. Complement factor H polymorphism and age-related macular degeneration. Science. 2005;308(5720):421–424.

121. Hageman GS, et al. A common haplotype in the complement regulatory gene factor H (HF1/CFH) predisposes individuals to age-related macular degeneration. Proc Natl Acad Sci U S A. 2005;102(20):7227–7232.

122. Haines JL, et al. Complement factor H variant increases the risk of age-related macular degeneration. Science. 2005;308(5720):419–421.

123. Thakkinstian A, et al. Systematic review and meta-analysis of the association between complement factor H Y402H polymorphisms and age-related macular degeneration. Hum Mol Genet. 2006;15(18):2784–2790.

124. Zareparsi S, et al. Strong association of the Y402H variant in complement factor H at 1q32 with susceptibility to age-related macular degeneration. Am J Hum Genet. 2005;77(1):149–153.

125. Alsenz J, et al. Structural and functional analysis of the complement component factor H with the use of different enzymes and monoclonal antibodies to factor H. Biochem J. 1985;232(3):841–850.

126. Pickering MC, et al. Uncontrolled C3 activation causes membranoproliferative glomerulonephritis in mice deficient in complement factor H. Nat Genet. 2002;31(4):424–428.

127. Johnson PT, et al. Individuals homozygous for the age-related macular degeneration risk-conferring variant of complement factor H have elevated levels of CRP in the choroid. Proc Natl Acad Sci U S A. 2006;103(46):17456–17461.

128. Duvall-Young J, et al. Fundus changes in mesangiocapillary glomerulonephritis type II: clinical and fluorescein angiographic findings. Br J Ophthalmol. 1989;73(11):900–906.

129. Duvall-Young J, MacDonald MK, McKechnie NM. Fundus changes in (type II) mesangiocapillary glomerulonephritis simulating drusen: a histopathological report. Br J Ophthalmol. 1989;73(4):297–302.

130. Raines MF, Duvall-Young J, Short CD. Fundus changes in mesangiocapillary glomerulonephritis type II: vitreous fluorophotometry. Br J Ophthalmol. 1989;73(11):907–910.

131. Leys A, et al. Fundus changes in membranoproliferative glomerulonephritis type II. A fluorescein angiographic study of 23 patients. Graefes Arch Clin Exp Ophthalmol. 1991;229(5):406–410.

132. Dewan A, et al. HTRA1 promoter polymorphism in wet age-related macular degeneration. Science. 2006;314(5801):989–992.

133. Ufret-Vincenty RL, et al. Transgenic mice expressing variants of complement factor H develop AMD-like retinal findings. Invest Ophthalmol Vis Sci. 2010;51(11):5878–5887.

134. Cashman SM, et al. Expression of complement component 3 (C3) from an adenovirus leads to pathology in the murine retina. Invest Ophthalmol Vis Sci. 2011;52(6):3436–3445.

135. Johnson LV, et al. A potential role for immune complex pathogenesis in drusen formation. Exp Eye Res. 2000;70(4):441–449.

136. Nozaki M, et al. Drusen complement components C3a and C5a promote choroidal neovascularization. Proc Natl Acad Sci U S A. 2006;103(7):2328–2333.

137. Graves DT, Jiang Y. Chemokines, a family of chemotactic cytokines. Crit Rev Oral Biol Med. 1995;6(2):109–118.

138. Murphy PM, et al. International union of pharmacology. XXII. Nomenclature for chemokine receptors. Pharmacol Rev. 2000;52(1):145–176.

139. Zlotnik A, Yoshie O. Chemokines: a new classification system and their role in immunity. Immunity. 2000;12(2):121–127.

140. Gupta N, Brown KE, Milam AH. Activated microglia in human retinitis pigmentosa, late-onset retinal degeneration, and age-related macular degeneration. Exp Eye Res. 2003;76(4):463–471.

141. van der Schaft TL, et al. Early stages of age-related macular degeneration: an immunofluorescence and electron microscopy study. Br J Ophthalmol. 1993;77(10):657–661.

142. Raoul W, et al. CCL2/CCR2 and CX3CL1/CX3CR1 chemokine axes and their possible involvement in age-related macular degeneration. J Neuroinflammation. 2010;7:87.

143. Chan CC, et al. Detection of CX3CR1 single nucleotide polymorphism and expression on archived eyes with age-related macular degeneration. Histol Histopathol. 2005;20(3):857–863.

144. Combadiere C, et al. CX3CR1-dependent subretinal microglia cell accumulation is associated with cardinal features of age-related macular degeneration. J Clin Invest. 2007;117(10):2920–2928.

145. Tuo J, et al. Murine ccl2/cx3cr1 deficiency results in retinal lesions mimicking human age-related macular degeneration. Invest Ophthalmol Vis Sci. 2007;48(8):3827–3836.

146. Yang X, et al. Polymorphisms in CFH, HTRA1 and CX3CR1 confer risk to exudative age-related macular degeneration in Han Chinese. Br J Ophthalmol. 2010;94(9):1211–1214.

147. Kuziel WA, et al. Severe reduction in leukocyte adhesion and monocyte extravasation in mice deficient in CC chemokine receptor 2. Proc Natl Acad Sci U S A. 1997;94(22):12053–12058.

148. Lu B, et al. Abnormalities in monocyte recruitment and cytokine expression in monocyte chemoattractant protein 1-deficient mice. J Exp Med. 1998;187(4):601–608.

149. Higgins GT, et al. Induction of angiogenic cytokine expression in cultured RPE by ingestion of oxidized photoreceptor outer segments. Invest Ophthalmol Vis Sci. 2003;44(4):1775–1782.

150. Jonas JB, et al. Monocyte chemoattractant protein 1, intercellular adhesion molecule 1, and vascular cell adhesion molecule 1 in exudative age-related macular degeneration. Arch Ophthalmol. 2010;128(10):1281–1286.

151. Yamada K, et al. Inhibition of laser-induced choroidal neovascularization by atorvastatin by downregulation of monocyte chemotactic protein-1 synthesis in mice. Invest Ophthalmol Vis Sci. 2007;48(4):1839–1843.

152. Tsutsumi C, et al. The critical role of ocular-infiltrating macrophages in the development of choroidal neovascularization. J Leukoc Biol. 2003;74(1):25–32.

153. Luhmann UF, et al. The drusenlike phenotype in aging Ccl2-knockout mice is caused by an accelerated accumulation of swollen autofluorescent subretinal macrophages. Invest Ophthalmol Vis Sci. 2009;50(12):5934–5943.

154. Ambati J, et al. An animal model of age-related macular degeneration in senescent Ccl-2- or Ccr-2-deficient mice. Nat Med. 2003;9(11):1390–1397.

155. Cardona AE, et al. Control of microglial neurotoxicity by the fractalkine receptor. Nat Neurosci. 2006;9(7):917–924.

156. Silverman MD, et al. Constitutive and inflammatory mediator-regulated fractalkine expression in human ocular tissues and cultured cells. Invest Ophthalmol Vis Sci. 2003;44(4):1608–1615.

157. Combadiere C, et al. Decreased atherosclerotic lesion formation in CX3CR1/apolipoprotein E double knockout mice. Circulation. 2003;107(7):1009–1016.

158. Jung S, et al. Analysis of fractalkine receptor CX(3)CR1 function by targeted deletion and green fluorescent protein reporter gene insertion. Mol Cell Biol. 2000;20(11):4106–4114.

159. Ross RJ, et al. Immunological protein expression profile in Ccl2/Cx3cr1 deficient mice with lesions similar to age-related macular degeneration. Exp Eye Res. 2008;86(4):675–683.

160. Mattapallil MJ, et al. The Rd8 mutation of the Crb1 gene is present in vendor lines of C57BL/6 N mice and embryonic stem cells, and confounds ocular induced mutant phenotypes. Invest Ophthalmol Vis Sci. 2012;53(6):2921–2927.

161. Jeffrey BG, Neuringer M. Age-related decline in rod phototransduction sensitivity in rhesus monkeys fed an n-3 fatty acid-deficient diet. Invest Ophthalmol Vis Sci. 2009;50(9):4360–4367.

162. Umeda S, et al. Early-onset macular degeneration with drusen in a cynomolgus monkey (Macaca fascicularis) pedigree: exclusion of 13 candidate genes and loci. Invest Ophthalmol Vis Sci. 2005;46(2):683–691.

163. Suzuki MT, Terao K, Yoshikawa Y. Familial early onset macular degeneration in cynomolgus monkeys (Macaca fascicularis). Primates. 2003;44(3):291–294.

164. Nicolas MG, et al. Studies on the mechanism of early onset macular degeneration in cynomolgus monkeys. II. Suppression of metallothionein synthesis in the retina in oxidative stress. Exp Eye Res. 1996;62(4):399–408.

165. Nicolas MG, et al. Studies on the mechanism of early onset macular degeneration in cynomolgus (Macaca fascicularis) monkeys. I. Abnormal concentrations of two proteins in the retina. Exp Eye Res. 1996;62(3):211–219.

166. Bellhorn RW, et al. Pigmentary abnormalities of the macula in rhesus monkeys: clinical observations. Invest Ophthalmol Vis Sci. 1981;21(6):771–781.

167. Dawson WW, et al. Macular disease in related rhesus monkeys. Doc Ophthalmol. 1989;71(3):253–263.

168. El-Mofty AA, et al. Retinal degeneration in rhesus monkeys. Macaca mulatta. Survey of three seminatural free-breeding colonies. Exp Eye Res. 1980;31(2):147–166.

169. Francis PJ, et al. Rhesus monkeys and humans share common susceptibility genes for age-related macular disease. Hum Mol Genet. 2008;17(17):2673–2680.

170. Hope GM, et al. A primate model for age related macular drusen. Br J Ophthalmol. 1992;76(1):11–16.

171. Jonas JB, Hayreh SS, Martus P. Influence of arterial hypertension and diet-induced atherosclerosis on macular drusen. Graefes Arch Clin Exp Ophthalmol. 2003;241(2):125–134.

172. Monaco WA, Wormington CM. The rhesus monkey as an animal model for age-related maculopathy. Optom Vis Sci. 1990;67(7):532–537.

173. Olin KL, et al. Trace element status and free radical defense in elderly rhesus macaques (Macaca mulatta) with macular drusen. Proc Soc Exp Biol Med. 1995;208(4):370–377.

174. Stafford TJ, Anness SH, Fine BS. Spontaneous degenerative maculopathy in the monkey. Ophthalmology. 1984;91(5):513–521.

175. Ulshafer RJ, et al. Macular degeneration in a community of rhesus monkeys. Ultrastructural observations. Retina. 1987;7(3):198–203.

176. Dawson WW, et al. Adult-onset macular degeneration in the Cayo Santiago macaques. P R Health Sci J. 1989;8(1):111–115.

177. El-Mofty A, et al. Macular degeneration in rhesus monkey (Macaca mulatta). Exp Eye Res. 1978;27(4):499–502.

178. Engel HM, et al. Degenerative changes in maculas of rhesus monkeys. Ophthalmologica. 1988;196(3):143–150.

179. Dawson WW, et al. Maculas, monkeys, models. AMD and aging. Vision Res. 2008;48(3):360–365.

180. Klein R, et al. The relationship of age-related maculopathy, cataract, and glaucoma to visual acuity. Invest Ophthalmol Vis Sci. 1995;36(1):182–191.

181. Group CR, et al. Ranibizumab and bevacizumab for neovascular age-related macular degeneration. N Engl J Med. 2011;364(20):1897–1908.

182. van Wijngaarden P, Qureshi SH, Inhibitors of vascular endothelial growth factor (VEGF) in the management of neovascular age-related macular degeneration: a review of current practice. Clin Exp Optom. 2008;91(5):427–437.

183. Campochiaro PA. Gene therapy for ocular neovascularization. Curr Gene Ther. 2007;7(1):25–33.

184. Edelman JL, Castro MR. Quantitative image analysis of laser-induced choroidal neovascularization in rat. Exp Eye Res. 2000;71(5):523–533.

185. Bora PS, et al. Immunotherapy for choroidal neovascularization in a laser-induced mouse model simulating exudative (wet) macular degeneration. Proc Natl Acad Sci U S A. 2003;100(5):2679–2684.

186. Economou MA, et al. Inhibition of VEGF secretion and experimental choroidal neovascularization by picropodophyllin (PPP), an inhibitor of the insulin-like growth factor-1 receptor. Acta Ophthalmol. 2008;86 Thesis 4:42–49.

187. Semkova I, et al. Investigation of laser-induced choroidal neovascularization in the rat. Invest Ophthalmol Vis Sci. 2003;44(12):5349–5354.

188. Ciulla MM, et al. Vascular network changes in the retina during ageing in normal subjects: a computerized quantitative analysis. Ital Heart J. 2000;1(5):361–364.

189. Ryan SJ. The development of an experimental model of subretinal neovascularization in disciform macular degeneration. Trans Am Ophthalmol Soc. 1979;77:707–745.

190. Tobe T, et al. Targeted disruption of the FGF2 gene does not prevent choroidal neovascularization in a murine model. Am J Pathol. 1998;153(5):1641–1646.

191. Campa C, et al. Effects of an anti-VEGF-A monoclonal antibody on laser-induced choroidal neovascularization in mice: optimizing methods to quantify vascular changes. Invest Ophthalmol Vis Sci. 2008;49(3):1178–1183.

192. Seo MS, et al. Dramatic inhibition of retinal and choroidal neovascularization by oral administration of a kinase inhibitor. Am J Pathol. 1999;154(6):1743–1753.

193. Campos M, et al. A novel imaging technique for experimental choroidal neovascularization. Invest Ophthalmol Vis Sci. 2006;47(12):5163–5170.

194. Ogata N, et al. Expression of basic fibroblast growth factor mRNA in developing choroidal neovascularization. Curr Eye Res. 1996;15(10):1008–1018.

195. Yamada H, et al. Cell injury unmasks a latent proangiogenic phenotype in mice with increased expression of FGF2 in the retina. J Cell Physiol. 2000;185(1):135–142.

196. Oshima Y, et al. Increased expression of VEGF in retinal pigmented epithelial cells is not sufficient to cause choroidal neovascularization. J Cell Physiol. 2004;201(3):393–400.

197. Shen WY, et al. Expression of cell adhesion molecules and vascular endothelial growth factor in experimental choroidal neovascularisation in the rat. Br J Ophthalmol. 1998;82(9):1063–1071.

198. Wada M, et al. Expression of vascular endothelial growth factor and its receptor (KDR/flk-1) mRNA in experimental choroidal neovascularization. Curr Eye Res. 1999;18(3):203–213.

199. Yi X, et al. Vascular endothelial growth factor expression in choroidal neovascularization in rats. Graefes Arch Clin Exp Ophthalmol. 1997;235(5):313–319.

200. Ando A, et al. Nitric oxide is proangiogenic in the retina and choroid. J Cell Physiol. 2002;191(1):116–124.

201. Berglin L, et al. Reduced choroidal neovascular membrane formation in matrix metalloproteinase-2-deficient mice. Invest Ophthalmol Vis Sci. 2003;44(1):403–408.

202. Lambert V, et al. Matrix metalloproteinase-9 contributes to choroidal neovascularization. Am J Pathol. 2002;161(4):1247–1253.

203. Zhu J, et al. Focal adhesion kinase signaling pathway participates in the formation of choroidal neovascularization and regulates the proliferation and migration of choroidal microvascular endothelial cells by acting through HIF-1 and VEGF expression in RPE cells. Exp Eye Res. 2009;88(5):910–918.

204. Sakurai E, et al. Macrophage depletion inhibits experimental choroidal neovascularization. Invest Ophthalmol Vis Sci. 2003;44(8):3578–3585.

205. Dobi ET, Puliafito CA, Destro M. A new model of experimental choroidal neovascularization in the rat. Arch Ophthalmol. 1989;107(2):264–269.

206. Zhang ZX, et al. Hypoxia specific SDF-1 expression by retinal pigment epithelium initiates bone marrow-derived cells to participate in Choroidal neovascularization in a laser-induced mouse model. Curr Eye Res. 2011;36(9):838–849.

207. Bora NS, et al. Complement activation via alternative pathway is critical in the development of laser-induced choroidal neovascularization: role of factor B and factor H. J Immunol. 2006;177(3):1872–1878.

208. Lima e Silva R, et al. Suppression and regression of choroidal neovascularization by polyamine analogues. Invest Ophthalmol Vis Sci. 2005;46(9):3323–3330.

209. Ciulla TA, et al. Intravitreal triamcinolone acetonide inhibits choroidal neovascularization in a laser-treated rat model. Arch Ophthalmol. 2001;119(3):399–404.

210. Kim SJ, Toma HS. Inhibition of choroidal neovascularization by intravitreal ketorolac. Arch Ophthalmol. 2010;128(5):596–600.

211. Olson JL, et al. Intravitreal anakinra inhibits choroidal neovascular membrane growth in a rat model. Ocul Immunol Inflamm. 2009;17(3):195–200.

212. Rennel ES, et al. A human neutralizing antibody specific to Ang-2 inhibits ocular angiogenesis. Microcirculation. 2011;18(7):598–607.

213. Olson JL, Courtney RJ, Mandava N. Intravitreal infliximab and choroidal neovascularization in an animal model. Arch Ophthalmol. 2007;125(9):1221–1224.

214. Zou Y, Xu X, Chiou GC. Effect of interleukin-1 blockers, CK112, and CK116 on rat experimental choroidal neovascularization in vivo and endothelial cell cultures in vitro. J Ocul Pharmacol Ther. 2006;22(1):19–25.

215. Fu Y, et al. Angiogenesis inhibition and choroidal neovascularization suppression by sustained delivery of an integrin antagonist, EMD478761. Invest Ophthalmol Vis Sci. 2007;48(11):5184–5190.

216. Pan CK, et al. Comparison of long-acting bevacizumab formulations in the treatment of choroidal neovascularization in a rat model. J Ocul Pharmacol Ther. 2011;27(3):219–224.

217. Reich SJ, et al. Small interfering RNA (siRNA) targeting VEGF effectively inhibits ocular neovascularization in a mouse model. Mol Vis. 2003;9:210–216.

218. Huang H, Shen J, Vinores SA. Blockade of VEGFR1 and 2 suppresses pathological angiogenesis and vascular leakage in the eye. PLoS One. 2011;6(6):e21411.

219. Saishin Y, et al. VEGF-TRAP(R1R2) suppresses choroidal neovascularization and VEGF-induced breakdown of the blood-retinal barrier. J Cell Physiol. 2003;195(2):241–248.

220. Takahashi K, et al. Intraocular expression of endostatin reduces VEGF-induced retinal vascular permeability, neovascularization, and retinal detachment. FASEB J;2003;17(8):896–898.

221. Balaggan KS, et al. EIAV vector-mediated delivery of endostatin or angiostatin inhibits angiogenesis and vascular hyperpermeability in experimental CNV. Gene Ther. 2006;13(15):1153–1165.

222. Lai CC, et al. Suppression of choroidal neovascularization by adeno-associated virus vector expressing angiostatin. Invest Ophthalmol Vis Sci. 2001;42(10):2401–2407.

223. Mori K, et al. AAV-mediated gene transfer of pigment epithelium-derived factor inhibits choroidal neovascularization. Invest Ophthalmol Vis Sci. 2002;43(6):1994–2000.

224. Ryan SJ. Subretinal neovascularization after argon laser photocoagulation. Albrecht Von Graefes Arch Klin Exp Ophthalmol. 1980;215(1):29–42.

225. Ryan SJ. Subretinal neovascularization. Natural history of an experimental model. Arch Ophthalmol. 1982;100(11):1804–1809.

226. Criswell MH, et al. The squirrel monkey: characterization of a new-world primate model of experimental choroidal neovascularization and comparison with the macaque. Invest Ophthalmol Vis Sci. 2004;45(2):625–634.

227. Ishibashi T, et al. Morphologic observations on experimental subretinal neovascularization in the monkey. Invest Ophthalmol Vis Sci. 1987;28(7):1116–1130.

228. Miller H, et al. Pathogenesis of laser-induced choroidal subretinal neovascularization. Invest Ophthalmol Vis Sci. 1990;31(5):899–908.

229. Criswell MH, et al. Anastomotic vessels remain viable after photodynamic therapy in primate models of choroidal neovascularization. Invest Ophthalmol Vis Sci. 2005;46(6):2168–2174.

230. Ohkura T, et al. Experimental study on expanded polytetrafluoroethylene (E-PTFE) for portal vein reconstruction with combined operation of the digestive tract. J Cardiovasc Surg (Torino). 1982;23(4):328–333.

231. Shen WY, et al. Preclinical evaluation of a phosphorothioate oligonucleotide in the retina of rhesus monkey. Lab Invest. 2002;82(2):167–182.

232. Goody RJ, et al. Optimization of laser-induced choroidal neovascularization in African green monkeys. Exp Eye Res. 2011;92(6):464–472.

233. Tolentino MJ, et al. Intravitreal injection of vascular endothelial growth factor small interfering RNA inhibits growth and leakage in a nonhuman primate, laser-induced model of choroidal neovascularization. Retina. 2004;24(4):660.

234. Zahn G, et al. Preclinical evaluation of the novel small-molecule integrin alpha5beta1 inhibitor JSM6427 in monkey and rabbit models of choroidal neovascularization. Arch Ophthalmol. 2009;127(10):1329–1335.

235. elDirini AA, Ogden TE, Ryan SJ. Subretinal endophotocoagulation. A new model of subretinal neovascularization in the rabbit. Retina. 1991;11(2):244–249.

236. Kiilgaard JF, et al. A new animal model of choroidal neovascularization. Acta Ophthalmol Scand. 2005;83(6):697–704.

237. Goldberg MF. Editorial: Bruch's membrane and vascular growth. Invest Ophthalmol. 1976;15(6):443–446.

238. Lassota N, et al. Surgical induction of choroidal neovascularization in a porcine model. Graefes Arch Clin Exp Ophthalmol. 2007;245(8):1189–1198.

239. Sarks SH. New vessel formation beneath the retinal pigment epithelium in senile eyes. Br J Ophthalmol. 1973;57(12):951–965.

240. Sarks JP, Sarks SH, Killingsworth MC. Morphology of early choroidal neovascularisation in age-related macular degeneration: correlation with activity. Eye (Lond). 1997;11(Pt 4):515–522.

241. Zhao L, et al. Translocation of the retinal pigment epithelium and formation of sub-retinal pigment epithelium deposit induced by subretinal deposit. Mol Vis. 2007;13:873–880.

242. Qiu G, et al. A new model of experimental subretinal neovascularization in the rabbit. Exp Eye Res. 2006;83(1):141–152.

243. Kleinman HK, Martin GR. Matrigel: basement membrane matrix with biological activity. Semin Cancer Biol. 2005;15(5):378–386.

244. Wang ZY, et al. Erythropoietin as a novel therapeutic agent for atrophic age-related macular degeneration. Med Hypotheses. 2009;72(4):448–450.

245. Tamai K, et al. Lipid hydroperoxide stimulates subretinal choroidal neovascularization in the rabbit. Exp Eye Res. 2002;74(2):301–308.

246. Baba T, et al. A rat model for choroidal neovascularization using subretinal lipid hydroperoxide injection. Am J Pathol. 2010;176(6):3085–3097.

247. Bora PS, et al. Role of complement and complement membrane attack complex in laser-induced choroidal neovascularization. J Immunol. 2005;174(1):491–497.

248. Lyzogubov VV, et al. Polyethylene glycol (PEG)-induced mouse model of choroidal neovascularization. J Biol Chem. 2011;286(18):16229–16237.

249. Grossniklaus HE, et al. Macrophage and retinal pigment epithelium expression of angiogenic cytokines in choroidal neovascularization. Mol Vis. 2002;8:119–126.

250. Oh H, et al. The potential angiogenic role of macrophages in the formation of choroidal neovascular membranes. Invest Ophthalmol Vis Sci. 1999;40(9):1891–1898.

251. Jo YJ, et al. Establishment of a new animal model of focal subretinal fibrosis that resembles disciform lesion in advanced age-related macular degeneration. Invest Ophthalmol Vis Sci. 2011;52(9):6089–6095.

252. Blaauwgeers HG, et al. Polarized vascular endothelial growth factor secretion by human retinal pigment epithelium and localization of vascular endothelial growth factor receptors on the inner choriocapillaris. Evidence for a trophic paracrine relation. Am J Pathol. 1999;155(2):421–428.

253. Miller JW, et al. Vascular endothelial growth factor/vascular permeability factor is temporally and spatially correlated with ocular angiogenesis in a primate model. Am J Pathol. 1994;145(3):574–584.

254. Kvanta A, et al. Subfoveal fibrovascular membranes in age-related macular degeneration express vascular endothelial growth factor. Invest Ophthalmol Vis Sci. 1996;37(9):1929–1934.

255. Lopez PF, et al. Transdifferentiated retinal pigment epithelial cells are immunoreactive for vascular endothelial growth factor in surgically excised age-related macular degeneration-related choroidal neovascular membranes. Invest Ophthalmol Vis Sci. 1996;37(5):855–868.

256. Okamoto N, et al. Transgenic mice with increased expression of vascular endothelial growth factor in the retina: a new model of intraretinal and subretinal neovascularization. Am J Pathol. 1997;151(1):281–291.

257. Kwak N, et al. VEGF is major stimulator in model of choroidal neovascularization. Invest Ophthalmol Vis Sci. 2000;41(10):3158–3164.

258. Takeda A, et al. CCR3 is a target for age-related macular degeneration diagnosis and therapy. Nature. 2009;460(7252):225–230.

259. Stewart MW. The expanding role of vascular endothelial growth factor inhibitors in ophthalmology. Mayo Clin Proc. 2012;87(1):77–88.

260. Meyer CH, Holz FG. Preclinical aspects of anti-VEGF agents for the treatment of wet AMD: ranibizumab and bevacizumab. Eye (Lond). 2011;25(6):661–672.

261. Bakri SJ, et al. Pharmacokinetics of intravitreal bevacizumab (Avastin). Ophthalmology. 2007;114(5):855–859.

262. Bakri SJ, et al. Pharmacokinetics of intravitreal ranibizumab (Lucentis). Ophthalmology. 2007;114(12):2179–2182.

263. Gaudreault J, et al. Preclinical pharmacokinetics of Ranibizumab (rhuFabV2) after a single intravitreal administration. Invest Ophthalmol Vis Sci. 2005;46(2):726–733.

264. Thaler S, et al. Toxicity testing of the VEGF inhibitors bevacizumab, ranibizumab and pegaptanib in rats both with and without prior retinal ganglion cell damage. Acta Ophthalmol. 2010;88(5):e170–e176.

265. Miki K, et al. Effects of intraocular ranibizumab and bevacizumab in transgenic mice expressing human vascular endothelial growth factor. Ophthalmology. 2009;116(9):1748–1754.

266. Maier P, et al. Intravitreal injection of specific receptor tyrosine kinase inhibitor PTK787/ZK222 584 improves ischemia-induced retinopathy in mice. Graefes Arch Clin Exp Ophthalmol. 2005;243(6):593–600.

267. Thumann G. Prospectives for gene therapy of retinal degenerations. Curr Genomics. 2012;13(5):350–362.

268. Chizzolini M, et al. Good epidemiologic practice in retinitis pigmentosa: from phenotyping to biobanking. Curr Genomics. 2011;12(4):260–266.

269. Inglehearn CF, et al. A linkage survey of 20 dominant retinitis pigmentosa families: frequencies of the nine known loci and evidence for further heterogeneity. J Med Genet. 1998;35(1):1–5.

270. Wang DY, et al. Gene mutations in retinitis pigmentosa and their clinical implications. Clin Chim Acta. 2005;351(1–2):5–16.

271. Thompson DA, et al. Rd9 is a naturally occurring mouse model of a common form of retinitis pigmentosa caused by mutations in RPGR-ORF15. PLoS One. 2012;7(5):e35865.

272. Ross JW, et al. Generation of an inbred miniature pig model of retinitis pigmentosa. Invest Ophthalmol Vis Sci. 2012;53(1):501–507.

273. Aguirre G. Retinal degenerations in the dog. I. Rod dysplasia. Exp Eye Res. 1978;26(3):233–253.

274. May CA, Lutjen-Drecoll E, Narfstrom K. Morphological changes in the anterior segment of the Abyssinian cat eye with hereditary rod-cone degeneration. Curr Eye Res. 2005;30(10):855–862.

275. Cheung N, Mitchell P, Wong TY. Diabetic retinopathy. Lancet. 2010;376(9735):124–136.

276. Robinson R, et al. Update on animal models of diabetic retinopathy: from molecular approaches to mice and higher mammals. Dis Model Mech. 2012;5(4):444–456.

277. Kern TS, et al. Comparison of three strains of diabetic rats with respect to the rate at which retinopathy and tactile allodynia develop. Mol Vis. 2010;16:1629–1639.

278. Sima AA, et al. The BB-rat—an authentic model of human diabetic retinopathy. Curr Eye Res. 1985;4(10):1087–1092.

279. Danis RP, Yang Y. Microvascular retinopathy in the Zucker diabetic fatty rat. Invest Ophthalmol Vis Sci. 1993;34(7):2367–2371.

280. Matsuura T, et al. Proliferative retinal changes in diabetic rats (WBN/Kob). Lab Anim Sci. 1999;49(5):565–569.

281. Miyamura N, Amemiya T. Lens and retinal changes in the WBN/Kob rat (spontaneously diabetic strain). Electron-microscopic study. Ophthalmic Res. 1998;30(4):221–232.

282. Goto Y, et al. Development of diabetes in the non-obese NIDDM rat (GK rat). Adv Exp Med Biol. 1988;246:29–31.

283. Yamada H, et al. Retinal neovascularisation without ischaemia in the spontaneously diabetic Torii rat. Diabetologia. 2005;48(8):1663–1668.

284. Makino S, et al. Breeding of a non-obese, diabetic strain of mice. Jikken Dobutsu. 1980;29(1):1–13.

285. Midena E, et al. Studies on the retina of the diabetic db/db mouse. I. Endothelial cell-pericyte ratio. Ophthalmic Res. 1989;21(2):106–111.

286. Barber AJ, et al. The Ins2Akita mouse as a model of early retinal complications in diabetes. Invest Ophthalmol Vis Sci. 2005;46(6):2210–2218.

287. Johnson MA, et al. Ocular structure and function in an aged monkey with spontaneous diabetes mellitus. Exp Eye Res. 2005;80(1):37–42.

3

PATHOGENESIS AND PATHOPHYSIOLOGY OF AGE-RELATED MACULAR DEGENERATION

ANA MACHÍN MAHAVE • ERNESTO ROMERA REDONDO
JOHN BARNWELL KERRISON

INTRODUCTION

Age-related macular degeneration (AMD) is the leading cause of severe visual acuity loss in the United States among people older than 60 years, representing 54% of legal blindness (1). In the general population, the number of people in this group is increasing. As a result, vision loss from macular degeneration is a growing problem. Ninety percent of AMD patients have dry AMD, and 10% of AMD patients have wet AMD. Currently, an estimated 8 million Americans are affected with early AMD, and over 1 million will develop advanced AMD within the next 5 years (2).

Many changes in the macula could be due to normal aging. The focus of study has been which aging processes are implicated in the pathogenesis of senile macular degeneration or at what stage they become pathologic (3). The critical question to be answered is "Is AMD a normal process of aging or is it a disease by itself?" (4–7). Most of the authors defend the theory in which AMD is an advanced stage or perturbation of the normal process of eye senescence (3,4,8,9).

The pathophysiology of AMD is incompletely understood, but genetic tools offer new insights into the development and progress of AMD (10).

RISK FACTORS

AMD is a multifactorial disease in which multiple genetic and environmental factors are involved.

Age: Age is the largest risk factor for AMD (11–17).

Smoking: The mechanism by which smoking might affect the retina is unknown; however, there exists a direct association between the risk of developing advanced AMD with the number of cigarettes smoked (18,19).

Sunlight exposure: Individuals who wore sunglasses regularly were less likely to develop soft drusen (20). Results from the Beaver Dam Study suggest that people who spent leisure time outdoors were at an increased risk of developing early AMD (21). On the other hand, some studies have shown little or no association between sunlight exposure and the risk of AMD (22–24).

White individuals: It is postulated that increased levels of melanin could increase the free radical scavenging potential of the retinal pigment epithelium (RPE) and Bruch's membrane (BrM), thereby protecting against the risk of advanced AMD (25–28).

Female sex: Female gender might be a risk factor in individuals older than 75 years (29), with double the risk of developing wet AMD in comparison with age-matched men. However, nonstatistically significant differences have been demonstrated (30).

Cholesterol levels, obesity, hypertension, cardiovascular disease, and increased dietary fat: These factors seem to be related to the risk of developing AMD, but different studies do not agree (31–37).

Genetics: Several studies show a genetic factor in the pathogenesis of the disease (38–41). The gene for apolipoprotein E (APOE) is the first identified susceptibility gene for AMD and has been also associated with other diseases of aging including Alzheimer's disease. APOE epsilon 2 allele is associated with a 50% increased risk of AMD (42); however, APOE epsilon 4 allele is associated with 57% reduction in risk of wet AMD (43). Several loci have been also associated with AMD, including two major loci in the complement factor H (CFH) gene on 1q32 and the ARMS2/HTRA1 locus on the 10q26 gene cluster (44,45).

In short, genes influence many biologic pathways, but genetic susceptibility can be modified by environmental factors. Together, they are greatly predictive of onset and progression of disease (46,47).

PATHOPHYSIOLOGY AND PATHOLOGY

The pathology of AMD is characterized by degenerative changes affecting outer retina (photoreceptors), RPE, BrM, and choriocapillaris. These structures, collectively called Ruysch's complex (4,48), provide an optimal environment for retinal function—high-resolution and color vision (cones), and peripheral vision and vision at dusk (rods).

AMD can be classified according to its onset, distinguishing early and late AMD. Early pathologic changes in AMD involve basal deposits (laminar and linear) (49) in BrM, which cannot be distinguished by clinical evaluation. Late-stage AMD shows loss of RPE, decreased choriocapillaris density, and decreased lumen diameter of the choriocapillaris. There is no neovascularization in atrophic or dry AMD. In wet AMD, neovascularization, exudative change, and disciform scar formation are observed (50).

THE RETINAL PIGMENT EPITHELIUM

The RPE is a central element in the pathogenesis of AMD. It is a postmitotic, cuboidal monolayer of pigmented cells, which improves visual resolution and neutralizes photo-oxidative stress. The RPE has a very high metabolic rate and is rich in mitochondria. It is located between the neural retina and choroid. Because of its neuroectodermal origin, the RPE is considered part of the retina. The inner boundary (apical membrane) interdigitates with the outer segments of photoreceptors. The outer boundary (basolateral

membrane) faces BrM forming the outer blood–retinal barrier (BRB). Functions of the RPE include regeneration of bleached visual pigments; formation and maintenance of two extracellular matrixes, the interphotoreceptor matrix and BrM; transport of nutrients, ions, and water between photoreceptors and the choriocapillaris; and phagocytosis of membranous discs of the outer segments of photoreceptors (51). Another pivotal function of the RPE is light absorption and protection against photo-oxidation. The RPE is also involved in the immune privilege of the eye through the secretion of immunosuppressant factors (52).

TRANSPORT

Transport through the RPE is bidirectional. From the subretinal space to choroid, the RPE transports electrolytes and water. From the blood to the photoreceptors, the RPE transports glucose and other nutrients.

Transport from blood to the photoreceptors encompasses glucose and other vital nutrients. The RPE absorbs glucose, retinol, ascorbic acid, and fatty acids in the blood and delivers them to the photoreceptor. For the transport of glucose, the RPE has high amounts of glucose transporter (GLUT) in both their apical and basolateral membranes. Another notable function of the RPE is transport of retinyl to ensure its supply to the retinal photoreceptors. In this process, many complex intermediate steps take place. A critical step involves an RPE enzyme that isomerizes all-trans-retinyl esters into 11-cis-retinal, which is essential for rod and cone function (33,53).

The delivery of the fatty acids such as docosahexaenoic acid and eicosapentaenoic acid to the photoreceptor is another important RPE function (54). These omega-3 fatty acids cannot be synthesized by the nervous tissue but are an essential component of the membranes of neurons and photoreceptors. They are synthesized in the liver from the precursor, linolenic acid, and are carried in the blood by plasma lipoproteins (33). In addition, docosahexaenoic acid is the precursor of the D1 neuroprotectin that protects RPE from oxidative stress (25,55). The main sources of omega-3 fatty acid are fish products. The Blue Mountain Eye Study and some case–control studies have found evidence of reduced risk of advanced AMD and in those who eat fish regularly (34,56,57).

Transport from photoreceptors to blood is important for ions and water. The RPE transports ions and water from the subretinal space (apical side) into the blood of the choroid (basolateral side). This process requires energy, and the Na (+)/K (+)-ATPase, on the apical membrane of the RPE, provides the energy (58). Tight junctions between RPE cells result in a barrier between the subretinal space and the choriocapillaris. Notably, paracellular resistance of this barrier is 10 times the transcellular resistance. For this reason, water cannot pass through the paracellular RPE pathway and passes mainly through the transcellular pathway via aquaporin-1 (59,60).

LIGHT ABSORPTION AND PROTECTION AGAINST OXIDATIVE STRESS

The retina is the only neural tissue in the body that is exposed to direct sunlight, which favors the oxidation of lipids and is toxic for the photoreceptors. Retina consumes proportionally more oxygen than other tissues, generating free radicals that are toxic to the cells of the retina. The RPE is essential to countering oxidative stress in the retina. The RPE cells contain pigments, such as melanin and lipofuscin, which absorb and filter the light. The RPE also produces antioxidant molecules including lutein, zeaxanthin, or ascorbate as well as enzymes, such as superoxide dismutase and catalase, that reduce reactive species (61).

PHAGOCYTOSIS

The RPE is a phagocytic system that is essential for the renewal of photoreceptors. Each photoreceptor has an inner and outer segment, the outer segment of each cone has a membrane folded 700 times, and the outer segment of every rod has about 1,000 discs (62).

The photoreceptors are often exposed to constant high light levels, which leads to accumulation of oxidized proteins and lipids. The concentration of photo-oxidized substances increases within the photoreceptors daily. The transduction of the light depends on the photoreceptor by appropriate functioning and structure of the proteins, retinyl, and cell membranes. Therefore, to maintain the excitability of the photoreceptor outer segments, they are undergoing constant renewal, reconstructed from its base. The tips of the outer segments of the photoreceptors, containing the highest concentration of free radicals, proteins, and photo-oxidized lipids, detach from the photoreceptors. Outer segments maintain a constant length through the coordinated release of its extremities and the formation of new discs. The discs detach from the outer segments and are phagocytosed by the RPE (63), which digest and deliver the essential molecules, such as docosahexaenoic acid and retinyl, back to the photoreceptors to rebuild their light-sensitive outer segments (32,64). Sometimes the content of the phagolysosomes are incompletely degraded, forming the residual bodies that are the substrates for lipofuscin formation. The residual bodies in the RPE accumulate with age, beginning as early as 16 months (65,66). The limited autophagocytic capacity of the RPE eventually results in an accumulation of metabolic waste in RPE cells throughout life. Dry AMD often begins in the parafoveal ring, where lipofuscin concentration is highest. However, lipofuscin disappears with cell death and a reduction in autofluorescent lipofuscin is a sign of progression toward late AMD.

SECRETION

RPE cells produce and secrete growth factors as well as essential factors for maintaining structural integrity of the retina and choroid. These molecules favor the photoreceptors' survival and ensure a structural integrity for optimal circulation and nutrient supply. RPE secretes pigment epithelium–derived factor (PEDF), vascular endothelial growth factor (VEGF), fibroblast growth factors (FGF-1, FGF-2, and FGF-5), transforming growth factor–β, insulin-like growth factor I, neuronal growth factor (NGF), growth factor derived from the brain, neurotrophin-3, ciliary neurotrophic factor, several interleukins, chemokines, tumor necrosis factor–α, colony-stimulating factors, and various types of metalloprotease tissue inhibitors (67,68).

The most important factors with regard to the pathophysiology of AMD are PEDF and VEGF. PEDF is a neuroprotection and antiangiogenic factor. PEDF inhibits endothelial cell proliferation and stabilizes choriocapillaris endothelium. It is important in embryonic eye development. Mice lacking PEDF develop more aggressive retinal vascularization in ischemia (69). VEGF is secreted in low concentrations during physiologic conditions, thereby preventing endothelial cell apoptosis. In addition, VEGF regulates vascular permeability, thus stabilizing endothelium fenestrations (70).

IMMUNE PRIVILEGE

The eye is an immune-privileged site, and the RPE cells have an important role in the maintenance of this immune privilege (71,72). In 1993, Liversidge et al. indicated how RPE cells could inhibit lymphocyte proliferation (73). Many pathways have been suggested to explain RPE immunosuppression (74). On the one hand, RPE inhibits T-cell proliferation through secretion of prostaglandins and immunosuppressive cytokines. On the other hand, apoptosis and phagocytosis properties have demonstrated both directly (decreasing T-cell number and clearing apoptotic lymphocytes) and indirectly (down-regulating proinflammatory cytokine secretion, such as IL-1b) (75,76).

Ambati et al. (77) in 2003 postulated in a study of mice that there is an accumulation of complement fragments that might damage RPE and induce VEGF production by RPE cells, resulting in the development of choroidal neovascularization (CNV). This study provides insight into the role of macrophages and complement in the pathophysiology of AMD (78).

BRUCH'S MEMBRANE

BrM is a complex pentalaminar extracellular matrix (ECM), located beneath the RPE, and includes three layers: a central elastic layer sandwiched between two collagenous layers. BrM is lined by the basement membranes of the RPE and the choriocapillaris (basal laminae). Apart from its structural support function, BrM is also highly permeable to fluid and small molecules like oxygen, glucose, and other molecules necessary to maintain retinal health and function (79). Proteoglycans play an important role in BrM (80). Their negative charge impairs the passage of positively charged macromolecules that are essential for maintenance of RPE.

Changes in BrM begin in the third or fourth decade of life (5,81,82). These changes include the accumulation of *membranous debris* on both sides of the elastic lamina, *drusen* between RPE basal lamina and inner collagenous layer of BrM, and *basal laminar deposits* that may occupy the same space as drusen or develop between the RPE cell and its basal lamina (79) and appears as an amorphous material. How drusen develop and why they can vary in location and features are unknown.

Drusen usually contain fragments of RPE cells (9), a core of glycoproteins, an outer dome of crystallins (83,84), chaperone proteins, APOE, vitronectin, and proteins related to inflammation (amyloid P, C5, and C5b–9 complement complex) (85). Drusen are classified as either hard or soft. Hard drusen look like small, yellow nodules and are not associated with AMD (86). Soft drusen appear as large, white or light yellow, dome-shaped elevations that can resemble localized serous RPE detachments.

BrM doubles in thickness and declines in elasticity between the ages of 10 and 90 years. It contains no lipids during the first 30 years of life, but lipid concentrations rise in later years (4). In addition to the structural alterations that take place in BrM during aging, its fluid permeability becomes substantially reduced. BrM acts as a scaffold for the choriocapillaris and RPE cells, regulating their survival. When this function is diminished, anoikis occurs. Anoikis is an apoptosis phenomenon resulting from incorrect cell adhesion, and this process takes place in photoreceptors, RPE cells, and possibly endothelial cells (4) of the choriocapillaris. The development of either excessive material in BrM or erosion of BrM has important consequences. It may lead to choroidal endothelial cell loss, instigate chronic local inflammation, and produce ischemic stress on the oxygen hungry photoreceptor cells.

CHORIOCAPILLARIS

Choriocapillaris is a plexus of capillaries with fenestrations on the side facing BrM and is part of the innermost layer in the choroid. The capillary network is designed in a lobular pattern for rapid blood flow to supply the high metabolic demand of the photoreceptors and RPE (82). In aging eyes, the lumina of the choriocapillaris and the choroidal thickness are reduced by half. The resulting hypoxia stabilizes hypoxia-inducible factor 1α, which activates genes encoding proteins such as erythropoietin that protect the photoreceptors (87). Hypoxia also increases the secretion of growth factors such as VEGF A within Ruysch's complex on the basal side of the RPE cells, causing development of choroidal neovascular membranes (4,88).

PATHOPHYSIOLOGY OF LATE AMD

Late-stage AMD shows the presence of RPE loss (cell death) or choriocapillaris attenuation without neovascularization in dry or atrophic AMD and exudative changes, neovascularization, or disciform scar in wet or neovascular AMD.

GEOGRAPHIC ATROPHY

Deposits of cellular debris in BrM alter the pathway of nutrient exchange between the RPE and choriocapillaris and lead to the downturn of RPE cells. At the same time, RPE cells overlying drusen are usually inflated and depigmented, and the adjacent photoreceptors are often damaged or dead (8). When the RPE degeneration is more advanced, thick basal laminar deposits take place in the BrM and obstruct nutrient exchange. These deposits may also decrease the adhesion of the RPE to the inner collagenous layer of BrM facilitating serous detachment of the RPE and retina (89,90).

Throughout their history, drusen reflect the state of the adjacent RPE cells. The greater the number of drusen and the larger they are, the greater the probability that the RPE cells will be damaged (8). Soft drusen easily became confluent and can reach a size that produces serous detachments of the RPE (91). Drusen sometimes disappear. Macrophages, pericytes, and choriocapillaris contribute to the removal, leading to their replacement by fibrous tissue.

By this time, RPE deterioration is critically advanced, and some cells may proliferate into small clumps, detach from BrM, and migrate into the retina. The final consequence of this process is geographic atrophy. Depigmentation exists in atrophic areas; however, at the edge of the lesions, pigmentation develops due to proliferation, hypertrophy, or phagocytosis of liberated melanin and lipofuscin (8,92). During the process of geographic atrophy, neural retina and damaged RPE cells disappear and the surviving rods and cones become shorter.

DISCIFORM SCAR

The main site of disturbance in neovascular AMD is BrM. However, the changes in BrM that predispose to neovascularization are unclear. With aging and as a consequence of membrane calcification, small fractures or gaps develop in BrM. Abnormal secretion from the deteriorating RPE cells might serve as attractant for endothelial cells, phagocytic cells, and lymphocytes, resulting in neovascularization.

Lipofuscin accumulation, RPE membrane thickening, and intracellular residual body increase help stimulate new vessel formation. Therefore, new vessels occur as a consequence of an imbalance in the stimulating and inhibiting influences of growth factors, and any disruption in the diffusion through BrM to choroid could alter this balance. Once established, the new vessels have tendency to leak and bleed. When this occurs, the fluid extends laterally beneath the RPE in the same plane where basal laminar deposit and soften drusen are located.

There are three types of pigment epithelial detachment (PED) associated with AMD: drusenoid, serous, and fibrovascular. Drusenoid PED is a confluence of several soft drusen. Fibrovascular PED is a form of occult CNV. Serous PED is not exactly a breakdown in the outer BRB, it seems to develop from a dysfunction in the complex RPE cells–BrM. Fluid moves from the retina into the BrM as a result of active movement of ions by the RPE cells. If BrM became hydrophobic, resistance to water flow could cause fluid to collect between RPE and BrM (74). Serous exudates and blood may enter the retinal space. The retinal detachment may extend beyond the zone of RPE detachment and result in a rapid destruction of the RPE and photoreceptors over an area much larger than the region of vascular invasion, so the loss of vision is more severe in neovascular AMD than it is in geographic atrophy. Hemorrhage under the RPE or retina stimulates proliferation of fibrous tissue that produces a disciform scar, increasing the size of the area of blindness.

CONCLUSION

The main features of the AMD are the formation of drusen; thickening and other signs of damage of BrM; depigmentation and RPE hyperplasia; and accumulation of basal laminar deposits beneath the RPE. However, these are not unique or pathognomonic of this disease as we often observe them in most eyes of elderly individuals (93–96). In summary, the main signs of AMD increase with age, but only in some persons, they progress to the stage of cell death and functional loss. According to this point of view, AMD is an advanced stage of a process that occurs in all eyes. It is part of a common and continuing process in which the transition between age and disease is marked by loss of vision (9).

In 1972, Hogan (97) described the role RPE plays in the macula and postulated the existence of a gradual decrease in the activity of RPE, which resulted in accumulation of metabolic waste in BrM and loss of permeability. Zarbin (10) summarized five key concepts:

1. AMD includes disorders of aging and pathologic events.
2. Oxidative stress plays an important role in the damage of the RPE and BrM.
3. The RPE damage results in chronic inflammation of BrM and the choroid.

4. Choriocapillaris and RPE injury lead to the formation of an abnormal ECM that produces an alteration in the diffusion of nutrients between the retina and the RPE, which in turn causes more damage.
5. RPE and choriocapillaris atrophy occurs as well as CNV growth.

It is hoped that in the future, better understanding of the pathophysiology and histopathology will lead to new treatments engaging different phases of the disease. Hopefully, vision loss can be delayed and/or even avoided in AMD.

REFERENCES

1. Congdon N, O'Colmain B, Klaver CC, et al. Causes and prevalence of visual impairment among adults in the United States. Arch Ophthalmol. 2004;122:477–485.
2. Age-related Eye Disease Study Research Group. Potential public health impact of age-related disease study results. Arch Ophthalmol. 2003;121:1621–1624.
3. Sharks SH. Ageing and degeneration in the macular region: a clinic-pathological study. Brit J Ophthalmol. 1976;60:324–341.
4. de Jong PT. Mechanisms of disease. N Engl J Med. 2006;355:1474–1485.
5. Hogan MJ, Alvarado J. Studies on the human macula. IV. Aging changes in Bruch's membrane. Arch Ophthalmol. 1967;77:410–420.
6. Peto R, Doll R. There is no such thing as aging. BMJ. 1997;315:1030–1032.
7. Powell DE. There is no such thing as ageing: ageing has been defined as to grow or make old. BMJ. 1998;316:1531.
8. Young RW. Pathophysiology of age-related macular degeneration. Surv Ophthalmol. 1987;31(5):291–306.
9. Zarbin MA. Current concept in the pathogenesis of age-related macular degeneration. Arch Ophthalmol. 2004;122:598–614.
10. Handa JT. New molecular histopathologic insights into the pathogenesis of age-related macular degeneration. Int Ophthalmol Clin. 2007;47(1):15–50.
11. Bird AC, Bressler NM, Bressler SB, et al. The International ARM Epidemiological Study Group. An international classification and grading system for age-related maculopathy and age related macular degeneration. Surv Ophthalmol. 1995;39:367–374.
12. Mitchell P, Smith W, Attebo K, et al. Prevalence of age-related maculopathy in Australia. Ophthalmology. 1995;102:1450–1460.
13. Klein R, Klein BE, Linton KL. Prevalence of age-related maculopathy. Ophthalmology. 1992;99:933–943.
14. Cruickshanks KJ, Hammar RF, Klein R, et al. The prevalence of age-related maculopathy by geographic region and ethnicity. Arch Ophthalmol. 1997;115:242–250.
15. Friedman DS, Katz J, Bressler NM, et al. Racial differences in the prevalence of age-related macular degeneration: the Baltimore eye survey. Ophthalmology. 1999;106:1049–1055.
16. Bressler NM, Bressler SB, West SK, et al. The grading and prevalence of macular degeneration in Chesapeake bay waterman. Arch Ophthalmol. 1989;107:847–852.
17. Van Newkirk MR, Nanjan MB, Wanh JJ, et al. The prevalence of age-related maculopathy: the visual impairment project. Ophthalmology. 2000;107:1593–1600.
18. Delcourt C, Diaz JL, Ponton-Sanchez A, et al. Smoking and age-related macular degeneration. Arch Ophthalmol. 1998;116:1031–1035.
19. Khan JC, Thurlby DA, Shahid H, et al. Smoking and age-related macular degeneration: the number of pack years of cigarette smoking is a major determinant of risk for both geographic atrophy and choroidal neovascularization. Br J Ophthalmol. 2006;90:75–80.
20. Delcourt C, Carriere I, Ponton-Sanchez A, et al. Light exposure and the risk of age-related macular degeneration: the POLA Study. Arch Ophthalmol. 2001;119:1463–1468.
21. Klein R, Klein BE, Jensen SC, et al. Sunlight and the 5-year incidence of early age-related maculopathy: the Beaver Dam Eye Study. Arch Ophthalmol. 2001;119:246–250.

22. The Age-Related Eye Disease Study Research Group. Risk factors associated with age-related macular degeneration: a case control study in the age-related eye disease study. Ophthalmology. 2000;107:2224–2232.

23. The Eye Disease Case-control Study Group. Risk factors for neovascular age-related macular degeneration. Arch Ophthalmol. 1992;110:1701–1708.

24. Klein R. Epidemiology. In: Berger JW, Fine SL, Maguire MG, eds. Age-related macular degeneration. St. Louis, MO: Mosby; 1999:31–55.

25. Coleman HR, Chan CH, Ferris III FL, et al. Age-related macular degeneration. Lancet. 2008;372:1835–1845.

26. Mukesh BN, Dimitrov PN, Leikin S, et al. Five year incidence of age-related maculopathy: visual impairment project. Ophthalmology. 2004;111:1176–1182.

27. Klein R, Klein BE, Jenson SC, et al. Age-related maculopathy in a multiracial United States population: the National Health and Nutrition Examination Survey III. Ophthalmology. 1999;106:1056–1065.

28. Schachat AP, Hyman L, Leske MC, et al. Features of age-related macular degeneration in a black population. Arch Ophthalmol. 1995;113:728–735.

29. Smith W, Assink J, Klein R, et al. Risk factors for age-related macular degeneration: pooled findings from three continents. Ophthalmology. 2001;108:697–704.

30. Mitchell P, Wang JJ, Foran S, et al. Five-year incidence of age-related maculopathy lesions: the Blue Mountain Eye Study. Ophthalmology. 2002;109:1092–1097.

31. Mares-Perlman JA, Brady WE, et al. Dietary fat and age-related maculopathy. Arch Ophthalmol. 1995;113:743–748.

32. Cho E, Hung S, Willet C, et al. Prospective study of dietary fat and the risk of age-related macular degeneration. Am J Clin Nutr. 2001;73:209–218.

33. Heuberger RA, Mares-Pearlman JA, Klein R, et al. Relationship of dietary fat to age-related maculopathy in the Third National Health and Nutrition Examination Survey. Arch Ophthalmol. 2001;119:1833–1838.

34. Seddon JM, Rosner B, Sperduto RD, et al. Dietary fat and risk for advanced age-related macular degeneration. Arch Ophthalmol. 2001;119:1191–1199.

35. Klein R, Klein BE, Tomany SC, et al. The association of cardiovascular disease with the long-term incidence of age-related maculopathy. Ophthalmology. 2003;110:1273–1280.

36. Fraser-Bell S, Wu J, Klein R, et al. Cardiovascular risk factors and age-related macular degeneration: the Los Angeles Latino Eye Study. Am J Ophthalmol. 2008;145:308–316.

37. Hogg RE, Woodside JV, Gilchrist SE, et al. Cardiovascular disease and hypertension are strong risk factors for choroidal neovascularization. Ophthalmology. 2008;115:1046–1052.

38. Traboulsi Ei. The challenges and surprises of studying the genetics of age-related macular degeneration. Am J Ophthalmol. 2005;139:908–911.

39. Piguet B, Wells JA, Palmvang IB, et al. Age-related Bruch's membrane change: a clinical study of the relative role of heredity and environment. Br J Ophthalmol. 1993;77:400–403.

40. Hamdi HK, Kenney C. Age-related macular degeneration: a new viewpoint, Front Biosci. 2003;8:305–314.

41. Zareparsi S, Reddick AC, Branham KE, et al. Association of apolipoprotein E alleles with susceptibility to age-related macular degeneration in a large cohort from a single center. Invest Ophthalmol Vis Sci. 2004;45:1306–1310.

42. Klaver CC, Kliffen M, Van Duijn CM, et al. Genetic association of apolipoprotein E with age-related macular degeneration. Am J Hum Genet. 1998;63:200–206.

43. Souied EH, Benlian P, Amouyel P, et al. The epsilon 4 allele of the apolipoprotein E gene as a potential protective factor of exudative age-related macular degeneration. Am J Ophthalmol. 1998;125:353–359.

44. Allikmets R. Simple and complex ABCR: genetic predisposition to retinal disease. Am J Hum Genet. 2000;67:793–799.

45. Weeks De, Conley YP, Tsai HJ, et al. Age-related maculopathy: a genome-wide scan with continued evidence of susceptibility loci within the 1q31, 10q26 and 17q25 regions. Am J Hum Genet. 2004;75(2):174–189.

46. Lim LS, Mitchell P, Seddon JM, et al. Age-related macular degeneration. Lancet. 2012;379:1728–1738.

47. Seddon JM, Reynolds R, Yu Y, et al. Risk models for progression to advanced age-related macular degeneration using demographic, environmental, genetic, and ocular factors. Ophthalmology. 2011;118:2203–2211.

48. Ruysch F. Asser primus: thesaurus anatomicus secundus. Amsterdam, The Netherlands: J.Waesbergios; 1722:3–14.

49. Green WR. Histopathology of age-related macular degeneration. Mol Vis. 1999;5:27.

50. Green WR, Enger C. Age-related macular degeneration histopathologic studies. The 1992 Lorenz E Zimmerman Lecture. Ophthalmology. 1993;100:1519–1535.

51. Thebault S. El epitelio pigmentario retiniano como componente de la barrera hematoretiniana: implicación en la retinopatía diabética. Revista Digital Universitaria [en línea]. 1 de marzo de. 2011;12(3). [Consultada: 2 de marzo de 2011]. Disponible en Internet: http://www.revista.unam.mx/vol.12/num3/art31/index.html. ISSN: 1607–6079.

52. Strauss O. The retinal pigment epithelium in visual function. Physiol Rev. 2005;85(3):845–881.

53. Redmon TM, Poliakov E, Yu S, et al. Mutation of key residues of RPE65 abolishes its enzymatic role as isomerohydrolase in the visual cycle. Proc Natl Acad Sci U S A. 2005;102:13658–13663.

54. Bazan NG, Gordon WC, Rodriguez de Turco EB. Docosahexaenoic acid uptake and metabolism in photoreceptors: retinal conservation by an efficient retinal pigment epithelial cell-mediated recycling process. Adv Exp Med Biol. 1992;318:295–306.

55. Bazan NG. Neurotrophins induce neuroprotective signaling in the retinal pigment epithelial cell by activating the synthesis of the anti-inflammatory and anti-apoptotic neuroprotectin D1. Adv Exp Med Biol. 2008;613:39–44.

56. SanGiovanni JP, Chew EY, Clemons TE, et al. The relationship of dietary lipid intake and age-related macular degeneration in a case–control study. Arch Ophthalmol. 2007;125:671–679.

57. Chua B, Flood V, Rochtchina E, et al. Dietary fatty acids and the 5-year incidence of age-related maculopathy. Arch Ophthalmol. 2006;124:981–986.

58. Marmorstein AD. The polarity of the retinal pigment epithelium. Traffic. 2001;2(12):867–872.

59. Erickson KK, Sundstrom JM, Antonetti DA. Vascular permeability in ocular disease and the role of tight junctions. Angiogenesis. 2007;10(2):103–117.

60. Verkman AS, Ruiz-Ederra J, Levin MH. Functions of aquaporins in the eye. Prog Retin Eye Res. 2008;27(4):420–433.

61. Girotti AW, Kriska T. Role of lipid hydroperoxides in photo-oxidative stress signaling. Antioxid Redox Signal. 2004;6(2):301–310.

62. Young RW. Shedding of discs from rod outer segments in the rhesus monkey. J Ultrastruct Res. 1971;34:190–203.

63. Young RW, Bok D. Participation of the retinal pigment epithelium in the rod outer segment renewal process. J Cell Biol. 1969;42:392–403.

64. Liu BF, et al. Low phagocytic activity of resident peritoneal macrophages in diabetic mice: relevance to the formation of advanced glycation end products. Diabetes. 1999;48(10):2074–2082.

65. Streeten BW. The sudanophilic granules of the human retinal pigment epithelium. Arch Ophthalmol. 1961;66:391–398.

66. Wing GL, Blanchard GC, Weiter JJ. The topography and age relationship of lipofuscin concentration in the retinal pigment epithelium. Invest Ophthalmol Vis Sci. 1978;17:601–607.

67. Witmer AN, et al. Vascular endothelial growth factors and angiogenesis in eye disease. Prog Retin Eye Res. 2003;22(1):1–29.

68. Stemfeld MD, et al. Cultured human retinal pigment epithelial cells express basic fibroblast growth factor and its receptor. Curr Eye Res. 1989;8(10):1029–1037.

69. Huang Q, et al. PEDF-deficient mice exhibit and enhanced rate of retinal vascular expansion and are more sensitive to hyperoxia-mediated vessel obliteration. Exp Eye Res. 2008;87(3):226–241.

70. Lu M, et al. Advanced glycation end products increase retinal vascular endothelial growth factor expression. J Clin Invest. 1998;101(6):1219–1224.

71. Streilein JW. Peripheral tolerance induction: lessons from immune privileges sites and tissues. Transplant Proc. 1996;28:2066–2070.

72. Wenkel H, Sreilein JW. Analysis of immune deviation elicited by antigens injected into the subretinal space. Invest Ophthalmol Vis Sci. 1998;39:1823–1834.

73. Liversidge J, McKay D, Mullen G, et al. Retinal pigment epithelial cells modulate lymphocyte function at the blood-retina barrier by autocrine PGE2 and membrane-bound mechanisms. Cell Immunol. 1993;149:315–330.

74. Carnota P, Bueno R, Rodriguez-Fontal M, et al. Pathophysiology of the blood-retinal barrier. In: Quiroz-Mercado H, ed. Macular surgery. 2nd ed. Philadelphia, PA: Lippincott Williams & Wilkins; 2011:17–28.

75. Willermain F, Caspers-Velu L, Nowak B, et al. Retinal pigment epithelial cell phagocytosis of T lymphocytes: possible implication in the immune privilege of the eye. Br J Ophthalmol. 2002;86:1417–1421.

76. Jorgensen A, Wiencke A, la Cour M, et al. Human retinal pigment epithelial cell-induced apoptosis in activated T cells. Invest Ophthalmol Vis Sci. 1998;39:1590–1599.

77. Ambati J, et al. An animal model of age related macular degeneration in senescence Ccl-2 or Ccr-2 deficient mice. Nat Med. 2003;9:1390–1397.

78. Tezel TH, Bora NS, Kaplan HJ. Pathogenesis of age-related macular degeneration. Trends Mol Med. 2004;10(9):417–420.

79. Mullins RF, Sohn EH. Bruch's membrane: the critical boundary in macular degeneration. In: Dr. Gui-Shuang Ying, ed. Degeneration, age related macular degeneration—the recent advances in basic research and clinical care. InTech; 2012. http://www.intechopen.com/books/age-related-macular-degeneration-the-recent-advances-in-basic-researchand-clinical-care/bruch-s-membrane-the-critical-boundary-in-amd. ISBN: 978-953-307-864-9.

80. Kliffen M, de Long PT, Luider TM. Protein analysis of human macula in relation to age-related maculopathy. Lab Invest. 1995;73:262–272.

81. Sarks SH. New vessels formation beneath the retinal pigment epithelium in senile eyes. Br J Ophthalmol. 1973;57:951–965.

82. Handa JT. Pathophysiology of the retinal pigmented epithelium and Choroid. In: Quiroz-Mercado H, ed. Macular surgery. 2nd Ed. Philadelphia, PA: Lippincott Williams & Wilkins; 2011:10–16.

83. Crabb JW, Miyagi M, Gu X, et al. Drusen proteome analysis: an approach to the etiology of age-related macular degeneration. Proc Natl Acad Sci U S A. 2002;99:14682–14687.

84. Hageman GS, Luther PJ, Victor Chong NH, et al. An integrated hypothesis that considers drusen as biomarkers of immunomediated processes at the RPE-Bruch's membrane interface in aging and age-related macular degeneration. Prog Retin Eye Res. 2001;20:705–732.

85. Umeda S, Suzuki MT, Okamoto H, et al. Molecular composition of drusen and possible involvement of anti-retinalautoimmunity in two different forms of macular degeneration in cynomolgus monkey (Macaca fascicularis). FASEB J. 2005;19:2088.

86. Geen WR, Enger C. Age-related macular degeneration histopathologic studies. The 1992 Lorenz E. Zimmerman lecture. Ophthalmology. 1993;100:1519–1535.

87. Grimm C, Wenzel A, Groszer M, et al. HIF-1-induced erythropoietin in the hypoxic retina protects against light induced retinal degeneration. Nat Med. 2002;8:718–724.

88. Dámore PA. Mechanisms of retinal and choroidal neovascularization. Invest Ophthalmol Vis Sci. 1994;35:3974–3979.

89. Braunstein RA, Gass JDM. Serous detachments of the retinal pigment epithelium in patients with senile macular disease. Am J Ophthalmol. 1979;88:652–660.

90. Gass JDM: Pathogenesis of disciform detachment of the neuroepithelium. III. Senile disciform macular degeneration. Am J Ophthalmol. 1967;63:617–644.

91. Green WR, Mc Donnell PJ, Yeo JH. Pathologic features of senile macular degeneration. Ophthalmology. 1985;92:615–627.

92. Burns RP, Feeney-Burns L. Clinico-morphologic correlations of drusen of Bruch´s membrane. Trans Am Ophthalmol Soc. 1980;78:206-223.

93. Feeney-Burns L, Eldred GE. Age-related changes in the ultrastructure of Bruch´s membrane. Am J Ophthalmol. 1985;100:686–697.

94. Green WR. Clinicopathologic studies of senile macular degeneration. In: Nicholson DH, ed. Ocular pathology update. Chicago, IL: Year Book Medical Publishers; 1982:115–144.

95. Hoshino M, Mizuno K, Ichikawa H. Aging alterations of retina and choroid of Japanese: light microscopic study of macular region of 176 eyes. Jpn J Ophthalmol. 1984;28:89–102.

96. Ring HG, Fugino T. Observation on the anatomy and pathology of the choroidal vasculature. Arch Ophthalmol. 1967;78:431–444.

97. Hogan MJ. Role of the retinal pigment epithelium in macular disease. Trans Am Acad Ophthalmol Otolaryngol. 1972;76(1):64–80.

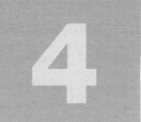

ETIOLOGY OF LATE AGE-RELATED MACULAR DISEASE

MAXIMILIANO OLIVERA

INTRODUCTION

Age-related macular disease (AMD) is a chronic, progressive disease of the retina, specifically the macula. AMD is an important cause of vision loss in the United States and all over the world. AMD, in all of its forms, has an overall prevalence of 6.5%, but some demographics, such as non-Hispanic White people, have a higher incidence (7.3%). Non-Hispanic Black people have a lower incidence rate (2.4%). The incidence of AMD increases with age. The incidence in individuals over 60 years old is 13.4% compared to an incidence in the 40- to 59-year-old group of 2.8% (1).

Like many other chronic diseases, it is important to understand its complex pathophysiology in order to develop screening and treatment strategies. Although we do not have a complete understanding of the complex pathophysiology of AMD, several studies over the last 20 years have identified many environmental and genetic risk factors. Identification of risk factors allows for the development of screening strategies in order to make a diagnosis as early as possible, improving the chances of a better visual outcome. For example, the understanding of pathophysiologic mechanisms involved in the development and progression of neovascular AMD, such as the role of the vascular endothelial growth factor (VEGF), permitted the design and development of anti-VEGF therapy for AMD. This has resulted in a radical change in the expectations for patients and physicians (2).

CLINICAL CLASSIFICATION OF AMD

AMD is not only about changes in the eye fundus examination. To diagnose AMD and determine what kind of AMD the patient has, it is important to consider the patient's symptoms.

In addition, it is important to understand that the aging eye is associated with certain changes (3). Most of these changes are almost clinically undetectable, and patients have no visual symptoms at all. These changes include the following:

- A decrease in density and distribution of photoreceptors
- Loss of melanin granules, lipofuscin accumulation, and residual body accumulation in the retinal pigment epithelium (RPE)
- Accumulation of basal lamellar deposits, formed by a lipid-rich granular material and collagen fibers, between the lamina basalis (plasma membrane) of the RPE cells and inner face of the basal membrane of RPE
- Changes in choriocapillaris

The characteristic physical sign of AMD is the presence of drusen. Drusen are small, rounded, yellowish lesions located beneath the RPE, inner to the Bruch's membrane. Drusen are classified by size: *small* (diameter less than 64 µm), *intermediate* (diameter between 64 and 124 µm), and *big* (diameter 125 µm or above). They may also be classified by the discreteness of their boundaries: *hard* (well defined), *soft* (not well defined), and *confluent* (contiguous limits between drusen).

In addition to drusen, other physical signs such as RPE hyper- and hypopigmentation, RPE atrophy, RPE detachments, choroidal neovascular membranes (CNVM), and hemorrhages give us information about the clinical status of the patient with AMD. Clinically, it is useful to classify AMD into early/late or dry/wet.

Early AMD

Early AMD is usually asymptomatic and clinically presents with drusen and RPE changes consisting of focal hyper- or hypopigmentation.

Late AMD

The main characteristic of late AMD is severe loss of vision.

The late stages of AMD have two different forms (dry and wet), although both forms may occur simultaneously in the same eye. Over time, dry AMD may develop to wet AMD.

Dry AMD

Patients with dry AMD have poor visual acuity, hyperpigmented RPE spots (usually juxtafoveal), and an area with visible choroidal vessels. Choroidal vessels are visible because the RPE cells over them have become atrophic. As these areas become confluent, they take on an appearance referred to as geographic atrophy. No neovascularization is present.

Wet AMD

Wet AMD is characterized by the presence of CNVM. Patients with wet AMD may experience a sudden onset of decreased visual acuity, metamorphopsia, and paracentral scotoma. Clinical findings include subretinal fluid, subretinal or sub-RPE hemorrhages, subretinal or intraretinal lipids, pigmentary subretinal ring, RPE irregularities and detachment, gray-white subretinal lesions, and cystoid macular edema (3).

▌EPIDEMIOLOGY

Incidence of AMD

According to the 2005–2008 NHANES (National Health and Nutrition Examination Survey) (1), the most AMD-compatible lesions were found in persons aged 60 or older in all the three ethnic groups studied (non-Hispanic Black, non-Hispanic White, and Mexican American). The incidence of early AMD is similar for non-Hispanic White persons aged 40 to 59 years (3%) and Mexican American persons aged 40 to 59 years (2.7%). The incidence of early AMD is lowest in non-Hispanic Black persons. Late AMD was more prevalent in non-Hispanic White persons.

The estimated total prevalence of any AMD in the US population aged 40 or older was 6.5%. Of a total of 7.2 million persons having any kind of AMD, 0.89 million (95% CI, 552,000–1.2 million) were estimated to have late AMD (see Ref. (1) for more details).

Risk Factors for AMD

The most important risk factor for AMD is age, but over the years, many factors, including genetic, demographic, behavioral, dietary, and other factors, have been studied as risk or protective factors for AMD. The AREDS (Age-Related Eye Disease Study) was a clinical trial sponsored by the National Eye Institute, one of the National Institutes of Health in the United States. The trial was designed to investigate the natural history and risk factors for AMD and cataracts and to evaluate the effect of high doses of antioxidants and zinc on the progression in patients with AMD. This study describes the demographic, behavioral, medical, and nonretinal factors associated with progression to neovascular AMD and central geographic atrophy (CGA).

Of all the studied factors, only a few were statistically associated with AMD. Subjects with advanced AMD, relative to the early AMD group, tend to be older, have fewer years of formal education, smoke more, have higher body mass index (BMI), have higher blood pressure, be myopic, have a history of angina, be more likely to have a lens opacity, and be less likely with hormone replacement therapy. Neovascular AMD was associated with white race and smoking more than 10 pack-years. CGA was associated with fewer years of formal education, being obese (higher BMI), smoking more than 10 pack-years, and not using antiacids (4).

There were also some other weak associations, such as diabetes, use of nonsteroidal anti-inflammatory agents, and hormone replacement therapy, that were reported in other studies (5–14) but not fully demonstrated on AREDS. Of note, hormone replacement therapy was reported to be a protective factor in some patients with specific polymorphisms in ARMS2 (HtrA serine peptidase 1) (15).

In contrast to risk factors for progression to neovascular AMD and CGA, black race (16,17); increased intake of docosahexaenoic acid (18), monounsaturated fatty acids (19), fish (20–22), and dark green leafy vegetables (23); and higher levels of serum carotenoids (24) were associated with a lower risk of progression.

▌GENETICS OF AMD

Patients with a positive familiar history of AMD have a higher risk of development of this disease (8,25,26). Late AMD is a polygenic disease. No single-gene defect accounts for disease. There are variations and defects in

Table 4.1	GENETIC LOCI ASSOCIATED TO AMD
ABCA4	ATP-binding cassette transporter; chr 1
APOE	Apolipoprotein E; chr 19
ARMS2/HTRA1	HtrA serine peptidase 1; chr 10
CF1	Complement factor 1; chr 4
C2	Complement component 2; chr 6
C3	Complement component 3; chr 19
CETP	Choleterylester transfer protein; chr 16
CFB	Complement factor B; chr 6
CFH	Complement factor H; chr 1
COL8A1	Collagen type 8 alpha 1 subunit; chr 3
FRK/COL10A1	Fyn-related kinase/alpha chain of type X collagen; chr 6
LIPC	Hepatic lipase; chr 15
TIMP3	Tissue inhibitor of metalloproteinase 3; chr 22
TLR3	Toll-like receptor 3; chr 4
TNFRSF10A	Tumor necrosis factor receptor superfamily 10a; chr 8
VEGF-A	Vascular endothelial growth factor A; chr 6

Adapted from Lim LS, Mitchell P, Seddon JM, et al. Age-related macular degeneration. Lancet. 2012;379:1728–1738.

genes functionally related to complement and immune processes, high-density lipoprotein (HDL) cholesterol, and mechanisms involving collagen formation, extracellular matrix production, and angiogenesis considered to be associated with the onset, progression, and bilateral involvement of early, intermediate, and advanced states of AMD (see Table 4.1 and Refs. (27–34) for more details) (35). Several pharmacogenetic studies found that variants in some genes are related to different treatment outcomes (Table 4.2) (36).

Genetic variations in genes encoding the complement proteins and regulators have been identified as protective or risk factors for AMD. Many of them are single nucleotide polymorphisms (SNPs), causing a change of a single amino acid in the polypeptide chain that could affect the binding affinity of the complement protein to its substrates. This suggests that certain individuals with some of these variations may be genetically predisposed to AMD. Variations of the complement system likely interact with environmental risk factors to determine overall risk.

Complement Factor H

Complement factor H (CFH), an important regulator of the alternative pathway, was the first complement protein to be implicated in the pathogenesis of AMD. Physiologically, CFH binds C3b and accelerates the decay of the alternative C3 convertase (C3bBb) and acts as cofactor for the inactivation of C3b by complement factor I (CFI) (37). CFH is produced locally in the eye by the RPE cells (38) and accumulates in the drusen, sub-RPE space, RPE, interphotoreceptor matrix, and choroid (38,39). Environmental factors vary CFH production by the RPE cells. In vitro studies show an increase in RPE CFH production by interferon gamma (40) and reduction in conditions of oxidative stress (38).

The CFH gene is located at chromosome position 1q23. Mutations of this gene manifest as dominant mendelian disorders (41). In 2005, three groups simultaneously (27,42,43) reported a nonsynonymous SNP in the CFH gene (rs1061170), resulting in a substitution of tyrosine by histidine at position 402 of the polypeptide (Y402H), which was important in the development of AMD. This change alters the ligand binding site of CRP (C-reactive protein), heparin, M protein, and glycosaminoglycans, probably leading to a reduced binding to cell surfaces and therefore impaired regulation of the alternative C3 convertase (44). A meta-analysis (45) suggested that this variant (Y402H) is a contributing factor in over half of all cases of AMD. Other SNPs throughout the CFH gene, including the SNP 162 V (38), resulting in substitution of isoleucine with valine residue within the C3b binding site, have been associated with AMD (32,38,41,46–50) and AMD progression (51–55).

Variations in VEGF Gene

Some authors (56–58) proposed that the SNP A/A in the allele rs3024997 and G/G re2010963 in the VEGF gene are associated with a better response to antiangiogenic (bevacizumab) therapy with regard to visual acuity outcomes. In a more recent study (59), using a multivariate data analysis and a higher number of patients, this SNP was not found to be associated with a different response to antiangiogenic therapy.

WHAT HAPPENS IN THE EYE WITH AMD?

In order to understand AMD, it is important to understand the physiologic aging of the eye. The age-related changes in the retina that predispose a person to AMD occur in the outer retina: the photoreceptors (PRs), the RPE, the Bruch's membrane, and the choriocapillaris. Most of these changes are not clinically detectable until a late stage, when they start to affect the visual function of the patients.

The Photoreceptors

PR cells translate light into electric activity that can be understood by the brain and central nervous system.

Table 4.2	PHARMACOGENETICS AND AMD		
Intervention	**Gene/locus**	**Variants**	**Results**
Photodynamic therapy	CFH	Rs1061170 (Y402H)	Controversial: Outcome for CC genotype lagged CT and TT; outcome for TT was poor; no genotype association
	LOC387715	Rs10490924 (A69S)	No significant genotype association
	VEGF	Rs2808635, Rs2146323	Anatomic outcome was strongly associated with SNPs.
	CRP	Rs2808635, Rs876538	Positive response was significantly associated with both variants.
	HTRA1	Rs11200638	No significant association
	FV	G1691A	Better outcome associated in patients carrying both genetic variants
	FII	G20210A	
	MTHFR	C677T	Better outcome associated with variants
	FXIIIA	G185T	Better outcome associated with variants
Intravitreal bevacizumab	CFH	Rs1061170 (Y402H)	CC genotype responded significantly better than TC and TT. CC genotype more likely to require reinjection
	LOC387715	Rs10490924 (A69S)	No significant association
Antioxidants and zinc	CFH	Rs1061170 (Y402H)	TT genotype responds better than CC.
	LOC387715	Rs10490924 (A69S)	No significant association

Adapted from Chen Y, Bedell M, Zhang K. Age-related macular degeneration: genetic and environmental factors of disease. Mol Interv. 2010;10(5):271–281.

Anatomically, PR cells have four different regions: the outer segment (OS), the inner segment, the cell body, and the synaptic terminal. The OS of the PR is composed of membranous disks, which have a high concentration of visual pigment. Rhodopsin, the visual pigment of rods, is a G protein–coupled receptor that when stimulated by a photon of light undergoes a conformational change initiating a series of biochemical steps leading to the onset of the electric activity (3). Numerous studies of the human and animal retina show that excessive light exposure leads to photochemical injury causing damage to the outer segment of the PR. Excessive light exposure is considered to be an environmental factor associated with AMD (60), but the magnitude of this risk is hard to evaluate and is controversial. Even under normal light conditions, the PR incurs significant oxidative stress, due to the great energy requirement for visual phototransduction (61). This stimulation increases the oxygen-reactive species, damaging DNA and other macromolecular complexes important for the PR survival (62,63). For a long-term survival of the PR cells, it is important to have a healthy RPE participating in the visual cycle, renewing the PR OSs and producing the interphotoreceptor cell matrix (3).

The Retinal Pigment Epithelium

The RPE is a postmitotic, cuboidal monolayer of cells located between the neural retina and the Bruch's membrane. Physiologically, it has a very high metabolic rate and performs several important functions for the retina. Of all the functions of the RPE, the most important for understanding AMD (64) are the following:

- Regeneration of bleached visual pigments (opsins)
- Formation and maintenance of the interphotoreceptor matrix and Bruch's membrane
- Transport of fluids and ions between PRs and choriocapillaris
- Phagocytosis

The reconstitution of the visual pigment rhodopsin occurs mainly in the RPE cells, through many intermediate steps. This mechanism has a key role for normal function of both cones and rods, transforming the all-trans-retinyl esters into 11-cis-retinal (65). As a phagocytic system, the RPE is essential for the renewal of PRs (66). Each PR has hundreds of disks in its outer segment. These disks are formed by plasma membrane, containing transmembrane protein rhodopsin, which is positioned in combination with four phospholipids and docosahexanoic acid. The OS disks of the PR cells are engulfed by the RPE. In the RPE, the disks fuse with lysosomes, forming phagolysosomes, where the contents are degraded. In young, healthy individuals, most of the disks are fully degraded, and lipofuscin accumulation is minimal, but over time, the self-limited phagocytic and degradative capacity of the RPE cells becomes more and more overloaded. This incompletely degraded membrane material accumulates in the form of lipofuscin in secondary lysosomes or residual bodies (67).

Lipofuscin is a yellow-brown, autofluorescent molecule that accumulates in all postmitotic cells, particularly the RPE (68–71). The presence of lipofuscin may act as a cellular aging indicator, and its quantity in tissues may be estimated by amounts of autofluorescence present. The autofluorescence from the eye fundus, mostly derived from lipofuscin, can be clinically and noninvasively quantified, allowing for an estimate of the aging degenerative process of the eye and a diagnostic and follow-up method for patients with AMD (72). Some factors increase (vitamin E deficiency) while others decrease (oxygen-free conditions and vitamin A deficiency) lipofuscin pigment formation.

The retinoid A2E is the major fluorophore of lipofuscin (73). Once it is synthesized, it cannot be eliminated by the RPE. Precursors of A2E, all-trans-retinal and ethanolamine, are formed within the PRs (74), but the fully synthesized A2E molecule arises from the phagolysosomal compartment of the RPE cells. When it reaches a critical concentration, the metabolism of phagocytized OS lipids by the RPE is impaired. Phagocytized and oxidized OS membranes are extruded by the RPE into the Bruch's membrane, contributing to drusen formation and membrane thickening.

A2E is toxic for the RPE. It inhibits the proton pump of lysosomes (75), causing leakage of the contents of the lysosomes into the cytoplasm of RPE cells. It inhibits phagolysosomal degradation of PR phospholipids (76) and can also damage the DNA of RPE cells. A2E also accumulates in the mitochondrial membranes, decreasing mitochondrial activity and enabling the translocation of cytochrome C and AIF (apoptosis-inducing factor) to the cytosol and nucleus, respectively. Functionally, the release of cytochrome C from the inner mitochondrial membrane generates oxidative stress and decreased electron flow, leading to impaired ATP synthesis. Both mechanisms are highly relevant for apoptosis by causing leakiness of the inner mitochondrial membrane and release of the propapoptotic proteins, activating the caspase cascade. AIF is a pro-apoptotic protein, which is strictly located in the mitochondria. Its translocation to the nucleus induces apoptosis, functionally independent from caspases (77). A2E also inhibits the normal activity of the enzyme RPE65 isomerohydrolase, a key enzyme of the visual cycle, which is responsible for the isomerization of all-trans-retinyl ester to 11-cis-retinol, the precursor of 11-cis-retinal (78). This inhibition could cause a disruption of 11-cis-retinal supply to the retina and result in PR dysfunction. A2E is known to perturb the cholesterol metabolism in the RPE cells, causing cholesterol accumulation within the late endosome/lysosome, inhibiting acid lipase and resulting in a feed-forward cycle of cholesterol accumulation in the RPE. This interferes with rhodopsin activation and PR membrane remodeling (79). A2E is also thought to be photosensitizing due to its broad light spectrum–absorbing capacities, particularly in the visible ranges, and thus generating reactive species of oxygen (80,81).

The Bruch's Membrane

The Bruch's membrane lies beneath the RPE and has three layers: two collagenous layers on the top and bottom and a central elastic layer (82). Proteoglycans are an important constituent of the Bruch's membrane (83). Their negative charges hinder the passage of the positively charged macromolecules necessary for RPE maintenance. Changes in the Bruch's membrane begin prior to the development of clinically significant AMD. As soon as the third decade of life, basal lamellar deposits and membranous debris, precursors of AMD, begin to appear (84,85).

Hard drusen appear between the basement membrane of the RPE and the inner collagenous layer of the Bruch's membrane in the third decade of life (86). It is not well understood how drusen develop. Drusen have a complex structure. They have a core of glycoproteins and an outer dome containing crystallins, chaperones, apolipoprotein E, vitronectin, inflammation-related proteins (as amyloid P, C5, C5b-9 complement complex), and fragments of RPE cells (87–91). Basal laminar deposits (BLD) contain granular electron-dense material, coated membrane bodies, and wide- or long-spaced fibrous collagen (92–96).

Vesicles and membranous debris, referred to as basal linear deposits, accumulate beneath the RPE basement membrane and correlate histopathologically to soft drusen (93,97).

Features of the normal aging of the Bruch's membrane include increased lipid concentration (99–104), calcification (98), and decreased concentration of metalloproteinases. The most common lipid in the aged Bruch's membrane deposits is the phospholipids, derived from local cells rather than blood (101). There is an age-related decrease in adhesion molecules, laminin and fibronectin, that is inversely correlated with the lipid content of the Bruch's membrane (100). In contrast, another study concluded that the main lipid component of these deposits was esterified cholesterol, similar to depositions in other membranes throughout the body that occur with age, suggesting a blood origin of these rather than cellular (105).

These changes contribute to the thickening of the Bruch's membrane, interfering in normal function of this membrane by decreasing the hydraulic conductivity. Thus, fluids pumped out by the RPE cells, toward the choroid, encounter the resistance provided by the thickened membrane, leading to the formation of serous RPE detachments. Such morphologic changes lead to alterations in cellular adhesion, which could cause the triggering of an apoptosis (106,107).

Choriocapillaris

The choriocapillaris is the vascular layer of the eye. Between the retina and the sclera, it is formed by an extensive fenestrated vascular network derived from the perforating ciliary arteries, branches of the ophthalmic artery. Its main role is to provide oxygen and macromolecules to the outer retina. Over the years, the choriocapillaris becomes less fenestrated and the lumina are reduced, causing less delivery of oxygen and macromolecules to the retina (98,108,109). This change results in hypoxia and activation in the transcription of genes such as erythropoietin (for PR protection) (110) and vascular endothelial growth factor A (VEGF-A) (111,112), causing the development of CNVM.

Choroidal Neovascular Membranes

CNVMs are fibrovascular complexes that arise from the choroid, penetrating the Bruch's membrane and proliferating in the sub-RPE and subretinal space. This complex is formed by two major components: neovascular sprouts and fibroblasts. Proliferation of this fibrovascular complex leads to disturbances in the normal architecture of the choriocapillaris, Bruch's membrane, RPE, photoreceptors, and retina.

Since the Macular Photocoagulation Study in the 1970s, CNVM was classified based on its localization relative to the fovea (extrafoveal, juxtafoveal, and parafoveal) and the pattern of dye leakage on fluorescein angiography (FA) (classic and occult). Advances in diagnostic techniques for CNVM, particularly indocyanine green angiography (ICGA) and optical coherence tomography (OCT), allowed determination of the retinal layer in which CNVMs are located.

A new classification for CNVM based on FA, OCT, and ICGA patterns includes type 1 (CNVM beneath RPE), type 2 (subretinal CNV), and type 3 (retinal angiomatous proliferation) (113).

UNDERSTANDING HOW ALL THESE CHANGES LEAD TO AMD

The aging process of the eye affects the PRs, the RPE, the Bruch's membrane, and the choriocapillaris. In these tissues, accumulation of substances, functional changes, and apoptosis may occur, and important pathophysiologic mechanisms are activated by these changes.

Angiogenesis

Angiogenesis, leading to the formation of CNVM, is one of the most important pathophysiologic features of late AMD. In angiogenesis, blood vessels grow in adult tissue from sprouts on preexisting vessels. This process involves several steps: cell migration, proliferation, and survival; vascular maturation; wall remodeling; and degradation of the extracellular matrix (114–116). Angiogenesis has a complex molecular regulation, representing a balance between the angiogenic and the antiangiogenic factors, affected by different pathologic states such as hypoxia, ischemia, or inflammation (2).

VEGF-A, Hypoxia, Inflammation, and Oxidative Stress

VEGF-A is a remarkable angiogenic factor. This homodimeric glycoprotein with a molecular weight of 45 kDa (117) has four major isoforms, distinguished by their molecular weight, acidity, and whether they are bounded to heparin.

VEGF-A is synthesized by RPE cells constitutively and is elevated in early forms of AMD and hypoxia. VEGF-A is highly selective for endothelial cells. It has diffusion characteristics that allow it to reach its target. It has several regulation mechanisms and affects the angiogenesis mechanism in different stages, including endothelial cell proliferation, survival, and migration, and also promotes the vascular hyperpermeability (118). VEGF receptors, VEGFR-1 (Flt-1), VEGFR-2 (Flk-1/KDR), and VEGFR-3 (Flt-4), are expressed predominantly in endothelial cells and to a lesser extent on monocytes and macrophages (119). Normal human choriocapillaris expresses all VEGF receptors in the choriocapillaris endothelium next to the RPE layer, suggesting a paracrine relation between RPE cells and the choriocapillaris (120). VEGF has also been shown to have survival function in the retina (121) and has a role in the maintenance of the adult choriocapillaris via stimulating the formation of fenestrations (122).

Hypoxia

The role of hypoxia on the pathogenesis of AMD is controversial. While some studies (123) showed that patients with AMD have decreased blood flow in the choriocapillaris, others (124) could not confirm a decrease in blood flow but found a decrease in pulse amplitude. It also has been theorized that the previously described age-related changes in the Bruch's membrane may limit the diffusion of oxygen and create an ischemic environment. Physiologically, pO_2 decreases linearly with distance from the choriocapillaris to the inner segment of the PRs. Under normal conditions, little of the O_2 in the choriocapillaris blood is extracted. Some studies have shown that as perfusion decreases, the oxygen extraction from the choriocapillaris increases (125), showing that there is significant reserve. This suggests that hypoxia is not the most important factor in causing an imbalance between angiogenic and antiangiogenic factors.

Inflammation

Studies of excised choroidal membranes and the growth patterns of CNVM suggest more is involved than just ischemia in driving neovascularization. Histologic studies of the

CNVM show vascular endothelium as well as a variety of inflammatory cells, such as lymphocytes, macrophages, and foreign body giant cells (126,127), similar to granulation tissue on a wound-repair response (128). Activated macrophages secrete proteolytic enzymes, collagenase, and elastase, which can erode an attenuated Bruch's membrane and thereby assist the migration of choroidal capillaries (129,130). Also, inflammatory cells produce cytokines such as interleukin-1, which induce VEGF, as shown in cultured choroidal fibroblasts (131). In one study (132), the amount of VEGF was found to be proportional to the number of macrophages in the specimen, suggesting that inflammation is important for the regulation of angiogenesis. Therefore, upregulation of VEGF may be the link between inflammation and promotion of new blood vessels in an eye with AMD.

Before the formation of the CNVM, there are signs of inflammation in an eye with AMD. Drusen deposits between the Bruch's membrane and RPE may contain bioactive fragments of complements (C3a and C5a) (133). These substances induce VEGF expression and have significant chemotactic activity that further invites inflammatory cells to the macular region (134). Another key actor of the complement system in AMD is the CFH. CFH binds and inactivates C3b deposited on intact host cells, allowing destruction of foreign or damaged cells (135). This is achieved through an important locus, domain 7 on the molecule (136–139). Domain 7 binds to heparin or sialic acid on host cells. Therefore, it is possible that alterations in domain 7 or the heparin/or sialic acid binding region of factor H could lead to or augment the destruction of normal or injured ocular cells as well as other foreign cells in an appropriate environment (44).

Extracellular drusen also contain advanced glycation end products (AGE), high levels of oxidized low-density lipoproteins (ox-LDL), and oxysterols (87,140,141). The receptor for AGE (RAGE), normally not markedly expressed in the retina, although highly accumulated in RPE cells, PRs, and choriocapillaris in advanced AMD (142,143), activates the nuclear factor kappa B (NFκB), master regulator of both innate and adaptive immunity. NFκB is a central regulator of IL-6, a cytokine that has been shown to be an important regulator of choroidal neovascularization (144–146), and VEGF. Damaged RPE and oxidized proteins and lipids in the Bruch's membrane have been postulated to activate and recruit dendritic cells from the choroid, enhancing the immune response in this area (88,147).

In a laser model of CNV, CD18 and ICAM-1 are expressed during development of CNV. Targeted disruption of either of these inhibits the development of CNVM. Animals models of CNV have been developed that mimic many aspects of CNVM in AMD. Mice expressing monocyte chemoattractant protein-1 (MCP-1) or its cognate, CC chemokine receptor-2, developed drusen, lipofuscin accumulation, geographic atrophy, and CNV (148). Depletion of the monocyte cell lines inhibits experimental CNV (149–151).

With time, the neovascularization appears to "burn out," leaving a cicatricial mass almost completely devoid of vessels. If ischemia is the only cause of neovascularization, one would expect these vessels to regress, which would increase the amount of ischemia present.

The Complement System

The complement system plays a fundamental role in host defense against pathogens, elimination of immune complexes and apoptotic cells, and adaptive immune responses. It consists of over 40 proteins and regulators found in the systemic circulation and some tissues. Three different activation pathways exist, each one with different triggers: the classical pathway (triggered by an antibody–antigen complex), the alternative pathway (triggered by binding to a host cell pathogen surface), and the lectin pathway (triggered by polysaccharides on microbial surfaces). These three pathways converge on the terminal complement complex (TCC), a multiprotein complex, formed from the binding of C5b to the plasma complement proteins C6, C7, C8, and C9 (152).

Components of the classic, alternative complement pathways and TCC have been found to be present in drusen (153), especially in older eyes with AMD.

Alterations of the complement system or its regulators can lead to damage of the tissues and is known to be implicated in a wide spectrum of diseases. Several studies suggest that complement plays a key role in the development of AMD (154).

Other Growth Factors Involved in Angiogenesis

Several other growth factors are involved in the regulation of angiogenesis in the eye. These mechanisms help us to understand why conventional therapies do not succeed in some cases and spur the development of new therapeutic strategies.

■ *Pigment epithelium–derived factor* (PEDF), produced by the RPE, is a neurotrophic PR growth factor and generally is thought to inhibit angiogenesis. It is the main anti-angiogenic cytokine in the eye. Under hypoxic conditions and wet AMD, secretion of PEDF is decreased, thereby allowing the endothelial mitogenic activity of VEGF to go unchecked (154–156). Some paradoxical effects have been identified (155,157).

■ *Platelet-derived growth factor* (PDGF) is involved in the development and differentiation of vessel walls. It is required to recruit pericytes and to promote maturation of the microvasculature. It is a potent chemoattractant, dedifferentiator, and mitogen for both fibroblasts and RPE cells (158–160). The potential therapeutic effect of anti-PDGF therapy still needs to be studied (161).

■ *Basic fibroblast growth factor* (bFGF) is a potent angiogenic molecule in vivo and is produced by a variety of cell types including vascular endothelial cells of the choriocapillaris, fibroblasts, astrocytes, and RPE cells (162,163). bFGF induces the secretion of VEGF and HGF by Müller glial cells and stimulates cell proliferation (163–165). One study comparing the antiangiogenic effect of bevacizumab (anti-VEGF) alone and combined with anti-bFGF antibodies observed that targeting bFGF in addition to VEGF could show synergistic effects in CNV treatment (166).

- *Angiopoietin-2*, detected in CNVM lesions (167), is upregulated by hypoxia and VEGF. It may facilitate hypoxia and VEGF-induced neovascularization by destabilizing existing vasculature (168,169).
- *Metalloproteinases* are enzymes that remodel the extracellular matrix in neovascular processes. They can be found in AMD CNVM lesions, and they are upregulated by the VEGF (170,171).

Oxidative Stress

Oxidative stress refers to a progressive cellular damage caused by reactive oxygen species (ROS) contributing to protein misfolding and evoking functional abnormalities during RPE cellular senescence (172). Light can induce the formation of reactive species, which in turn can lead to the formation of dysfunctional or toxic molecules of lipids and proteins or damage the DNA. Oxidized molecules are formed in the PR OSs as a normal part of daily life. Over the years, the amount of these molecules increases because the mechanisms needed to clear the reactive species out of the cells become insufficient (173). Oxidative stress also interferes with the capacity of the heat shock proteins and the ubiquitin–proteasome way to repair or degrade damaged proteins (174–176).

Aging primarily influences the oxidative balance between oxidizing factors and antioxidants. Other factors, such as cigarette smoking and alcohol consumption, aggravate oxidative imbalance and DNA damage (177). Antioxidant genes (178) and variants of the CFH gene influence the role of oxidative stress in AMD (179).

A wide variety of oxidative lesions to DNA have been described, including single- and double-stranded DNA breaks and the development of cross-linked lesions (180,181). The cell responds to genomic damage through repair processes employing a large number of proteins. The cell may turn off growth and replication until the repair process is complete (182). Responding to the Samurai law of biology (better dead than wrong), those cells unable to repair their DNA damage undergo apoptosis.

To help protect against inappropriate oxidation, there are basically three levels of protection: molecular, cellular, and tissue. On the molecular level, the cell has antioxidant vitamins and enzymes. These include vitamins C and E, superoxide dismutase, catalase, glutathione transferase (183), glutathione reductase, and glutathione peroxidase. The antioxidants may limit inappropriate oxidation in the first place or may terminate propagation reactions. On a cellular level, two main responses may occur. The cell may try to adapt to the oxidative stress by increased activation of transcription factors and proteins (184) that helps control gene expression of antioxidant enzymes. The cell could also start the apoptosis mechanism. Tissue mechanisms for responding or protecting against oxidative stress include complex intercellular signaling pathways as discussed below.

Scavenger receptors (185,186), in particular CD36, are present on the RPE cell and participate in phagocytosis of spent OSs. It is possible that ordinary everyday exposure of CD36 receptor to oxidized lipids in the PR OS helps maintain the constitutive secretion of VEGF by RPE cells. Excessive secretion of VEGF by RPE cells is supposed to be one factor responsible for the initiation of CNV. This raises the possibility that excessive exposure to oxidative damage may lead the RPE cells to secrete excessive VEGF. Armstrong et al. (187) have shown that injection of lipid peroxide derivate into the vitreous cavity caused retinal neovascularization that persisted for 4 weeks. After the injection, there was a cascade of cytokines secreted, including VEGF. The Bruch's membrane has an exponential increase in lipids with age. The lipids preferentially accumulate in the same region where the neovascularization grows. The Bruch's membrane has no known intrinsic mechanism to protect against oxidative damage to lipids, which accumulate over time. This mechanism could be important in the formation of CNVM in AMD.

Lipid peroxides not only accumulate in the Bruch's membranes but also accumulate in atherosclerotic plaques. In atherosclerotic vessels, the body mounts an aggressive cell-mediated mechanism to contain the oxidized material (188,189), principally using vascular endothelial cells and macrophages also stimulating the production of VEGF by these cells. The body has a number of defined strategies and methods for dealing with degenerating cells and tissue. Many of the same strategies and methods that are used in atherosclerosis of vessel walls are also used in the eye. Injection of these lipids has led to ocular neovascularization in the rabbit (190–192).

As discussed, the accumulation of oxidative damage may be a cause of neovascularization, but the same oxidative damage may also induce a senescent aging phenotype (193), with possible apoptosis. Oxidative damage can lead to an increased accumulation of lipofuscin within RPE cells, a finding linked to the development of geographic atrophy.

CONCLUSION

In this chapter, we discussed the etiology of age-related macular disease. Epidemiologic and genetic factors, clinical classification, anatomical changes, and how these changes affected the development and evolution of the AMD were discussed. While a complete understanding of AMD and its pathophysiology is still lacking, new evidence and understanding are rapidly accumulating. There is not a single gene defect or a single molecular disturbance that causes AMD.

It is a complex, multifactorial disease that may require a variety of treatment strategies to preserve vision for our patients.

REFERENCES

1. Klein R, Chou CF, Klein B, et al. Prevalence of age-related macular degeneration in the US Population. Arch Ophthalmol. 2011;129(1):75–80.

2. Bressler SB. Introduction: understanding the role of angiogenesis and antiangiogenic agents in age-related macular degeneration. Ophthalmology. 2009;116:S1–S7.

3. American Academy of Ophthalmology. Retina and Vitreous. Basic and Clinical Science Course Section 12. 2011–2012.

4. Age-Related Eye Disease Study Research Group. Risk factors for the incidence of advanced age-related macular degeneration in the Age-Related Eye Disease Study (AREDS) AREDS Report No. 19. Ophthalmology. 2005;112(4):533–539.

5. Klein R. Epidemiology. In: Berger JW, Fine SL, Maguire MG, eds. Age-related macular degeneration. St. Louis, MO: Mosby; 1999:31–55.

6. Seddon J. Epidemiology of age-related macular degeneration. In: Schachat AR, ed. Medical retina, vol 2, 3rd Ed. St. Louis, MO: Mosby; 2001:1039–1050.

7. Smith W, Assink J, Klein R, et al. Risk factors for age-related macular degeneration: pooled findings from three continents. Ophthalmology. 2001;108:697–704.

8. Hyman LG, Lilienfeld AM, Ferris FL III, et al. Senile macular degeneration: a case-control study. Am J Epidemiol. 1983;118:213–227.

9. Christen WG, Glynn RJ, Ajani UA, et al. Age-related maculopathy in a randomized trial of low-dose aspirin among US physicians. Arch Ophthalmol. 2001;119:1143–1149.

10. Klein R, Klein BE, Moss SE. Diabetes, hyperglycemia, and age-related maculopathy. The Beaver Dam Eye Study. Ophthalmology. 1992;82:1527–1534.

11. Smith W, Mitchell P, Wang JJ. Gender, oestrogen, hormone replacement and age-related macular degeneration: results from the Blue Mountains Eye Study. Aust N Z J Ophthalmol. 1997;25(Suppl):S13–S15.

12. Smith W, Mitchell P, Leeder SR, et al. Plasma fibrinogen levels, other cardiovascular risk factors, and age-related maculopathy: the Blue Mountains Eye Study. Arch Ophthalmol. 1998;116:583–587.

13. Tomany SC, Wang JJ, van Leeuwen R, et al. Risk factors for incident age-related macular degeneration. Pooled findings from 3 continents. Ophthalmology. 2004;111:1280–1287.

14. Snow KK, Cote J, Yang W, et al. Association between reproductive and hormonal factors and age- related maculopathy in postmenopausal women. Am J Ophthalmol. 2002;134:842–848.

15. Edwards DR, Gallins P, et al. Inverse association of female hormone replacement therapy with age-related macular degeneration and interactions with ARMS2 polymorphisms. Invest Ophthalmol Vis Sci. 2010;51(4):1873–1879.

16. Chumbley LC. Impressions of eye diseases among Rhodesian Blacks in Mashonaland. S Afr Med J 1977;52:316–318.

17. Gregor Z, Joffe L. Senile macular changes in the black African. Br J Ophthalmol. 1978;62:547–550.

18. Cho E, Hung S, Willet WC, et al. Prospective study of dietary fat and the risk of age-related macular degeneration. Am J Clin Nutr. 2001;73:209–218.

19. Parekh N, Voland RP, et al; CAREDS Research Study Group. Association between dietary fat intake and age-related macular degeneration in the Carotenoids in Age-Related Eye Disease Study (CAREDS): an ancillary study of the Women's Health Initiative. Arch Ophthalmol. 2009;127(11):1483–1493.

20. Seddon JM, Rosner B, Sperduto RD, et al. Dietary fat and the risk for advanced age-related macular degeneration. Arch Ophthalmol. 2001;119:1191–1199.

21. Seddon JM, Cote J, Rosner B. Progression of age-related macular degeneration: association with dietary fat, transunsaturated fat, nuts and fish intake. Arch Ophthalmol. 2003;121:1728–1737.

22. Smith W, Mitchell P, Leeder SR. Dietary fat and fish intake and age-related maculopathy. Arch Ophthalmol. 2000;118:401–404.

23. Seddon JM, Ajani UA, Sperduto RD, et al. Dietary carotenoids, vitamins A, C, and E, and advanced age-related macular degeneration. Eye Disease Case Control Study Group. JAMA. 1994;272:1413–1420.

24. Guymer RH, Chong EW. Modifiable risk factors for age-related macular degeneration. Med J Aust. 2006;184(9):455–458.

25. Klaver CC, Wolfs RC, Assink JJ, et al. Genetic risk of age-related maculopathy. Population-based familial aggregation study. Arch Ophthalmol. 1998;116;1646–1651.

26. Smith W, Mitchell P. Family history and age-related maculopathy: the Blue Mountains Eye Study. Aust N Z J Ophthalmol. 1998;26:203–206.

27. Klein RJ, Zeiss C, Chew EY, et al. Complement factor H polymorphism in age-related macular degeneration. Science. 2005;308:385–389.

28. Maller JB, Fagerness JA, Reynolds RC, et al. Variation in complement factor 3 is associated with risk of age-related macular degeneration. Nat Genet. 2007;39:1200–1201.

29. Fagerness JA, Maller JB, Neale BM, et al. Variation near complement factor I is associated with risk of advanced AMD. Eur J Hum Genet. 2009;17:100–104.

30. Reynolds R, Rosner B, Seddon JM. Serum lipid biomarkers and hepatic lipase gene associations with age-related macular degeneration. Ophthalmology. 2010;117:1989–1995.

31. Neale BM, Fagerness J, Reynolds R, et al. Genome-wide association study of advanced age-related macular degeneration identifies a role of the hepatic lipase gene (LIPC). Proc Natl Acad Sci U S A. 2010;107:7395–7400.

32. Chen W, Stambolian D, Edwards AO, et al. Genetic variants near TIMP3 and high-density lipoprotein-associated loci influence susceptibility to age-related macular degeneration. Proc Natl Acad Sci U S A. 2010;107:7401–7406.

33. McKay GJ, Patterson CC, Chakravarthy U, et al. Evidence of association of APOE with age-related macular degeneration—a pooled analysis of 15 studies. Hum Mutat. 2011;32:1407–1416.

34. Yu Y, Bhangale TR, Fagerness J, et al. Common variants near FRK/COL10A1 and VEGFA are associated with advanced age-related macular degeneration. Hum Mol Genet. 2011;20:3699–3709.

35. Lim LS, Mitchell P, Seddon JM, et al. Age-related macular degeneration. Lancet. 2012;379:1728–1738.

36. Chen Y, Bedell M, Zhang K. Age-related macular degeneration: genetic and environmental factors of disease. Mol Interv. 2010;10(5):271–281.

37. Pangburn MK. Host recognition and target differentiation by factor H, a regulator of the alternative pathway of complement. Immunopharmacology. 2000;49:149–157.

38. Hageman GS, Anderson DH, Johnson LV, et al. A common haplotype in the complement regulatory gene factor H (HF1/CFH) predisposes individuals to age-related macular degeneration. Proc Natl Acad Sci U S A. 2005;102:7227–7232.

39. Chen M, Forrester JV, Xu H. Synthesis of complement factor H by retinal pigment epithelial cells is down-regulated by oxidized photoreceptor outer segments. Exp Eye Res. 2007;84:635–645.

40. Kim YH, He S, Kase S, et al. Regulated secretion of complement factor H by RPE and its role in RPE migration. Graefes Arch Clin Exp Ophthalmol. 2009;247:651–659.

41. Klein ML, Schultz DW, Edwards A, et al. Age-related macular degeneration. Clinical features in a large family and linkage to chromosome 1q. Arch Ophthalmol. 1998;116:1082–1088.

42. Edwards AO, Ritter R III, Abel KJ, et al. Complement factor H polymorphism and age-related macular degeneration. Science. 2005;308:421–424.

43. Haines JL, Hauser MA, Schmidt S, et al. Complement factor H variant increases the risk of age-related macular degeneration. Science. 2005;308:419–421.

44. Khandhadia S, Cipriani V, Yates JRW, et al. Age-related macular degeneration and the complement system. Immunobiology. 2012;217:127–146.

45. Thakkinstian A, Han P, McEvoy M, et al. Systematic review and meta-analysis of the association between complement factor H Y402H polymorphisms and age-related macular degeneration. Hum Mol Genet. 2006;15:2784–2790.

46. Li M, Atmaca-Sonmez P, Othman M, et al. CFH haplotypes without the Y402H coding variant show strong association with susceptibility to age-related macular degeneration. Nat Genet. 2006;38:1049–1054.

47. Francis PJ, Schultz DW, Hamon S, et al. Haplotypes in the complement factor H (CFH) gene: associations with drusen and advanced age-related macular degeneration. PLoS One. 2007;2:e1197.

48. Seddon JM, Reynolds R, Maller J, et al. Prediction model for prevalence and incidence of advanced age-related macular degeneration based on genetic, demographic, and environmental variables. Invest Ophthalmol Vis Sci. 2009;50:2044–2053.

49. Gibson J, Cree A, Collins A, et al. Determination of a gene and environment risk model for age-related macular degeneration. Br J Ophthalmol. 2010;94:1382–1387.

50. Kopplin LJ, Igo RP Jr, Wang Y, et al. Genome-wide association identifies SKIV2L and MYRIP as protective factors for age-related macular degeneration. Genes Immun. 2010;11:609–621.

51. Despriet DD, Klaver CC, Witteman JC, et al. Complement factor H polymorphism, complement activators, and risk of age-related macular degeneration. JAMA. 2006;296:301–309.

52. Boekhoorn SS, Vingerling JR, Hofman A, et al. Alcohol consumption and risk of aging macular disorder in a general population: the Rotterdam Study. Arch Ophthalmol. 2008;126:834–839.

53. Schaumberg DA, Christen WG, Kozlowski P, et al. A prospective assessment of the Y402H variant in complement factor H, genetic variants in C-reactive protein, and risk of age-related macular degeneration. Invest Ophthalmol Vis Sci. 2006;47:2336–2340.

54. Seddon JM, Francis PJ, George S, et al. Association of CFH Y402H and LOC387715 A69S with progression of age-related macular degeneration. JAMA. 2007;297:1793–1800.

55. Farwick A, Wellmann J, Stoll M, et al. Susceptibility genes and progression in age-related maculopathy: a study of single eyes. Invest Ophthalmol Vis Sci. 2010;51:731–736.

56. Haines JL, Schnetz-Boutaud N, Schmidt S, et al. Functional candidate genes in age-related macular degeneration: significant association with *VEGF, VLDLR*, and *LRP6*. Invest Ophthalmol Vis Sci. 2006;47:329–335.

57. Churchill AJ, Carter JG, Lovell HC, et al. VEGF polymorphisms are associated with neovascular age-related macular degeneration. Hum Mol Genet. 2006;15:2955–2961.

58. Lin JM, Wan L, Tsai YY, et al. Vascular endothelial growth factor gene polymorphisms in age-related macular degeneration. Am J Ophthalmol. 2008;145:1045–1051.

59. Boltz A, Ruiß M, Jonas JB, et al. Role of vascular endothelial growth factor polymorphisms in the treatment success in patients with wet age-related macular degeneration. Ophthalmology. 2012;119:1615–1620.

60. Taylor HR, West S, Munoz B, et al. The long-term effects of visible light on the eye. Arch Ophthalmol. 1992;110:99–104.

61. Kagan VE, Shvedova AA, Novikov KN, et al. Light-induced free radical oxidation of membrane lipids in photoreceptors of frog retina. Biochim Biophys Acta. 1973;330:76–79.

62. Organisciak DT, Vaughan DK. Retinal light damage: mechanisms and protection. Prog Retin Eye Res. 2010;29:113–134.

63. Rodriguez-Rocha H, Garcia-Garcia A, Panayiotidis MI, et al. DNA damage and autophagy. Mutat Res. 2011;711:158–166.

64. De Jong PTVM. Age-related macular degeneration. N Engl J Med. 2006;355:1474–1485.

65. Redmond TM, Poliakov E, Yu S, et al. Mutation of key residues of RPE65 abolishes its enzymatic role as isomerohydrolase in the visual cycle. Proc Natl Acad Sci U S A. 2005;102:13658–13663.

66. Young RW, Bok D. Participation of the retinal pigmentary epithelium in the rod outer segment renewal process. J Cell Biol. 1969;42:392–403.

67. Eldred GE, Lasky MR. Retinal age pigments generated by self-assembling lysosomotropic detergents. Nature. 1993;25(361):724–726.

68. Wolf G. Lipofuscin, the age pigment. Nutr Rev. 1993;51:205–206.

69. Boulton M, Marshall J. Effects of increasing number of phagocytic inclusions on human retinal pigment epithelial cells in culture: a model for aging. Br J Ophthalmol. 1986;70:808–815.

70. Feeney-Burns L, Berman ER, Rothman H. Lipofuscin of human retinal pigment epithelium. Am J Ophthalmol. 1980;90:783–791.

71. Wing GL, Blanchard GC, Weiter JJ. The topography and age relationship of lipofuscin concentration in the retinal pigment epithelium. Invest Ophthalmol Vis Sci. 1978;17:601–607.

72. Delori FC, Dorey CK, Staurenghi G, et al. In vivo fluorescence of the ocular fundus exhibits retinal pigment epithelium lipofuscin characteristics. Invest Ophthalmol Vis Sci. 1995;36:718–729.

73. Eldred GE. Lipofuscin fluorophore inhibits lysosomal protein degradation and may cause early stages of macular degeneration. Gerontology. 1995;42:(Suppl 2)15–28.

74. Mata NL, Weng J, Travis GH. Biosynthesis of a major lipofuscin fluorophore in mice and humans with ABCR-mediated retinal and macular degeneration. Proc Natl Acad Sci U S A. 2000;97:7154–7159.

75. Bergmann M, Schutt F, Holz FG, et al. Inhibition of the ATP-driven proton pump in RPE lysosomes by the major lipofuscin fluorophore A2-E may contribute to the pathogenesis of age-related macular degeneration. FASEB J. 2004;18:562–564.

76. Finnemann SC, Leung LW, Rodriguez-Boulan E. The lipofuscin component A2E selectively inhibits phagolysosomal degradation of photoreceptor. Proc Natl Acad Sci U S A. 2002;99:6:3842–3847.

77. Suter M, Reme C, Grimm C, et al. Age-related macular degeneration: the lipofuscin component N-retinyl-N-retinylidene ethanolamine detaches proapoptotic proteins from mitochondria and induces apoptosis in mammalian retinal pigment epithelial cells. J Biol Chem. 2000;275:39625–39630.

78. Moiseyev G, Nikolaeva O, Chen Y, et al. Inhibition of the visual cycle by A2E through direct interaction with RPE63 and implications in Stargardt disease. Proc Natl Acad Sci U S A. 2010;107:41:17551–17556.

79. Lakkaraju A, Finnemann S, Rodriguez-Boulan E. The lipofuscin fluorophore A2E perturbs cholesterol metabolism in retinal pigment epithelial cells. Proc Natl Acad Sci U S A. 2007;104:26:11026–11031.

80. Sparrow JR, Zhou J, Cai B. DNA is a target of the photodynamic effects elicited in A2E-laden RPE by blue-light illumination. Invest Ophthalmol Vis Sci. 2003;44:2245–2251.

81. Sparrow JR, Fishkin N, Zhou J, et al. A2E, a byproduct of the visual cycle. Vision Res. 2003;43:2983–2990.

82. Hewitt AT, Nakazawa K, Newsome DA. Analysis of newly synthesized Bruch's membrane proteoglycans. Invest Ophthalmol Vis Sci. 1989;30:478–486

83. Kliffen M, de Jong PT, Luider TM. Protein analysis of human maculae in relation to age-related maculopathy. Lab Invest. 1995;73:267–272.

84. Hogan MJ, Alvarado J. Studies on the human macula. IV. Aging changes in Bruch's membrane. Arch Ophthalmol. 1967;77:410–420.

85. van der Schaft TL, de Bruijn WC, Mooy CM, et al. Is basal laminar deposit unique for age-related macular degeneration? Arch Ophthalmol. 1991;109:420–425.

86. van der Schaft TL, Mooy CM, de Bruijn WC, et al. Histologic features of the early stages of age-related macular degeneration: a statistical analysis. Ophthalmology. 1992;99:278–286.

87. Crabb JW, Miyagi M, Gu X, et al. Drusen proteome analysis: an approach to the etiology of age-related macular degeneration. Proc Natl Acad Sci U S A. 2002;99:14682–14687.

88. Hageman GS, Luthert PJ, Victor Chong NH, et al. An integrated hypothesis that considers drusen as biomarkers of immune-mediated processes at the RPE-Bruch's membrane interface in aging and age-related macular degeneration. Prog Retin Eye Res. 2001;20:705–732.

89. Rudnew A. Ueber die Entstehung, der sogenannten Glaskoerper der Choroides des menschlichen Auges und über das Wesen der hyalinen Degeneration der Gefässe derselben. Arch Pathol Anat Phyiol Klin Med. 1871;53:455–465.

90. Nakata K, Crabb JW, Hollyfield JG. Crystallin distribution in Bruch's membrane-choroid complex from age-related macular degeneration and age-matched donor eyes. Exp Eye Res. 2005;80:821–826.

91. Umeda S, Suzuki MT, Okamoto H, et al. Molecular composition of drusen and possible involvement of anti-retinal autoimmunity in two different forms of macular degeneration in cynomolgus monkey (*Macaca fascicularis*). FASEB J. 2005;19:2088.

92. Green WR, Enger C. Age-related macular degeneration histopathologic studies. The 1992 Lorenz E. Zimmerman Lecture. Ophthalmology. 1993;100:1519–1535.

93. Green WR. Histopathology of the age related macular degeneration. Mol Vis. 1999;3;5–27.

94. Grossniklaus HE, Green WR. Histopathologic and ultrastructural findings of surgically excised choroidal neovascularization. Submacular Surgery Trials Research Group. Arch Ophthalmol. 1998;116:745–749.

95. Ishibashi T, Sorgente N, Patterson R, et al. Aging changes in Bruch's membrane of monkeys: an electron microscopy study. Ophthalmologica. 1986;192:179–190.

96. Van der Schaft TL, Mooy CM, de Brujin WC, et al. Immunohistochemical light and electron microscopy of basal laminar deposit. Graefes Arch Clin Exp Ophthalmol. 1994;232:40–46.

97. Sarks JP, Sarks SH, Killingsworth MC. Evolution of soft drusen in age-related macular degeneration. Eye. 1994;8(Pt 3):269–283.

98. Ramrattan RS, van der Schaft TL, Mooy CM, et al. Morphometric analysis of Bruch's membrane, the choriocapillaris, and the choroid in aging. Invest Ophthalmol Vis Sci. 1994;35:2857–2864.

99. Bird AC, Marshall J. Retinal pigment epithelial detachments in the elderly. Trans Ophthalmol Soc U K. 1986;105:674–682.

100. Pauleikhoff D, Harper CA, Marshall J, et al. Aging changes in Bruch's membrane: a histochemical and morphologic study. Ophthalmology. 1990;97:171–178.

101. Holz FG, Sheraidah G, Pauleikhoff D, et al. Analysis of lipid deposits extracted from human macular and peripheral Bruch's membrane. Arch Ophthalmol. 1994;112:402–406.

102. Marshall J, Hussain AA, Starita C, et al. Aging and Bruch's membrane. In: Marmor MF, Wolfensberger TJ, eds. The retinal pigment epithelium: function and disease. New York: Oxford University Press; 1998:669–692.

103. Lyda W, Eriksen N, Krishna N. Studies of Bruch's membrane: flow and permeability studies in a Bruch's membrane-choroid preparation. Am J Ophthalmol. 1957;44:362–369.

104. Starita C, Hussain AA, Pagliarini S, et al. Hydrodynamics of ageing Bruch's membrane: implications for macular disease. Exp Eye Res. 1996;62:565–572.

105. Curcio CA, Millican CL, Bailey T, et al. Accumulation of cholesterol with age in human Bruch's membrane. Invest Ophthalmol Vis Sci. 2001;42:265–274.

106. Gilmore AP. Anoikis. Cell Death Differ. 2005;12:(Suppl 2):1473–1477.

107. Bertrand K. Survival of exfoliated epithelial cells: a delicate balance between anoikis and apoptosis. J Biomed Biotech. 2011;2011:1–9.

108. Sarks SH. Changes in the region of the choriocapillaris in ageing and degeneration. In: Shimizu K, ed. XXIII Concilium Ophthalmologicum, Kyoto 1978, Acta, vol 1. Amsterdam, The Netherlands: Excerpta Medica; 1979:228–238.

109. Korte GE, Reppucci V, Henkind P. RPE destruction causes choriocapillary atrophy. Invest Ophthalmol Vis Sci. 1984;25:1135–1145.

110. Grimm C, Wenzel A, Groszer M, et al. HIF-1-induced erythropoietin in the hypoxic retina protects against light-induced retinal degeneration. Nat Med. 2002;8:718–724.

111. D'Amore PA. Mechanisms of retinal and choroidal neovascularization. Invest Ophthalmol Vis Sci. 1994;35:3974–3979.

112. Spilsbury K, Garrett KL, Shen WY, et al. Overexpression of vascular endothelial growth factor (VEGF) in the retinal pigment epithelium leads to the development of choroidal neovascularization. Am J Pathol. 2000;157:1413.

113. Feund KB, Zweifel SA, Engelbert M. Do we need a new classification for choroidal neovascularization in age-related macular degeneration?. Retina. 2010;30:9:1333–1349.

114. Ferrara N, Kerbel RS. Angiogenesis as a therapeutic target. Nature. 2005;438:967–974.

115. Pepper MS. Manipulating angiogenesis. From basic science to the bedside. Arterioscler Thromb Vasc Biol. 1997;17:605–619.

116. Bernanke DH, Velkey JM. Development of the coronary blood supply: changing concepts and current ideas. Anat Rec. 2002;269:198–208.

117. Ferrara N, Gerber HP, LeCouter J. The biology of VEGF and its receptors. Nat Med 2003;9:669–676.

118. Wang F, Rendahl KG, Manning WC, et al. AAV-mediated expression of vascular endothelial growth factor induces choroidal neovascularization in rat. Invest Ophthalmol Vis Sci. 2003;44:781–790.

119. Terman BI, Dougher-Vermazen M, Carrion ME, et al. Identification of the KDR tyrosine kinase as a receptor for vascular endothelial cell growth factor. Biochem Biophys Res Commun. 1992;187:1579–1586.

120. Blaauwgeers HGT, Holtkamp GM, Rutten H. et al. Polarized vascular endothelial growth factor secretion by human retinal pigment epithelium and localization of vascular endothelial growth factor receptors on the inner choriocapillaris: evidence for a trophic paracrine relation. Am J Pathol. 1999;155:421–428.

121. Shima DT, Nishijima K, Jo N, et al. VEGF-mediated neuroprotection in ischemic retina. Invest Ophthalmol Vis Sci. 2004;45:3270.

122. Kim I, Ryan A, Rohan R, et al. Constitutive expression of VEGF, VEGFR-1, and VEGFR-2 in normal eyes. Invest Ophthalmol Vis Sci. 1999;40:2115–2121.

123. Grunwald JE, Hariprasad SM, DuPont J, et al. Foveolar choroidal blood flow in age-related macular degeneration. Invest Ophthalmol Vis Sci. 1998;39:385–390.

124. Mori F, Konno S, Hikichi T, et al. Pulsatile ocular blood flow study; decreases in exudative age related macular degeneration. Br J Ophthalmol. 2001;85:531–533.

125. Lisenmeier RA, Braun RD. Oxygen distribution and consumption in the cat retina during normoxia and hypoxemia. J Gen Physiol. 1992;99:177–197.

126. Penfold PI, Killingsworth MC, Sarks SH. Senile macular degeneration: the involvement of immunocompetent cells. Graefes Arch Clin Exp Ophthalmol. 1985;223:69–76.

127. Penfold PI, Killingsworth MC, Sarks SH. Senile macular degeneration. The involvement of giant cells in atrophy of the retinal pigment epithelium. Invest Ophthalmol Vis Sci. 1986;27:364–371.

128. Spraul CW, Lang GE, Grossniklaus HE, et al. Histologic and morphometric analysis of the choroid, Bruch's membrane, and retinal pigment epithelium in postmortem eyes with age-related macular degeneration and histologic examination of surgically excised choroidal neovascular membranes. Surv Ophthalmol. 1999;44(Suppl):S10–S32.

129. Werb Z, Gordon S. Secretion of a specific collagenase by stimulated macrophages. J Exp Med. 1975;142:346–360.

130. Unanue ER, Beller DI, Calderon J, et al. Regulation of immunity and inflammation by mediators from macrophages. Am J Pathol. 1976;85:465–478.

131. Kvanta A, Algvere PV, Berglin L, et al. Subfoveal fibrovascular membranes in age-related macular degeneration express vascular endothelial growth factor. Invest Ophthalmol Vis Sci. 1996;37:1929–1934.

132. Ku HH, Sohal RS. Comparison of mitochondrial pro-oxidant generation and antioxidant defenses between rat and pigeon: possible basis of variation in longevity and metabolic potential. Mech Ageing Dev. 1993;72:67–76.

133. Nozaki M, Raisler BJ, Sakurai E, et al. Drusen complement components C3a and C5a promote choroidal neovascularization. Proc Natl Acad Sci U S A. 2006;103:2328–2333.

134. Kijlstra A, La HE, Hendrikse F. Immunological factors in the pathogenesis and treatment of age-related macular degeneration. Ocul Immunol Inflamm. 2005;13:3–11.

135. Donoso LA, Kim D, Frost A, et al. The role of inflammation in the pathogenesis of age-related macular degeneration. Surv Ophthalmol. 2006;51:137–152.

136. Giannakis E, Male DA, Ormsby RJ, et al. Multiple ligand binding sites on domain seven of human complement factor H. Int Immunopharmacol. 2001;1:433–443.

137. Goldberg AF, Molday RS. Defective subunit assembly underlies a digenic form of retinitis pigmentosa linked to mutations in peripherin/rds and rom-1. Proc Natl Acad Sci U S A. 1996;93:13726–13730.

138. Goodrich DW, Lee WH. The molecular genetics of retinoblastoma. Cancer Surv. 1990;9:529–554.

139. Gordon DL, Kaufman RM, Blackmore TK, et al. Identification of complement regulatory domains in human factor H. J Immunol. 1995;155:348–356.

140. Ishibashi T, Murata T, Hangai M, et al. Advanced glycation end products in age-related macular degeneration. Arch Ophthalmol. 1998;116:1629–1632.

141. Javitt NB, Javitt JC. The retinal oxysterol pathway: a unifying hypothesis for the cause of age-related macular degeneration. Curr Opin Ophthalmol. 2009;20:151–157.

142. Yamada Y, Ishibashi K, Ishibashi K, et al. The expression of advanced glycation end-product receptors in rpe cells associated with basal deposits in human maculas. Exp Eye Res. 2006;82:840–848.

143. Howes KA, Liu Y, Dunaief JL, et al. Receptor for advanced glycation end-products and age-related macular degeneration. Invest Ophthalmol Vis Sci. 2004;45:3713–3720.

144. Izumi-Nagai K, Nagai N, Ozawa Y, et al. Interleukin-6 receptor-mediated activation of signal transducer and activator of transcription-3 (STAT3) promotes choroidal neovascularization. Am J Pathol. 2007;170:2149–2158.

145. Koto T, Nagai N, Mochimaru H, et al. Eicosapentaenoic acid is anti-inflammatory in preventing choroidal neovascularization in mice. Invest Ophthalmol Vis Sci. 2007;48:4328–4334.

146. Paimela T, Ryhanen T, Mannermaa E, et al. The effect of 17b-estradiol on IL-6 secretion and NF-jB DNA-binding activity in human retinal pigment epithelial cells. Immunol Lett. 2007;110:139–144.

147. Johnson LV, Leitner WP, Staples MK, et al. Complement activation and inflammatory processes in drusen formation and age related macular degeneration. Exp Eye Res. 2001;73:887–896.

148. Ambati J, Anand A, Fernandez S, et al. An animal model of age-related macular degeneration in senescent Ccl2- or Ccr2deficient mice. Nat Med. 2003;9:1390–1397.

149. Espinosa-Heidmann DG, Suner IJ, Hernandez EP, et al. Macrophage depletion diminishes lesion size and severity in experimental choroidal neovascularization. Invest Ophthalmol Vis Sci. 2003;44:3586–3592.

150. Sakurai E, Anand A, Ambati BK, et al. Macrophage depletion inhibits experimental choroidal neovascularization. Invest Ophthalmol Vis Sci. 2003;44:3578–3585.

151. Ishida S, Usui T, Yamashiro K, et al. VEGF164-mediated inflammation is required for pathological, but not physiological, ischemia induced retinal neovascularization. J Exp Med. 2003;198:483–489.

152. Comp Zhou W, Marsh JE, Sacks SH. Intrarenal synthesis of complement. 2011. http://www.nature.com/ki/journal/v59/n4/fig tab/4492147f1.html.

153. Mullins RF, Russell SR, Anderson DH, et al. Drusen associated with aging and age-related macular degeneration contain proteins common to extracellular deposits associated with atherosclerosis, elastosis, amyloidosis, and dense deposit disease. FASEB J. 2000;14:835–846.

154. Anderson DH, Mullins RF, Hageman GS, et al. A role for local inflammation in the formation of drusen in the aging eye. Am J Ophthalmol. 2002;134:411–431.

155. Dawson DW, Volpert OV, Gillis P, et al. Pigment epithelium-derived factor: a potent inhibitor of angiogenesis. Science. 1999;285:245–248.

156. Spranger J, Osterhoff M, Reimann M, et al. Loss of the antiangiogenic pigment epithelium-derived factor in patients with angiogenic eye disease. Diabetes. 2001;50:2641–2645.

157. Holekamp NM, Bouck N, Volpert O. Pigment epithelium-derived factor is deficient in the vitreous of patients with choroidal neovascularization due to age-related macular degeneration. Am J Ophthalmol. 2002;134:220–227.

158. Ek ET, Dass CR, Choong PF. Pigment epithelium-derived factor: a multimodal tumor inhibitor. Mol Cancer Ther. 2006;5:1641–1646.

159. Campochiaro PA, Glaser BM. Platelet-derived growth factor is chemotactic for human retinal pigment epithelial cells. Arch Ophthalmol. 1985;103:576–579.

160. Choudary P, Chen W, Hunt R. Production of platelet-derived growth factors by interleukin-1b and transforming growth factor-b stimulate RPE cells and leads to contraction of collagen gels. Invest Ophthalmol Vis Sci. 1997;38:824–833.

161. De Oliveira Dias JR, Buchele Rodrigues E, Maia M, et al. Cytokines in neovascular age-related macular degeneration: fundamentals of targeted combination therapy. Br J Ophthalmol. 2011;95:1631–1637.

162. Martin TA, Mansel R, Jiang WG. Hepatocyte growth factor modulates vascular endothelial-cadherin expression in human endothelial cells. Clin Cancer Res. 2001;7:734–737.

163. Rosenthal R, Malek G, Salomon N, et al. The fibroblast growth factor receptors, FGFR-1 and FGFR-2, mediate two independent signalling pathways in human retinal pigment epithelial cells. Biochem Biophys Res Commun. 2005;337:241–247.

164. García M, Vecino E. Role of Müller glía in neuroprotection and regeneration in the retina. Histol Histopathol. 2003;18:1205–1218.

165. Hollborn M, Jahn K, Limb GA, et al. Characterization of the basic fibroblast growth factor-evoked proliferation of the human Müller cell line, MIO-M1. Graefes Arch Clin Exp Ophthalmol. 2004;242:414–422.

166. Stahl A, Paschek L, Martin G, et al. Combinatory inhibition of VEGF and FGF2 is superior to solitary VEGF inhibition in an in vitro model of RPE-induced angiogenesis. Graefes Arch Clin Exp Ophthalmol. 2009;247:767–773.

167. Hera R, Keramidas M, Peoc'h M, et al. Expression of VEGF and angiopoietins in subfoveal membranes from patients with age-related macular degeneration. Am J Ophthalmol. 2005;139:589–596.

168. Pichiule P, Chavez JC, LaManna JC. Hypoxic regulation of angiopoietin-2 expression in endothelial cells. J Biol Chem. 2004;279:12171–12180.

169. Maisonpierre PC, Suri C, Jones PF, et al. Angiopoietin-2, a natural antagonist for Tie2 that disrupts in vivo angiogenesis. Science. 1997;277:55–60.

170. Hoffmann S, He S, Ehren M, et al. MMP-2 and MMP-9 secretion by RPE is stimulated by angiogenic molecules found in choroidal neovascular membranes. Retina. 2006;26:454–461.

171. Tatar O, Adam A, Shinoda K, et al. Matrix metalloproteinases in human choroidal neovascular membranes excised following verteporfin photodynamic therapy. Br J Ophthalmol. 2007;91:1183–1189.

172. Beatty S, Koh H, Phil M, et al. The role of oxidative stress in the pathogenesis of age-related macular degeneration. Surv Ophthalmol. 2000;45:115–134.

173. Jarrett SG, Boulton ME. Consequences of oxidative stress in age-related macular degeneration. Mol Aspects Med. 2012;33:399–417.

174. Kaarniranta K, Elo M, Sironen R, et al. Hsp70 accumulation in chondrocytic cells exposed to high continuous hydrostatic pressure coincides with mRNA stabilization rather than transcriptional activation. Proc Natl Acad Sci U S A. 1998;95:2319–2324.

175. Kaarniranta K, Salminen A, Eskelinen E, et al. Heat shock proteins as gatekeepers of proteolytic pathways—implications for age-related macular degeneration (AMD). Ageing Res Rev. 2009;8:128–139.

176. Kaarniranta K, Salminen A. Age-related macular degeneration: activation of innate immunity system via pattern recognition receptors. J Mol Med. 2009;87:117–123.

177. Venza I, Visalli M, Oteri R, et al. Combined effects of cigarette smoking and alcohol consumption on antioxidant/oxidant balance in age-related macular degeneration. Aging Clin Exp Res. 2012;24:530–536.

178. Hunter A, Spechler PA, Cwanger A, et al. DNA methylation is associated with altered gene expression in AMD. Invest Ophthalmol Vis Sci. 2012;53:2089–2105.

179. Shaw PX, Zhang L, Zhang M, et al. Complement factor H genotypes impact risk of age-related macular degeneration by interaction with oxidized phospholipids. Proc Natl Acad Sci U S A. 2012;109:13757–13762.

180. Nilsson I, Shibuya M, Wennstrom S. Differential activation of vascular genes by hypoxia in primary endothelial cells. Exp Cell Res. 2004;299:471–485.

181. Hasty P, Campisi J, Hoeijimakers J, et al. Aging and genome maintenance: lessons from the mouse?. Science. 2003;299:1355–1359.

182. Soussi T. The p53 tumor suppressor gene: from molecular biology to clinical investigation. Ann N Y Acad Sci. 2000;910:121–137.

183. Singhal SS, Godley BF, Chandra A, et al. Induction of glutathione S transferase hGST 5.8 is an early response to oxidative stress in RPE cells. Invest Ophthalmol Vis Sci. 1999;40:2652–2659.

184. Sasaki H, Ray PS, Zhu L, et al. Oxidative stress due to hypoxia/reoxygenation induces angiogenic factor VEGF in adult rat myocardium: possible role of NFkappaB. Toxicology. 2000;30(155):27–35.

185. Duncan KG, Bailey KR, Kane JP, et al. Human retinal pigment epithelial cells express scavenger receptors BI and BII. Biochem Biophys Res Commun. 2002;292:1017–1022.

186. Ryeom SW, Sparrow JR, Silverstein RL. CD36 participates in the phagocytosis of rod outer segments by retinal pigment epithelium. J Cell Sci. 1996;109:387–395.

187. Armstrong D, Ueda TO, Ueda TA, et al. Lipid peroxide stimulates retinal neovascularization in rabbit retina through expression of TNFa, VEGF and PDGF. Angiogenesis. 1998;2:174–184.

188. Terpstra V, Bird DA, Steinberg D. Evidence that the lipid moiety of oxidized low density lipoprotein plays a role in its interaction with macrophage receptors. Proc Natl Acad Sci U S A. 1998;17(95):1806–1811.

189. Boullier A, Bird DA, Chang MK, et al. Scavenger receptors, oxidized LDL and atherosclerosis. Ann N Y Acad Sci. 2001;947:214–222.

190. Ueda TO, Ueda TA, Fukuda S, et al. Lipid peroxide undiced TNFa, VEGF and neovascularization in the rabbit cornea, effect of TNF inhibition. Angiogenesis. 1998;2:174–184.

191. Tamai K, Spaide RF, Ellis EA, et al. Lipid hydroperoxide stimulates subretinal choroidal neovascularization in the rabbit. Exp Eye Res. 2002;74:301–308.

192. Honda S, Hjelmeland LM, Handa JT. Senescence associated beta galactosidase activity in human retinal pigment epithelial cells exposed to mild hyperoxia in vitro. Br J Ophthalmol. 2002;86:159–162.

193. Zhang C, Baffi J, Cousins SW, et al. Oxidant induced cell death in retinal pigment epithelium cells mediated through release of apoptosis-inducing factor. J Cell Sci. 2003;116:1915–1923.

5

HISTOPATHOLOGY OF AGE-RELATED MACULAR DEGENERATION

MARIANA INGOLOTTI • ERIC P. JABLON
JOHN BARNWELL KERRISON • HUGO QUIROZ-MERCADO
D. VIRGIL ALFARO III

INTRODUCTION

Age-related macular degeneration (AMD) is the leading cause of central vision loss in the over-65 population in developed countries. It is a bilateral, degenerative, and chronic disease limited to the macula so that the peripheral retinal function is relatively preserved. Progressive histopathologic changes (Fig. 5.1) in the retinal pigment epithelium (RPE), retina photoreceptor cell layer, Bruch's membrane (BM), and choriocapillaris are seen in these patients.

The most common histologic findings in nonneovascular or dry AMD are drusen; a thickened and basophilic BM; and geographic atrophy, hypertrophy, and hyperplasia of the RPE. Choroidal neovascularization (CNV), pigment epithelial detachment (PED), and disciform scar are important features of neovascular or wet AMD. The purpose of this chapter is to give a detailed description of the histopathologic findings encountered in AMD with emphasis on the ultrastructure, composition, and formation of different lesions.

NORMAL AGING OF THE RETINA

In discussing the histopathology of AMD, one must consider normal aging changes in the outer retina, a major risk factor for the development of this disease. The photoreceptor layer, RPE, BM, and choriocapillaris constitute the Ruysch's complex (1). This complex suffers age-associated changes that commence at approximately the age of 20.

Certainly, the RPE shows ultrastructural changes seen in electron microscopy. Its melanin granules migrate to the basal portion of the cell, and the amount of lipofuscin granules increases as a result of the phagocytosis of the rod and cone outer segments. With age, the efficacy of rod and cone outer segment digestion reduces, and they can be extruded into the BM and in the space between the basement membrane of the RPE and its cellular membrane where they accumulate. Lipids from the digestion of organelles like mitochondria and endoplasmic reticulum can also deposit here (2).

Lipofuscin is an autofluorescent pigment formed through the oxidation of unsaturated fatty acids. In short, it is an undigestable residue of cytoplasmic catabolism. Studies showed that content of lipofuscin in the cells increases with age. On the contrary, melanin content decreases showing an inverse relation between these two compounds not only in their final concentration but also in their topographical distribution. This interesting finding may suggest a protective mechanism in the formation of lipofuscin (3).

Thickened BM is another alteration that occurs over time. Histologically, there is an increase in basophilia with hematoxylin and eosin (H&E) stain because of progressive calcium salt and lipid deposition in both inner and outer collagenous zones (4). Moreover, studies have shown that a large portion of the lipids found in this tissue are lipoprotein-like particles that increase with advancing age. These deposits were found to increase in the inner collagenous and elastic layers, but not in the outer collagenous layer. Authors have related these findings to the formation of a hydrophobic barrier within the BM that altered the filtration capacity through the area (5). These deposits may also be related to small granules, another major deposit found at the BM by Huang et al. They suggested there could be an interaction between this two inclusion types, but the identity of these small granules could not be determined (6). In addition, the accumulation of cholesterol esters with advancing age can be compared to accumulation of cholesterol esters in the intima of large arteries in

atherosclerosis (7). Finally, there is an increase in collagen cross-linking in the inner portion of this membrane causing a negative effect on its permeability. This cross-linkage provides strength and density to the collagen network together with the loss of flexibility, elasticity, and filtration properties. Therefore, the RPE collagenases become less effective in the removal of other BM components considering this tight network is blocking their way (8).

The photoreceptor layer manifests a different response to aging. Immunohistochemical analysis concludes that the cone photoreceptor population shows more anomalies compared with rod photoreceptor population in non-AMD retinas. Nevertheless, the signs of degeneration have an early onset in cones, but rods appear to die more promptly. Cones can prolapse into the outer plexiform layer and

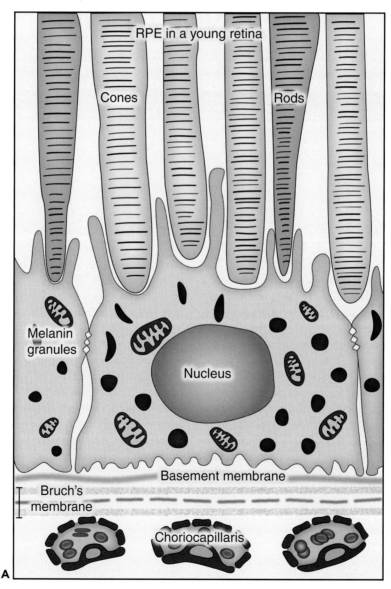

Figure 5.1 ■ Histopathological changes in the two main forms of AMD. This diagram is showing the structural and functional changes of a normal RPE cell when developing dry or wet AMD. **A.** The RPE in a young retina has a homogenous distribution of the melanin granules, a BM without deposits, and a preserved function.

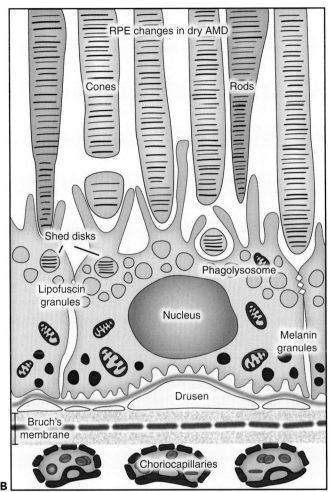
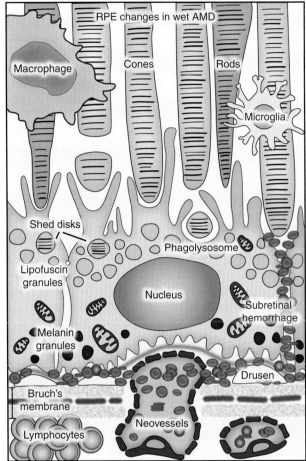

Figure 5.1 ■ (*Continued*) **B.** In dry AMD, the RPE melanin granules are localized basally, and lipofuscin granules increase in number while the efficacy of the disks digestion reduces. Note the formation of drusen between the basement membrane of the RPE and the inner collagen layer of the BM and the thickened BM. **C.** In wet AMD, CNV develops, and an inflammatory response develops with an influx of lymphocytes and macrophages to the scene. These fragile new vessels leak and lead to subretinal hemorrhage.

subretinal space and lose their synaptic contact without succumbing to cell death as do rods (9).

Some authors consider AMD to be an accentuation of normal aging changes. Age is a key factor in its pathogenesis. Nevertheless, many people maintain an excellent vision in spite of advancing age and its consequences.

DRY/NONNEOVASCULAR AMD

Drusen

Drusen are deposits of extracellular matrix localized between the basement membrane of the RPE and the inner collagen layer of the BM. They can extend to the outer collagenous zone if there is discontinuity in the central band of elastic fibers (10,11). They are often seen in the aging retina, as a hereditary condition (dominantly inherited drusen) or secondary to a variety of intraocular processes including inflammation, trauma, and chronic retinal detachment (2). However, an increase in number, size, and confluence was

established as a risk factor for the development of AMD (12). Because of this, it is important to distinguish which yellow deposits will lead to atrophy of the RPE or CNV. The American Academy of Ophthalmology proposed the following classification according to the size of the drusen (13):

■ Small (less than 64 μm of diameter)
■ Intermediate (64–124 μm of diameter)
■ Large (≥125 μm of diameter)

Immunohistochemical and proteomic studies of drusen composition have revealed different proteins other than RPE remnants (lipofuscin) like immunoglobulins, class II antigens, acute-phase proteins (e.g., fibrinogen, C-reactive protein, and vitronectin), components of the complement cascade and its inhibitors, apolipoproteins B and E, and lipids (e.g., cerebrosides), among others (8,14,15). These deposits are collectively known as drusen, but they are not all alike. Drusen main types are hard, soft, and diffuse or confluent, although authors have also described several others subtypes such as basal, nodular, mixed, and calcified regressing drusen (11).

Hard drusen are pinpoint-sized, sharp-edged yellowish retinal lesions easily seen on ophthalmoscopic exam. They are hyperfluorescent in the early stages of the fluorescein angiography and stain late without leakage. Histopathologically, hard drusen are hyaline-like, dense, rounded, homogenous bodies restricted to the basement membrane of the RPE and BM. They consist of a uniform periodic acid-Schiff-positive material and are eosinophilic on the H&E stain (Fig. 5.2A and B) until they start accumulating calcium and consequently become basophilic (16). They also stain lightly positive with special staining technique for lipid (2). On the electron microscopy, they are finely granular or amorphous nodules with similar electrodensity to the basal membrane of the RPE. They may also contain pale vesicles, tubular structures, curly membranes, and wide-banded collagen (15). The overlying RPE is thinned due to degenerative changes as described in Ulshafer et al. (17) electron microscopy studies. There are several hypotheses concerning the formation of hard drusen. Some authors have shown that the main initiating event in their development is the shedding of portions of RPE cells into the BM that are then hyalinized during the apoptosis process (18,19). Others have demonstrated that they are formed by lipidization and degeneration of single cells (20,21). This matter is still uncertain.

In contrast, soft drusen have less well-defined boundaries and tend to become confluent. Histologically, they are composed of a pale-staining amorphous more irregular and granular material located in the thickened inner layer of the BM. Green et al. (16) pointed out that they represent a serous detachment of the thickened inner aspect of the BM along with the RPE. On electron microscopy, this thickened area consists of vesicles, membranous debris, and wide-spaced collagen associated with the basal laminar deposits (22).

The basal deposits represent one of the earliest morphologic changes in the AMD. The two main types of basal deposits are basal laminar deposits (*BLamDs*) and basal linear deposits (*BLinDs*) (23). *BLamDs* are seen as soft granular eosinophilic material or extensive plaques that elevate the atrophic RPE from the inner surface of BM. On electron microscopy, these deposits are found to be limited to the plasma membrane and the basement membrane of the RPE and are comprised of extracellular matrix material with wide-spaced collagen (24). These deposits contain laminin, collagen type IV, vitronectin, extracellular matrix–modulating metalloproteinases, activated complement, glycoproteins, heparan sulfate, cholesterol, carbohydrates, and apolipoproteins B and E (8,25). In contrast, *BLinDs* are located in the thickened inner layer of the BM and appear to be electron dense rich in lipid material. These deposits represent what many authors have described as "diffuse drusen" (26). With progressive death of pigment epithelial cells, drusen start to fade by decreasing in size and becoming what some authors called calcified drusen (27). In fact, RPE atrophy, represented by hypopigmentary changes on clinical exam, is seen concomitantly with calcified or refractile drusen in histopathologic studies (28).

In summary, soft drusen along with basal linear deposits reveal an RPE dysfunction that influences the development of CNV (29,30). It has been reported that the thickening due to these deposits predisposes the BM to splitting and consequent complications such as retinal PED, neovascularization, and scarring (31).

Geographic Atrophy

Geographic or areolar atrophy also called advanced "dry" AMD involves an extensive degeneration (150 μm or larger) of the RPE and the overlying receptors that are metabolically dependent upon the RPE. It is labeled as "geographic" because the areas of atrophic RPE are

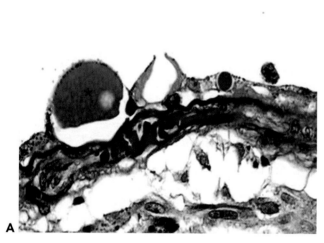 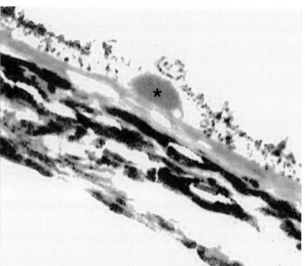

Figure 5.2 ■ Histopathologic section of drusen (*asterisk*) showing atrophy of the overlying pigment epithelium and photoreceptors. **A.** Masson trichrome digital stain 40×. **B.** H&E stain 20× (Courtesy Zárate JO, Alvarado M© 2011. Unpublished data.)

well demarcated and not related to any specific anatomy structure (32). Some authors describe a nongeographic atrophy in cases where atrophic areas are noncontiguous or manifest as speckled depigmented areas (13). On funduscopic examination, geographic atrophy is seen as a sharply demarcated round or oval hypopigmented spot, frequently found either juxtafoveal or parafoveal, that allows an enhanced view of the underlying large choroidal vessels (1,33). On fluorescein angiography, geographic atrophy demonstrates an early hyperfluorescent area due to the window defect in the RPE. The loss of epithelium transmits fluorescein brightly, but the extent of the lesion does not change in the late phases.

On microscopy, areas of geographic atrophy lack photoreceptors and RPE cells, and the outer plexiform layer is adherent to the BM (Fig. 5.3A and B) (4). This is seen as hypopigmented or atrophic areas overlying a diffusive thickened inner aspect of the BM (26). Calcified or retractile drusen, as previously described, are also observed (28). The RPE demonstrates other changes such as hypertrophy and hyperplasia, which are clinically seen as focal hyperpigmentation (23). Clumps of pigmented cells in the subretinal space and the outer retinal layers may also be observed histologically (26).

Studies performed by Schatz et al. demonstrated that in addition to RPE atrophy, one may also observe atrophy of the choriocapillaris. During fluorescein angiography, the choriocapillaris fills more slowly than normal indicating an ultrastructural damage (32). It is not understood if the choriocapillaris atrophy is secondary to RPE deterioration or vice versa. In fact, there is direct in vitro evidence that RPE cells may support the survival of the choriocapillaris endothelial cells by both insoluble molecules and growth factors such as basic fibroblast growth factor (bFGF). In other words, without them, the cells become apoptotic (34). Therefore, the absence of RPE or anything that can reduce its availability, like deposits in BM, produces choriocapillaris atrophy. An alternative theory postulated by Ciulla et al. (35) supporting the vascular pathogenesis of AMD hypothesizes that there is a primary vascular alteration in the choroid, which eventually causes a collateral effect on the RPE. This issue requires further research.

Even though at one time it was assumed patients with geographic atrophy were not at risk of developing exudative complications, it is now well known that neovascular changes can occur (16). It has been established that this new vessel formation depends on the viability of the RPE so that it can only grow in the edges of the lesion where the pigment epithelium remains intact or hypertrophic (27). Furthermore, Kliffen et al. illustrated this event with a light microscopic image and demonstrated that the junctional zone was comprised of hypertrophic RPE cells and basal laminar deposits. They assumed that if neovascularization was present, this was where it was supposed to be found in association with macrophages and giant cells (36). Also, geographic atrophy can coexist with subretinal neovascularization or be followed by serous detachment of the RPE (11).

Pigment Epithelial Detachment

After a while, basal laminar deposits enlarge and coalesce providing a larger cleavage plane in BM, which is no longer seen as soft drusen but as a serous PED. Indeed, this appears to be a key event in the evolution to the development of subretinal neovascularization (16).

The inner aspect of the BM also suffers from rip or tears as a common complication of PEDs. The clinical and fluorescein angiographic aspects of these lesions were first described by Hoskin et al. in 1981. They determined that the tear always took place at the edge of the PED and that the remaining detached pigment epithelium retracted, leaving an area of nude BM. The retracted epithelium was folded parallel to the edge of the rip and, in some cases, reattached afterward to the BM at a new site. There was no modification on the overlying retina. Moreover, in the fluorescein angiogram, the nude BM made the choroidal vessels be seen in the first frame prior to hyperfluorescence within 2 seconds. There was no leakage into the subretinal fluid, but some late dye accumulation was identified subretinally as well as dark hypofluorescent folds of residual detached pigment epithelium (37). Tears may also develop after laser photocoagulation or antiangiogenic therapy in patients with neovascular AMD (38,39).

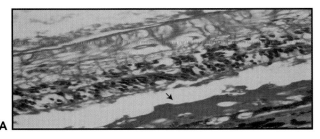
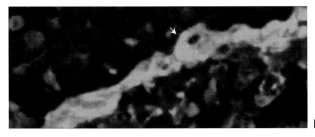

Figure 5.3 ■ Geographic atrophy. **A.** Retinal and choroidal tissue. Photoreceptor lesion with fibrosis (*arrow*) H&E stain 20×. **B.** Macular retinal atrophy and fibrosis (*arrow*). Masson trichrome digital stain 60×. (Courtesy Zárate JO, Alvarado M© 2011. Unpublished data.)

WET/EXUDATIVE/NEOVASCULAR AMD

Choroidal Neovascularization

Choroidal also known as subretinal neovascularization (CNV) is one of the main features of wet AMD. The new vessel formation extends from the choroid into the thickened portion of the BM or from the margins of the optic nerve head (40). Studies have confirmed that a prior break in the BM is not necessary for vessel proliferation because the new vessels can make their way through it by themselves (41). CNV is often seen in retinas in which softening and confluence of drusen have taken place (42). In histologic sections, Albert et al. (11) described the following findings: (a) breaks in BM; (b) a granulomatous inflammatory pattern with macrophages, lymphocytes, and fibroblasts; (c) basal laminar deposits and soft drusen; and (d) RPE depigmentation, hypertrophy, hyperplasia, and folding. On electron microscopy, both mature and newly formed capillaries have fenestrations similar to their choriocapillaris precursors. They also have high permeability to fluorescein and may cause leakage or fluorescein blockage (43). Even though they are initially very small, are nondetectable, and have capillary characteristics, they acquire arterial and venous features with time. Ophthalmoscopically, they can either be seen through the atrophic RPE or hidden underneath fibrous grayish tissue or RPE hypertrophy. CNV can be localized to the macula, peripapillary retina, or peripheral retina. CNV can be restricted to the BM (Fig. 5.4A and B) or trespass the RPE and grow into the subsensory space associated with fibroblastic RPE metaplasia and migration of macrophages (33). Anastomosis between choroidal and retinal vessels can develop. This characteristic is often seen in late stages of AMD when the disciform scar is well established (2). The neovascular membranes can be recognized in the fluorescein angiogram as a fine network of vessels with early filling, associated with exudation and subretinal hemorrhage. These specific elements are toxic for the RPE and photoreceptors, and they may lead to RPE detachment, proliferation of fibrous tissue, cystoid macular edema, and occasional circinate retinopathy (33,44,45). In this setting, fibroblasts can be identified invading the hematoma. Also,

the surviving RPE cells are transformed into elongated spindly cells while the overlying photoreceptor atrophy resulting in a submacular nodule, plaque, or fibroglial scar tissue that contracts and distorts the retina (40).

Sometimes, the boundaries of subretinal membranes may appear obscure in the fluorescein angiography but can be better defined using indocyanine green angiography (ICG). Viewing specific characteristics of the membranes is crucial while making treatment decisions. There are two main types of membranes: classic (well-defined) membranes and occult (poorly defined) ones. Classic membranes are well-demarcated, hyperfluorescent areas in early phases of the angiogram with blurry boundaries in late phases. They are located in the subretinal space where they are observed as an inverted layer of refractive RPE on the external aspect of the membrane (46). In contrast to classic membranes, occult membranes are poorly defined because they grow within sub-RPE deposits where there is not enough space for the pooling of the dye causing the so-called angiographic term late fluorescence of undetermined source (33). They are firmly adherent to the RPE and BM and have no potential plane of cleavage that allows surgical removal without destroying the overlying retina (46).

The pathogenesis of this process remains unclear. Although it has been proposed that vascular proliferation is a response to outer retinal ischemia, the lack of retinal neovascularization, typical outer ischemic retina atrophy, and absence of choriocapillaris occlusion render this hypothesis weak (2).

Retinal Angiomatous Proliferation

Retinal angiomatous proliferation (RAP) is a distinct form of CNV in the paramacular area in exudative AMD. The concept of RAP was first established by Yannuzzi et al. (47) in 2001 due to three elements: (a) early appearance of neovascularization, (b) a contiguous telangiectasia in the retina, and (c) the variable or late onset of retinal–choroidal anastomosis. It had already been described, despite some inconsistencies, by several authors (48–50).

In RAP, new retinal vessels expand toward the inner retina and below the RPE. Three stages of the disease have

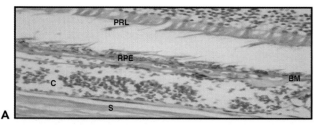
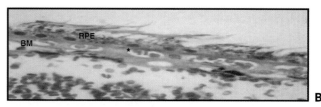

Figure 5.4 ■ Wet AMD. **A.** Histologic section shows CNV at the BM. Retinal pigment epithelium (RPE), choroid (C), and sclera (S). H&E stain 40×. **B.** Magnified view of the choroidal neovessels (*asterisk*). H&E stain 60× (Courtesy Zárate JO, Alvarado M© 2011. Unpublished data.)

been established based on clinical biomicroscopic examination, fluorescein angiography, ICG, and optical coherence tomography. Its histopathologic correlation has been obviated (51). Immunohistochemical studies performed in neovascular membranes obtained by surgical excision demonstrated hypoxia inducible factor one (HIF-1) alpha and HIF-2 alpha expression in vascular endothelial cells in the neovascularization. This suggests that RAP tissue is in a hypoxic state predisposing it to VEGF expression. Valuable data regarding RAP pathogenesis were provided by this study. Migration of CD68-positive macrophages expressing hypoxia factors in the area of neovascularization was observed, suggesting that ischemic *and* inflammatory factors are associated with the development and progression of RAP (52).

Disciform Scar

The formation of a disciform scar represents the end stage of AMD. As previously described, the CNV fragile endothelium is associated with leakage and bleeding, leading to RPE detachments. In the process of reorganizing the damaged tissue, a fibrovascular disciform scar is generated.

The major histopathologic components of this scar are mounds of dense collagenous connective tissue on the inner surface of the BM (24). It is generally associated with the loss of neural tissue (photoreceptors) in the outer retina. As a general rule, the thinner and smaller the scar's diameter, the greater the photoreceptor survival (33). In spite of this, morphometric studies confirmed that the ganglion cell and inner nuclear layers are relatively preserved (53). Cystoid degeneration and lamellar and full-thickness macular holes are other examples of possible degenerative changes (4). RPE proliferation, hyperplasia, and fibrous metaplasia have been reported. These epithelial cells are responsible for the production of large quantities of extracellular matrix material. The disciform lesions can be partially pigmented because of melanin and hemosiderin presence and may be difficult to differentiate from nevi, malignant melanoma, or pigment epithelium tumors (45). Vascular supply is provided by choroidal vessel in most cases, rarely by retinal vessels (4).

A rare but devastating complication of this condition is a massive subretinal hemorrhage. It has been documented by Wood et al. (54) that neovascular tissue present within the macular disciform lesions was the source of such bleedings after a complete retinal detachment occurred. Other studies suggest that anticoagulant medication, widely used among the AMD age group, can be a risk factor for developing this unfortunate outcome. Therefore, the authors recommend that anticoagulant therapy should be prescribed in cases only when it is indicated (55). Moreover, another complication known as senile Coats' response can also develop, resulting in extensive exudation in and under the retina with lipid and cholesterol deposition (16).

REFERENCES

1. de Jong PT. Age-related macular degeneration. N Engl J Med. 2006;355(14):1474–1485.

2. Spencer WH; American Academy of Ophthalmology. Ophthalmic pathology: an atlas and textbook. 4th ed. Philadelphia, PA: W.B. Saunders; 1996.

3. Weiter JJ, et al. Retinal pigment epithelial lipofuscin and melanin and choroidal melanin in human eyes. Invest Ophthalmol Vis Sci. 1986;27(2):145–152.

4. Hampton GR, Nelsen PT. Age-related macular degeneration: principles and practice. New York: Raven Press; 1992:300.

5. Huang JD, Curcio CA, Johnson M. Morphometric analysis of lipoprotein-like particle accumulation in aging human macular Bruch's membrane. Invest Ophthalmol Vis Sci. 2008;49(6):2721–2727.

6. Huang JD, et al. Age-related changes in human macular Bruch's membrane as seen by quick-freeze/deep-etch. Exp Eye Res. 2007;85(2):202–218.

7. Curcio CA, et al. Accumulation of cholesterol with age in human Bruch's membrane. Invest Ophthalmol Vis Sci. 2001;42(1):265–274.

8. Booij JC, et al. The dynamic nature of Bruch's membrane. Prog Retin Eye Res. 2010;29(1):1–18.

9. Shelley EJ, et al. Cone degeneration in aging and age-related macular degeneration. Arch Ophthalmol. 2009;127(4):483–492.

10. Farkas TG, Sylvester V, Archer D. The ultrastructure of drusen. Am J Ophthalmol. 1971;71(6):1196–1205.

11. Albert DM, Jakobiec FA. Principles and practice of ophthalmology. 3rd Ed. Philadelphia, PA: Elsevier Saunders; 2007.

12. Bressler SB, et al. Relationship of drusen and abnormalities of the retinal pigment epithelium to the prognosis of neovascular macular degeneration. The Macular Photocoagulation Study Group. Arch Ophthalmol. 1990;108(10):1442–1447.

13. Regillo CD, Holekamp N, Johnson MW, et al. Basic and clinical science course section 12. Retina and vitreous 2008-2009. San Francisco, CA:The Foundation of the American Academy of Ophthalmology; 2008:124–136.

14. Nowak JZ. Age-related macular degeneration (AMD): pathogenesis and therapy. Pharmacol Rep. 2006;58(3):353–363.

15. Schmack I, Kang SJ, Grossniklaus HE. Histopatologia de la degeneracion macular asociada a la edad. Mones J, Gomez-Ulla F, eds. Degeneracion macular asociada a la edad. Barcelona: Proust Science; 2005:73–84.

16. Green WR, McDonnell PJ, Yeo JH. Pathologic features of senile macular degeneration. Ophthalmology. 1985;92(5):615–627.

17. Ulshafer RJ, et al. Scanning electron microscopy of human drusen. Invest Ophthalmol Vis Sci. 1987;28(4):683–689.

18. Burns RP, Feeney-Burns L. Clinico-morphologic correlations of drusen of Bruch's membrane. Trans Am Ophthalmol Soc. 1980;78:206–225.

19. Hogan MJ. Role of the retinal pigment epithelium in macular disease. Trans Am Acad Ophthalmol Otolaryngol. 1972;76(1):64–80.

20. Fine BS. Lipoidal degeneration of the retinal pigment epithelium. Am J Ophthalmol. 1981;91(4):469–473.

21. el Baba F, et al. Clinicopathologic correlation of lipidization and detachment of the retinal pigment epithelium. Am J Ophthalmol. 1986;101(5):576–583.

22. Sassani JW. Ophthalmic pathology with clinical correlations. Philadelphia, PA: Lippincott-Raven; 1997:337.

23. Green WR. Histopathology of age-related macular degeneration. Mol Vis. 1999;5:27.

24. Eagle RC. Eye pathology: an atlas and basic text. Philadelphia, PA: W.B. Saunders; 1999:306.

25. Lommatzsch A, et al. Are low inflammatory reactions involved in exudative age-related macular degeneration? Morphological and immunohistochemical analysis of AMD associated with basal deposits. Graefes Arch Clin Exp Ophthalmol. 2008;246(6):803–810.

26. Bressler NM, et al. Clinicopathologic correlation of drusen and retinal pigment epithelial abnormalities in age-related macular degeneration. Retina. 1994;14(2):130–142.

27. Sarks JP, Sarks SH, Killingsworth MC. Evolution of geographic atrophy of the retinal pigment epithelium. Eye (Lond). 1988;2(Pt 5):552–577.

28. Cukras C, et al. Natural history of drusenoid pigment epithelial detachment in age-related macular degeneration: Age-Related Eye Disease Study Report No. 28. Ophthalmology. 2010;117(3):489–499.

29. Zarbin MA, Age-related macular degeneration: review of pathogenesis. Eur J Ophthalmol. 1998;8(4):199–206.

30. Jager RD, Mieler WF, Miller JW. Age-related macular degeneration. N Engl J Med. 2008;358(24):2606–2617.

31. Kenyon KR, et al. Diffuse drusen and associated complications. Am J Ophthalmol. 1985;100(1):119–128.

32. Schatz H, McDonald HR. Atrophic macular degeneration. Rate of spread of geographic atrophy and visual loss. Ophthalmology. 1989;96(10):1541–1551.

33. Hamilton AMP, Gregson R, Fish GE. Text atlas of the retina. Boston, Oxford: Butterworth-Heinemann; Martin Dunitz; 1998:417.

34. Liu X, et al. Extracellular matrix of retinal pigment epithelium regulates choriocapillaris endothelial survival in vitro. Exp Eye Res. 1997;65(1):117–126.

35. Ciulla TA, et al. Color Doppler imaging discloses reduced ocular blood flow velocities in nonexudative age-related macular degeneration. Am J Ophthalmol. 1999;128(1):75–80.

36. Kliffen M, et al. Morphologic changes in age-related maculopathy. Microsc Res Tech. 1997;36(2):106–122.

37. Hoskin A, Bird AC, Sehmi K. Tears of detached retinal pigment epithelium. Br J Ophthalmol. 1981;65(6):417–422.

38. Gass JD. Pathogenesis of tears of the retinal pigment epithelium. Br J Ophthalmol. 1984;68(8):513–519.

39. Gelisken F, et al. Retinal pigment epithelial tears after single administration of intravitreal bevacizumab for neovascular age-related macular degeneration. Eye (Lond). 2009;23(3):694–702.

40. Lucas DR, Greer CH. Greer's ocular pathology. 4th Ed. Oxford, Boston: Blackwell Scientific Publications; 1989:339.

41. Heriot WJ, et al. Choroidal neovascularization can digest Bruch's membrane. A prior break is not essential. Ophthalmology. 1984;91(12):1603–1608.

42. Sarks SH. Council Lecture. Drusen and their relationship to senile macular degeneration. Aust J Ophthalmol. 1980;8(2):117–130.

43. Miller H, Miller B, Ryan SJ. Newly-formed subretinal vessels. Fine structure and fluorescein leakage. Invest Ophthalmol Vis Sci. 1986;27(2):204–213.

44. Green WR, Key SN III. Senile macular degeneration: a histopathologic study. Trans Am Ophthalmol Soc. 1977;75:180–254.

45. Apple DJ, Rabb MF. Ocular pathology: clinical applications and self-assessment. 5th Ed. St. Louis, MO: Mosby; 1998:705.

46. Grossniklaus HE, Gass JD. Clinicopathologic correlations of surgically excised type 1 and type 2 submacular choroidal neovascular membranes. Am J Ophthalmol. 1998;126(1):59–69.

47. Yannuzzi LA, et al. Retinal angiomatous proliferation in age-related macular degeneration. Retina. 2001;21(5):416–434.

48. Hartnett ME, et al. Classification of retinal pigment epithelial detachments associated with drusen. Graefes Arch Clin Exp Ophthalmol. 1992;230(1):11–19.

49. Slakter JS, et al. Retinal choroidal anastomoses and occult choroidal neovascularization in age-related macular degeneration. Ophthalmology. 2000;107(4):742–753; discussion 753–754.

50. Lafaut BA, et al. Clinicopathological correlation of deep retinal vascular anomalous complex in age related macular degeneration. Br J Ophthalmol. 2000;84(11):1269–1274.

51. Yannuzzi LA, Freund KB, Takahashi BS. Review of retinal angiomatous proliferation or type 3 neovascularization. Retina. 2008;28(3):375–384.

52. Shimada H, et al. Clinicopathological findings of retinal angiomatous proliferation. Graefes Arch Clin Exp Ophthalmol. 2007;245(2):295–300.

53. Kim SY, et al. Morphometric analysis of the macula in eyes with geographic atrophy due to age-related macular degeneration. Retina. 2002;22(4):464–470.

54. Wood WJ, Smith TR. Senile disciform macular degeneration complicated by massive hemorrhagic retinal detachment and angle closure glaucoma. Retina. 1983;3(4):296–303.

55. Tilanus MA, et al. Relationship between anticoagulant medication and massive intraocular hemorrhage in age-related macular degeneration. Graefes Arch Clin Exp Ophthalmol. 2000;238(6):482–485.

6

CLASSIFICATION OF EXUDATIVE AGE-RELATED MACULAR DEGENERATION

MICHELLE L. CROUSE • WISSAM CHARAFEDDIN
GERARDO GARCIA-AGUIRRE • GABRIELA E. GRANELLA
D. VIRGIL ALFARO III • JOHN BARNWELL KERRISON
ERIC P. JABLON

■ INTRODUCTION

Age-related macular degeneration (AMD) has been subject to many divisions, namings, and classification schemes since it was first described by Haab in 1885 (1). The disease has since been subdivided into two major forms: nonexudative (dry AMD) and exudative (wet AMD). In nonexudative AMD, visual loss develops as the result of geographic atrophy involving the foveal center (2,3). In exudative AMD, visual loss develops secondary to choroidal neovascularization (CNV), which leads to bleeding, exudation, and eventual scar formation (4). Exudative AMD is distinguished from nonexudative AMD when the integrity of the Bruch's membrane–retinal pigment epithelium (RPE) complex separates and forms a pigment epithelial detachment (PED). While nonexudative AMD has not been subject to subdivisions, exudative AMD has several subclassifications. In the past, exudative AMD has been most commonly divided into *occult* and *classic* types, based on characteristic lesion formation. In classic exudative AMD, lesion boundaries were well demarcated on fluorescein angiography (FA), while occult lesions had irregular boundaries and stippled hyperfluorescence. Other classifications have been based on the grading systems of various studies and clinical trials (5).

In 1995, based on postoperative results in patients with CNV, Gass (6,7) suggested a shift in the classification of exudative AMD using the anatomic localization rather than the appearance on FA as was proposed in the Macular Photocoagulation Study (MPS) (8,9). Such classification was limited by the lack of imaging available at the time but can now be used due to multimodal imaging, employing the use of FA, optical coherence tomography (OCT), and indocyanine green (ICG) angiography.

A new classification scheme proposed by Freund et al. (10) builds on the Gass model, dividing neovascularization into four types depending on location: type 1, located under the RPE; type 2, above the RPE, in the subretinal space; type 3, characterized by intraretinal neovascularization (IRN), also known as retinal angiomatous proliferation (RAP); and type 4, polypoidal choroidal vasculopathy (PCV), considered by some to be type 1 neovascularization. While PCV is a sub-RPE vascular lesion, it does not have the clinical, structural, and angiographic characteristics of type 1 lesions. This method of classification would not rely on only one imaging technology as in the past with FA but also on imaging techniques that emerged in recent years, refining our understanding of the disease.

TYPE 1 NEOVASCULARIZATION

Gass defined type 1 neovascularization histologically as neo-vascularization occurring beneath the RPE monolayer. It is by far the most common form of neovascularization in AMD. In a study by Cohen et al. (11), occult CNV with or without PED represented 56.6% of the 207 cases studied. With FA, these vessels are usually described as occult or poorly defined. In a study by Lafaut et al. (12), occult membranes were analyzed after surgical excision. All cases consisted of thin fibrovascular membranes in the sub-RPE space. Only in two of the ten specimens was an additional smaller fibrovas-cular component found in the subretinal space.

FA terminology applied to type 1 lesions includes "late leakage of undetermined source" or vascularized PED. ICG was found to be useful in detecting choroidal neovascular membranes (CNVMs), especially if FA cannot reveal a well-defined neovascular membrane (Figs. 6.1A and 6.2A). ICG is a complementary imaging study in the diagnosis of occult lesions where masking phenomena may prevent

the visualization of the neovascular net. ICG is less dependent on leakage as ICG dye bound to albumin is kept in the intravascular space (13,14). This relatively new technique helped in deciding the eligibility of treatment with photodynamic therapy (PDT) in some occult CNV cases (15). Yannuzzi and Slakter (16,17) found that 39% and 44%, respectively, of patients with occult CNV by FA showed well-demarcated hyperfluorescence by ICG angiography. The ICG pattern of type 1 neovascularization can be classified into three types depending on the size of the hyperfluo-rescent area: focal spots, plaques, or a combination of both (18). In a postmortem histopathologic study of an eye with ICG plaque, Chang et al. (19) confirmed the localization of plaques documented by ICG to be between the RPE and an intact Bruch's membrane.

Spectral-domain optical coherence tomography (SD-OCT) allows visualization of intraretinal structures as well as RPE morphology (Figs. 6.1B and 6.2B). It identifies RPE detachment and CNV-related infiltration. According to Malamos et al. (14), with the use of the RPE map, it is

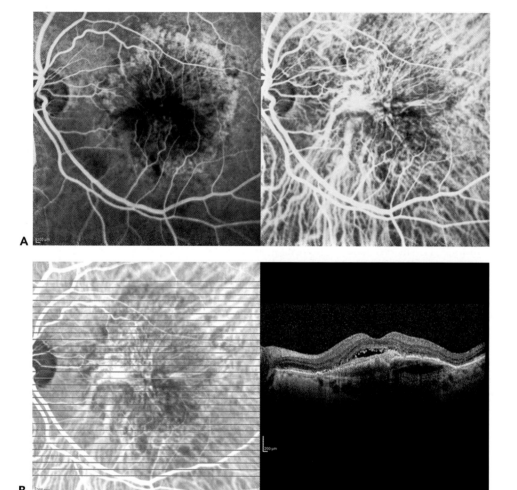

Figure 6.1 ■ **A.** Type 1 CNVM. **Left.** FA showing leakage of undetermined origin. **Right.** ICG angiography showing arteriolized pattern of choroidal neovascularization. **B.** Type 1 CNVM. **Left.** ICG angiography showing arteriolized pattern of CNV. **Right.** Macular OCT showing a visible large pigment epithelium detachment (PED).

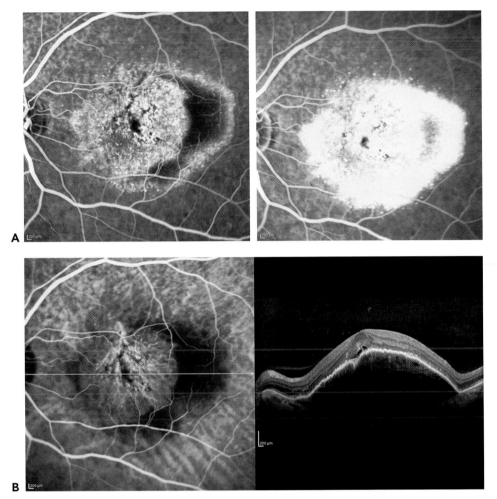

Figure 6.2 ■ **A.** Type 1 CNVM. Early- and late-phase FA: Leakage of undetermined origin. PED is visible. **B.** Type 1 CNVM. **Left.** ICG: Bushy appearance of CNVM apparent with ICG. **Right.** OCT of the same case. Pigment epithelium detachment with minimal subretinal fluid.

possible to identify the location of the occult CNVM. If a membrane is hidden under the RPE, the latter appears slightly prominent, flat at the top, and slowly declining at the margins. These lesions are usually ill defined and convex with irregular surfaces. SD-OCT can be more informative than is FA and allows better identification and classification of membranes with occult components that may not be easily detected and delineated. The 3D surface maps of the RPE further clarify the exact level of the lesion and its microscopic morphology in combination with B-scan morphology.

Type 1 membranes are the most common type associated with AMD, while type 2 membranes are associated with focal lesions affecting the Bruch's membrane and the RPE in diseases such as high myopia with lacquer cracks, ocular histoplasmosis syndrome, serpiginous choroiditis, and choroidal ruptures (20). In disorders like AMD, lipid-rich material, such as cuticular drusen, contains numerous complement components that accumulate between the Bruch's membrane and the RPE. Type 1 neovascularization grows in the presence of such material and is not seen in disorders with focal disturbances of the RPE–Bruch's

membrane complex such as multifocal choroiditis and panu-veitis, myopia, and choroidal rupture (10). Type 1 pattern is rarely seen in disorders like Best disease, vitelliform macular dystrophy, and pseudoxanthoma elasticum where material accumulates above and below the RPE monolayer (10).

Unlike classic lesions, occult-type lesions rarely cause visual symptoms promptly, allowing some lesions to grow to a large size before being detected clinically. They tend to have a variable and less aggressive natural course based on the presenting acuities and long-term natural history. In the MARINA study (21), patients with occult neovascular lesions presented better initial visual acuities than in the ANCHOR study (22) patients who had classic lesions. This was also observed in the VIP and TAP trials where many minimally classic lesions and occult lesions with no classic component had relatively acceptable visual acuity (23). According to Grossniklaus et al. (24), this benign course may relate to the theory that in some eyes, type 1 neovascularization may grow as a compensatory mechanism to provide nutritional support to the ischemic outer retina by recapitulating the normal choriocapillaris. In his study,

Engelbert et al. (25) observed that only one eye out of eighteen eyes with type 1 neovascularization (6%) developed geographic atrophy overlying affected areas.

The exudation in type 1 neovascularization is predominantly in the form of subretinal fluid. Subretinal fluid is less clinically aggressive than is cystoid macular edema (CME). The presence of CME portends a poor prognosis, in that it presumably indicates damage to the outer retinal barrier in the form of RPE dysfunction and disruptions in the tight junctions that contribute to the external limiting membrane (ELM) band on SD-OCT (3). However, in some cases, type 1 neovascularization may follow an aggressive course and cause a decrease in visual acuity. These vessels may also erode through the RPE giving rise to type 2 neovascularization. In the TAP study, approximately 40% of eyes progressed from minimally classic to predominantly classic lesions with 24% converting in the first 3 months (26). This was also confirmed by Schneider et al. (27) when 23% of eyes with occult lesions having no classic components progressed to predominantly classic membranes over a period of 6 to 12 months. Overall, the conversion rate from occult with no classic to classic neovascularization at 1 year was 46% (39%–54%); no conversion in the reverse direction was ever described (28).

The response to treatment with intravitreal anti–vascular endothelial growth factor (VEGF) therapy may be less than the response observed in type 2 or type 3 neovascularization. Eyes with these type of neovessels may often continue to manifest extrafoveal subretinal fluid. Type 1 neovascularization may be less responsive to anti-VEGF treatment; nevertheless, the antipermeability effects of these drugs are often sufficient to resolve most, if not all, of the fluid above the RPE monolayer and may limit the continued growth of these vessels. Despite the incomplete clearance of subretinal fluid, and sometimes the CME, many eyes maintain stable visual acuity for up to 5 years on monthly anti-VEGF treatment with no eyes experiencing sight-threatening submacular hemorrhages (25).

It was described by Spaide (29) that vessels may be detected by SD-OCT as hyperreflective material lining the undersurface of the elevated RPE. The contraction of this neovascular tissue, spontaneously or in response to intravitreal anti-VEGF treatment, could produce dehiscence and tears in the RPE layer. Such possibility can be predicted by the linear diameter of the PED as well as the maximal PED height (30).

TYPE 2 NEOVASCULARIZATION

As mentioned previously, the type 2 pattern predominates in macular disorders where there is a focal alteration of the RPE–Bruch's membrane complex such as pathologic myopia with lacquer cracks (Fig. 6.3A and B), punctate inner choroidopathy, multifocal choroiditis and panuveitis, histoplasmosis, and choroidal rupture. It is seen also in entities where material is deposited above the RPE such as

vitelliform macular dystrophies, Best's disease, Stargardt's disease, subretinal drusenoid deposits (reticular pseudodrusen), and pseudoxanthoma elasticum (10).

Type 2 lesions usually start as type 1 neovascularization and then can penetrate the RPE–Bruch's membrane complex to proliferate in the subretinal space above the RPE monolayer to give the type 2 appearance (28).

Histopathology studies show that predominantly classic neovascularization is mainly subretinal or combined subretinal with sub-RPE components. Classic membranes were seen to contain not just capillaries but also larger caliber vessels, whereas occult membranes contained predominantly, or only, capillaries (12).

According to MPS criteria, CNV was considered well defined or classic when a net of new vessels was identified at an early stage of FA with progressive leakage in later stages (Fig. 6.4A and B). They fluoresce intensively against a relatively dark background due to attenuation of the choroidal fluorescence by the intervening RPE (Fig. 6.5A). About 17% (11) of all CNVM show exclusively classic membranes, but it is possible that many of these harbor small areas of type 1 vessels that are undetectable by FA alone (10). Occult lesions are sometimes underestimated due to overlying classic membranes, but a PED seen on OCT can explain the presence of an occult membrane. Classic membranes can also be seen with ICG as an area of hyperfluorescence without marked leakage activity. ICG images may underestimate the dimension of the neovascular complex compared to morphologic imaging by SD-OCT (31).

On OCT, a high level of correlation was found between areas of classic CNV seen on FA and the volume of subretinal tissue (32). It is possible to differentiate a classic CNV using SD-OCT. The retinal thickness map specifically shows a well-defined lesion with steep borders and a craterlike central depression (14). Leakage and staining can be easily differentiated with this imaging technique where hyperreflectivity represents visualization of fibrotic tissue and not edema. With OCT, type 2 membranes can be localized above the RPE and beneath the photoreceptor outer segments (10) (Fig. 6.5B).

The hyperreflective line, anterior to the RPE line, represents the inner segment–outer segment junction of the photoreceptors (33). Disorganization of this layer, overlying the inner segment–outer segment (IS/OS) junction, is often accompanied by intraretinal cystic spaces. Intraretinal fluid rather than subretinal fluid predominates in type 2 lesions and usually is associated with decreased visual acuity (34,35). The differentiation between these two types of leakage can be easily seen with OCT but is not possible with FA (10).

In patients with classic lesions, most vision loss occurs within the first 6 months with little vision loss after the first year. Predominantly classic lesions included in the TAP trial were found to be smaller in size than the occult (type 1) lesions included in the VIP trial. It is suggested that predominantly classic lesions almost always cause visual symptoms promptly, perhaps allowing identification

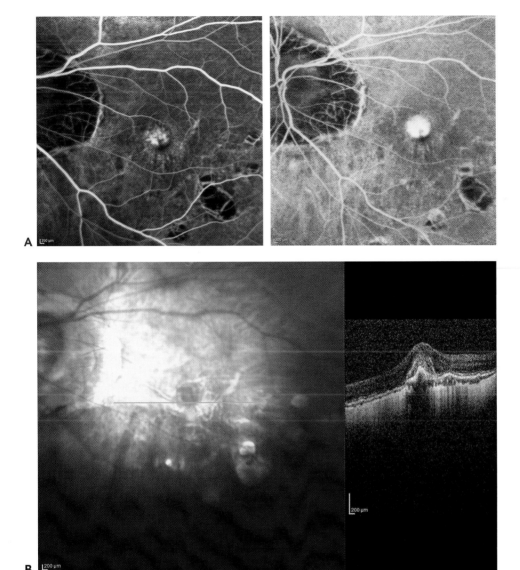

Figure 6.3 ■ **A.** Type 2 membrane in a case with high myopia. FA (early and late phases) showing leak in a classic pattern. **B.** OCT of the same case. Disruption of the RPE is observed as well as a hyperreflective area anterior to the RPE that corresponds to a type 2 CNVM.

of smaller lesion sizes, whereas occult lesions may or may not cause prompt visual symptoms, which allows them to grow to larger sizes (23,28).

Early in their evolution, type 2 vessels appear to be exquisitely sensitive to intravitreal anti-VEGF agents. There may be a decrease in the volume of subretinal fluid and fibrovascular tissue. In larger and more mature lesions, the abnormal vessels remain as a hyperreflective band (subretinal fibrosis) causing disorganization and thinning of the overlying receptors. This is seen as a disruption of the IS/OS junction, loss of the ELM, and thinning of the outer nuclear layer on SD-OCT. These eyes may continue to manifest intraretinal fluid despite frequent treatment, presumably due to the loss of the outer blood–retinal barrier in the form of RPE damage and disruption of the tight junctions that contribute to ELM band on the OCT (10).

Even in eyes with early lesions, the disruption of the IS/OS layer may be indicative of the future visual result, and visual recovery may be limited in these eyes because of the initial assault to the photoreceptors (33).

TYPE 3: RETINAL ANGIOMATOUS PROLIFERATION

It was a long-held belief that all neovascularizations in AMD originated from the choroidal circulation. In 2001, Yannuzzi et al. (36) challenged this traditional dogma based on the presumed origin and evolution of the neovascularization process. They believed that IRN originating from the inner retinal circulation produced a surrounding telangiectatic compensatory response to accommodate an increase in

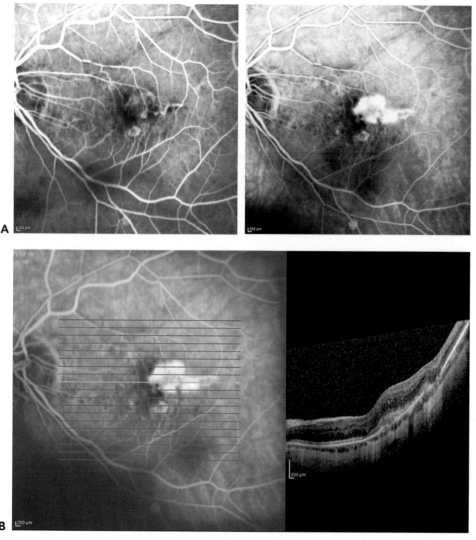

Figure 6.4 ■ **A.** FA showing CNVM (early and late phase) with leakage in a classic pattern. **B.** OCT of the same case: Intact RPE with an overlying hyperreflective lesion representing a type 2 CNVM.

vascular perfusion, and they termed this variant "retinal angiomatous proliferation" (RAP). Thereafter, and due to a lingering uncertainty as to the origin of these lesions, Freund et al. (37) have proposed naming this vascular lesion "type 3 neovascularization" to distinguish and emphasize the location of the neovascularization (intraretinal) independent of its origin. Type 3 neovascularization, or RAP, indicates proliferating vessels within and below the retina itself. The origin of this neovascular subtype can be from either circulation and may originate from both circulations simultaneously in the form of a retinal–choroidal anastomosis (RCA). The presence of an RCA gives this entity many of its characteristic clinical, SD-OCT, and angiographic features including intraretinal hemorrhages and CME. Type 3 lesions have been observed originating in areas with substantial photoreceptors, bringing the deep retinal vasculature in close proximity to the underlying RPE, Bruch's membrane, and choriocapillaries. Typically, the angiogenic response occurs overlying a focal drusen/basal laminar

deposit that may already be infiltrated by type 1 vessels. Presumably, loss of or erosion through the intervening RPE and an appropriate angiogenic milieu would allow the retinal and choroidal circulations to merge in the form of RCA with a continued proliferative response. As these lesions originate from both the retinal and choroidal circulations, they never originate within the foveal avascular zone.

RAP is further subdivided into three stages, which describe the disease progression. Stage I indicates the earliest clinical manifestations, in which RAP begins in the deep retinal complex forming IRN. As the vessels evolve, they extend beneath the neurosensory retina, becoming subretinal neovascularization (SRN), or stage II. In stage III, an RCA is formed as SRN merges with choroidal circulation, forming CNV (38–41) and the potential for a vascularized pigment epithelium detachment (PED). FA is useful in revealing the presence of the angiomatous intraretinal vascular complex and the extension of the associated PED. However, other diagnostic techniques, such as indocyanine

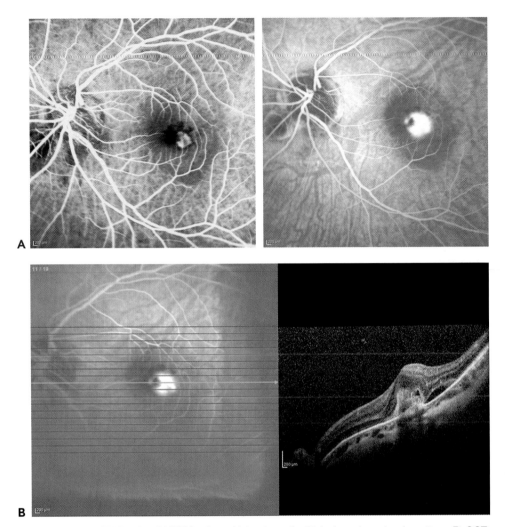

Figure 6.5 ■ **A.** FA showing CNVM (early and late phases) with leakage in a classic pattern. **B.** OCT of the same eye showing disruption of the RPE with an overlying hyperreflective lesion associated with subretinal fluid.

green (ICG) angiography and OCT, have now proven to be as useful—or even more—to demonstrate the presence of the RAP lesion.

Treating RAP has proven difficult due to the unique nature of the disease and a lack of clinical trials focused on this form of neovascularization. To date, only prospective and observational studies have been conducted, often with small sample sizes, and no standard of treatment has been established. As with other forms of neovascularization, the main treatment options for RAP include anti-VEGF agents, PDT, focal laser, transpupillary thermotherapy, and surgical ablation, or various combinations of these. To date, PDT with intravitreal triamcinolone provided the most promising results initially, but by 12 months, many of the effects had faded (42). Anti-VEGF agents may be beneficial in decreasing vasogenic drive and retinal edema, when followed by PDT (43). ICG-guided focal laser obliteration as salvage treatment may be an option, as proposed by Bearelly et al. (44).

TYPE 4: POLYPOIDAL CHOROIDAL VASCULARIZATION

Polypoidal choroidal vascularization (PCV) is recognized as a subset of type 1 CNV due to the location of PCV abnormalities, below the RPE. The various clinical manifestations of PCV are shown in Figure 6.6. PCV is most frequently characterized by a branching network of choroidal vessels and orange-red polypoidal lesions (45). PCV vascular abnormalities lie between the RPE and Bruch's membrane (46); therefore, PED is often seen in patients with PCV (47,48). PCV has often been misdiagnosed as other forms of exudative AMD due to similarities in clinical appearance on OCT and FA (49). Both PCV and CNV cause hemorrhages and other signs of exudation, leading to scarring and fibrosis, and have similar genetic markers; however, PCV has significant differences from CNV in epidemiology, pathophysiology, clinical course, and treatment response.

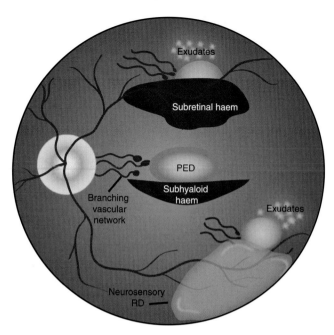

Figure 6.6 ■ Common presentations of PCV, including branching vascular network, PED, exudation, and subretinal hemorrhage. Illustration by Mariana Ingolotti.

When PCV was first described, it was thought rare and was once recognized as a disease that primarily affected black women (50). It is now known that PCV affects people of all races, although at varying rates. PCV diagnoses are given most frequently within Asian populations (51), where PCV is thought to be as common as wet AMD is in Caucasian populations (48,52,53). Although they are less affected by PCV, two studies focusing on Caucasian patients indicate that PCV is not specific to "pigmented races" (54,55) and

that Caucasian patients, especially those with extramacular lesions, should be examined for PCV (53,54). The age of diagnosis for PCV is typically younger than that for exudative AMD, between the ages of 60 and 70 years (56).

PCV, with its varying presentations and response to treatment, is in need of its own classification system. Several possible schemes have been proposed (Table 6.1). The first scheme divides PCV into three groups, relating it to CNV. In group one, the most common type, choroidal vascular abnormalities are observed beneath the RPE. In group two, PCV and CNV are present, expanding beneath the RPE with polypoidal lesions developing at vessel termini. And, in group three, CNV develops secondary to radiation treatment (60). A second scheme is based on polyp size, location, formation, and number of polyps (57). The third scheme divides the disease into exudative and hemorrhagic groups. The exudative group is characterized by a serous PED associated with intraretinal lipid deposits in the macula. It mimics chronic central serous chorioretinopathy in the elderly. The hemorrhagic group is characterized by hemorrhagic PED and subretinal hemorrhage, mimicking exudative AMD (58). All of these schemes are designed to better explain the clinical course of the disorder and tailor treatment options to individuals.

Genetic research may eventually lead to a more objective classification scheme for PCV and the other forms of macular degeneration. Genetic studies have found that PCV and AMD have similar genotypes and major alleles in both Japanese and Caucasian patients. The major loci associated with AMD and their haplotype-tagging alleles (CFH, CFB/C2, and ARMS2/HTRA1 with rs547154, rs1061170, rs1410996, and rs10490924) were also significantly associated with PCV (59,61–63). While genetic studies

Table 6.1	PROPOSED SCHEMES FOR THE SUBCLASSIFICATION OF PCV			
Location of vascular abnormalities (57)	**Group 1** ■ Choroidal vascular abnormalities beneath the RPE	**Group 2** ■ PCV and CNV present ■ Expands below the RPE ■ Polypoidal lesions develop at vessel termini.		**Group 3** ■ CNV develops secondary to radiation treatment.
Polyp classification scheme (58)	**Location of polyps** ■ Extrafoveal ■ Subfoveal ■ Juxtafoveal ■ Parapapillary	**Number of discrete polyp areas** ■ Multiple discrete areas ■ Single discrete area	**Largest polyp size** ■ Larger lesion size requires more aggressive treatment. ■ Average largest lesion size was 207 μm.	**Formation of polyps** ■ Single polyp ■ Cluster of polyps ■ String of polyps
Exudation vs. hemorrhage (59)	**Exudative group** ■ Serous RPE detachment ■ Intraretinal lipid deposits ■ Mimics chronic central serous chorioretinopathy in the elderly		**Hemorrhagic group** ■ Hemorrhagic PED ■ Subretinal hemorrhage ■ Mimics exudative AMD	

demonstrate similarities between the two disorders, many differences are seen in tissue studies.

Examinations of PCV tissue have been small in number but provide many clues into the pathogenesis of PCV and its relationship to CNV. Most histology studies have focused on vasculature, specifically the branching vascular networks unique to PCV. These analyses have been unable to determine the pathogenesis of this characteristic. Two theories seem plausible: (a) The vessels stem from new CNV, and (b) the vessels are existing choroidal vessels that have dilated abnormally. Histologic findings show that vascular endothelial cells within PCV specimens were negative for VEGF (48,64). As VEGF is primary to CNV development, its absence may suggest that the dilated vessels stem from existing choroidal vessels (64).

Vessel pathology shows large choroidal arterioles and venules, with the arterioles having an inner elastic layer, a feature not present in CNV. These arterioles are located below the Bruch's membrane and may explain the pulsation often observed in ICG angiography (65), a characteristic of PCV that distinguishes it from CNV (46,66,67). Pulsation may represent an abnormality of inner choroidal

vasculature, increased intravascular pressure, and greater physical stress on the vessel wall (55). Pulsatile lesions have a different pathophysiologic mechanism and, therefore, may respond differently to treatment (68). Another distinct vascular characteristic of PCV is the hyalinization of choroidal vessels with arteriosclerotic changes (Fig. 6.7A and B). This is unique to PCV, as hyalinization has not been reported in eyes with CNV (69).

Other histologic findings link PCV with CNV. In some PCV eyes, fibrovascular membranes have been located within the Bruch's membrane (70,71). In one case, clusters of thin-walled dilated vessels correlated with polypoidal structures on ophthalmoscopy and ICG angiography, indicating that the fibrovascular complex was subretinal CNV. However, this eye had previously undergone radiation for a subretinal neovascular membrane, making radiation associated choroidal neovasculopathy a possibility (72).

Nakashizuka et al. (69) found that PCV and CNV can be found simultaneously in the same eye, either by chance or, as they speculate, secondary to a wound repair reaction. Massive exudation of fibrin and blood plasma from dilated hyalinized choroidal vessels may raise choroidal tissue

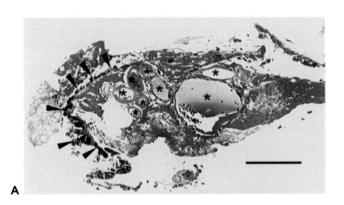

A

Retinal Angiomatous Proliferation

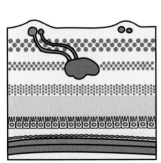
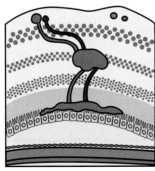
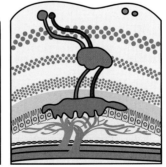

Stage 1	Stage 2	Stage 3
intraretinal angioma	subretinal capillary extension	retinal-choroidal anastomosis

B

Figure 6.7 ■ **A.** Photomicrograph showing dilated vessels (*asterisk*) beneath the RPE (*arrowheads*) that were thickened and hyalinized. (Lafaut BA, Aisenbrey S, Broecke C, et al. Polypoidal choroidal vasculopathy pattern in age-related macular degeneration. A clinicopathologic correlation. Retina. 2000;20:650–654; Nakashizuka H, Mitsumata M, Okisaka S, et al. Clinicopathologic findings in polypoidal choroidal vasculopathy. IOVS. 2008;49(11):4729–4726.) **B.** Illustration of dilated and hyalinized vessels, shown in **(A)**, as they are located between the Bruch's membrane and the RPE. Illustration by Mariana Ingolotti.

pressure, leading to protrusion of choroidal tissues through the RPE and Bruch's membrane. These cases resulted in a classic CNV pattern on FA.

Histologic studies, OCT, FA, and ICG angiography have all demonstrated distinctions between PCV and other forms of exudative AMD. Many of these studies have led researchers to conclude that PCV is caused by inner choroidal abnormalities, not CNV (1,40,51,60,73).

In 1999, OCT was first used to examine PCV. Iijima et al. (74) showed that cross-sectional OCT images of the retina accurately located polypoidal structures seen on ICG angiograms. Since then, other studies have proven that choroidal hyperreflectivity on OCT tomograms can accurately locate the choroidal abnormalities demonstrated on ICG and aid in the diagnosis of PCV (75,76), as shown in Figure 6.8. In particular, PED, branching vascular networks, and polypoidal lesions can be located (78,79). SD-OCT reveals the Bruch's membrane as a line of high reflectivity beneath vascular abnormalities caused by PCV (80). For some patients with PCV, a double-layer sign,

consisting of the RPE and another hyperreflective layer, is seen on OCT in the area of network vessels, particularly in eyes with serous retinal detachment (81). OCT scans have been used to compare the macular and choroidal thickness in PCV eyes to those with other forms of exudative AMD. Koizumi et al. (82) used spectral-domain OCT and found thickening in the choroid of PCV eyes. When subfoveal choroidal thickness measured greater than 300 μm, patients were 5.6 times more likely to have PCV. These results suggest that there may be significant structural differences in the PCV choroid as compared to typical exudative AMD, most likely stemming from dilation of choroidal vessels or choroidal vascular hyperpermeability as seen on ICG. Enhanced depth imaging OCT also demonstrated choroidal thickening in patients with PCV and showed that in exudative AMD, choroidal thinning was more likely to occur (83).

Due to the location of PCV lesions, below the RPE, FA is not useful as a diagnostic tool for PCV. A patient examined with FA only may appear to have classic CNV (84).

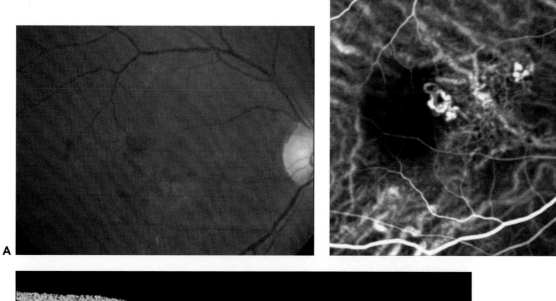

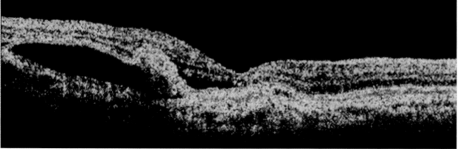

Figure 6.8 ■ PCV in a 75-year-old man. **A.** Funduscopic examination shows two reddish orange nodules (*arrows*) with serous PED. **B.** ICG shows branching vascular network (*arrowhead*) terminating in polypoidal lesions (*arrows*). Temporal polypoidal lesion accompanies serous PED. OCT images. **C.** show branching vascular network (*arrowheads*) terminating in polypoidal lesion (*arrows*). (Tsujikawa A, Sasahara M, Otani A, Gotoh N, et al. Pigment epithelial detachment in polypoidal choroidal vasculopathy. Am J Ophthalmol. 2007;143: 102–111.) (Ref. 77).

Although FA is rarely used to diagnose PCV, it can demonstrate differences between the two disease types. The late FA phase staining characteristic of CNV is not seen in PCV vascular lesions (60). Unlike other forms of exudative AMD, PCV is characterized in FA by low incidence of subretinal fibrovascular proliferation, slow progression of vascular abnormality, and minimal association with CNV (51).

ICG dye has a higher retention in the choroid than fluorescein dye, and it allows for better imaging of the choroidal circulation and greater understanding of disease pathology (48). ICG has shown that branching vascular networks give rise to polypoidal lesions (85). In 2005, Yuzawa et al. (60) used high-speed ICG to demonstrate that the branching vascular networks seen in most PCV eyes fill simultaneously with the surrounding choroidal arteries, with some vessels showing focal dilation, constriction, and tortuosity. These results led the research team to conclude that PCV is caused by inner choroidal vascular abnormalities, not CNV.

ICG conducted on PCV eyes has shown one significant difference from ICG conducted on eyes with other forms of exudative AMD. In PCV, a characteristic late phase geographic hyperfluorescence is seen on ICG (Fig. 6.9), occurring approximately 10 minutes after injection of the ICG dye. This was noted by Kang et al. (86) in a 2009 angiographic study. Angiography showed late-phase hyperfluorescence in 100% of eyes with PCV, but in other forms of exudative AMD, only 7.5% demonstrated this characteristic (87). Hyperfluorescence in late-phase ICG indicates greater vascular permeability in PCV than in other types of CNV. This vascular characteristic may lead to the PED often present in PCV eyes (48).

ICG allows for better imaging, which in turn can lead to better understanding of the nature of the disease, its potential causes, and earlier diagnosis. Distinguishing PCV from other similar diseases is necessary not only to determine the course of disease but also to choose the best treatment option.

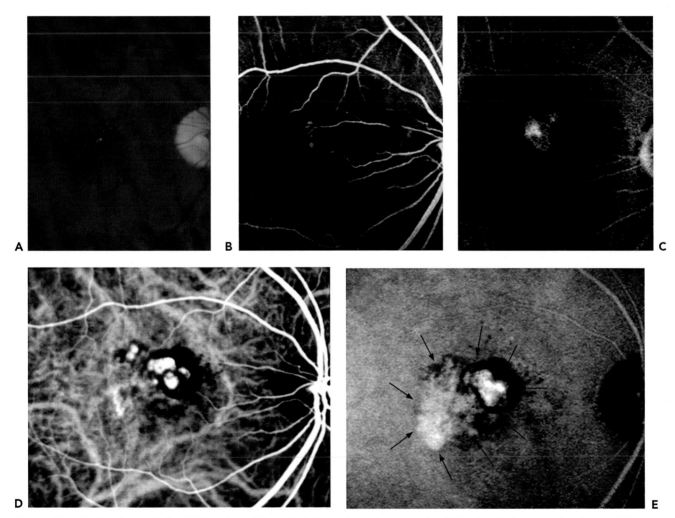

Figure 6.9 ■ Series demonstrating PCV as viewed through photography and angiography. **A.** Fundus photography showing exudation. **B.** Early-phase FA. **C.** Late-phase FA. **D.** Early-phase ICG indicates typical PCV. **E.** Late geographic hyperfluorescence (*black arrows*) in ICG. (Stangos A, Gandhi JS, Nair-Sahni J, Heimann H, et al. Polypoidal choroidal vasculopathy masquerading as neovascular age-related macular degeneration refractory to ranibizumab. Am J Opthalmol. 2010;150:666–673; Kang SW, Chung SE, Shin WJ, et al. Polypoidal choroidal vasculopathy and late geographic hyperfluorescence on ICG angiography. Br J Opthalmol. 2009;93:759–764.)

Given its relationship to type 1 CNV, the attempted treatments for PCV have mirrored those for CNV, but the two diseases have responded differently. Although ranibizumab and bevacizumab show good short-term results in reducing subretinal or intraretinal fluid in PCV, anti-VEGF treatments were not successful in reversing the choroidal vascular changes that are characteristic of the disease (87–89). This difference in treatment response may be due to the role VEGF plays within the diseased tissue. The exact role of VEGF in the pathogenesis of PCV is yet to be determined; however, current research indicates that the development of PCV stems from choroidal vascular abnormalities and is less dependent on VEGF pathways (46,48,64).

PDT was an early treatment for exudative AMD, and its efficacy in treating PCV has been evaluated in numerous clinical trials. Findings show that PDT for polypoidal lesions leads to improvement in the short term, but branching vascular networks do not respond to treatment; therefore, polypoidal lesions can reoccur (90–92). Combining PDT and anti-VEGF therapy has achieved stabilization of PCV lesions, decreased the size of PCV lesions, decreased macular thickness, and required fewer maintenance treatments of PDT (58,92). The diagnosis of PCV is not always segregated from type 1 to type 2 CNV (93). This overlap of presentations may explain why some PCV eyes respond well to treatment while others do not.

SUMMARY

The classification of exudative AMD has changed markedly since the imaging techniques OCT and ICG have joined FA as diagnostic standards. These tools have illuminated the various disease pathologies within exudative AMD and have allowed for the creation of a more accurate classification system. With current imaging tools, Gass's proposed location-based classification scheme has been realized. The inclusion of RAP and PCV expands the original Gass classification of exudative AMD from two to four types. Accurate classification of exudative AMD is not only significant for diagnostic accuracy but also necessary for predicting the course of the disease and evaluating treatment options. Although the same treatment options are available for all four types of exudative AMD, their response to treatment varies; therefore, accurate diagnosis is the first step in providing efficacious care.

REFERENCES

1. Sarks SH. Ageing and degeneration in the macular region: a clinico-pathological study. Br J Ophthalmol. 1976;60:324–340.

2. Bressler NM, Bressler SB, Fine SL. Age-related macular degeneration. Surv Ophthalmol. 1988;32:375–413.

3. West SK. Looking forward to 20/20: a focus on the epidemiology of eye diseases. Epidemiol Rev. 2007;22:64–70.

4. Green WR, Enger C. Age-related macular degeneration histopathologic studies. The 1992 Lorenz E. Zimmerman Lecture. Ophthalmology. 1993;100:1519–1535.

5. Thompson W. Classification of age-related macular degeneration. In: Alfaro DV, ed. Age-related macular degeneration: a comprehensive textbook. Philadelphia, PA: Lippincott Williams & Wilkins; 2006:44–52.

6. Gass JDM. Biomicroscopic and histopathologic considerations regarding the feasibility of surgical excision of subfoveal neovascular membranes. Am J Ophthalmol. 1994;118(3):285–298.

7. Glaussniklaus HE, Gass JDM. Clinicopathologic correlations of surgically excised Type 1 and Type 2 submacular choroidal neovascular membranes. Am J Ophthalmol. 1998;126(1):59–69.

8. Macular Photocoagulation Study Group. Laser photocoagulation of subfoveal neovascular lesion in age-related macular degeneration: results of a randomized clinical trial. Arch Ophthalmol. 1991;109:1220–1231.

9. Macular Photocoagulation Study Group. Occult choroidal neovascularization. Influence on visual outcome in patients with age-related macular degeneration. Arch Ophthalmol. 1996;114:400–412.

10. Freund KB, Zweifel SA, Engelbert M. Do we need a new classification for choroidal neovascularization in age-related macular degeneration? Retina. 2010;30(9):1333–1349.

11. Cohen SY, Creuzot-Garcher C, Darmon J, et al. Types of choroidal neovascularisation in newly diagnosed exudative age-related macular degeneration. Br J Ophthalmol. 2007;91:1173–1176.

12. Lafaut BA, Bartz-Schmidt KU, Vanden Broecke C, et al. Clinicopathological correlation in exudative age related macular degeneration: histological differentiation between classic and occult choroidal neovascularization. Br J Ophthalmol. 2000;84(3):239–243.

13. Obana A, Gohto Y, Matsumoto M, et al. Indocyanine green angiographic features prognostic of visual outcome in the natural course of patients with age related macular degeneration. Br J Ophthalmol. 1999;83(4):429–437.

14. Malamos P, Sacu S, Georgopoulos M, et al. Correlation of high-definition optical coherence tomography and fluorescein angiography imaging in neovascular macular degeneration. Invest Ophthalmol Vis Sci. 2009;50(7):4926–4933.

15. Haddad WM, Coscas G, Soubrane G. Eligibility for treatment and angiographic features at the early stage of exudative age related macular degeneration. Br J Ophthalmol. 2002;86(6):663–669.

16. Yannuzzi LA, Slakter JS, Sorenson JA, et al. Digital indocyanine green videoangiography and choroidal neovascularization. Retina. 1992;12(3):191–223.

17. Slakter JS, Yannuzzi LA, Sorensen JA, et al. A pilot study of indocyanine green videoangiography-guided laser photocoagulation of occult choroidal neovascularization in age-related macular degeneration. Ophthalmology. 1995;102(4):465–472.

18. Guyer DR, Yannuzzi LA, Slakter JS, et al. Classification of choroidal neovascularization by digital indocyanine green videoangiography. Ophthalmology. 1996;103(12):2054–2060.

19. Chang TS, Freund KB, de la Cruz Z, et al. Clinicopathologic correlation of choroidal neovascularization demonstrated by indocyanine green angiography in a patient with retention of good vision for almost four years. Retina. 1994;14(2):114–124.

20. Gass JDM. Stereoscopic atlas of macular disease: diagnosis and treatment. 3rd Ed. St. Louis, MO: Mosby; 1997.

21. MARINA Study Group. Ranibizumab for neovascular age-related macular degeneration. N Engl J Med. 2006;355(14):1419–1431.

22. ANCHOR Study Group. Ranibizumab versus Verteporfin for neovascular age-related macular degeneration. N Engl J Med. 2006;355(14):1432–1444.

23. Treatment of Age-Related Macular Degeneration with Photodynamic Therapy and Verteporfin in Photodynamic Therapy Study Groups. Effect of lesion size, visual acuity, and lesion composition on visual acuity change with and without Verteporfin therapy for choroidal neovascularization secondary to age-related macular degeneration: TAP and VIP report No.1. Am J Ophthalmol. 2003;136(3):407–418.

24. Grossniklaus HE, Green WR. Choroidal neovascularization. Am J Ophthalmol. 2004;137(3):496–503.

25. Engelbert M, Zweifel SA, Freund KB, et al. Long-term follow-up for type 1 (subretinal pigment epithelium) neovascularization using a modified treat and extend dosing regimen of intravitreal antivascular endothelial growth factor therapy. Retina. 2010;30(9):1368–1375.

26. Treatment of Age-Related Macular Degeneration with Photodynamic Therapy (Tap) Study Group. Photodynamic therapy of subfoveal choroidal neovascularization in age-related macular degeneration with verteporfin: one-year results of 2 randomized clinical trials—TAP report 1. Arch Ophthalmol. 1999;117(10):1329–1345.

27. Schneider U, Gelisken F, Inhoffen W. Natural course of occult choroidal neovascular in age-related macular degeneration: development of classic lesions in fluorescein angiography. Acta Ophthalmol Scand. 2005;83(2):141–147.

28. Shah AR, Del Priore LV. Natural history of predominantly classic, minimally classic, and occult subgroups in exudative age-related macular degeneration. Ophthalmology. 2009;116(10):1901–1907.

29. Spaide RF. Enhanced depth imaging optical coherence tomography of retinal pigment epithelial detachment in age-related macular degeneration. Am J Ophthalmol. 2009;147(4):644–652.

30. Chiang A, Chang LK, Sarraf D. Predictors of anti-VEGF associated retinal pigment epithelial tear using fluorescein angiography and optical coherence tomography analysis. Retina. 2008;28(9):1265–1269.

31. Sulzbacher F, Kiss C, Munk M, et al. Diagnostic evaluation of type 2 (classic) choroidal neovascularization: optical coherence tomography, indocyanine green angiography, and fluorescein angiography. Am J Ophthalmol. 2011;152:799–806.

32. Sadda SR, Liakopoulos S, Keane PA, et al. Relationship between angiographic and optical coherence tomographic (OCT) parameters for quantifying choroidal neovascular lesions. Graefes Arch Clin Exp Ophthalmol. 2010;248(2):175–184.

33. Witkin AJ, Vuong LN, Srinivasan VJ, et al. High-speed ultrahigh optical coherence tomography before and after ranibizumab for age-related macular degeneration. Ophthalmology. 2009;116(5):956–963.

34. Akagi-Kurashige Y, Tsujikawa A, Oishi A, et al. Relationship between retinal morphological findings and visual function in age-related macular degeneration. Graefes Arch Clin Exp Ophthalmol. 2012;250(8):1129–1136.

35. Ting TD, Oh M, Cox TA, et al. Decreased visual acuity associated with cystoid macular edema in neovascular age-related macular degeneration. Arch Ophthalmol. 2002;120:731–737.

36. Yannuzzi LA, Negrão S, Iida T, et al. Retinal angiomatous proliferation in age-related macular degeneration. Retina. 2001;21:416–434.

37. Freund KB, Ho IV, Barbazetto IA, et al. Type 3 neovascularization: the expanded spectrum of retinal angiomatous proliferation. Retina. 2008;28:201–211.

38. Hartnett ME, Weiter JJ, Gardts A. Classification of retinal pigment epithelial detachments associated with drusen. Graefes Arch Clin Exp Ophthalmol. 1992;230:11–19.

39. Kuhn D, Meunier I, Soubrane G, et al. Imaging of chorioretinal anastomosis in vascularized retinal pigment epithelium detachments. Arch Ophthalmol. 1995;113:1392–1398.

40. Yannuzzi LA, Wong DWK, Sforzolini BS, et al. Polypoidal choroidal vasculopathy and neovascularized age-related macular degeneration. Arch Ophthalmol. 1999;117:1503–1510.

41. Brancato R, Introini U, Pierro L, et al. Optical coherence tomography (OCT) angiomatous proliferation (RAP) in retinal. Eur J Ophthalmol. 2002;12:467–472.

42. Saito M, Shiragami CH, Shiraga F, et al. Comparison of intravitreal triamcinolone acetonide with photodynamic therapy and intravitreal bevacizumab with photodynamic therapy for retinal angiomatous proliferation. Am J Ophthalmol. 2010;149:472–481.

43. Saito M, Iida T, Kano M. Combined intravitreal ranibizumab and photodynamic therapy for retinal angiomatous proliferation. Am J Ophthalmol. 2012;153(3):504–514.

44. Bearelly S, Espinosa-Heidmann DG, Cousins SW. The role of dynamic indocyanine green angiography in the diagnosis and treatment of retinal angiomatous proliferation. Br J Ophthalmol. 2008;92:191–196.

45. Yannuzzi LA, Sorenson J, Spaide RF, et al. Idiopathic polypoidal choroidal vasculopathy. Retina. 1990;10:1–8.

46. Park DH, Kim IN. Asymptomatic extramacular abnormal choroidal lesions in eyes with macular polypoidal choroidal vasculopathy. Jpn J Ophthalmol. 2010;54:48–54.

47. Musashi K, Tsujikawa A, Hirami Y, et al. Microrips of the retinal pigment epithelium in polypoidal choroidal vasculopathy. 2007;143:883–885.

48. Imamura Y, Engelbert M, Iida T, et al. Polypoidal choroidal vasculopathy: a review. Surv Ophthalmol. 2010;55:501–515.

49. Ahuja R, Stanga P, Vingerling J, et al. Polypoidal choroidal vasculopathy in exudative and haemorrhagic pigment epithelial detachments. Br J Ophthalmol. 2000;84:479–484.

50. Stern RM, Zakov N, Zegarra H, et al. Multiple recurrent serosanguineous retinal pigment epithelial detachments in black women. Am J Ophthalmol. 1985;100:560–569.

51. Sho K, Takahashi K, Yamada II, et al. Polypoidal choroidal vasculopathy: incidence, demographic features, and clinical characteristics. Arch Ophthalmol. 2003;121:1392–1396.

52. Byeon SH, Lee SC, Oh HS, et al. Incidence and clinical patterns of polypoidal choroidal vasculopathy in Korean patients. Jpn J Ophthalmol. 2008;52:57–62.

53. Maruko I, Iida T, Saito M, et al. Clinical characteristics of exudative age-related macular degeneration in Japanese patients. Am J Ophthalmol. 2007;144:15–22.

54. Lafaut BA, Leys AM, Snyers B, et al. Polypoidal choroidal vasculopathy in caucasians. Graefes Arch Clin Exp Ophthalmol. 2000;238:752–759.

55. Scassellati-Sforzolini B, Mariotti C, Bryan R, et al. Polypoidal choroidal vasculopathy in Italy. Retina. 2001;21:121–125.

56. Lim TH, Laude A, Tan CSH. Polypoidal choroidal vasculopathy: an angiographic discussion. Eye. 2010;24:483–490.

57. Cackett P, Wong D, Yeo I. A classification system for polypoidal choroidal vasculopathy. Retina. 2009;29:187–191.

58. Uyama M, Wada M, Nagai Y, et al. Polypoidal choroidal vasculopathy: natural history. Am J Ophthalmol. 2002;133:639–648.

59. Lima L, Schubert C, Ferrara D, et al. Three major loci involved in age-related macular degeneration are also associated with polypoidal choroidal vasculopathy. Ophthalmology. 2010;117:1567–1570.

60. Yuzawa M, Mori R, Kawamura A. The origins of polypoidal choroidal vasculopathy. Br J Ophthalmol. 2005;89:602–607.

61. Sakurada Y, Kubota T, Imasawa M, et al. Role of complement factor H I62V and age-related maculopathy susceptibility 2 A69S variants in the clinical expression of polypoidal choroidal vasculopathy. Ophthalmology. 2011;118:1402–1407.

62. Sakurada Y, Kubota T, Imasawa M, et al. Angiographic lesion size associated with LOC387715 A69S genotype in subfoveal polypoidal choroidal vasculopathy. Retina. 2009;29:1522–1526.

63. Sakurada Y, Kubota T, Mabuchi F, et al. Association of LOC387715 A69S with vitreous hemorrhage in polypoidal choroidal vasculopathy. Am J Ophthalmol. 2007;145:1058–1062.

64. Nakajima M, Yuzawa M, Shimada H, et al. Correlation between indocyanine green angiographic findings and histopathology of polypoidal choroidal vasculopathy. Jpn J Ophthalmol. 2004;48:249–255.

65. Kuroiwa S, Tateiwa H, Hisatomi T, et al. Pathological features of surgically excised polypoidal choroidal vasculopathy membranes. Clin Exp Ophthalmol. 2004;32:297–302.

66. Okubo A, Ito M, Sameshima M, et al. Pulsatile blood flow in the polypoidal choroidal vasculopathy. Ophthalmology. 2005;112:1436–1441.

67. Akaza E, Matsumoto Y, Yuzawa M. Pulsation in polypoidal choroidal vasculopathy. Nippon Ganka Gakkai Zasshi. 2006;110:288–292.

68. Byeon SH, Lew YJ, Lee SC, et al. Clinical features and follow-up results of pulsating polypoidal choroidal vasculopathy treated with photodynamic therapy. Acta Ophthalmol. 2010;88:660–668.

69. Nakashizuka H, Mitsumata M, Okisaka S, et al. Clinicopathologic findings in polypoidal choroidal vasculopathy. IOVS. 2008;49(11):4729–4726.

70. Terasaki H, Miyake Y, Suzuki T, et al. Polypoidal choroidal vasculopathy treated with macular translocation: clinical pathological correlation. Br J Ophthalmol. 2002;86:321–327.

71. Lafaut BA, Aisenbrey S, Broecke C, et al. Polypoidal choroidal vasculopathy pattern in age-related macular degeneration. A clinicopathologic correlation. Retina. 2000;20:650–654.

72. Spaide RF, Leys A, Herrmann-Delemazure B, et al. Radiation-associated choroidal neovasculopathy. Ophthalmology. 1999;106:2254–2260.

73. Moorthy RS, Lyon AT, Rabb MF, et al. Idiopathic polypoidal choroidal vasculopathy of the macula. Ophthalmology. 1995;105:1380–1385.

74. Iijima H, Imai M, Gohdo T, et al. Optical coherence tomography of idiopathic polypoidal choroidal vasculopathy. Am J Ophthalmol. 1999;127:301–305.

75. Giovannini A, Amato GP, D'Altobrando E, et al. Optical coherence tomography (OCT) in idiopathic polypoidal choroidal vasculopathy (IPCV). Doc Ophthalmol. 1999;97:367–371.

76. Sa HS, Yoon Cho H, Woong Kang S. Optical coherence tomography of idiopathic polypoidal choroidal vasculopathy. Korean J Ophthalmol. 2005;29:275–280.

77. Tsujikawa A, Sasahara M, Otani A, et al. Pigment epithelial detachment in polypoidal choroidal vasculopathy. Am J Ophthalmol. 2007;143:102–111.

78. Iijima H, Iida T, Imai M, et al. Optical coherence tomography of orange-red subretinal lesions in eyes with idiopathic polypoidal choroidal vasculopathy. Am J Ophthalmol. 2000;129:21–26.

79. Kameda T, Tsujikawa A, Otani A, et al. Polypoidal choroidal vasculopathy examined with en face optical coherence tomography. Clin Exp Ophthalmol. 2007;35:596–601.

80. Ojima Y, Hangai M, Sakamoto A, et al. Improved visualization of polypoidal choroidal vascularization. Retina. 2009;29:52–59.

81. Sato T, Kishi S, Watanabe G, et al. Tomographic features of branching vascular networks in polypoidal choroidal vasculopathy. Retina. 2007;27:589–594.

82. Koizumi H, Yamagishi T, Yamazaki T, et al. Subfoveal choroidal thickness in typical age-related macular degeneration and polypoidal choroidal vasculopathy. Graefes Arch Clin Exp Ophthalmol. 2011;249:1123–1128.

83. Chung SE, Kang SW, Lee JH, et al. Choroidal thickness in polypoidal choroidal vasculopathy and exudative age-related macular degeneration. Ophthalmology. 2011;118:840–845.

84. Mori F, Eguchi S. Polypoidal choroidal vasculopathy: from the viewpoint of an Asian ophthalmologist. Br J Ophthalmol. 2007;91:1104–1105.

85. Zuo CG, Wen F, Huang SZ, et al. Angiographic leakage of polypoidal choroidal vasculopathy on indocyanine angiography. Clin Med J. 2010;123(12):1548–1552.

86. Kang SW, Chung SE, Shin WJ, et al. Polypoidal choroidal vasculopathy and late geographic hyperfluorescence on indocyanine green angiography. Br J Ophthalmol. 2009;93:759–764.

87. Stangos A, Gandhi JS, Nair-Sahni J, et al. Polypoidal choroidal vasculopathy masquerading as neovascular age-related macular degeneration refractory to ranibizumab. Am J Ophthalmol. 2010;150:666–673.

88. Matsumiya W, Honda S, Bessho H, et al. Early responses to intravitreal ranibizumab in typical neovascular age-related macular degeneration and polypoidal choroidal vasculopathy. J Ophthalmol. 2011;150: 674–682.

89. Hikichi T, Ohtsuka H, Higuchi M, et al. Improvement of angiographic findings of polypoidal choroidal vasculopathy after intravitreal injection of ranibizumab monthly for 3 months. Am J Ophthalmol. 2010;150:675–682.

90. Otani A, Sasahara M, Yodoi Y, et al. Indocyanine green angiography: guided photodynamic therapy for polypoidal choroidal vasculopathy. Am J Ophthalmol. 2007;144:7–14.

91. Wakabayashi T, Gomi F, Sawa M, et al. Marked vascular changes of polypoidal choroidal vasculopathy after photodynamic therapy. Br J Ophthalmol. 2008;92:936–940.

92. Akaza E, Yuzawa M, Mori R. Three-year follow-up results of photodynamic therapy for polypoidal choroidal vasculopathy. Jpn J Ophthalmol. 2011;55:39–44.

93. Tomohiro I. Polypoidal choroidal vasculopathy with an appearance similar to classic choroidal neovascularisation on fluorescein angiography. Br J Ophthalmol. 2007;91:1103–1104.

7

POLYPOIDAL CHOROIDAL VASCULOPATHY

GISELA BARCAT ANGELELLI • D. VIRGIL ALFARO III
LAWRENCE YANNUZZI • RICHARD J. ANTCLIFF

■ INTRODUCTION HISTORY

Polypoidal choroidal vasculopathy (PCV) is a distinct clinical entity characterized by a branching choroidal vascular network with polypoidal vascular dilations at the border of that network (1).

It was first described by Yannuzzi et al. (2) as a variant of choroidal neovascularization (CNV) in African American women in the peripapillary area, and they proposed the term "idiopathic polypoidal choroidal vasculopathy."

Kleiner et al. (3) later described a similar group of patients in a presentation entitled "Posterior Uveal Bleeding Syndrome."

Subsequently Stern et al. (4) described recurrent, multiple, bilateral, asymmetric, serosanguineous retinal pigment epithelium (RPE) detachments in a group of black women.

Yannuzzi et al. described these vessels as a distinct abnormality of the choroidal vasculature with two demonstrable components: (i) dilated and branching inner choroidal vessels, and (ii) terminal reddish-orange, spheroid aneurysmal-like, definitions which were called "polyp-like" (1).

This new clinical description led to Yannuzzi and collaborators dropping the word "idiopathic" and introducing the term polypoidal choroidal vasculopathy or PCV in 1990 (1).

Since then, with the advent of diagnostic techniques, such as indocyanine green angiography (ICGA), the spectrum

of the vasculopathy has been better illustrated by the longer wavelengths used to excite the indocyanine molecule, providing a more detailed representation of choroidal circulation (5).

Knowledge and understanding of PCV has increased over the last two decades, but there are still some pathogenic mechanisms that need further study.

This chapter focuses on providing a guide to clinical manifestations, diagnosis, and treatment strategies for patients with PCV based on the findings of clinical trials.

■ EPIDEMIOLOGY

In pigmented races, such as African Americans and Asians, PCV is the main vascular component of neovascular maculopathies.

Also known to occur in white-race patients with or without concomitant drusen, this form of neovascularization is characteristically distributed from the peripapillary area to the peripheral fundus.

The age of diagnosis can range from the 20s to the 80s, but PCV is most commonly diagnosed between 60 and 70 years of age (6).

In Asian races, PCV is the most common form of macular disease in adults and elderly people (7,8), including Korean (9) (mean age 64.6 years), Chinese (10) (mean age 65.4 years), and Japanese (11) people (mean age 72.8 years).

Initially PCV had been thought to be a condition exclusively found in women (4). Subsequent studies have shown that while there is a female preponderance in Caucasian races (75%), in Asian races there is a male preponderance (71%).

PCV can affect both eyes, having a considerable likelihood of developing lesions in a fellow eye. Several studies in Asian and European populations showed that the incidence of bilateral lesions is 24.1% in Koreans (9), 18.4% in Japanese (11), 24.7% (12) in Chinese (10), and 25% in Europeans (13).

The typical soft drusen of age-related macular degeneration (AMD) are not usually present particularly in highly pigmented individuals, but they may be seen in white patients. Furthermore, their distribution is generally in the central macula area in highly pigmented individuals, while Caucasian patients more typically have involvement in the peripapillary area.

Yannuzzi et al. (14) showed that drusen were observed in 63 (70%) of 90 fellow eyes with unilateral macular degeneration compared with only one (16.7%) of six fellow eyes with polypoidal CNV. Among Japanese patients with PCV, 23% showed soft drusen in the central macula in conjunction with the polypoidal vascular abnormality (15).

The distribution of the lesions also appears to be different in pigmented and Caucasian races. While in African Americans and Asians the lesions are generally in the macular area, in Caucasians these lesions are more typically located in the peripapillary area (13).

It is unclear what the reasons for these differences are, but evidence suggests that susceptibility genes for PCV may be different between pigmented races and white patients (13,16,17).

GENETICS AND BIOMARKERS

Genetic studies suggest that PCV is a type of CNV. HTRA1 is a membrane serine peptidase 1 found to be associated with both neovascular AMD (12,18) and PCV (19–21).

This gene is thought to regulate degradation of extracellular matrix proteoglycan. Overexpression of HTRA1 caused by a single-nucleotide mutation may alter the integrity of Bruch's membrane, and facilitate the expansion of abnormal choroidal capillaries (20).

Furthermore, both in Asian and white populations, PCV has been shown to share certain risk and protective alleles related to the complement system. Polymorphism for genes of complement factor H (CFH), complement component 2, and factor B were investigated in PCV, and a significant association was noted with CFH variants rs3753394 and rs800292 (6,22).

On the other hand, the Y204H variant of CFH (rs1061170) and the BF and C2 variants were not significantly associated with PCV (23).

Coding variant I62V in the CFH gene (24) and the variants of ARMS2 (LOC387715), a gene coding mitochondrial

protein in photoreceptors (25,26), were found to be associated in Japanese patients with PCV (19).

Another study using a Japanese population showed that there was no significant difference in the incidence of CFH Y402H and HTRA rs11200638 between eyes with typical exudative AMD and with PCV (27).

Recent genetic studies have demonstrated an association between genotype and outcomes in the treatment of PCV. Polyp regression and resolution of leakage were found to be significantly better in particular genotypes of the LOC387715 and HTRA1 genes following combination therapy with verteporfin PDT and bevacizumab (28,29).

No specific serum biomarker for PCV has been identified yet (6,22).

CLINICAL MANIFESTATIONS

The principal clinical manifestations of PCV are seen in the posterior segment. The presence of orange-red nodule–like structures beneath the RPE associated with an adjacent serous pigment epithelial detachment or overlying neurosensory detachment (Fig. 7.1A), subretinal hemorrhage (Fig. 7.1B), and lipid exudates (Fig. 7.1C) is considered the clinical hallmark of PCV. In some patients, progressive subretinal fibrosis and atrophic scarring can be observed (Fig. 7.1D).

PCV has been classified clinically (30) as (i) quiescent, polyps in the absence of subretinal or intraretinal fluid or hemorrhage; (ii) exudative, exudation without hemorrhage, which includes variously neurosensory retinal thickening, neurosensory detachment, PED, and subretinal lipid exudation; and (iii) hemorrhagic, any subretinal or sub-RPE hemorrhage with or without other exudative characteristics. This clinical classification described the primary features of the disease, but the evidence regarding its correlation with prognosis or treatment selection is limited.

The typical manifestations in a patient who is symptomatic for less than 3 months are extensive subretinal exudation and bleeding with minimal cystic change in the retina and a surprisingly good visual acuity (VA). This discrepancy between the severity of the serosanguineous detachments and good visual acuity is best explained by the minimal intraretinal changes. For patients with symptoms longer than 3 months, there are considerable lipid depositions from protein leakage from active aneurysmal elements in the polypoidal vascular abnormalities (6) (Fig. 7.1C).

The morphology of PCV can be distributed into three groups (i) single polyp (Fig. 7.2A); (ii) cluster: more than two polyps in a group (Fig. 7.2B); and (iii) string: three or more polyps in a line (Fig. 7.2C).

Cackett et al. (31) found cluster formation in 66.7% of the cases, single in 27.5%, and string in 5.8% in a retrospective study of 123 patients.

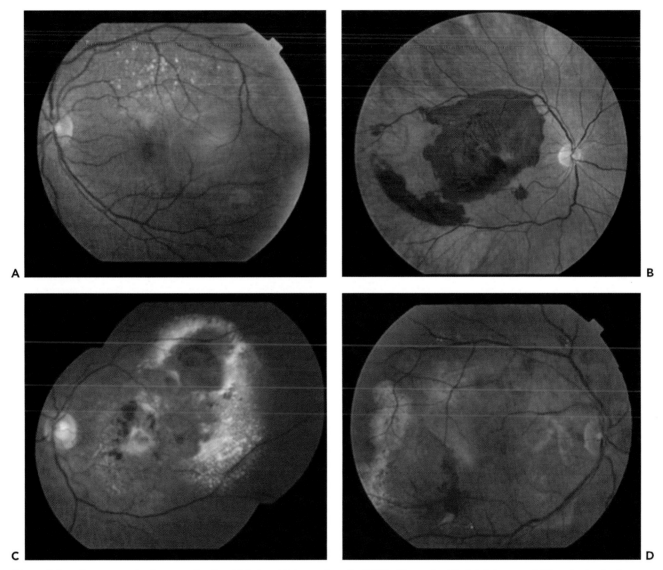

Figure 7.1 ■ Representative images of polypoidal choroidal vasculopathy (PCV). Pigment epithelial detachment **(A)** and subretinal hemorrhage **(B)** are common manifestations. **C.** Subretinal lipid is often observed. **D.** In some patients, progressive subretinal fibrosis can be observed. (Reprinted from Imamura Y, Engelbert M, Iida T, et al. Polypoidal choroidal vasculopathy: a review. Surv Ophthalmol. 2010;55(6):501–515. doi: 10.1016/j.survophthal.2010.03.004. Epub 2010 Sep 20, with permission.)

Uyama et al. (32) found that PCV lesions resembling a cluster of grapes had marked bleeding and leakage and high risk of severe visual loss.

It therefore seems that clusters are associated with an increased frequency of massive hemorrhage resulting in poorer visual outcomes.

NATURAL HISTORY OF THE DISEASE

The natural history of PCV depends on factors including location (peripapillary vs. macular), size of the lesion, and associated bleeding and exudation—which may resolve or progress, sometimes to extensive subretinal fibrosis. The evolution of this condition is probably heavily influenced by the racial background and individual genetic makeup. In Japanese patients, PCV is a chronic disease with a variable course. The risk factors seen in CNV secondary to AMD, including soft confluent drusen and focal hyperpigmentation, are not notable findings in patients with PCV.

Despite having recurrent leakage and bleeding, not all patients develop disciform scars, and others may retain useful vision for years. Some patients, however, experience severe visual loss from a combination of extensive bleeding, exudation, and macular damage.

In a study of the natural history of patients with PCV, Uyama et al. (32) reported that half of the study eyes had

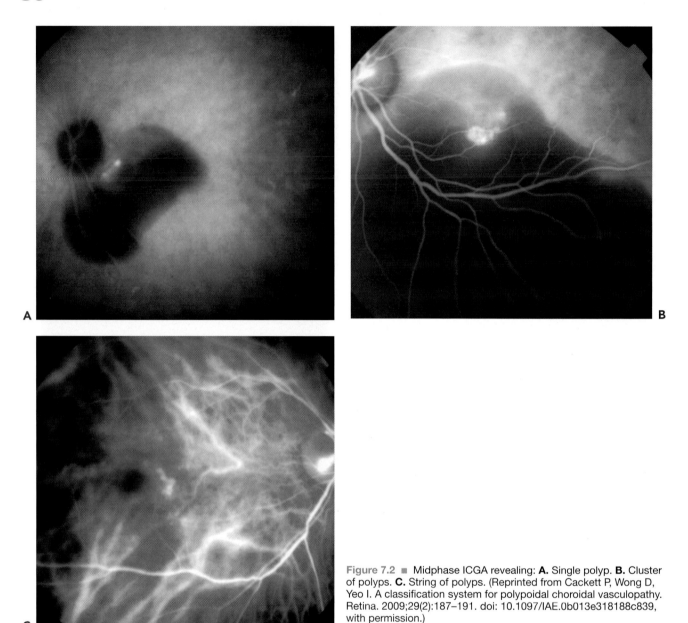

Figure 7.2 ■ Midphase ICGA revealing: **A.** Single polyp. **B.** Cluster of polyps. **C.** String of polyps. (Reprinted from Cackett P, Wong D, Yeo I. A classification system for polypoidal choroidal vasculopathy. Retina. 2009;29(2):187–191. doi: 10.1097/IAE.0b013e318188c839, with permission.)

hemorrhagic episodes, recurrent leakage, or severe RPE atrophy after a long follow-up period (24–54 months) (33). Following the spontaneous resolution of the acute serosanguineous complications, there may be signs of subretinal fibrosis, pigment epithelial hyperplasia, and atrophic degeneration (34) (Fig. 7.1D). The incidence of sub-RPE hemorrhage or subretinal hemorrhage described in patients with PCV is high (30%–64%) (35,36).

On the other hand, Uyama et al. (32) described stabilization of visual acuity and regression of neovascular lesion with good visual prognosis in 50% of eyes with polypoidal CNV in the posterior pole that were followed for at least 2 years.

PCV has been described in association with other macular abnormalities, such as central serous chorioretinopathy (37,38), typical neovascular (type 1 or 2) AMD (39), sickle

cell retinopathy (40), melanocytoma of the optic nerve (41), circumscribed choroidal hemangioma (42), tilted disk syndrome (43), pathological myopia (43), choroidal osteoma (44), and angioid streaks in pseudoxanthoma elasticum (45).

DIAGNOSIS

Imaging such as fluorescein angiography (FA), ICGA, and high-resolution optical coherence tomography (OCT) is important for the diagnosis of PCV.

The EVEREST study was the first to include a set of well-defined criteria for PCV diagnosis.

This study defined PCV as the presence of early subretinal focal ICGA hyperfluorescence (appearing within the first 6 minutes after injection of indocyanine green) and in addition, at least one of the following angiographic or clinical criteria: (i) association with a branching vascular network (BVN) seen in ICGA; (ii) presence of pulsatile polyp seen in dynamic ICGA; (iii) nodular appearance when viewed stereoscopically; (iv) presence of hypofluorescent halo (in first 6 minutes); (v) orange subretinal nodules in stereoscopic color fundus photograph (polyp corresponding to ICGA lesions); or (vi) association with massive submacular hemorrhage (defined as size of hemorrhage of at least 4 disk areas) (33).

Fundus Autofluorescence

Fundus autofluorescence (FAF) photography is used to visualize lipofuscin, which accumulates in RPE and provides information about RPE metabolism and function.

Yamagishi et al. (46), studied the incidence and distribution of hypoautofluorescence comparing Japanese patients with PCV and typical neovascular AMD.

In affected eyes with PCV, the sites of the neovascular lesions showed two distinct FAF patterns: (i) confluent hypoautofluorescence at the polypoidal lesions and (ii) granular hypoautofluorescence at the branching choroidal vascular networks.

Confluent hypoautofluorescence was defined as a manifestation of a homogeneous lack of autofluorescence that was well demarcated and clearly distinguishable from the other adjacent lesions. Granular hypoautofluorescence was defined as a heterogeneous mixed finding of the hypoautofluorescence lesion at the various levels.

The confluent hypoautofluorescence pattern was seen in 80.4% eyes with PCV, while it was seen in no eyes with AMD, suggesting that it is a pattern exclusively of PCV. The granular hypoautofluorescence pattern was seen in both PCV (98.9%) and AMD (87.1%) (46).

Overall the incidence of hypoautofluorescence was higher in the PCV group.

Fluorescein Angiography

The difficulty in precisely delineating structures under the RPE has limited the usefulness of FA in studying and diagnosing the disease.

However, typical findings show mottled hyperfluorescence in the early stage of the angiogram with late staining of the polyps (47), associated with serous or serosanguineous pigment epithelial detachment (PED). Serous PED in the early arteriovenous phase of the angiogram demonstrates progressive, uniform hyperfluorescence with late, intense pooling of fluorescein, while hemorrhagic PED blocks fluorescence and the normal choroid. Alternatively, PCV can be obscured by greater fluorescence from staining serous PED or blocked by serosanguineous PED, making it impossible to determine the exact boundary of the lesion.

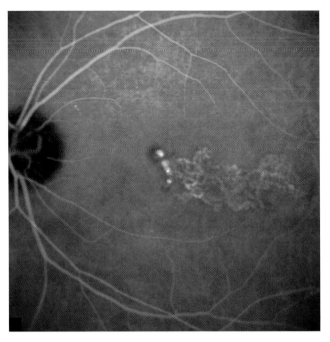

Figure 7.3 ■ ICGA corresponding with large BVN ending in string polypoidal lesion. Identification of a BVN is not an absolute requirement for a diagnosis of PCV because it is not always clearly visualized by ICGA. (Reprinted from Koh AH, et al. Polypoidal choroidal vasculopathy: evidence-based guidelines for clinical diagnosis and treatment. Retina. 2013;33(4):686–716. doi: 10.1097/IAE.0b013e3182852446, with permission.)

This serosanguineous detachment may or may not be vascularized (48).

In many clinical trials, FA is performed to determine CNV activity.

FA, however, cannot show BVN with terminating polyps related to PCV, whereas they can be visualized with ICGA, which provides a more reliable diagnostic tool than conventional FA (49) (Fig. 7.3).

Indocyanine Green Angiography

ICGA is essential for a definitive diagnosis of PCV (1,6,50). The longer wavelengths used in this imaging system penetrate more deeply. The ICG molecule is stimulated by the absorption of infrared light in the range from 790 to 805 nm. The RPE and the choroid absorbs up to 75% of the blue-green light used for FA, but only up to 38% of the near infrared light used for ICG. The higher transmittance of light above 800 nm and the strong intravascular retention of the ICG molecule allow better resolution of the choroidal vasculature.

PCV is defined as the presence of single or multiple focal areas of hyperfluorescence arising from the choroidal circulation within the first 6 minutes after injection of indocyanine green, with or without an associated BVN.

The recommended time window in which the polyps of PCV appear after injection of indocyanine green is given as 6 minutes, as used by the EVEREST trial.

In the early phases of the ICGA, dye is visible within the vascular network of the PCV lesion, before it is visible in the retinal vessels. Several seconds after the network vessels are seen to fill with dye, small hyperfluorescent "polyps" became visible. These vascular polypoidal structures usually occur at the termini of vessels at the edge of the vascular network. The area within and immediately surrounding the network remains hypofluorescent compared to the uninvolved choroid. The polypoidal structures can show leakage of ICG dye, with the dye collecting initially in the core of the polypoidal structure. In the late phase, the core of the polypoidal structure becomes relatively hypofluorescent because of the washout of the dye, producing a ring-like staining of the polyps. This finding may help in distinguishing between the polyps that are actively leaking, which will become visible as a ring of hyperfluorescence, and those that are not, which will appear as hypofluorescent rings (51).

Lesion size seems to influence the fluorescence pattern. Lesions smaller than half a disk diameter appear to have intense uniform fluorescence, whereas internal details seem to be visible in larger polypoidal lesions, suggesting the presence of an internal architecture.

The appearance of vessels in PCV often depend on their location in the fundus. In juxtapapillary lesions, the vascular channels may follow a radial, arching pattern and may be interconnected with smaller spanning branches more evident and numerous at the edges of the lesion. When PCV is limited to the macula, a vascular network often follows an oval distribution. With macular and juxtapapillary involvement, vessels in the network usually course in an irregular latticework and do not follow the lobular pattern of choroidal vasculature.

Because the choriocapillaris cannot be clearly visualized with ICGA, the precise location of the polypoidal structures in relation to the choriocapillaris cannot be stated with certainty.

Optical Coherence Tomography

Higher-resolution OCT images provide considerably better delineation of sub-RPE lesions (15,52).

Both time- and spectral-domain OCT (SD-OCT) have confirmed that pathologic vascular lesions of PCV are located beneath the RPE. They appear on OCT scans as abnormalities in the contour of the highly reflective line representing the RPE (53,54). The polypoidal lesions appear as sharp protrusions of the RPE with moderate reflectivity beneath the RPE line (27,55).

Using SD-OCT, moderate reflectivity has been noted in the space between undulating RPE and straight Bruch's membrane lines. These areas seem to correspond with BVN.

In conventional OCT scans, BVN were represented by one or two highly reflective blurred lines, where the outer reflective layer is believed to represent the inner boundary of the Bruch's membrane–choriocapillaris complex.

In some of these eyes, cross-sectional images through the PCV lesions resembled the appearance of "pearls on a string" as described by Freund et al. (56), however, polyp structures are not always visible by OCT (6) (Fig. 7.4A and B).

The PCV lesions can be found both at the margin and within the associated type 1 neovascular lesions (6). The PCV lesions are localized to just below the hyperreflective RPE band near the anterior surface of the associated type 1 neovascular tissue (56).

Sato et al. (57) described the presence of these two highly reflective layers (the RPE and a sub-RPE layer) as the "double-layer sign" within the area of the network of vessels in PCV (Fig. 7.4C).

They hypothesized that the "double-layer" sign occurs when the RPE and its basement membrane ("inner reflective layer") become separated from the remainder of Bruch's membrane and the inner choroid ("outer reflective layer") by fluid.

Abe et al. (58) demonstrated that the OCT "double-layer" sign is most prominent in areas where ICGA shows "abnormal blood vessel networks" in association with larger PCV lesions.

Khan et al. (56) described a "triple-layer sign" when part of the Bruch's membrane had detached from the underlying choroid (Fig. 7.4D); this separation creates a second hyporeflective space beneath the elevated remainder of Bruch's membrane, suggesting that the polyps and BVN are more adherent to the basal surface of the RPE than to the underlying choroid, which supports the hypothesis that PCV represents a form of neovascular tissue rather than alterations of the native choroidal vasculature.

Microrips of RPE and RPE tears may occur at the margin of the serosanguineous PED (59). However, they often disappear spontaneously (60).

■ TREATMENT

PCV may be considered as active if there is clinical OCT or FA evidence of any one of the following that is attributable to PCV: Vision loss ≥5 letters (Early Treatment Diabetic Retinopathy Study) or equivalent, subretinal fluid or intraretinal fluid, PED, subretinal or sub-RPE hemorrhage, and fluorescein leakage. Active PCV can be symptomatic or asymptomatic: treatment should be initiated for active and symptomatic PCV and can be considered for active, asymptomatic PCV (30).

Photocoagulation

Direct thermal laser photocoagulation still has a role in the treatment of extrafoveal polyps. The ICGA-guided thermal laser photocoagulation may be considered for extrafoveal polyps. However, direct thermal laser photocoagulation is not recommended for the initial therapy of active juxtafoveal or subfoveal PCV given the destructive nature of this treatment modality (30).

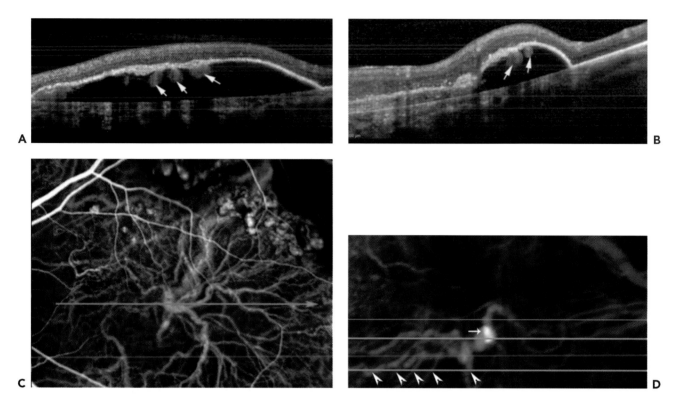

Figure 7.4 ■ **A, B.** SD-OCT B-scan shows multiple polyps structures adherent to the undersurface of a RPE detachment (*arrows*) creating "pearls on a string." **C.** SD-OCT B-scan shows PCV lesions (*arrows*) located between the RPE and Bruch's membrane creating a "double-layer sign." **D.** SD-OCT B-scan shows multiple PCV lesions adherent to the undersurface of a RPE detachment. The *arrow* shows part of the Bruch's membrane that remains attached to the undersurface of the PCV lesions, creating a "triple-layer sign." (Reprinted from Khan S, Engelbert M, Imamura Y, et al. Polypoidal choroidal vasculopathy: simultaneous indocyanine green angiography and eye-tracked spectral domain optical coherence tomography findings. Retina. 2012;32(6):1057–1068. doi: 10.1097/IAE.0b013e31823beb14, with permission.)

In 2003, Yuzawa et al. (61) noted that total lesion ablation provided better outcomes compared with laser ablation of the vascular polyps alone. They evaluated the efficacy of photocoagulation in 47 eyes of PCV. Of the 10 eyes undergoing photocoagulation of whole lesions, 9 showed absorption of exudate and/or blood and maintained or improved visual acuity. However, of the 37 eyes undergoing laser photocoagulation of only the polypoidal component, 20 (54%) showed decreased visual acuity because of recurrent or persistent exudation or due to foveal atrophy.

They concluded that photocoagulation is recommended only if it is feasible to treat the entire polypoidal lesion.

Photodynamic therapy

Photodynamic therapy (PDT) is currently the most successful treatment reported.

In the EVEREST trial, 61 Asian patients with symptomatic PCV were treated with verteporfin PDT monotherapy, 0.5 mg ranibizumab monotherapy, or a combination of these treatments. The primary endpoint was the proportion of patients with ICGA-assessed complete regression of polyps at 6th month. The secondary endpoints included mean change in best-corrected visual acuity (BCVA) at 6th month and safety.

PDT was administered according to the treatment protocol of the Age-Related Macular Degeneration with Photodynamic Therapy study (62); patients were infused with verteporfin (6 mg/m^2), and 15 minutes after the start of infusion, PDT at standard fluence (light dose, 50 J/cm^2; dose rate, 600 mW/cm^2; wavelength, 689 nm) was applied to the study eye for 83 seconds. The laser spot size was derived by adding 1,000 mm to the greatest linear dimension. Thus, both BVN and polyps were included in the verteporfin PDT treatment area.

They showed that at 6 months, verteporfin combined with ranibizumab or alone was superior to ranibizumab monotherapy achieving complete polyp regression (77.8%, 71.4%, and 28.6%, respectively). Also, they showed that mean change (±standard deviation) in best-corrected visual acuity was 10.9 (±10.9) for the verteporfin PDT + ranibizumab group, 7.5 (±10.6) for verteporfin PDT alone, and 9.2 (±12.4) for ranibizumab monotherapy. They concluded that verteporfin PDT combined with ranibizumab 0.5 mg or alone were superior to ranibizumab monotherapy in achieving complete regression of polyps. Because the study was not designed to demonstrate a difference between verteporfin PDT plus ranibizumab combination therapy and verteporfin PDT monotherapy, the evidence supports the use of either therapy (30).

Yannuzzi et al. (48) evaluated the efficacy of "selective PDT" with ICGA-guided PDT with verteporfin for PCV.

They used ICGA because it provides improved imaging of the true extent of the PCV lesion without obscuration by blood or leakage at the site of serous pigment epithelial elevations. This method avoided treating the nonvascular components of the lesion mandated by standard FA-based techniques. In addition, the smaller PDT spot size minimized the possibility of choroidal ischemic changes and, therefore, stimulation of vascular endothelial growth factor (VEGF) (63–66).

They applied standard PDT with verteporfin with a spot size of 200 μm around the active component adding 400 μm to the greatest linear dimension. They avoided the fovea if it was not affected.

PDT with verteporfin was applied using the same parameters as for the treatment of neovascular AMD in the Treatment of Age-Related Macular Degeneration with Photodynamic Therapy Study (62). Retreatment was performed under ICGA guidance when leakage was present in FA.

Their outcomes were improvement of vision ≥3 ETDRS lines in 15 eyes (50%), decrease of vision with a loss of ≥3 ETDRS lines in 6 eyes (20%), and stable vision in 9 eyes (30%).

They suggested that the better outcomes were due to reducing collateral choroidal damage and secondary up-regulation of VEGF, which may predispose to subsequent recurrent neovascularization (48,63).

Among described complications with PDT, subretinal hemorrhage is the most common (35,67).

Occasionally it can be massive and could lead to vitreous hemorrhage and a poor visual prognosis (35,53,62).

Massive subretinal hemorrhage has been treated by pars plana vitrectomy, with poor visual outcomes (53).

Recurrent bullous detachment and chorioretinal anastomosis have been reported (68,69), and PDT is also known to cause choroidal infarction and ischemia (64).

Retinal function as assessed by multifocal electroretinograms can be disturbed by PDT; however, retinal sensitivity in the macular area of eyes with subfoveal PCV improved shortly after PDT (70).

Intravitreal bevacizumab or ranibizumab for PCV

Although PCV appears likely to be refractory to anti-VEGF therapy, the exact role of VEGF in the pathogenesis of PCV remains to be elucidated. The first findings in surgical specimens of PCV demonstrated positive immunohistochemical staining for VEGF in the RPE and vascular endothelial cells. However, recent studies showed negative immunostaining in vascular cells for VEGF (71).

In another study, Tong et al. (72) found that the VEGF levels in aqueous humor in PCV were significantly lower than those in neovascular AMD.

Moreover, recent studies analyzing PCV lesions refractory to anti-VEGF therapy suggest that the development of PCV is less likely to be dependent on a VEGF-related pathway than is more typical type 1 neovascularization (73).

Available data indicate that anti-VEGF agents may reduce leakage associated with PCV but are ineffective for complete regression of the polypoidal dilatations (74,75).

A recent report showed that ranibizumab leads to stabilization of vision, resolution of subretinal hemorrhage, and decrease in the PCV-associated macular edema. However, polypoidal complexes decreased in only 33% of the patients (76).

In the EVEREST study ranibizumab monotherapy group, the visual acuity improved in spite of the presence of polyps. This finding may be attributed to the antipermeability effects of ranibizumab, thereby resolving retinal thickening and exudate accumulation. These findings are consistent with those reported earlier with other anti-VEGF therapies.

Cho et al. (77) compared the effectiveness of intravitreal injection of bevacizumab and ranibizumab in 121 patients with PCV. Patients received three or more injections of 1.25 mg intravitreal bevacizumab, or 0.5 mg intravitreal ranibizumab, and outcomes were assessed after 12 months. They found no significant differences between both study groups in BCVA outcomes or central foveal thickness improvement. Polyp regression was also similar in both groups, with a regression rate of 24% in bevacizumab patients and 23% in the ranibizumab group.

There are no currently published studies comparing aflibercept (Eylea) with ranibizumab or bevacizumab.

Combination therapy

It is well known that PDT induced up-regulation of VEGF. Therefore, treatment with both PDT, to resolve the polypoidal lesions, and anti-VEGF agents, to control up-regulation of VEGF, may be a reasonable strategy to maintain or improve the visual acuity and the anatomic changes in patients with PCV.

In the EVEREST study, the results showed the superior efficacy of intravitreal ranibizumab and PDT in achieving complete regression of polypoidal lesions (primary outcome), and BCVA (secondary outcomes).

Saito et al. (78) reported the efficacy of ranibizumab combined with PDT for patients with PCV for improving visual acuity and decreasing retinal and choroidal thickness without adverse events over 12 months. Recently, Ruamviboonsuk et al. (79) also reported the efficacy of combination therapy in 12 patients with PCV.

The ideal interval between intravitreal injection of anti-VEGF agents and PDT is controversial. Saito and collaborators administered PDT 1 or 2 days after intravitreal ranibizumab injection. Sato et al. (80) administered PDT 7 days after intravitreal bevacizumab, whereas Gomi et al. (81) administered PDT 1 day after intravitreal bevacizumab.

Currently, several groups have started to investigate combination therapy with PDT.

ASSESSMENTS AND RETREATMENT

Efficacy assessments include the evaluation of anatomical endpoints (ICGA-assessed polyp regression based on polyp area and total lesion area, OCT-measured CRT, leakage assessed by FA) and functional changes (assessed BCVA).

In the EVEREST Study, ICGA was performed at baseline and at months 3, 4, 5, and 6 to evaluate the polyp area. The researchers measured the area of the best-fit circles around all individual polyps excluding the hypofluorescent halo.

Patients were placed into one of four groups based on the polyp regression seen on ICGA: (i) Complete regression: no polyps seen on the imaging; (ii) partial regression: >10% decrease in polyp area compared with screening; (iii) no change: ≤10% change of polyp area compared with screening; and (iv) increase: >10% increase in polyp area compared with screening.

Immediately after the completion of ICGA, FA was performed through dilated pupils to assess presence of leakage and to obtain fundus photographs at baseline and at months 3, 4, 5, and 6. Changes in CRT were determined by OCT measurements at baseline and at months 1 to 6 (33).

Patients with partial or no polyp regression after the initial 3 months were retreated with their assigned therapy. Patients with complete polyp regression by ICGA and leakage on FA were retreated with verteporfin PDT (or sham), and those with a decrease in BCVA of ≥5 letters were retreated with ranibizumab (or sham) (33).

We would suggest a protocol similar to that of Saito et al. (78) of follow-up examinations including evaluation of OCT every month, FA and ICGA every 3 months until the polypoidal lesions show complete regression, and then treatment restart if new exudative changes or subretinal hemorrhages are seen on fundus examination or OCT (Fig. 7.5).

If polypoidal lesions are seen on ICGA, administer combined therapy of one intravitreal ranibizumab injection and PDT (Fig. 7.5).

For patients with residual or new exudative changes in the BVN vessels but with complete regression of the polypoidal lesions on ICGA, administer intravitreal ranibizumab (Fig. 7.5).

CONCLUSIONS

PCV is a distinct entity, clinically characterized by red nodule-like structures beneath the RPE, associated with serosanguineous RPE detachment or a neural retina detachment and subretinal hemorrhage.

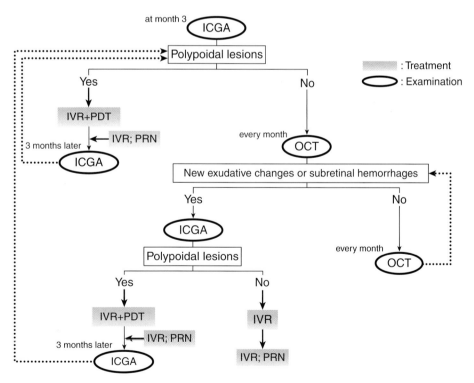

Figure 7.5 ■ Graph shows retreatment criteria after month tree treatment. Follow-up examinations included evaluation of the OCT images every month. (IVR, intravitreal ranibizumab injection. IVR + PDT, intravitreal ranibizumab injection plus PDT; PRN, pro re nata.) (Reprinted from Saito M, Iida T, Kano M. Combined intravitreal ranibizumab and photodynamic therapy for polypoidal choroidal vasculopathy. Retina. 2012;32(7):1272–1279. doi: 10.1097/IAE.0b013e318236e624, with permission.)

PCV has a varied evolutionary pathway; it could develop disciform scars, resulting in a severe visual impairment, or retain useful vision for many years (about 50% of patients in this group). Compared to exudative AMD, PCV has a better visual prognosis.

It has been observed that pigmented races have a higher incidence of PCV, and even in Asians PCV is the most common form of macular disease.

Diagnosing and staging of PCV has always been very challenging, but with the evolution of the newest diagnostic techniques such as OCT and ICGA it has become easier and much more accurate. Nowadays ICGA is considered to be the gold standard technique diagnosing PCV, especially due to its advantages over other techniques such as IVFA in obtaining images of vascular abnormalities covered by blood or other tissues.

PDT is currently the best treatment. In spite of becoming outmoded as a single therapy because of not completing polyp closure, anti-VEGF therapy is now being studied and developed as part of a combined therapy with PDT. This combined therapy has been shown to be more effective than single PDT therapy.

In conclusion, PCV has not been completely elucidated; more studies searching for prognostic and genetic clues are needed to develop better treatments and more accurate clinical follow-ups.

REFERENCES

1. Yannuzzi LA, Sorenson J, Spaide RF, et al. Idiopathic polypoidal choroidal vasculopathy (IPCV). Retina. 1990;10:1–8.

2. Ciardella AP, Donsoff IM, Huano SJ, et al. Polypoidal choroidal vasculopathy. Surv Ophthalmol. 2004;49(1):25–37.

3. Kleiner RC, Brucker AJ, Johnston RL. The posterior uveal bleeding syndrome. Retina. 1990;10(1):9–17.

4. Stern RM, Zakov ZN, Zegarra H, Gutman FA. Multiple recurrent serosanguineous retinal pigment epithelial detachments in black women. Am J Ophthalmol. 1985;100:560–569.

5. Yannuzzi LA, Slakter JS, Sorenson JA, et al. Digital indocyanine green videoangiography and choroidal neovascularization. Retina. 1992;12:191–223.

6. Imamura Y, Engelbert M, Iida T, et al. Polypoidal choroidal vasculopathy: a review. Surv Ophthalmol. 2010;55(6):501–515.

7. Uyama M, Matsubara T, Fukushima I, et al. Idiopathic polypoidal choroidal vasculopathy in Japanese patients. Arch Ophthalmol. 1999;117(8):1035–1042.

8. Yannuzzi LA, Ciardella A, Spaide RF, et al. The expanding clinical spectrum of idiopathic polypoidal choroidal vasculopathy. Arch Ophthalmol. 1997;115:478–485.

9. Byeon SH, Lee SC, Oh HS, et al. Incidence and clinical patterns of polypoidal choroidal vasculopathy in Korean patients. Jpn J Ophthalmol. 2008;52:57–62.

10. Liu Y, Wen F, Huang S, et al. Subtype lesions of neovascular age-related macular degeneration in Chinese patients. Graefes Arch Clin Exp Ophthalmol. 2007;245:1441–1445.

11. Maruko I, Iida T, Saito M, et al. Clinical characteristics of exudative age-related macular degeneration in Japanese patients. Am J Ophthalmol. 2007;144:15–22.

12. Dewan A, Liu M, Hartman S, et al. HTRA1 promoter polymorphism in wet age-related macular degeneration. Science. 2006;314(5801):989–992.

13. Lafaut BA, Leys AM, Snyers B, et al. Polypoidal choroidal vasculopathy in Caucasians. Graefes Arch Clin Exp Ophthalmol. 2000;238:752–759.

14. Yannuzzi LA, Wong DWK, Sforzolini BS, et al. Polypoidal choroidal vasculopathy and neovascular age-related macular degeneration. Arch Ophthalmol. 1999;117(11):1503–1510.

15. Iwama D, Tsujikawa A, Sasahara M, et al. Polypoidal choroidal vasculopathy with drusen. Jpn J Ophthalmol. 2008;52(2):116–21.

16. Ahuja RM, Stanga PE, Vingerling JR, et al. Polypoidal choroidal vasculopathy in exudative and haemorrhagic pigment epithelial detachments. Br J Ophthalmol. 2000;84:479–484.

17. Scassellati-Sforzolini B, Mariotti C, Bryan R, et al. Polypoidal choroidal vasculopathy in Italy. Retina. 2001;21:121–125.

18. Yang Z, Camp NJ, Sun H, et al. A variant of the HTRA1 gene increases susceptibility to age-related macular degeneration. Science. 2006;314(5801):992–993.

19. Kondo N, Honda S, Ishibashi K, et al. LOC387715/HTRA1 variants in polypoidal choroidal vasculopathy and age-related macular degeneration in a Japanese population. Am J Ophthalmol. 2007;144(4):608–612.

20. Lee KY, Vithana EN, Mathur R, et al. Association analysis of CFH, C2, BF, and HTRA1 gene polymorphisms in Chinese patients with polypoidal choroidal vasculopathy. Invest Ophthalmol Vis Sci. 2008;49(6):2613–2619.

21. Lima LH, Schubert C, Ferrara DC, et al. Three major loci involved in age-related macular degeneration are also associated with polypoidal choroidal vasculopathy. Ophthalmology 2010;117(8):1567–1570.

22. Freund KB, Zweifel SA, Engelbert M. Do we need a new classification for choroidal neovascularization in age-related macular degeneration? Retina. 2010;30(9):1333–1349.

23. Moorthy RS, Lyon AT, Rabb MF, et al. Idiopathic polypoidal choroidal vasculopathy of the macula. Ophthalmology. 1998;105(8):1380–1385.

24. Kondo N, Honda S, Kuno S, et al. Coding variant I62V in the complement factor H gene is strongly associated with polypoidal choroidal vasculopathy. Ophthalmology. 2009;116(2):304–310.

25. Gotoh N, Nakanishi H, Hayashi H, et al. ARMS2 (LOC387715) variants in Japanese patients with exudative age-related macular degeneration and polypoidal choroidal vasculopathy. Am J Ophthalmol. 2009;147(6):1037–1041.

26. Kanda A, Chen W, Othman M, et al. A variant of mitochondrial protein LOC387715/ARMS2, not HTRA1, is strongly associated with age-related macular degeneration. Proc Natl Acad Sci USA. 2007;104(41):16227–16232.

27. Gotoh N, Yamada R, Nakanishi H, et al. Correlation between Y402H and HTRA1 rs11200638 genotype to typical exudative age-related macular degeneration and polypoidal choroidal vasculopathy phenotype in the Japanese population. Clin Experiment Ophthalmol. 2008;36(5):437–442.

28. Nakata I, Yamashiro K, Yamada R, et al. Genetic variants in pigment epithelium-derived factor influence response of polypoidal choroidal vasculopathy to photodynamic therapy. Ophthalmology. 2011;118:1408–1415.

29. Park DH, Kim IT. LOC387715/HTRA1 variants and the response to combined photodynamic therapy with intravitreal bevacizumab for polypoidal choroidal vasculopathy. Retina. 2012;32:299–307.

30. Koh AH; Expert PCV Panel. Polypoidal choroidal vasculopathy: evidence-based guidelines for clinical diagnosis and treatment. Retina. 2013;33(4):686–716.

31. Cackett P, Wong D, Yeo I. A classification system for polypoidal choroidal vasculopathy. Retina. 2009;29(2):187–191.

32. Uyama M, Wada M, Nagai Y, et al. Polypoidal choroidal vasculopathy: natural history. Am J Ophthalmol. 2002;133:639–648.

33. Koh A, Lee WK, Chen LJ, et al. EVEREST study: efficacy and safety of verteporfin photodynamic therapy in combination with ranibizumab or alone versus ranibizumab monotherapy in patients with symptomatic macular polypoidal choroidal vasculopathy. Retina. 2012;32:1453–1464.

34. Sho K, Takahashi K, Yamada H, et al. Polypoidal choroidal vasculopathy: incidence, demographic features, and clinical characteristics. Arch Ophthalmol. 2003;121:1392–1396.

35. Akaza E, Mori R, Yuzawa M. Long-term results of photodynamic therapy of polypoidal choroidal vasculopathy. Retina. 2008;28:717–722.

36. Costa RA, Navajas EV, Farah MF, et al. Polypoidal choroidal vasculopathy: angiographic characterization of the network vascular elements and a new treatment paradigm. Prog Retin Eye Res. 2005;24(5):560–586.

37. Yannuzzi LA, Freund KB, Goldbaum M, et al. Polypoidal choroidal vasculopathy masquerading as central serous chorioretinopathy. Ophthalmology. 2000;107:767–777.

38. Ahuja RM, Downes SM, Stanga PE, et al. Polypoidal choroidal vasculopathy and central serous chorioretinopathy. Ophthalmology. 2001;108:1009–1010.

39. Tamura H, Tsujikawa A, Otani A, et al. Polypoidal choroidal vasculopathy appearing as classic choroidal neovascularization on fluorescein angiography. Br J Ophthalmol. 2007;91(9):1152–1159.

40. Smith RE, Wise K, Kingsley RM. Idiopathic polypoidal choroidal vasculopathy and sickle cell retinopathy. Am J Ophthalmol. 2000;129:544–546.

41. Bartlett HM, Willoughby B, Mandava N. Idiopathic polypoidal choroidal vasculopathy in a patient with melanocytoma of the optic nerve. Retina. 2001;21:396–399.

42. Li H, Wen F, Wu D. Polypoidal choroidal vasculopathy in a patient with circumscribed choroidal hemangioma. Retina. 2004;24:629–631.

43. Mauget-Faÿsse M, Cornut PL, Quaranta El-Maftouhi M, et al. Polypoidal choroidal vasculopathy in tilted disk syndrome and high myopia with staphyloma. Am J Ophthalmol. 2006;142:970–975.

44. Fine HF, Ferrara DC, Ho I-V, et al. Bilateral choroidal osteomas with polypoidal choroidal vasculopathy. Retin Cases Brief Rep. 2008;2:15–17.

45. Baillif-Gostoli S, Quaranta-El Maftouhi M, Mauget-Faÿsse M. Polypoidal choroidal vasculopathy in a patient with angioid streaks secondary to pseudoxanthoma elasticum. Graefes Arch Clin Exp Ophthalmol. 2010;248:1845–1848.

46. Yamagishi T, Koizumi H, Yamazaki T, et al. Fundus autofluorescence in polypoidal choroidal vasculopathy. Ophthalmology. 2012;119(8):1650–1657.

47. Rosa RH Jr, Davis JL, Eifrig CW. Clinicopathologic reports, case reports, and small case series: clinicopathologic correlation of idiopathic polypoidal choroidal vasculopathy. Arch Ophthalmol. 2002;120(4):502–508.

48. Eandi CM, Ober MD, Freund KB, Slakter JS, Yannuzzi LA. Selective photodynamic therapy for neovascular age-related macular degeneration with polypoidal choroidal neovascularization. Retina. 2007;27(7):825–831.

49. Spaide RF, Yannuzzi LA, Slakter JS, Sorenson J, Orlach DA. Indo-cyanine green videoangiography of idiopathic polypoidal choroidal vasculopathy. Retina. 1995;15:100–110.

50. Shiraga F, Matsuo T, Yokoe S, et al. Surgical treatment of submacular hemorrhage associated with idiopathic polypoidal choroidal vasculopathy. Am J Ophthalmol. 1999;128:147–154.

51. Kwok AK, Lai TY, Chan CW, et al. Polypoidal choroidal vasculopathy in Chinese patients. Br J Ophthalmol. 2002;86:892–897.

52. Iijima H, Iida T, Imai M, et al. Optical coherence tomography of orange-red subretinal lesions in eyes with idiopathic polypoidal choroidal vasculopathy. Am J Ophthalmol. 2000; 129(1): 21–26.

53. Gomi F, Ohji M, Sayanagi K, et al. One-year outcomes of photodynamic therapy in age-related macular degeneration and polypoidal choroidal vasculopathy in Japanese patients. Ophthalmology. 2008;115:141–146.

54. Gotoh N, Kuroiwa S, Kikuchi T, et al. Apolipoprotein E polymorphisms in Japanese patients with polypoidal choroidal vasculopathy and exudative age-related macular degeneration. Am J Ophthalmol. 2004;138(4):567–573.

55. Honda S, Imai H, Yamashiro K, et al. Comparative assessment of photodynamic therapy for typical age-related macular degeneration and polypoidal choroidal vasculopathy: a multicenter study in Hyogo prefecture. Japan Ophthalmologica. 2009; 223(5):333–338.

56. Khan S, Engelbert M, Imamura Y, et al. Polypoidal choroidal vasculopathy: simultaneous indocyanine green angiography and eye-tracked spectral domain optical coherence tomography findings. Retina. 2012;32:1057–1068.

57. Sato T, Kishi S, Watanabe G, et al. Tomographic features of branching vascular networks in polypoidal choroidal vasculopathy. Retina. 2007; 27:589–594.

58. Abe S, Yamamoto T, Haneda S, et al. Three-dimensional features of polypoidal choroidal vasculopathy observed by spectral-domain OCT. Ophthalmic Surg Lasers Imaging. 2010; 9:1–6.

59. Tsujikawa A, Hirami Y, Nakanishi H, et al. Retinal pigment epithelial tear in polypoidal choroidal vasculopathy. Retina. 2007;27(7):832–838.

60. Musashi K, Tsujikawa A, Hirami Y, et al. Microrips of the retinal pigment epithelium in polypoidal choroidal vasculopathy. Am J Ophthalmol. 2007;143(5):883–885.

61. Yuzawa M, Mori R, Haruyama M. A study of laser photocoagulation for polypoidal choroidal vasculopathy. Jpn J Ophthalmol. 2003;47(4):379–384.

62. Treatment of Age-Related Macular Degeneration with Photodynamic Therapy (TAP) Study Group. Photodynamic therapy of subfoveal choroidal neovascularization in age-related macular degeneration with verteporfin: one-year results of 2 randomized clinical trials—TAP Report 1. Arch Ophthalmol. 1999;117:1329–1345.

63. Schmidt-Erfurth U, Schlotzer-Schrehard U, Cursiefen C, et al. Influence of photodynamic therapy on expression of vascular endothelial growth factor (VEGF), VEGF receptor 3, and pigment epithelium-derived factor. Invest Ophthalmol Vis Sci. 2003;44:4473–4480.

64. Klais CM, Ober MD, Freund KB, et al. Choroidal infarction following photodynamic therapy with verteporfin. Arch Ophthalmol. 2005;123:1149–1153.

65. Lafaut BA, Aisenbrey S, Broecke CV, Bartz-Schmidt KU. Clinicopathological correlation of deep retinal vascular anomalous complex in age-related macular degeneration. Br J Ophthalmol. 2000;84:1269–1274.

66. Schmidt-Erfurth U, Hasan T. Mechanism of action of photo- dynamic therapy with verteporfin for the treatment of age-related macular degeneration. Surv Ophthalmol. 2000; 45: 195–214.

67. Tano Y. Ophthalmic PDT Study Group. Guidelines for PDT in Japan. Ophthalmology. 2008;115:585–585.e6.

68. Prakash M, Han DP. Recurrent bullous retinal detachment from photodynamic therapy for idiopathic polypoidal choroidal vasculopathy. Am J Ophthalmol. 2006;142(6):1079–1081.

69. Yodoi Y, Tsujikawa A, Otani A, et al. Chorioretinal anastomosis after photodynamic therapy for polypoidal choroidal vasculopathy: CRA after PDT for PCV. Int Ophthalmol. 2007;28(4):297–299.

70. Yodoi Y, Tsujikawa A, Kameda T, et al. Central retinal sensitivity measured with the microperimeter 1 after photodynamic therapy for polypoidal choroidal vasculopathy. Am J Ophthalmol. 2007;143(6):984–994.

71. Terasaki H, Miyake Y, Suzuki T, et al. Polypoidal choroidal vasculopathy treated with macular translocation: clinical pathological correlation. Br J Ophthalmol. 2002;86:321–327.

72. Tong JP, Chan WM, Liu DT, et al. Aqueous humor levels of vascular endothelial growth factor and pigment epithelium-derived factor in polypoidal choroidal vasculopathy and choroidal neovascularization. Am J Ophthalmol. 2006;141(3): 456–462.

73. Gomi F, Sawa M, Sakaguchi H, et al. Efficacy of intravitreal bevacizumab for choroidal vasculopathy. Br J Ophthalmol. 2008;92(1):70–73.

74. Lai TY, Chan WM, Liu DT, et al. Intravitreal bevacizumab (Avastin) with or without photodynamic therapy for the treatment of polypoidal choroidal vasculopathy. Br J Ophthalmol. 2008;92:661–666.

75. Cheng CK, Peng CH, Chang CK, et al. One-year outcomes of intravitreal bevacizumab (avastin) therapy for polypoidal choroidal vasculopathy. Retina. 2011;31:846–856.

76. Kokame GT, Yeung L, Lai JC. Continuous anti-VEGF treatment with ranibizumab for polypoidal choroidal vasculopathy: 6-month results. Br J Ophthalmol. 2010;94:297–301.

77. Cho HJ, Kim JW, Lee DW, et al. Intravitreal bevacizumab and ranibizumab injections for patients with polypoidal choroidal vasculopathy. Eye (Lond). 2012;26(3):426–433.

78. Saito M, Iida T, Kano M. Combined intravitreal ranibizumab and photodynamic therapy for polypoidal choroidal vasculopathy. Retina. 2012;32(7):1272–1279.

79. Ruamviboonsuk P, Tadarati M, Vanichvaranont S, et al. Photodynamic therapy combined with ranibizumab for polypoidal choroidal vasculopathy: results of a 1-year preliminary study. Br J Ophthalmol. 2010;94:1045–1051.

80. Sato T, Kishi S, Matsumoto H, et al. Combined photodynamic therapy with verteporfin and intravitreal bevacizumab for polypoidal choroidal vasculopathy. Am J Ophthalmol. 2010;149:947–954.

81. Gomi F, Sawa M, Wakabayashi T, et al. Efficacy of intravitreal bevacizumab combined with photodynamic therapy for polypoidal choroidal vasculopathy. Am J Ophthalmol. 2010;150: 48–54.

8

RETINAL ANGIOMATOUS PROLIFERATION IN AGE-RELATED MACULAR DEGENERATION

GABRIELA E. GRANELLA • ERIC P. JABLON

INTRODUCTION

It is known that choroidal neovascularization (CNV) in age-related macular degeneration (AMD) may erode through the retinal pigment epithelium (RPE), infiltrate the neurosensory retina, and communicate with the retinal circulation in what has been referred to as a retinal–choroidal anastomosis (RCA). This is extremely common in the end stage of disciform disease (1). The reverse is also possible, as angiomatous proliferation originates from the retina and extends posteriorly into the subretinal space, eventually communicating in some cases with choroidal new vessels. This form of neovascular AMD, termed retinal angiomatous proliferation (RAP), can be confused with CNV. RAP begins in the deep retinal complex forming intraretinal neovascularization (IRN), which may subsequently progress to extend beneath the neurosensory retina, forming subretinal neovascularization (SRN) and a vascularized pigment epithelium detachment (PED). In the advanced stages of the process, there may be an RCA. Clinical features of RAP include intraretinal hemorrhages, cystoid macular edema (CME), and associated vascularized PED. Fluorescein angiography (FA) is useful in revealing the presence of the angiomatous intraretinal vascular complex and the extension of the associated PED. However, other diagnostic techniques, such as indocyanine green (ICG) angiography and optical coherence tomography (OCT), have now proven to be as useful—or even more—to demonstrate the presence of the RAP lesion.

HISTORY

Oeller (2), nearly 110 years ago, predicted the presence of retinal vascular communications in the predisciform stage of AMD in his classic, chorioretinal atlas. Later in 1985, Sorenson et al. (3) reported a communication between the retinal and choroidal circulation as a cause of recurrent CNV and eventual failure of thermal laser treatment. The retina itself was the source of the recurrent vascular ingrowth, which was subretinal rather than subpigment epithelial or CNV.

In 1992, Hartnett et al. (4), in a landmark article, were the first to describe retinal neovascularization as an early finding in neovascular AMD, preceding the disciform scarring stage of the disease. In a clinical and fluorescein angiographic description of 125 patients with neovascular AMD and an associated serous PED, they found nine patients (7.3%) to have retinal vascular abnormalities, which were described as "retinal angiomatous lesions." Eight of these nine eyes underwent thermal laser photocoagulation and eventually had recurrent CNV and progressive disciform scar formation. In 1995, Kuhn et al. (5) first clearly identified an RCA as a potential manifestation of this form of neovascular AMD. They specifically addressed the development of an RCA to an associated vascularized PED. Utilizing ICG angiography, this group found evidence for an RCA in 50 of 186—or 28%—of AMD patients with an associated vascularized PED. Indeed, they termed this form of neovascular AMD "retinal–choroidal anastomosis." The outcome of laser photocoagulation treatment in these individuals was poor. Hartnett et al. (6), in a subsequent report in 1996 on 13 patients with this form of neovascular AMD and an associated serous PED, suggested that the neovascularization was in the deep retina; furthermore, an anastomosis connecting the retinal circulation to a deep retinal vascular abnormality was characteristic of the disorder. This subgroup of cases was termed "deep retinal vascular anomalous complex," and the authors described other important associated macular abnormalities, including localized intraretinal hemorrhages and capillary telangiectasia. Support and validation of these clinical impressions were made possible by the work of Lafaut et al. (7). These investigators reported on clinical–pathologic correlations in six patients who had macular translocation surgery for this form of neovascular AMD. They found that IRN and SRN with detachment of the neurosensory retina were the most conspicuous findings. They also believed that the initiating vasogenic events were IRN and SRN, as reported by Slakter et al. (15).

In current terminology, it is known as RAP. It was first classified and named as a subset of AMD by Yannuzzi et al. (8) in 2001, who chose to name the condition RAP indicating the early appearance and origin of the neovascularization in the retina, the contiguous circumferential telangiectatic changes surrounding the core of new vessels, the development of IRN, the progression of new vessels into the subretinal space, and the variable as well as late onset of an RCA. In 2008, this form of neovascularization that originates from the retinal circulation has been demonstrated in a clinicopathologic correlation; Monson et al. (9) investigated the histopathologic features of RAP in an 87-year-old woman and reported an intraretinal angiomatous complex within the outer layer of the neurosensory retina overlaying a large PED with no CNV and no break in the Bruch's membrane.

EPIDEMIOLOGY

Patients with RAP are similar clinically to patients with neovascular AMD from classic CNV or occult CNV (10). RAP has been estimated to account for 12% to 15% of newly diagnosed neovascular AMD (11) and is believed to have a different natural course and response to therapy compared with standard CNV (12). The patients with RAP tend to be female by a ratio of more than 2:1 and elderly at the time of initial diagnosis (80 years old). RAP is most frequently seen in Caucasians and uncommonly seen in Asians, and to date, it has not been described in Blacks. This racial predilection differentiates RAP from polypoidal CNV, which has a predisposition for pigmented races and the peripapillary area (13).

The initial lesion itself is always extrafoveal, presumably because of the perifoveal capillary-free zone, and it has never been reported to occur in the peripapillary area or peripheral fundus for reasons that are not known (14). Patients with RAP also exhibited a marked tendency toward bilateral and symmetric neovascular disease (15). In the study presented by Yannuzzi et al. (8), it was not possible to determine with reasonable assurance the presenting neovascular nature of bilateral cases with disciform disease in one eye. Patients who presented with unilateral RAP and subsequently developed neovascular changes in the fellow eye had an identical form of neovascular AMD without exception. Gross et al. (16) have reported that, in patients with unilateral RAP, a neovascular event in the fellow eye occurs at an annual and accumulative rate that far exceeds that for other forms of neovascular AMD, with a bilateral involvement in 100% of cases within 3 years. These findings, although considered well established, differ from those presented by Campa et al. (17) who showed that the incidence of RAP in the fellow eye is much lower (36.4% at 3 years) compared with previous report; however, these results have several limitations related to the retrospective nature and the small number of patients.

CLASSIFICATION

It was a long-held belief that all neovascularization in AMD originated from the choroidal circulation. In 2001, Yannuzzi et al. (8) challenged this traditional dogma based on the presumed origin and evolution of the neovascularized process. They believed that IRN originating from the inner retinal circulation produced a surrounding telangiectatic compensatory response to accommodate an increase in vascular perfusion, and they termed this variant "retinal angiomatous proliferation". Thereafter, and due to a lingering uncertainty as to the origin of these lesions, Freund (11) has proposed naming this vascular lesion "type 3 neovascularization" to distinguish and emphasize the location of the neovascularization (intraretinal) independent of its origin.

Type 3 neovascularization (RAP) is now part of a logical extension of the original classification proposed by Gass (18) in his classic text on macular diseases. This classification is based upon the anatomic position of the abnormal vessels in relation to the monolayer RPE. Type 1 implies neovascularization located external or beneath the RPE. FA of eyes with these vessels commonly shows a pattern that is "poorly defined" with minimal leakage, also described as occult CNV. Type 2 neovascularization implies vessels that have penetrated the RPE layer to proliferate in the subneurosensory space. FA of this form of neovascularization will typically show a "well-defined" pattern with intense leakage, also referred to as classic CNV. The type 3 neovascularization or RAP therefore indicates proliferating vessels within and below the retina itself. The origin of this neovascular subtype can be from either circulation and may originate from both circulations simultaneously in the form of an RCA. The presence of an RCA gives this entity many of its characteristic clinical, spectral-domain optical coherence tomography (SD-OCT), and angiographic features including intraretinal hemorrhages and CME. Type 3 lesions have been observed originating in areas with substantial photoreceptor loss that has brought the deep retinal vasculature in close proximity to the underlying RPE, Bruch's membrane, and choriocapillaris. Typically, the angiogenic response occurs overlying a focal drusen/basal laminar deposit that may already be infiltrated by type 1 vessels. Presumably, loss of or erosion through the intervening RPE and an appropriate angiogenic milieu would allow the retinal and choroidal circulations to merge in the form of RCA with a continued proliferative response. As these lesions originate from both the retinal and choroidal circulations, they never originate within the foveal avascular zone.

A three-stage classification was proposed to characterize the clinical manifestations and progressive changes. The clinical appearance of the earliest manifestations was termed "stage I" (Fig. 8.1). As these vessels evolved, they appeared to extend beneath the neurosensory retina to become SRN termed "stage II" (Fig. 8.2A and B) and eventually merged with the choroidal circulation proliferating beneath the RPE as CNV, or stage III, to form an RCA (Fig. 8.3). The original interpretation of this angiogenic sequence was based on reports of atypical forms of neovascularization in AMD (4,5,13), particularly with the use of combined FA and ICG angiography and the first-generation OCT imaging system (OCT–1, Carl Zeiss, Meditec, Inc., Dublin, CA, USA) available at that time (19).

Stage I: Intraretinal Neovascularization

Capillary proliferation within the retina, originating from the deep capillary plexus in the paramacular area, is the earliest manifestation detected in any patient with RAP. In this stage, there is usually a nodular mass of angiomatous tissue in the middle and inner retina. As this lesion progresses, there is a predominantly vertical extension of the IRN to the anterior and posterior boundaries of the retina. The neovascularization also may show a lateral extension of the vessels in an irregular stellate configuration. This is characterized by projections of capillaries tangentially and obliquely from the primary neovascularized area, resembling the appearance of a sea urchin. One or more prominently dilated perfusing arterioles or draining venules could be seen early in this stage, communicating with the core of the IRN. Evidence also demonstrates a retinal–retinal anastomosis (RRA). Some medium-sized capillaries projecting from the core of angiomatous proliferation have been noted to communicate with the larger, dilated inner retinal vessels. A few intraretinal hemorrhages and intraretinal edema could be seen clinically surrounding the IRN. The FA reveals a focal area of intraretinal staining with an indistinct border corresponding to the IRN and surrounding intraretinal edema. ICG reveals a focal area of intense hyperfluorescence within the retina or a so-called hot spot at the site of the IRN. Matsumoto et al. (20) showed with SD-OCT the origin of the IRN in nine eyes with untreated RAP. Retinal edema was always observed around the IRN in eyes with stage I. The frequency of retinal edema around the IRN and the low incidence of serous retinal detachment (SRD) suggest the intraretinal origin of neovascularization in RAP. The IRN was outside the avascular fovea in all eyes and appeared as a highly reflective mass that originated at the outer plexiform layer (OPL) and extended to the deeper retinal layers. In eyes at stage I, the highly reflective mass at the OPL corresponding to IRN disappeared, but drusenoid PED remained unchanged after repeated intravitreal bevacizumab (IVB) in SD-OCT, which lends further support to the postulation of intraretinal origin of RAP. The disruption of the RPE beneath the IRN is often seen in stage I. Although Freund et al. (11) interpreted the disrupted RPE as intraretinal invasion of CNV in early-stage RAP, it may reflect the drusenoid PED with attached IRN.

Stage II: Subretinal Neovascularization

Stage II is present when the IRN extends posteriorly beyond the photoreceptor layer of the retina into the subretinal space, forming SRN. At this point, there is a

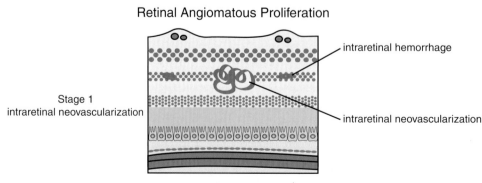

Retinal Angiomatous Proliferation

Stage 1
intraretinal neovascularization

intraretinal hemorrhage

intraretinal neovascularization

Figure 8.1 ■ Stage I: Intraretinal neovascularization.

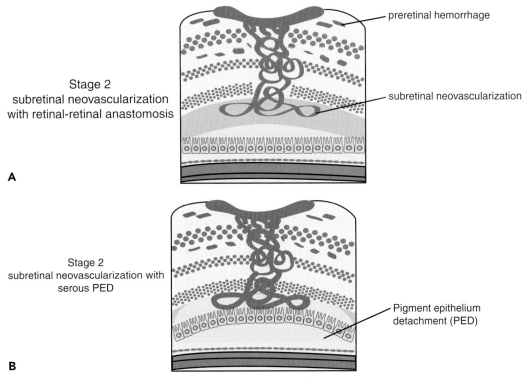

Figure 8.2 ■ **A.** Stage II: subretinal neovascularization with a retinal–retinal anastomosis. **B.** Stage II: subretinal neovascularization with a serous PED.

broader, tangential vascular proliferation under the retina. There is also a localized neurosensory retinal detachment, an increase in the intraretinal edema, and multiple small intraretinal hemorrhages that extend circumferentially to the limits of the macular detachment, but not beyond. Although there could be a slight thickening of the surface of the retina from the neovascularization, new vessels do not extend detectably into the preretinal space. As the RAP expands within the retina, and in particular beneath the retina, the dilated perfusing or draining retinal vessels could be seen clinically to decussate posteriorly toward the SRN. In stage II, a clear RRA could be seen, with a perfusing retina arteriole and draining venule communicating in some eyes with a "hairpin loop" within the core of the SRN.

An associated serous PED also could be seen as the SRN reached or fused with the RPE. In FA, the SRN appears to have a small area of classic CNV predominantly within the occult lesion. The ICG angiogram reveals a hot spot at the site of the neovascularization within and beneath the retina. There is also some late extension of leakage in the retina from the IRN. Although this stage of classification assumes the presence of new subretinal vessels originating from the retinal vasculature, a choroidal vascular component could not be ruled out on the basis of the clinical and angiographic examinations. At this stage, SD-OCT shows major retinal edema around the IRN in comparison to stage I. SD-OCT can also show hemorrhagic or nonhemorrhagic PED, although Matsumoto et al. (20) demonstrated that no

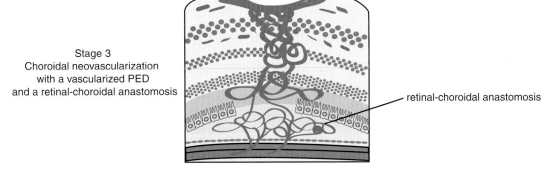

Figure 8.3 ■ Stage III: choroidal neovascularization with a vascularized PED and a RCA.

hemorrhagic PED was observed in the six eyes with stage II disease with PED. RRA and disrupted RPE beneath the IRN are also present. SRD is less frequent.

Stage III: Choroidal Neovascularization

A more common and definitive documentation of stage III is made when there is clinical and angiograph evidence of a vascularized PED or a predisciform scar. The ICG angiogram, however, is most helpful in determining the presence of CNV: Only the vascular components—IRN, SRN, and CNV—will be hyperfluorescent, and they can be distinguished as contrast is enhanced from the hypofluorescent exudative spaces. Identification of a clearly distinct and documentable RCA is rare. In a few cases, a connection between the two circulations could be identified, constituting an RCA. Otherwise, it can only be assumed that there is a communicating network of vessels between the two circulations.

A dilated retinal venule is particularly conspicuous in stage III, as perfusion of the SRN and CNV appears to be predominantly from the choroidal circulation with notable drainage into the retina. In these cases, the retinal and subretinal neovascularized components are noticeably smaller in lateral dimensions, compared to the more aggressive CNV beneath a distinctly larger vascularized PED. In fact, some patients have only a small area of IRN and SRN cascading above a large, placoid area of CNV. In a study by Krebs et al. (21) comparing the morphologic findings of the SD-OCT (Cirrus) to the time-domain OCT (Stratus), the authors reported the presence of RPE breaks only in eyes with RAP stage III. In OCT, the detection of a band of tissue protruding in the PED may be indicative of an accompanying CNV when FA or ICG fails to demonstrate it.

With the advent of new technology such as the SD-OCT, Freund et al. (22) do not see a value in the current staging system for RAP (or type 3 neovascularization), as it was based on observations of eyes with relatively long-standing lesions and does not accurately describe the evolution of these lesions. They argue that the advent of SD-OCT has helped explain one of the confusing aspects of this entity.

In the past, it was difficult to understand how a PED could occur in an eye with an RCA because, with the older time-domain OCT systems, one rarely saw evidence of vascular tissue bridging the space beneath the PED. These observations led some investigators to conclude that the neovascularization must have originated within the neurosensory retina. They believe that the RCA does persist after the elevation of the RPE monolayer in the form of type 1 vessels lining the undersurface of the RPE that maintain the connection to the choroidal circulation. These vessels are more readily detected with SD-OCT as hyperreflective material directly beneath the elevated hyperreflective RPE band.

TREATMENT

A range of alternative treatment options have been reported in case series with limited evidence of efficacy, from intravitreal treatments alone or, in combination with laser, to surgical excision of neovascularization in RAP, with variable success rates (16,23–38). Unfortunately, no randomized controlled data have been published to date. Treatment studies include thirty observational studies that had more than 3 months of follow-up and seven prospective studies. The main treatment options included inhibitors of vascular endothelial growth factor (anti-VEGF agents), photodynamic therapy (PDT) alone or in combination with intravitreal triamcinolone (IVTA) or anti-VEGF agents, focal laser, transpupillary thermotherapy (TTT), and surgical ablation alone or in combination with other agents. A few studies investigated the response of various stages of RAP, but the numbers are limited, and the prognosis (depending on the stage when treatment is started, the sooner the better) is currently considered to be poor.

Anti-VEGF Agents

These factors are thought to have a strong effect on RAP because an overexpression of VEGF is known to be the trigger of the deep retinal neovascularization in this condition (8). All three anti-VEGF agents available for treatment of neovascular AMD (pegaptanib sodium (39), ranibizumab, and bevacizumab) have demonstrated, in most of the studies, the capability to reduce vascular leakage and improve the visual outcome in patients with RAP. The protocols used for treatment in the available studies varied between them, and most investigators evaluated effect of as-needed dosing schedule based on visual acuity (VA) and retinal morphology. The VA recordings were converted to Early Treatment Diabetic Retinopathy Study (ETDRS) letters for analysis of mean change in visual acuity, resulting in +4 ETDRS letters at 3 months, +1.5 ETDRS at 6 months, and +3 ETDRS at 12 months. The change in VA was associated with a decrease in central retinal thickness. Nevertheless, persistence of activity of lesion was noted in nearly all patients at the end of follow-up (30,40–45). Only one eye experienced injection-related inflammation, which subsequently resolved with appropriate treatment (42). From the studies available, bevacizumab had the best response in all stages of RAP lesion with maximum efficacy at 3 months, sustained over 12 months. However, the results should be interpreted with caution as most of the studies used bevacizumab and did not include RAP stage, lesion size, and location. The sample sizes were also small.

Laser Photocoagulation

Direct laser photocoagulation of the neovascular process is a standardized treatment for extrafoveal CNV (46). The most appropriate modality of laser beam delivery for RAP lesions is unknown, although several investigators have used this treatment modality in extrafoveal RAPs. Focal laser ablation of RAP lesions was described previously by Hartnett et al. (6). Direct treatment with focal laser stabilizes most of the RAP lesion, although there is no statistical significant in visual outcome (28,29,47,48). In twelve eyes treated by Bottoni et al. (47) by retinal feeder vessel treatment, a closure rate of 25% was noted at the end of 23.4 months. As with other retinal vascular pathologies treated with feeder vessel treatment, reperfusion of the occluded vasculature is common. The same group reported 9/24 eyes achieving complete closure after a grid laser treatment. Using modified TTT and modified diode laser (two consecutive, superimposed, subthreshold spots of 3 and 1.2 mm), Bottoni et al. (47) achieved a closure rate of 40% with scarring previously reported following TTT, which has limited success. The use of ICG imaging allows differentiation of the intraretinal and subretinal components of neovascularization associated with stage II RAP lesions and selective ablation of only the intraretinal component of the neovascularization. FA is limited in its ability to detect RAP lesions for laser treatment.

Two studies provided the outcome of the combination of laser photocoagulation to the hot spot on ICG combined with IVTA (Krieglstein et al. (48) and Roth et al. (29)). Concomitant use of IVTA may also decompress the PED when present and suppress the neovascular drive, as observed by Krieglstein et al. (48) and Roth et al. (29). However, the effect of focal laser treatment is short lived. This effect could be due to either incomplete treatment with previous focal laser or early treatment for reperfusion leading to a prolonged effect. In addition, the use of micropulse laser may reduce associated collateral damage (29). In micropulse diode laser treatment, the laser energy is delivered with a series of repetitive short pulses (typically of 0.1–0.3 ms) so the duration of exposure is typically 0.1 to 0.5 second, and thus, there are minimum heat transfer and damage to overlying neural retina and limited collateral damage.

Photodynamic Therapy

It is difficult to predict stabilization of RAP neovascular lesion with PDT application because PDT targets CNV and not retinal vessels, the source of neovascularization in RAP. In addition, the risks of acute retinal tears are higher in RAP when associated with PED (24). Treatment with PDT was FA (and ICG) guided, and the standard protocol for PDT recommended by the verteporfin in photodynamic therapy (VIP) study group was used in all studies. Cumulative evidence from observational studies on PDT alone in RAP indicates a mean change of VA of –2 ETDRS letters at 3 months, –10 ETDRS letters at 6 months, and –1 ETDRS letters at 12 months.

Combination Treatment of PDT with Other Agents

Corticosteroids have been effective mainly due to their ability to control the inflammatory cascade. IVTA causes short-term VA benefit due to reduced exudation from the neovascular process and the resultant decrease in subretinal fluid but not from a permanent cessation of neovascular growth. It has been postulated that IVTA probably has a beneficial role in RAP lesions as an adjunctive therapy because of its ability to reduce the macular fluid, ensuring anatomic stability and improved visual outcome. The studies that assessed the effects of the combination of IVTA and PDT used different protocols. The mean change of VA was +6 ETDRS at 3 months, +10 ETDRS at 6 months, and +5 ETDRS letters at 12-month follow-up. Most of the studies report stabilization by 6 months although IVTA is also associated with increased incidence of raised pressure and cataract formation. However, Saito et al. (35) showed that combined treatment of IVB plus PDT significantly improved the VA and reduced the number of treatments in patients with RAP compared with combined treatment of IVTA plus PDT during a 12-month follow-up.

A year later, Saito et al. (37) also studied the combination of anti-VEGF and PDT by retrospectively reviewing 20 treatment-naïve eyes of 16 patients, treated with three consecutive monthly intravitreal injections of ranibizumab and PDT and followed up for at least 12 months. PDT was applied 1 or 2 days after the initial injection. Retreatment was performed as a combined therapy of a single intravitreal ranibizumab injection and PDT. The mean best-corrected visual acuity (BCVA) levels significantly improved from 0.24 at baseline to 0.43 at 12 months (2.51 lines). The BCVA, for the same period, improved in ten eyes (by 3 lines or more) and was stable (defined as a loss of less than 3 lines of vision) in 10 eyes. No patient had a decrease in the BCVA of three lines or more during the follow-up, and they concluded that further evaluation requires a larger patient sample and a long-term controlled study to compare treatment efficacy with anti-VEGF monotreatment.

Comparison of Visual Outcomes of Different Treatment Modalities

The combination of PDT and IVTA provided the best results at 6 months. However, the effects faded by 12 months with a high incidence of cataract. No therapy, either alone or in combination, seems to be effective for this complex disease process. Looking at all the available evidence, the suggested treatment option that may most lead to benefit is three monthly injections of anti-VEGF agents to decrease the vasogenic drive and concomitant retina edema, followed by PDT. In case of reoccurrence, ICG-guided focal laser obliteration as salvage treatment may be an option, as proposed by Bearelly et al. (49).

Response of Various Stages of RAP

Few studies subclassified RAP into the various stages to understand the treatment response at each stage of the disease. Understandably, the earlier the disease process is identified and treated, the better the prognosis.

SUMMARY

The natural history of RAP is characterized by a rapid loss of vision and progression to stage II (with or without associated pigment epithelial detachment) leading to a very high risk of a worse outcome in short time (12). It is important for clinicians to realize that this form of neovascular AMD is not uncommon, and it may have its own clinical course and prognostic parameters that differ distinctly from other forms of neovascular AMD originating from CNV. Given the presence of neovascular AMD and the suspicion of occult CNV or minimally classic CNV on FA, an ICG angiogram should be considered to rule out RAP. Above all, the physician should be aware of this form of neovascularization so that a proper diagnosis can be made and an appropriate treatment, when available, be administered.

Finally, clinical knowledge and recognition of RAP are important as this form of neovascular AMD may have a natural course, visual prognosis, and response to treatment distinct from other forms of neovascularization in AMD. Because RAP may present simply as IRN or progress to be complicated by SRN with or without a serous PED, and with or without CNV and an RCA, different forms of treatment may be preferable for each stage of the disorder.

None of the available options provide a satisfactory response compared with the outcome on CNV in neovascular AMD. There is no single treatment that is equally effective in all stages of RAP. Early recognition and treatment are crucial for this condition. Combination therapy using PDT and IVTA seems to be the best option to provide short-term benefit. It is important to conduct treatment trials comparing available options for this condition to better inform retinal specialists on the optimum treatment protocols at various stages of this condition.

REFERENCES

1. Green WR, Gass JDM. Senile disciform degeneration of the macula. Arch Ophthalmol. 1971;86:487–494.

2. Oeller's J. Atlas of rare ophthalmoscopic conditions and supplementary plates to the atlas of ophthalmoscopy [Snowball T, trans]. Wiesbaden, Germany: JF Bergman; 1904, Part C.

3. Sorenson JA, Yannuzzi LA, Shakin JL. Recurrent subretinal neovascularization. Ophthalmology. 1985;92:1059–1074.

4. Hartnett ME, Weiter JJ, Gardts A, et al. Classification of retinal pigment epithelial detachments associated with drusen. Graefes Arch Clin Exp Ophthalmol. 1992;230:11–19.

5. Kuhn D, Meunier I, Soubrane G, et al. Imaging of chorioretinal anastomosis in vascularized retinal pigment epithelium detachments. Arch Ophthalmol. 1995;113:1392–1398.

6. Hartnett ME, Weiter JJ, Staurenghi G, et al. Deep retinal vascular anomalous complexes in advanced age-related macular degeneration. Ophthalmology. 1996;103:2042–2053.

7. Lafaut BA, Aisenbrey S, Broecke CV, et al. Clinicopathological correlation of deep retinal vascular anomalous complex in age-related macular degeneration. Br J Ophthalmol. 2000;84:1269–1274.

8. Yannuzzi LA, Negrão S, Iida T, et al. Retinal angiomatous proliferation in age-related macular degeneration. Retina. 2001;21:416–434.

9. Monson DM, Smith JR, Klein ML, et al. Clinicopathologic correlation of retinal angiomatous proliferation. Arch Ophthalmol. 2008;126:1664–1668.

10. Yannuzzi LA, Hope–Ross M, Slakter JS, et al. Analysis of vascularized pigment epithelial detachments using indocyanine green videography. Retina. 1994;14:99–113.

11. Freund KB, Ho IV, Barbazetto IA, et al. Type 3 neovascularization: the expanded spectrum of retinal angiomatous proliferation. Retina. 2008;28:201–211.

12. Viola F, Massacesi A, Orzalesi N, et al. Retinal angiomatous proliferation: natural history and progression of visual loss. Retina. 2009;29:732–739.

13. Yannuzzi LA, Wong DWK, Sforzolini BS, et al. Polypoidal choroidal vasculopathy and neovascularized age-related macular degeneration. Arch Ophthalmol. 1999;117:1503–1510.

14. Yannuzzi LA, Freund KB, Takahashi BS, et al. Review of retinal angiomatous proliferation or type 3 neovascularization. Retina. 2008;28(3):375–384.

15. Slakter JS, Yannuzzi LA, Schneider U, et al. Retinal choroidal anastomoses and occult choroidal neovascularization in age-related macular degeneration. Ophthalmology. 2000;107:742–754.

16. Gross NE, Aizman A, Brucker A, et al. Nature and risk of neovascularization in the fellow eye of patients with unilateral retinal angiomatous proliferation. Retina. 2005;25:713–718.

17. Campa C, Harding SP, Pearce IA, et al. Incidence of neovascularization in the fellow eye of patients with unilateral retinal angiomatous proliferation. Eye (Lond). 2010;24:1585–1589.

18. Gass JD. Stereoscopic atlas of macular diseases. 4th Ed. St. Louis, MO: CV Mosby; 1997:26–30.

19. Brancato R, Introini U, Pierro L, et al. Optical coherence tomography (OCT) angiomatous proliferation (RAP) in retinal. Eur J Ophthalmol. 2002;12:467–472.

20. Matsumoto H, Sato T, Kishi S. Tomographic features of intraretinal neovascularization in retinal angiomatous proliferation. Retina. 2010;30(3):425–430.

21. Krebs I, Glittenberg C, Hagen S, et al. Retinal angiomatous proliferation: morphological changes assessed by Stratus, Cirrus OCT. Ophthalmic Surg Lasers Imaging. 2009;40:285–289.

22. Freund KB, Zweifel SA, Engelbert M. Do we need a new classification for choroidal neovascularization in age-related macular degeneration?. Retina. 2010;30(9):1333–1349.

23. Borrillo JL, Sivalingam A, Martidis A, et al. Surgical ablation of retinal angiomatous proliferation. Arch Ophthalmol. 2003;121:558–561.

24. Boscia F, Furino C, Sborgia L, et al. Photodynamic therapy for retinal angiomatous proliferation and pigment epithelium detachment. Am J Ophthalmol. 2004;138:1077–1079.

25. Shimada H, Mori R, Arai K, et al. Surgical excision of neovascularization in retinal angiomatous proliferation. Graefes Arch Clin Exp Ophthalmol. 2005;243:519–524.

26. Nakata M, Yuzawa M, Kawamura A, et al. Combining surgical ablation of retinal inflow and outflow vessels with photodynamic therapy for retinal angiomatous proliferation. Am J Ophthalmol. 2006;141:968–970.

27. Freund KB, Klais CM, Eandi CM, et al. Sequenced combined intravitreal triamcinolone and indocyanine green angiography-guided photodynamic therapy for retinal angiomatous proliferation. Arch Ophthalmol. 2006;124:487–492.

28. Johnson TM, Glaser BM. Focal laser ablation of retinal angiomatous proliferation. Retina. 2006;26:765–772.

29. Roth DB, Scott IU, Gloth JM, et al. Micropulsed laser photocoagulation and intravitreal triamcinolone acetonide injection for the treatment of retinal angiomatous proliferation. Retina. 2007;27:1201–1204.

30. Lai TY, Chan WM, Liu DT, et al. Ranibizumab for retinal angiomatous proliferation in neovascular age-related macular degeneration. Graefes Arch Clin Exp Ophthalmol. 2007;245:1877–1880.

31. Krebs I, Binder S, Stolba U, et al. Subretinal surgery and transplantation of autologous pigment epithelial cells in retinal angiomatous proliferation. Acta Ophthalmol. 2008;86:504–509.

32. Engelbert M, Zweifel SA, Freund KB. "Treat and extend" dosing of intravitreal antivascular endothelial growth factor therapy for type 3 neovascularization/retinal angiomatous proliferation. Retina. 2009;29:1424–1431.

33. Gharbiya M, Allievi F, Recupero V, et al. Intravitreal bevacizumab as primary treatment for retinal angiomatous proliferation. Twelve-month results. Retina. 2009;29:740–749.

34. Lo Giudice G, Gismondi M, De Belvis V, et al. Single-Session photodynamic therapy combined with intravitreal bevacizumab for retinal angiomatous proliferation. Retina. 2009;29:949–955.

35. Saito M, Shiragami CH, Shiraga F, et al. Comparison of intravitreal triamcinolone acetonide with photodynamic therapy and intravitreal bevacizumab with photodynamic therapy for retinal angiomatous proliferation. Am J Ophthalmol. 2010;149:472–481.

36. Atmani K, Voigt M, Le Tien V, et al. Ranibizumab for retinal angiomatous proliferation in age-related macular degeneration. Eye (Lond). 2010;24:1193–1198.

37. Saito M, Iida T, Kano M. Combined intravitreal ranibizumab and photodynamic therapy for retinal angiomatous proliferation. Am J Ophthalmol. 2012;153(3):504–514.

38. Nakano S, Honda S, Oh H, et al. Effect of photodynamic therapy (PDT), posterior subtenon injection of triamcinolone acetonide with PDT, and intravitreal injection of ranibizumab with PDT for retinal angiomatous proliferation. Clin Ophthalmol. 2012;6:277–282.

39. Mahmood S, Kumar N, Lenfestey PM, et al. Early response of retinal angiomatous proliferation treated with intravitreal pegaptanib: a retrospective review. Eye (Lond). 2009;23:530–535.

40. Gragoudas ES, Adamis AP, Cunningham ET Jr, et al. Pegaptanib for neovascular age-related macular degeneration. N Engl J Med. 2004;351:2805–2816.

41. Rosenfeld PJ, Brown DM, Heier JS, et al. Ranibizumab for neovascular age-related macular degeneration. N Engl J Med. 2006;355:1419–1431.

42. Kang JH, Park KA, Chung SE, et al. Retinal angiomatous proliferation and intravitreal bevacizumab injection. Korean J Ophthalmol. 2007;21:213–215.

43. Costagliola C, Romano MR, Dell'Omo R, et al. Intravitreal bevacizumab for the treatment of retinal angiomatous proliferation. Am J Ophthalmol. 2007;144:449–451.

44. Ghazi NG, Knape RM, Kirk TQ, et al. Intravitreal bevacizumab (Avastin) treatment of retinal angiomatous proliferation. Retina. 2008;28:689–695.

45. Amselem L, Llopis M, Cervera E, et al. az-[Intravitreal injection of bevacizumab (Avastin) for retinal angiomatous proliferation]. Arch Soc Esp Oftalmol. 2008;83:53–56.

46. Argon laser photocoagulation for senile macular degeneration. Results of a randomized clinical trial. Arch Ophthalmol. 1982;100:912–918.

47. Bottoni F, Massacesi A, Cigada M, et al. Treatment of retinal angiomatous proliferation in age-related macular degeneration: a series of 104 cases of retinal angiomatous proliferation. Arch Ophthalmol. 2005;123:1644–1650.

48. Krieglstein TR, Kampik A, Ulbig M. Intravitreal triamcinolone and laser photocoagulation for retinal angiomatous proliferation. Br J Ophthalmol. 2006;90:1357–1360.

49. Bearelly S, Espinosa-Heidmann DG, Cousins SW. The role of dynamic indocyanine green angiography in the diagnosis and treatment of retinal angiomatous proliferation. Br J Ophthalmol. 2008;92:191–196.

9

DIFFERENTIAL DIAGNOSIS OF AGE-RELATED MACULAR DEGENERATION

GABRIELA PAPA-OLIVA • MONICA RODRIGUEZ-FONTAL
D. VIRGIL ALFARO III

◼ INTRODUCTION

The diagnosis of age-related macular degeneration (AMD) can be challenging, particularly when the patient is in the age group commonly affected by AMD. Nonneovascular AMD is the most common type of AMD, observed in 90% of cases. Nonneovascular AMD demonstrates chorioretinal atrophy that may be difficult to differentiate from retina changes associated with other pathologies. The other major form of AMD, neovascular AMD, occurs with loss of visual acuity secondary to choroidal neovascularization (CNV). An extensive number of conditions can predispose the macula to develop CNV (1).

This chapter examines the differential diagnosis of age-related macular degeneration.

◼ NONNEOVASCULAR AGE-RELATED MACULAR DEGENERATION

It is well known that aging produces changes at the level of the outer retina, retinal pigment epithelium (RPE), Bruch's membrane, and choriocapillaris (2). These changes are microscopic, are sometimes not visible on clinical examination, and should be distinguished from clinically visible changes found in patients with nonneovascular AMD. Among these changes are drusen and alterations of the RPE.

Drusen are histologically defined as abnormal thickening of the inner face of the Bruch's membrane and clinically defined as yellow or yellowish-white deposits at the level of the retina. They are classified by size (small less than 64 μm, 64–124 μm intermediate, and large greater than 125 μm), by type (soft and hard), by distribution (greater clinical significance if located in the macula inner circular area of 3,000 μm in diameter), and by the extent of fundus involvement (3,4).

◼ DIFFERENTIAL DIAGNOSIS OF NONNEOVASCULAR AGE-RELATED MACULAR DEGENERATION

The most common diseases that can present changes similar to nonneovascular AMD are central serous chorioretinopathy (CSC), pattern dystrophy, dominant drusen, chloroquine toxicity, central areolar choroidal dystrophy, and cuticular drusen (Table 9.1).

Cuticular Drusen

Cuticular drusen or basal laminar drusen (BLD) were described by Gass in 1977 (5). Patients with BLD have

Table 9.1	DIFFERENTIAL DIAGNOSIS OF NONNEOVASCULAR AMD

Central serous chorioretinopathy
Pattern dystrophy
Dominant drusen
Chloroquine toxicity
Central areolar choroidal dystrophy
Cuticular drusen

numerous, small, uniformly sized, round, slightly raised, yellow, subretinal lesions on ocular fundus examination. These lesions are grouped into small clusters and usually span the macula between the arcades (Fig. 9.1A). The drusen are hyperfluorescent during fluorescein angiography and fade in later-phase frames (Fig. 9.1B). The lesions may develop a yellowish vitelliform material anterior to RPE. As it progresses, it clears and develops a marked or minimal geographic atrophy. The vitelliform material can block choroidal fluorescence in early stages of fluorescein angiography and stain in the later phase. The staining in later frames may mimic the appearance of type 1 occult CNV.

Initially, the term BLD was used to distinguish these drusen from drusen associated with AMD (6). Subsequent histologic analysis demonstrated that both types of drusen were indistinguishable. Both the BLD and the drusen associated with AMD are located between the basement membrane of the RPE and the inner collagenous layer of the Bruch's membrane (7). Furthermore, both types of drusen were shown to be histologically indistinct using light and electron microscopy. This entity should not be confused with the histopathologic terms "basal lamellar deposits" or "basal linear deposits." Although the visual prognosis for cuticular drusen is better than the visual prognosis for patients with AMD, the possibility of CNV exists in both diseases and is associated with worse visual acuity outcomes (8).

Central Serous Chorioretinopathy

This idiopathic disease is most common in Caucasian, Hispanic, and Asian patients between the second and fifth decade of their lives. More often, it is diagnosed in patients with type A personality, high stress levels, or use of corticosteroids (inhaled, topical, or systemic). CSC clinically presents as a sensory retinal detachment that may also be associated with RPE serous retinal detachment. The diagnostic challenge is significant for older age groups with changes in the RPE due to multifocal serous detachments (9,10). In some cases, the formation of "gutter–like" distribution of RPE atrophy in the absence of drusen may help make the diagnosis (Fig. 9.2).

Patients with chronic or recurrent CSC may have decreased visual acuity as a result of RPE dysfunction, subretinal precipitates, and subretinal CNV. The presence of CNV and subretinal fluid in a patient with CSC may be difficult to distinguish from neovascular AMD. Diagnostic clues include absence of drusen, absence of hemorrhage, patches of RPE atrophy in a gutter–like distribution, and the presence of multiple pigmented epithelium detachments (Fig. 9.3).

Pattern Dystrophy

The term "pattern dystrophy" represents a group of related conditions inherited in an autosomal dominant fashion. These macular dystrophies are relatively benign disorders. They are characterized by an abnormality at the level of RPE with hyperpigmentation and variably shaped yellow or gray deposits (Fig. 9.4A and B). The patients are asymptomatic and usually have normal vision. The classic appearance of pattern dystrophy demonstrates the pigmented lesions in the shape of a butterfly. The lesions are clearly seen in the fluorescein angiography. Typically, the lesions are hypofluorescent with a surrounding hyperfluorescent rim (Fig. 9.4C and D). This configuration helps to differentiate them from soft drusen of AMD (11–13). Other pattern dystrophies that we need to have

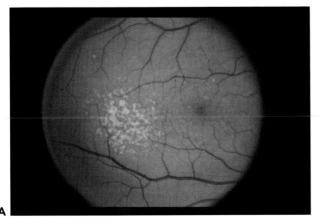
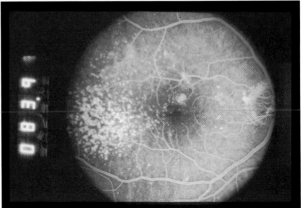

Figure 9.1 ■ **A.** Basal laminar drusen. **B.** Fluorescein angiography showing starry-night pattern.

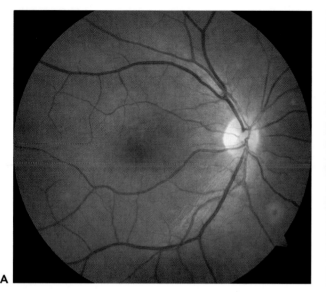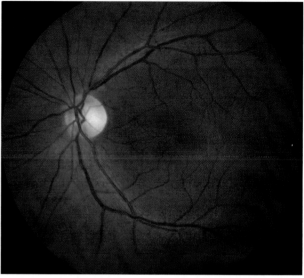

Figure 9.2 ■ Central serous chorioretinopathy. **A.** Fundus photograph, right eye, showing RPE changes from CSC. **B.** Fundus photograph, left eye, showing RPE changes from CSC.

in mind are reticular dystrophy of Sjögren and macroreticular dystrophy.

Chloroquine Toxicity

Chloroquine has high affinity with melanin and is deposited in the RPE. The toxic damage is initiated by the degeneration of the photoreceptors, with subsequent degeneration of other retinal cells and the RPE. RPE mottling and nongeographic atrophy may be seen in the macular area in patients with toxic changes. The absence of drusen and a

positive history of drug ingestion are essential to make the diagnosis (14) (Fig. 9.5A and B).

Dominant Drusen

This entity is inherited in an autosomal dominant fashion, affecting individuals between the second and third decade of their lives, and it is best observed on fluorescein angiography. Drusen may become confluent after the fourth decade. Initially, patients are asymptomatic. Eventually, central vision loss correlates with macular involvement,

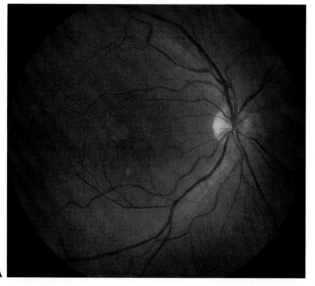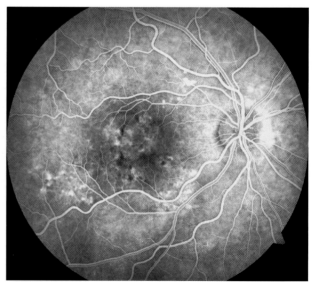

Figure 9.3 ■ Central serous chorioretinopathy. **A.** Fundus photograph, right eye, showing RPE changes from multifocal serous detachments. **B.** Fluorescein angiography showing leakage.

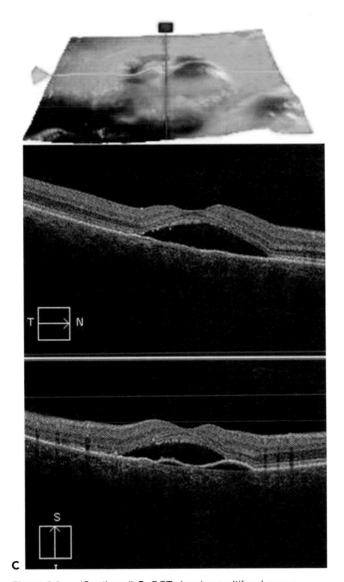

Figure 9.3 ■ *(Continued)* **C.** OCT showing multifocal serous pigmented epithelium detachments and subretinal fluid.

NEOVASCULAR AGE-RELATED MACULAR DEGENERATION

The term CNV refers to ingrown fibrovascular tissue from the choroidal circulation into or underneath the retina. This fibrovascular tissue can progress to a disciform scar and cause irreversible vision loss. Any pathologic process that disturbs the RPE and choroid, leading to the disruption of the Bruch's membrane, can be associated with CNV (17). There are different causes of CNV; some of those more frequently found are age-related macular degeneration, ocular histoplasmosis, multifocal choroiditis, myopia, and trauma.

CNV has been divided in two types: type I and type II. Type I CNV is characterized by a neovascular growth between the inner and outer aspects of the Bruch's membrane, and it is more frequent in AMD. In type II CNV, neovascular growth occurs within the subsensory retinal space. Type II CNV is more frequent in young patients (18–20). Clinically, we suspect the presence of age-related CNV, typically type I, when a patient older than 60 years complains of metamorphopsia or scotoma and the ocular fundus reveals fluid or blood in the subretinal space. An RPE detachment and intraretinal blood are also possible indicators of this condition. Intravenous fluorescein angiography and optical coherence tomography (OCT) are needed to evaluate the presence of CNV and are helpful in assessing the differential diagnosis of the causes of the CNV.

DIFFERENTIAL DIAGNOSIS OF NEOVASCULAR AGE-RELATED MACULAR DEGENERATION

There are multiple clinical entities that can mimic neovascular AMD (Table 9.2). We discuss in this section some of the most important entities.

Retinal Arteriolar Macroaneurysms

Retinal arteriolar macroaneurysms are present in more than 75% of patients with arterial hypertension over 60 years old. Significantly fewer are associated with retinal vein occlusions. Clinical features of retinal arteriolar macroaneurysm include focal dilation of a retinal artery with hemorrhages in all anatomic compartments (subretinal, intraretinal, or vitreous), retinal edema, and circinate lipid exudates. When the hemorrhage or associated lipid extends into the macula, it may be confused with CNV. Fluorescein angiography findings will differentiate the two entities. Macroaneurysms will demonstrate focal hyperfluorescence in the early frames, with late staining of the damaged vascular wall. Often, an area of capillary nonperfusion surrounds the lesion. The neighboring vasculature

and it can be distinguished from AMD only on the basis of family history (15) (Fig. 9.6).

Central Areolar Choroidal Atrophy

The mean age at onset of visual loss is the fourth decade of life, with subsequent gradual deterioration in visual acuity. At early stages, the disease presents no symptoms associated with symmetric fine mottled areolar depigmentation of the fovea. In later stages, the depigmented area develops a sharply demarcated geographic atrophy that involves photoreceptors, RPE, and choriocapillaris (Fig. 9.7). In the elderly patient, central areolar choroidal atrophy may be confused with AMD (16).

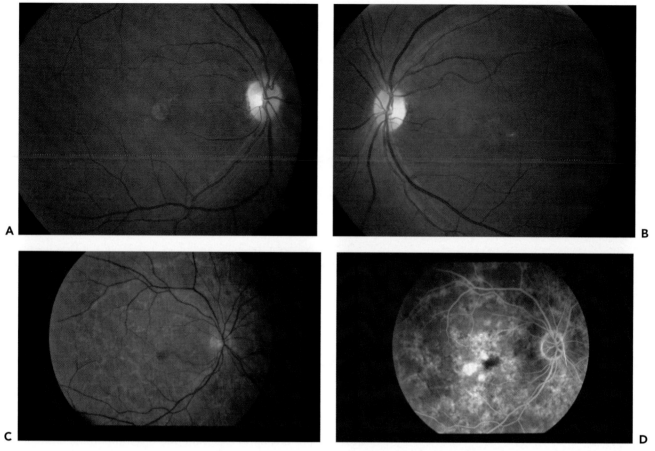

Figure 9.4 ■ **A,B.** Pattern dystrophy of the RPE, right and left eye. **C.** Fluorescein angiogram, right eye, reveals central hypofluorescence surrounded by hyperfluorescence. **D.** Fluorescein angiogram, left eye, showing central staining.

may exhibit microaneurysms and intra-arterial collateral formation (21–23) (Fig. 9.8).

Vitelliform Dystrophy

The presence of a vitelliform material, as in adult-onset foveomacular vitelliform dystrophy, can mimic an occult CNV in the late phase of a fluorescein angiography. Also, vitelliform lesions in adults can have fundus features that

can be mistaken for a pigmented epithelium detachment (24) (Fig. 9.9).

Acquired Juxtafoveal Telangiectasia

Juxtafoveal telangiectasia is a term that describes entities presenting with incompetence, ectasia, and/or irregular dilations of the capillary network affecting only the parafoveal region of one or both eyes. The term idiopathic

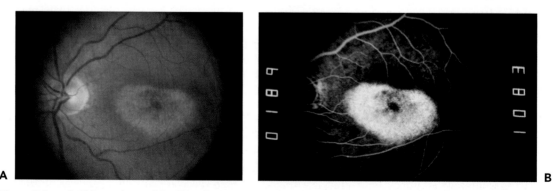

Figure 9.5 ■ **A.** Chloroquine toxicity. Note the lack of drusen and presence of retinal pigment epithelial changes similar to nonneovascular age-related macular degeneration. **B.** Fluorescein angiography of the same fundus.

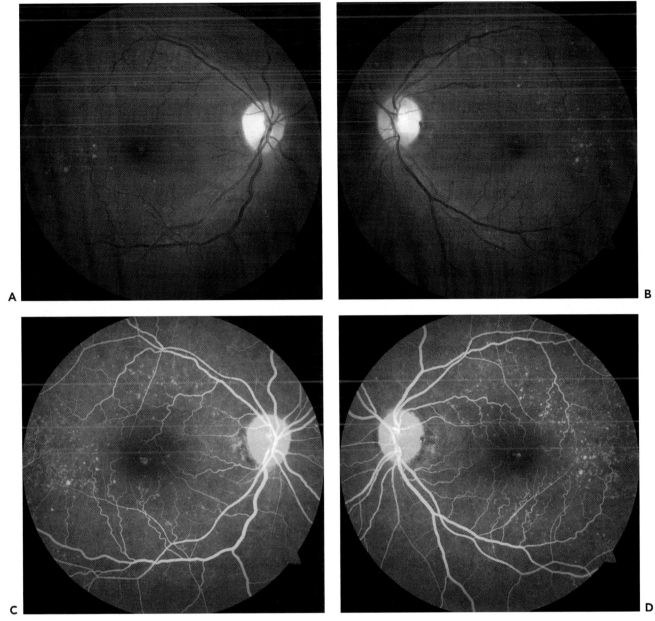

Figure 9.6 ■ **A,B.** Fundus photo showing dominant drusen syndrome. **C,D.** Fluorescein angiography of the same eyes.

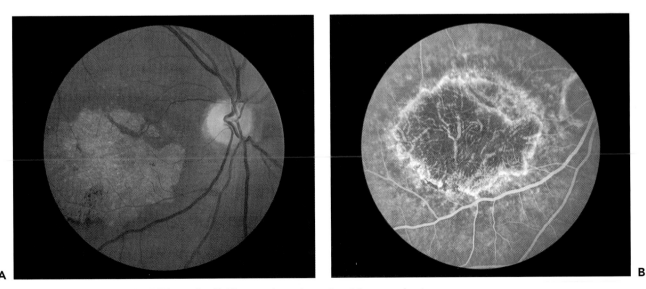

Figure 9.7 ■ **A.** Central areolar RPE atrophy. **B.** Fluorescein angiography of the same fundus.

Table 9.2 DIFFERENTIAL DIAGNOSIS OF NEOVASCULAR AMD

Not Associated with CNV
Retinal arteriolar macroaneurysms
Vitelliform dystrophy
Acquired juxtafoveal telangiectasis
Central serous chorioretinopathy
Inflammatory conditions: choroiditis, Harada's disease, posterior scleritis

Associated with CNV
Degenerative and Hereditary Conditions
Age-related macular degeneration
Myopic degeneration
Angioid streaks
Best's disease
Fundus flavimaculatus
Idiopathic juxtafoveal retinal telangiectasia
Membranoproliferative glomerulonephritis type II
Choroideremia

Inflammatory and Infectious Conditions
Ocular histoplasmosis syndrome
Multifocal choroiditis
Serpiginous choroiditis
Vogt-Koyanagi-Harada syndrome
Birdshot chorioretinopathy
Punctate inner choroidopathy
Acute multifocal posterior placoid pigment epitheliopathy

Multiple evanescent white dot syndrome (MEWDS)
Behcet's syndrome
Sarcoidosis
Toxoplasma retinochoroiditis
Toxocariasis
Rubella
Endogenous Candida endophthalmitis
Sympathetic ophthalmia

Trauma
Choroidal rupture
Intense photocoagulation
Intraocular foreign body

Tumor
Choroidal nevus
Choroidal melanoma
Choroidal hemangioma
Metastatic choroidal tumors
Hamartomas of the RPE
Choroidal osteoma

Miscellaneous
Idiopathic
Anterior ischemic optic neuropathy
Idiopathic CSC
Radiation retinopathy
Chronic papilledema

juxtafoveolar retinal telangiectasias (IJFT) was coined by Gass and Oyakawa in 1982 (25). They proposed the first classification of these entities into four groups based largely on their clinical and fluorescein angiographic features. In 1993, Gass and Blodi (26) further updated this classification by subdividing IJFT into three distinct groups, 1, 2, and 3, based on demographic difference or clinical severity. In this section, we discuss two subgroups of IJFT that may resemble neovascular AMD,

especially when pigmentary changes and fibrovascular scarring are present.

Group 1B (unilateral idiopathic juxtafoveal telangiectasias) is congenital and found in males in the fourth decade of life. The fovea avascular zone may be significant smaller and almost completely vascularized (Fig. 9.10).

Group 2A (bilateral acquired juxtafoveal telangiectasias) is an acquired form and is the most common type. Affected patients are middle-aged or older (mean 55 years). Males

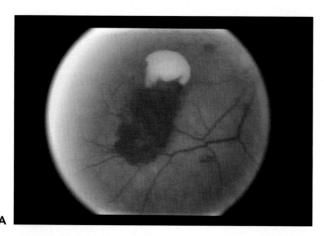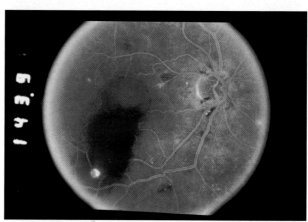

Figure 9.8 ■ **A.** Retinal macroaneurysm. The presence of hemorrhage and exudates extending into the macula may lead to a diagnosis of CNV. **B.** Fluorescein angiography demonstrates the early filling of the macroaneurysm.

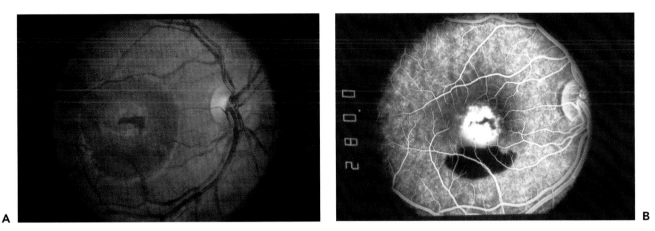

Figure 9.9 ■ **A.** Vitelliform dystrophy. **B.** Fluorescein angiography of the same fundus. Unlike CNV, this material shows early hypofluorescence and a ring of irregular hyperfluorescence surrounding the hypo- or nonfluorescent area.

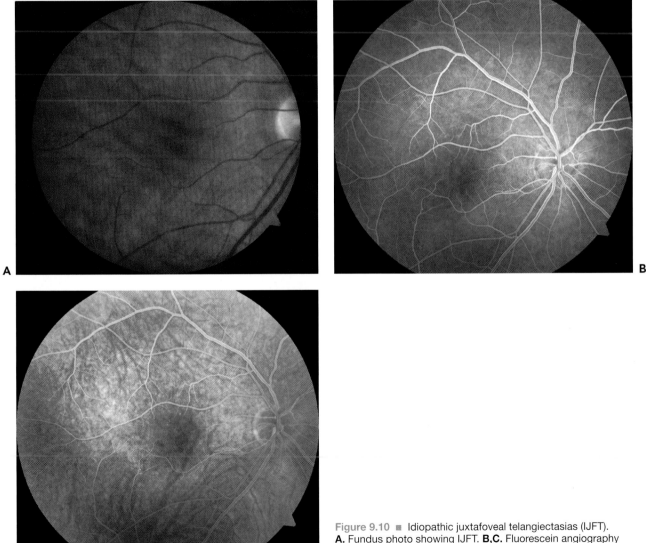

Figure 9.10 ■ Idiopathic juxtafoveal telangiectasias (IJFT).
A. Fundus photo showing IJFT. **B,C.** Fluorescein angiography demonstrating early and late frames of the same eye.

and females are equally affected. This disorder is bilateral and may be asymmetric. The entire juxtafoveal network may be involved. The macular pigment plaques with subretinal fluid and subretinal vascularization may be mistaken for age-related macular degeneration, but drusen and pigment epithelial detachment are generally absent in IJFT 2A.

Conditions Associated with Choroidal Neovascularization

CNV is associated with many ocular conditions, including inflammatory, infectious, degenerative, hereditary, and congenital disorders; ocular tumors; trauma; and a few miscellaneous disorders with specific clinical signs (Table 9.2). The recognition of these ocular conditions is important for determining prognosis and management. The clinical presentation of the most common disorder associated with CNV is reviewed in this section.

Ocular Histoplasmosis Syndrome

Ocular histoplasmosis syndrome (OHS) is an inflammatory disease secondary to a systemic dissemination of *Histoplasma capsulatum* fungus that occurs after inhalation of fungal spore into the lungs. The fungus is endemic to the Mississippi and Ohio River Valley areas. Maculopathy does not usually develop until patients are 20 to 50 years of age. The diagnosis is made by the presence of the clinical triad: peripapillary choroidal atrophy, histo spots, and CNV without vitreous inflammation (Fig. 9.11). CNV typically begins at the site of histo spots in the macula area (27,28).

Other inflammatory conditions such as multifocal choroiditis and punctate inner choroidopathy must be ruled out. Multifocal choroiditis has chorioretinal scars similar to those in the OHS, but they have a low incidence of positive

histoplasmin skin test reactions and calcified granulomata on chest x-ray films. Also, anterior chamber inflammation and vitreous inflammation are frequently found. Punctate inner choroidopathy affects mainly young myopic healthy women with small yellow spots. Those lesions resemble those seen in multifocal choroiditis, but they are smaller and without vitreous inflammation. Both inflammatory diseases can present with CNV; however, they are not as aggressive as CNV secondary to AMD (29).

Pathologic Myopia

A peripapillary myopic crescent that extends into the macula is the hallmark ophthalmoscopic finding in pathologic myopia. Pathologic myopia may present with posterior staphylomas, lacquer cracks, Fuchs' spots, and CNV. Myopia is the most common cause of CNV in young patients, accounting for up to 60% of CNV in patients younger than 50 years old. CNV is the most common vision-threatening macular complication in pathologic myopia, present in 4% to 11% of the affected eyes (Fig. 9.12).

Treatment of CNV due to pathologic myopia is controversial. Different treatments have been evaluated in different consecutive prospective or retrospective interventional series, including direct laser photocoagulation, photodynamic therapy (PDT), surgical removal, macular translocation, and anti–vascular endothelial growth (VEGF) therapy. PDT, surgical removal, and intravitreal anti-VEGF factor are associated with better visual outcomes than natural history (30–33).

Angioid Streaks

Angioid streaks (AS) are irregular linear breaks in the Bruch's membrane that typically emanate from the optic disk and may extend into the macula. They are light, red-orange to dark, red-brown color. The vision loss in patients with AS is caused by the presence of CNV. Fluorescein

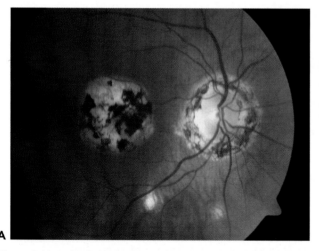
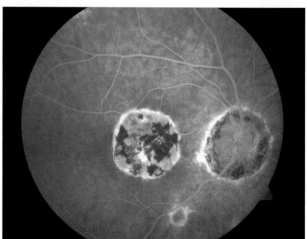

Figure 9.11 ■ Ocular histoplasmosis syndrome. **A.** Fundus photo showing macular lesion, punched-out histo spots, and peripapillary atrophy. **B.** Fluorescein angiography of the same eye.

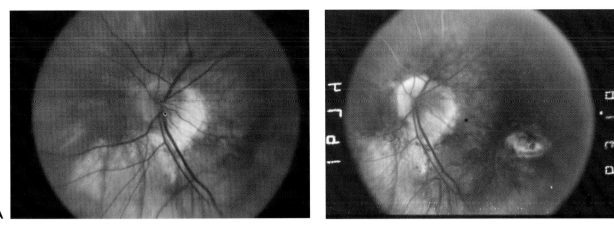

Figure 9.12 ■ **A.** Myopic degeneration with characteristic tilted optic disk, peripapillary chorioretinal atrophy, and lacquer cracks. **B.** Fluorescein angiography of the same fundus with a Fuchs spot representing RPE hyperplasia associated with a small, nonprogressing area of CNV.

angiography shows slightly hyperfluorescent, vessel-like streaks in early exposures not associated with dye filling or leakage, unless CNV is present (Fig. 9.13). The natural course of the CNV is poor, usually resulting in foveal involvement and central visual loss. AS are associated with a variety of systemic disorders such as pseudoxanthoma elasticum, Ehlers-Danlos syndrome, Paget disease, and sickle cell anemia.

The treatment of macular CNV in patients with AS has remained a challenge. Laser photocoagulation, PDT, submacular surgery, and anti-VEGF drugs have been used with variable results (34,35).

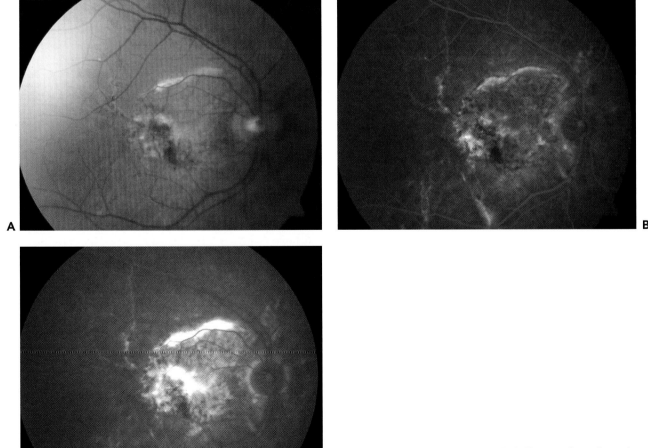

Figure 9.13 ■ **A.** Angioid streaks. **B,C.** Fluorescein angiography showing AS associated to CNV.

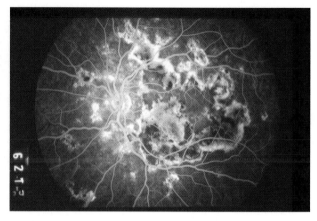

Figure 9.14 ■ **A.** CNV in a patient with serpiginous choroiditis. **B.** Fluorescein angiography of the same fundus.

Serpiginous Choroiditis

Serpiginous choroiditis is a bilateral inflammatory disorder of the RPE and the choroid. It is a recurrent, bilateral, inflammatory, chronic, and progressive disease. It is reported to start with irregular gray-white patches representing subretinal infiltration, which show a propensity to development near the optic disk or in the posterior pole. The serpentine shape of the lesions starts in the peripapillary area and tends to spread centrifugally, hence its name. The main cause of decreased vision is macular involvement with development of CNV (Fig. 9.14). The CNV associated with serpiginous choroiditis is distinguished from CNV secondary to AMD based on the presence of an inflammatory component in the former and drusen in the latter. Serial examination at regular intervals is needed to monitor the disease progression, recurrences, and involvement of the other eye. Improvement in vision and resolution of lesions threatening the fovea in patients with serpiginous choroiditis can occur with a combination therapy of systemic steroids and immunosuppressive agents. Recurrences could not be prevented in spite of the treatment given (36–38).

Idiopathic CNV

This condition should be considered a diagnosis of exclusion in the absence of any other fundus abnormality or associated condition (39). Serum inflammatory factors in patients with idiopathic CNV, such as VEFG factor and IgE, may play a role in the formation of idiopathic CNV. PDT and intravitreal anti-VEGF drugs may be used to treat idiopathic CNV (40,41).

REFERENCES

1. Iyer M, Mieler WF. Differential diagnosis of age-related macular degeneration. In: Alfaro V, ed. Age-Related Macular Degeneration. 1st Ed. New York: Springer; 2006:73–85.

2. American Academy of Ophthalmology. Retina y vitreo. Barcelona, Spain: Elsevier; 2009:408.

3. Klein R, Davis MD, Magli YL, et al. The Wisconsin age-related maculopathy grading system. Ophthalmology. 1991;98(7):1128–1134.

4. Schachat AP, Hyman L, Leske MC, et al. Features of age-related macular degeneration in a black population. The Barbados Eye Study Group. Arch Ophthalmol. 1995;113(6):728–735.

5. Gass J. Stereoscopic atlas of macular disease: diagnosis and treatment. 2nd Ed. St. Louis, MO: Mosby; 1977.

6. Gass JD, Jallow S, Davis B. Adult vitelliform macular detachment occurring in patients with basal laminar drusen. Am J Ophthalmol. 1985;99:445–459.

7. Russell SR, Mullins RF, Schneider BL, et al. Location, substructure, and composition of basal laminar drusen compared with drusen associated with aging and age-related macular degeneration. Am J Ophthalmol. 2000;129:205–214.

8. Cohen SY, Meunier I, Soubrane G, et al. Visual function and course of basal laminar drusen combined with vitelliform macular detachment. Br J Ophthalmol. 1994;78:437–440.

9. Yannuzzi LA, Shakin JL, Fisher YL, et al. Peripheral retinal detachments and retinal pigment epithelial atrophic tracts secondary to central serous pigment epitheliopathy. Ophthalmology. 1984;91:1554–1572.

10. Spaide RF, Campeas L, Haas A, et al. Central serous chorioretinopathy in younger and older adults. Ophthalmology. 1996;103:2070–2079; discussion 2079–2080.

11. Gass JDM. A clinicopathologic study of a peculiar foveomacular dystrophy. Trans Am Ophthalmol Soc. 1974;72:139–156.

12. Marmor MF, Byers B. Pattern dystrophy of the pigment epithelium. Am J Ophthalmol. 1977;84:32–44.

13. Hsieh RC, Fine BS, Lyons JS. Patterned dystrophies of the retinal pigment epithelium. Arch Ophthalmol. 1977;95:429–435.

14. Michael F, Marmor MD, Ronald E, et al. Recommendations on screening for chloroquine and hydroxychloroquine retinopathy: a report by the American Academy of Ophthalmology. Ophthalmology. 2002;109(7):1377–1382.

15. Deutman AF, Jansen LMAA. Dominantly inherited drusen of Bruch's membrane. Br J Ophthalmol. 1979;82:84.

16. Leveille AS, Morse PH, Kiernan JP. Autosomal dominant central pigment epithelial and choroidal degeneration. Ophthalmology. 1982;89(12):1407–1413.

17. Klein R, Klein BE, Knudtson MD, et al. Fifteen-year cumulative incidence of age-related macular degeneration: the Beaver Dam Eye Study. Ophthalmology. 2007;114(2):253–262.

18. Gass JD. Biomicroscopic and histopathologic considerations regarding the feasibility of surgical excision of subfoveal neovascular membranes. Am J Ophthalmol. 1994;118(3):285–298.

19. Macular Photocoagulation Study Group. Subfoveal neovascular lesions in age-related macular degeneration. Guidelines for evaluation and treatment in the macular photocoagulation study. Arch Ophthalmol. 1991;109(9):1242–1257.

20. Weisz JM, O'Connell SR, Bresseler NM. Treatment guidelines for age-related macular degeneration based upon results from the macular photocoagulation study. In: Quiroz-Mercado H, ed. Macular surgery. 1st Ed. Philadelphia, PA: Lippincott Williams & Wilkins; 2000:201–211.

21. Lavin MJ, Marsh RJ, Peart S, et al. Retinal arterial macroaneurysms: a retrospective study of 40 patients. Br J Ophthalmol. 1987;71(11):817–825.

22. Moosavi RA, Fong KC, Chopdar A. Retinal artery macroaneurysms: clinical and fluorescein angiographic features in 34 patients. Eye (Lond). 2006;20(9):1011–1020.

23. Panton RW, Goldberg MF, Farber MD. Retinal arterial macroaneurysms: risk factors and natural history. Br J Ophthalmol. 1990;74:595–600.

24. Jaffe GJ, Schatz H. Histopathologic features of adult-onset foveomacular pigment epithelial dystrophy. Arch Ophthalmol. 1988;106:958–960.

25. Gass JD, Oyakawa RT. Idiopathic juxtafoveolar retinal telangiectasis. Arch Ophthalmol. 1982;10:769–780.

26. Gass JD, Blodi BA. Idiopathic juxtafoveolar retinal telangiectasis. Update of classification and follow-up study. Ophthalmology. 1993;100:1536–1546.

27. Parnell JR, Jampol LM, Yannuzzi LA, et al. Differentiation between presumed ocular histoplasmosis syndrome and multifocal choroiditis with panuveitis based on morphology of photographed fundus lesions and fluorescein angiography. Arch Ophthalmol. 2001;119(2):208–212.

28. Dreyer RF, Gass DJ. Multifocal choroiditis and panuveitis. A syndrome that mimics ocular histoplasmosis. Arch Ophthalmol. 1984;102(12):1776–1784.

29. Essex RW, Wong J, Fraser-Bell S, et al. Punctate inner choroidopathy: clinical features and outcomes. Arch Ophthalmol. 2010;128(8):982–987.

30. Brancato R, Pece A, Avanza P, et al. Photocoagulation scar expansion after laser therapy for choroidal neovascularization in degenerative myopia. Retina. 1990;10:239–243.

31. Verteporfin in Photodynamic Therapy Study Group. Photodynamic therapy of subfoveal choroidal neovascularization in pathologic myopia with verteporfin. 1-year results of a randomized clinical trial—VIP report no. 1. Ophthalmology. 2001;108:841–852.

32. Uemura A, Thomas MA. Subretinal surgery for choroidal neovascularization in patients with high myopia. Arch Ophthalmol. 2000;118:344–350.

33. Lalloum F, Souied EH, Bastuji-Garin S, et al. Intravitreal ranibizumab for choroidal neovascularization complicating pathologic myopia. Retina. 2010;30(3):399–406.

34. Artunay O, Yuzbasioglu E, Rasier R, et al. Combination treatment with intravitreal injection of ranibizumab and reduced fluence photodynamic therapy for choroidal neovascularization secondary to angioid streaks: preliminary clinical results of 12-month follow-up. Retina. 2011;31(7):1279–1286.

35. Finger RP, Charbel Issa P, Schmitz-Valckenberg S, et al. Long-term effectiveness of intravitreal bevacizumab for choroidal neovascularization secondary to angioid streaks in pseudoxanthoma elasticum. Retina. 2011;31(7):1268–1278.

36. Abrez H, Biswas J, Sudharshan S. Clinical profile, treatment, and visual outcome of serpiginous choroiditis. Ocul Immunol Inflamm. 2007;15(4):325–335.

37. Marcuello Melendo B, Torrón Fernández-Blanco C, Pérez Oliván S, et al. Serpiginous choroiditis: clinical course and treatment. Arch Soc Esp Oftalmol. 2004;79(5):237–242.

38. Christmas NJ, Oh KT, Oh DM, et al. Long-term follow-up of patients with serpiginous choroiditis. Retina. 2002;22(5):550–556.

39. Ho AC, Yannuzzi LA, Pisicano K, et al. The natural history of idiopathic subfoveal choroidal neovascularization. Ophthalmology. 1995;102(5):782–789.

40. Zhang H, Liu ZL, Sun P, et al. Intravitreal bevacizumab for treatment of subfoveal idiopathic choroidal neovascularization: results of a 1-year prospective trial. Am J Ophthalmol. 2012;153(2):300–306.

41. Giansanti F, Virgili G, Varano M, et al. Photodynamic therapy for choroidal neovascularization in pediatric patients. Retina. 2005;25(5):590–596.

10

FLUORESCEIN ANGIOGRAPHY

GISELA BARCAT ANGELELLI • ERIC P. JABLON
RICHARD B. ROSEN • D. VIRGIL ALFARO III

INTRODUCTION

In 1871, the sodium fluorescein molecule was synthesized by Baeyer and used as an early ophthalmic research tool (1). Ninety years later, Novotny and Alvis introduced the concept of serial fundus photography after intravenous injection of sodium fluorescein dye to study the retinal and choroidal circulation. This was the first human fluorescein angiogram, what they called "a method of photographing fluorescein circulating in blood vessels (2)."

Their initial observations were of diabetic and hypertensive patients, but it was not long before this novel technique was used to study age-related macular degeneration (AMD). Currently, fluorescein angiography (FA) is the gold standard for the differential diagnosis of neovascular AMD and determination of lesion characteristics (3).

This chapter focuses on the application of the powerful tool of FA for AMD, the classification system that has developed as a result of detailed observations, and the findings of clinical trials, which have used FA in directing treatment and retreatment of choroidal neovascularization (CNV).

FA PRINCIPLES AND TECHNIQUES

FA represents an application of the physical phenomenon of luminescence. Luminescence is the emission of light in the visible spectrum from any source that has been stimulated by electromagnetic radiation. It occurs when energy in the form of electromagnetic radiation is absorbed at a shorter wavelength, shifted, and reemitted at a longer visible wavelength. The process involves decay from a wavelength of higher energy to a wavelength at a lower energy state, causing free electrons in an excited state to emit energy in the form of light when returning to a lower state.

Fluorescence is the luminescence maintained in response to continuous excitation; therefore, fluorescence is present only if the excitation is present. Thus, retinal angiography is possible because of these chemical and physical properties of sodium fluorescein.

Sodium fluorescein ($C_{20}H_{12}O_5Na$) is a water-soluble hydrocarbon that emits green-yellow light having a wavelength 520 to 530 nm after excitation with blue light of wavelength 465 to 490 nm. In other words, if a blue light is projected as an exciting light from a camera into the eye, the sodium fluorescein circulating inside the eye will absorb and discharge a green-yellow reemission, or responder light, that will come toward the camera. Because these frequencies are within the visible spectrum of light, conventional photographic devices and techniques are able to capture angiographic images. This small molecule with a weight of 376.27 Da—compared to 775 Da for indocyanine green (ICG)—readily diffuses through the fenestrated vessels of the choriocapillaris but does not cross the intercellular tight junctions between the retinal pigment epithelium (RPE) and retinal vascular endothelium (RVE). Consequently, any condition that compromises the intact blood–retinal barrier, obstructs blood flow, or changes the normal pigmentation of the retina or pigment epithelium can cause abnormalities on angiography allowing the physiology of the fundus to be studied (4).

Maximal fluorescence of sodium fluorescein occurs at a pH of 7.4, ideal for human blood (5). It is relatively inert, making intravenous injection safe with minimal adverse reactions (6). When mixed with human blood, fluorescein becomes 80% bound to plasma proteins (compared to near-total binding of ICG to serum globulins), while 20% is unbound or free. Only this 20% of sodium fluorescein not bound to protein will fluoresce.

Before the angiogram, the patient should be informed of the nature and side effects of the study. After signing a consent form, the patient is seated in front of the camera with one forearm extended.

First, stereo color and red-free photographs are taken of the macula. Then, 5 to 10 mL of fluorescein dye is injected intravenously.

There are a few immediate side effects associated with fluorescein injection, particularly nausea and vomiting.

After fluorescein injection, angiophotography commences in 10 to 12 seconds. Immediately after the injection of dye, six rapid-sequence photos are taken of the primary macula during the filling phase (7). This is followed by a stereo pair of the primary macula at approximately 30, 40, 60, 90, and 180 seconds postinjection. Late stereophotos are taken between 5 and 10 minutes postinjection (8).

The first fluorescein angiograms in the late 1960s were made with the classic black body Zeiss fundus camera, equipped with a Contax camera, which advanced the film with a circular turning knob and recycled the photographic flash every 1 to 3 seconds, depending on its intensity (9,10). Novotny and Alvis (2) then modified the Zeiss fundus camera about which they noted in their original article that the main limitation of this prototype was the flash apparatus causing a 12-second delay between photographs. Advances in the original angiography system included modifications of the power pack and flash unit, addition of dual camera backs for ease in performing color fundus photography and FA, use of a motor drive for rapid and motionless film advancement, and a stereo separator for stereophotography (7).

Since their introduction in the mid-1980s, digital angiographic systems have gained widespread use in the ophthalmic community and have undergone technical improvements that have advanced their ability to provide high-resolution images (9,10).

The advent of digital imaging allows the physician to determine appropriate patient diagnosis and treatment options immediately in comparison to the patient's previous imaging studies. This is accomplished using digital overlay techniques that allow for precise evaluation of changes in fundus abnormalities detected on the angiographic studies (9,10).

Technicians are able to make adjustments in gain, focus, and flash intensity on a real time; assess the quality of the study as it is ongoing; and allow for immediate feedback and training with the physician.

Another advantage to digital imaging is in the area of patient education. Digital imaging allows the physician to manipulate and display the angiographic study while explaining diagnostic and treatment options to the patients on a real-time basis (10). Advantages of such systems also include immediate image processing compared to the development time of film and ease in file storage, file transfer, and file incorporation into electronic medical record systems.

A generation of newly created and defined medical retinal specialists was dedicated to acquire, interpret, and archive these images as a guide for treatment, lasers, vitreoretinal surgery, and pharmacotherapeutic advances (10).

In the Macular Photocoagulation Study (MPS), the photographs used for treatment were obtained 72 to 96 hours prior to treatment (8). Based on findings of the Treatment of AMD with Photodynamic Therapy (TAP) study, treatment for subfoveal CNV with verteporfin photodynamic therapy (PDT) should be performed within a week. In grading the FA, the distance of the neovascular lesion to the center of the fovea, the membrane size, and the leakage characteristics are noted using a stereo viewer. For film angiography, a ration of reticule measurement to the camera magnification factor is used to measure the lesion dimensions. Many digital angiography systems contain measurement software for exact measurements and automatic conversion for different camera settings, yet an enlarged early- or mid-frame FA image is invaluable during thermal laser treatment to ensure adequate coverage of the CNV. Utilization of microfilm reader, angiogram projector, or a digital display to guide laser treatment suite offers the best usage of the angiogram study.

The patients should be properly informed of later effects of FA like temporary yellow skin color, fluorescent urine, and photosensitivity for 24 hours, and they should be informed of the rare but potentially serious risks like hives, asthmatic symptoms, and laryngeal edema (6–11).

These can usually be managed by intravenous administration of cortisone. Any facility that performs FA should be equipped with a proper resuscitation kit and have in place a care plan and adequately trained personnel in the event of an adverse reaction (7).

FA INTERPRETATION

AMD is a retinal disease in which all of the various abnormal FA patterns can be observed (Fig. 10.1). These angiographic abnormalities are broadly classified as those leading to decreased fluorescence (hypofluorescence) or abnormally increased fluorescence (hyperfluorescence) (12). Hypofluorescence represents either blocked fluorescence or a vascular filling defect. Pertaining to AMD, blocked fluorescence is typically due to intraretinal/subretinal/subpigment epithelial hemorrhage or pigment proliferation/clumping. The depth of a lesion can be determined by relating the level of the blocked fluorescence to details of the retinal circulation. In advanced nonneovascular AMD, hypofluorescence can develop from choroidal vascular atrophy, and retinal vascular occlusion can occur after thermal laser or verteporfin PDT.

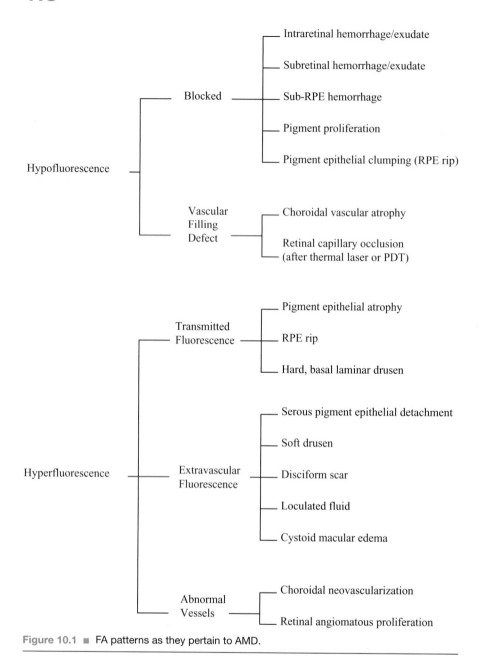

Figure 10.1 ■ FA patterns as they pertain to AMD.

Hyperfluorescence in AMD can be the result of loss of the normal barrier to background choroidal fluorescence known as transmitted fluorescence. Examples include hard drusen, nongeographic atrophy (non-GA) of the RPE in which abnormal background fluorescence fades during the course of the study (window defect), and geographic atrophy (GA) of the RPE in which atrophy of the choriocapillaris reveals the staining of the underlying sclera (13). Leakage of dye into a confined space is characterized by progressive, uniform hyperfluorescence known as pooling, which can be seen with soft drusen and serous RPE detachment. Abnormal blood vessels are noteworthy for their lack of intercellular tight junctions allowing permeability to fluorescein. CNV and intraretinal neovascularization (IRN) in AMD lead to early and progressive hyperfluorescence with late leakage.

▌INDICATIONS FOR FA IN AMD

While FA is an integral part in the care process of AMD, it does not replace history and careful ophthalmic examination in assessing a patient, and it is not required for all patients or at each visit (9). FA is indicated for any patient with AMD and vision loss, metamorphopsia, or new scotoma in which CNV is suspected (14,15). Because not all patients with neovascular AMD are symptomatic, those at high risk for developing CNV should be carefully examined for signs of such changes (16). While stereoscopic slit lamp ophthalmoscopy can usually detect evidence of CNV (including subretinal fluid, hard exudate, blood, pigment epithelial elevation, or a gray-green membrane), angiography is needed to detect the size, exact location, and leakage characteristics of the lesion (17). CNV may be undetectable by clinical examination alone. In patients with clinical signs of advanced nonneovascular AMD, FA may be helpful in assessing progression of pigment epithelial atrophy, particularly if vision changes are reported.

Because of the increasing incidence of AMD with age, elderly patients with media opacity that may limit careful macular examination, such as cataracts or keratopathy, may benefit from FA (13). Angiography may reveal neovascular or nonneovascular changes that might alter the treatment recommendations or preoperative counseling regarding cataract extraction or corneal transplantation.

FA is a crucial part of the postoperative assessment in patients with CNV who have undergone thermal laser photocoagulation or verteporfin PDT because of the greater sensitivity in detecting CNV, revealing a significant percentage of recurrent lesions not suspected on clinical examination (18). Based on the MPS, for treatment of classic CNV including well-demarcated boundaries with thermal laser, the initial postoperative FA is indicated between 2 and 4 weeks to confirm that the entire CNV lesion has been treated and is obliterated. If adequate treatment is present, repeat FA should be performed in 4 to 6 weeks followed by intervals at the discretion of the treating physician (9). According to the TAP and Verteporfin in Photodynamic Therapy (VIP) studies following verteporfin PDT, the evidence suggests repeat FA should be performed at 3-month intervals with retreatment as indicated (19). Like the MPS, TAP, and VIP, similar angiography protocols should be used, including early-, mid-, and late-phase 30-degree film stereophotos centered on the macula after rapid (less than 6 seconds) injection of 5 mL of 10% of sodium fluorescein solution (10).

Over the past two decades, a great deal of effort and expense has gone into the study of new treatments for neovascular AMD. These studies could not be carried out without the ability of FA to objectively document treatment response. Ongoing trials with injected anti-angiogenic drugs, non–verteporfin PDT, prophylactic laser to high-risk nonneovascular AMD, transpupillary thermotherapy, radiation therapy, selective feeder vessel laser therapy, serum apheresis, submacular surgery, and macular translocation all include FA in their pretreatment and posttreatment protocol. Currently, there are insufficient data to direct the use of FA after these unproven treatments (9).

ANGIOGRAPHIC PATTERNS IN AMD

Nonneovascular AMD

The majority of patients with AMD have the nonneovascular form, which consists of drusen and RPE abnormalities. Several types of drusen exist that differ histopathologically and angiographically. Hard drusen are small (63 µm), round discrete deposits on ophthalmoscopy that correspond to lipidized RPE or accumulation of hyaline material in the inner and outer collagenous zones of the Bruch's membrane (20). In FA, hard drusen typically appear as transmission defects due to overlying RPE thinning or depigmentation (21). Angiography often reveals a greater number of hard drusen than can be seen clinically (22).

Soft drusen are larger (greater than 63 µm) with irregular, poorly defined borders and the propensity to coalesce and become confluent. FA of soft drusen shows progressive hyperfluorescence and dye pooling without leakage beyond its margin (Fig. 10.2). Histopathologically, soft drusen are localized detachments between the RPE and (a) basal laminar deposit in an eye with diffuse basal laminar deposit, (b) basal linear deposit in an eye with diffuse basal linear deposit, or (c) localized accumulation of basal linear deposit in an eye without diffuse basal linear deposit (20–24). Studies have also identified vascularization of soft drusen, which may account for a component of the hyperfluorescence (21).

When soft drusen coalesce, the resulting irregular, shallow elevation of the RPE is referred to as drusenoid RPE detachment (23). Unlike a serous RPE detachment, where FA staining uniformly increases during the study and remains bright in the late phases, drusenoid RPE detachment is less fluorescent and either stains faintly or fades in the late phases of the study (13) (Figs. 10.2 and 10.3).

Basal laminar drusen represent angiographically and histologically distinct deposits, which appear as innumerable, small, round, semitranslucent, yellow lesions on fundus biomicroscopy. FA reveals early, discrete hyperfluorescence and late fading that has been described as "stars in the sky" (25) (Fig. 10.4). Histopathology reveals basal laminar drusen to be nodularity of a diffusely thickened inner Bruch's membrane (25).

In addition to drusen, nonneovascular AMD is defined by the presence of RPE abnormalities, including hyperpigmentation, non-GA, and GA. All forms of RPE change may be present in the same eye over time or simultaneously. Focal hyperpigmentation appears as a blocked fluorescence on FA and is characterized by focal RPE hypertrophy and pigment migration into the subretinal space and outer retina (21). Focal hyperpigmentation is often associated with soft drusen, GA, or neovascular AMD but may appear alone (Fig. 10.2).

RPE atrophy is a common feature in AMD and has been documented to replace regressed drusen or follow collapse of a serous RPE detachment (20–26). Non-GA and GA share the common histopathologic feature of RPE loss. However, in GA, this loss is more extensive, and there is associated atrophy of the overlying retina and underlying choriocapillaris leading to the difference in fluorescein appearance (Fig. 10.5). Non-GA typically appears as mottled early hyperfluorescence, which fades late consistent with window defect. Conversely, GA does not hyperfluoresce early because of the loss of underlying

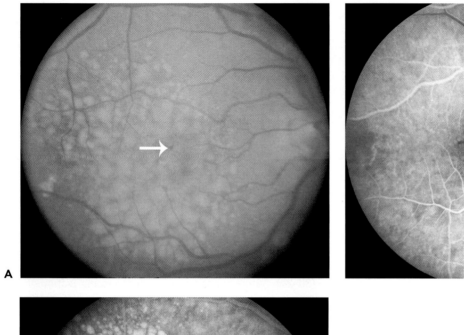

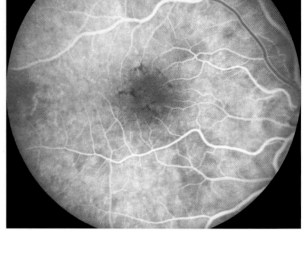

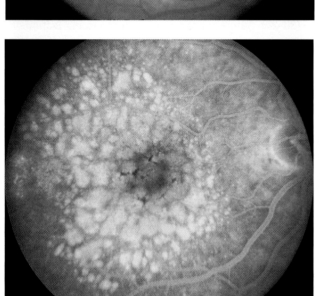

Figure 10.2 ■ Soft drusen and drusenoid RPE detachment. **A.** Fundus photograph. Early **(B)** and late **(C)** angiogram demonstrating progressive hyperfluorescence from dye pooling. Arrow indicates an area of focal hyperpigmentation.

choriocapillaris; only larger choroidal vessels are apparent. Late in the FA, well-defined hyperfluorescence from staining of the exposed deep choroid and sclera is apparent (13).

NEOVASCULAR AMD

The term neovascular AMD refers to the presence of abnormal blood vessels, serous or hemorrhagic detachment of the pigment epithelium, lipid exudation, subretinal fibrosis, or disciform scar formation. The growth of abnormal blood vessels from the choroid into the Bruch's membrane, as well as under and into the neurosensory retina, is known as CNV and accounts for the majority of severe vision loss in AMD. Angiographic criteria of classic and occult CNV were defined in the MPS.

This fluorescein-based classification was applied for the purpose of determining which patients would benefit from thermal laser photocoagulation intended to eradicate the entire neovascular lesion. Clearly distinguished boundaries were deemed essential to determine the location of the lesion and the distance from the lesion border to the center of the foveal avascular zone.

The interpretation of CNV evolved during the course of the MPS and later investigations into the following system described. The MPS has defined the term lesion component as the area of the retina containing CNV or interfering with the ability to define the boundaries of CNV. A neovascular lesion represents the entire complex of lesion components and may include the CNV and the features that block the view of the boundaries (27).

Classic or well-defined CNV is an area of early hyperfluorescence with well-demarcated boundaries and progressive

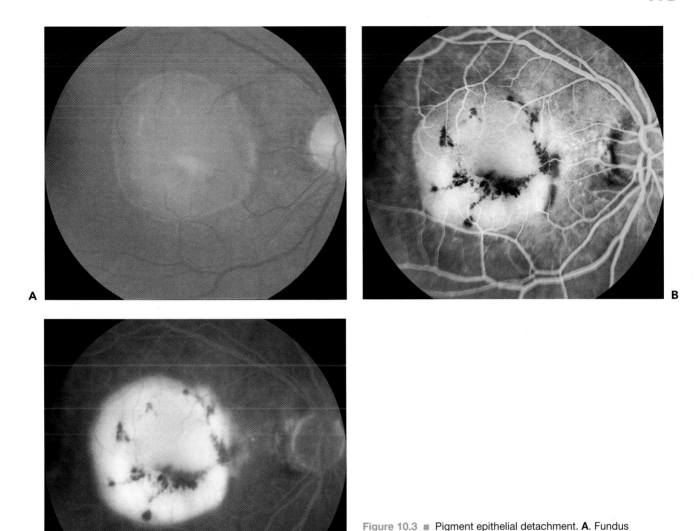

Figure 10.3 ■ Pigment epithelial detachment. **A**. Fundus photograph. Early **(B)** and late **(C)** angiographs demonstrating the uniform progressive hyperfluorescence, unlike a drusenoid retinal PED, which is less fluorescent and stains faintly in the late phases of the study (see Fig. 10.2).

pooling of dye leakage in the overlying subretinal space in the later phases of the angiogram that usually obscures the boundaries of the CNV (28).

Initially, the boundaries are well demarcated, allowing the clinician to accurately determine the location of the lesion and the distance from the lesion border to the center of the foveal avascular zone. Occasionally, the capillaries of the CNV appear as a lacy cartwheel network in the early phase. Because the new vessels leak, progressive hyperfluorescence and blurring of the lesion edge continue during the course of the FA (Fig. 10.6). This leakage may pool in the subretinal space if a neurosensory retinal detachment is present or may collect in the outer plexiform layer in the form of cystic retinal edema. Dye pooling well demarcated in a confined space of a localized sensory retinal detachment or within intraretinal cystic spaces has been termed loculated fluid (29). Loculated fluid was a common finding in patients with new subfoveal

CNV in the MPS and may confuse the treating physician as to the boundary of the lesion. A variant of classic CNV has been described in which new vessel filling is slower and the boundaries are not distinguished until approximately 2 minutes after dye injection. Despite a slow fill, the boundaries present initially correspond to the area of leakage in the late frames (8). Classic CNV has been further categorized based on location with respect to the fovea: (a) Extrafoveal CNV is greater than 200 μm from the foveal center, (b) juxtafoveal CNV is located between 1 and 199 μm from the foveal center, and (c) subfoveal CNV is located under the center of the fovea. In the TAP and VIP studies, lesion component proportions were further delineated. A neovascular lesion in which the CNV component is greater than 50% of the total lesion size is defined as predominately classic. Lesions in which the classic CNV component comprises less than 50% of the total area are referred to as minimally classic (30).

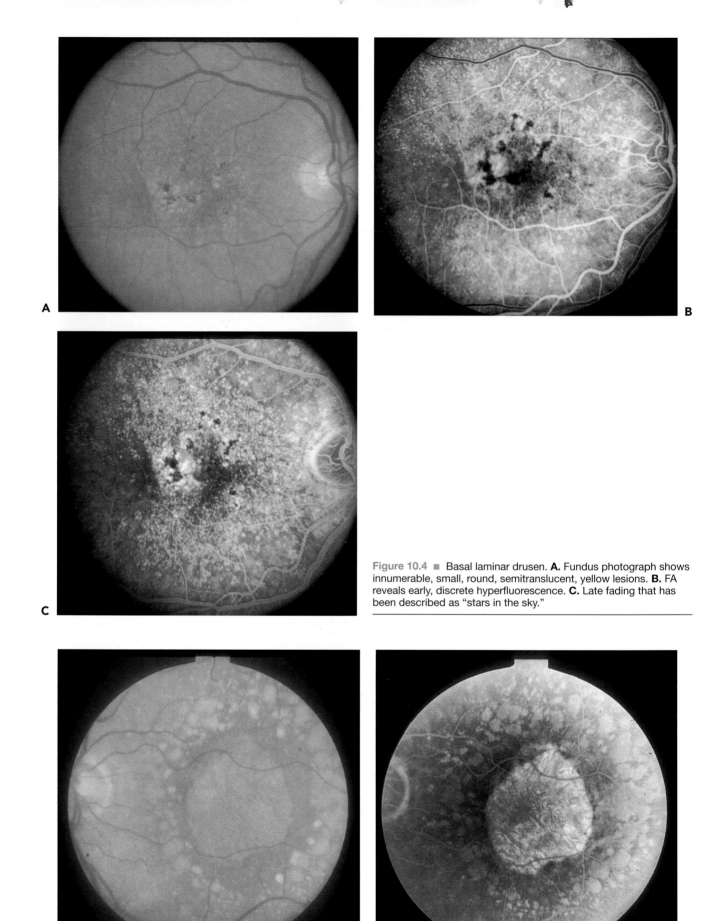

Figure 10.4 ■ Basal laminar drusen. **A.** Fundus photograph shows innumerable, small, round, semitranslucent, yellow lesions. **B.** FA reveals early, discrete hyperfluorescence. **C.** Late fading that has been described as "stars in the sky."

Figure 10.5 ■ Geographic atrophy of the RPE. **A.** Fundus photograph demonstrating loss of RPE with sharp borders and surrounding large drusen. **B.** Angiograph reveals well-defined hyperfluorescence from staining of the exposed deep choroid and sclera.

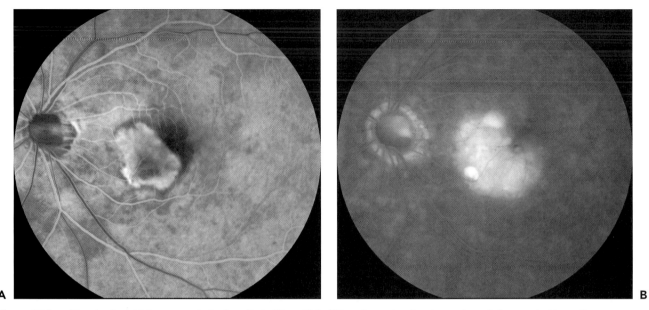

Figure 10.6 ■ Classic choroidal neovascularization. Early **(A)** and late **(B)** angiographs showing early well-demarcated hyperfluorescence with late leakage.

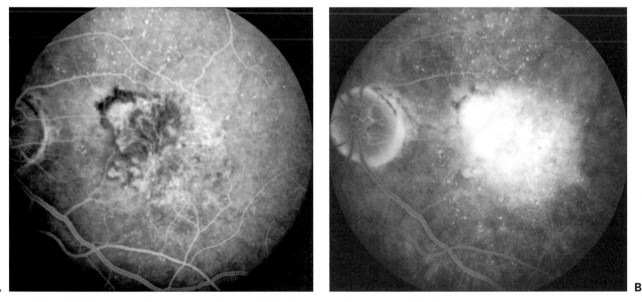

Figure 10.7 ■ Mid **(A)** and late **(B)** angiogram of occult CNV in the form of fibrovascular PED. There is stippled hyperfluorescence apparent 1 to 2 minutes after fluorescein injection with ill-defined leakage in the late frames.

Occult or poorly defined forms of CNV are classified in two distinct patterns of hyperfluorescence, fibrovascular pigment epithelial detachment (PED) and late-phase leakage of undetermined source (28). Fibrovascular PED is defined as an irregular elevation of the RPE detected on stereoangiography associated with stippled hyperfluorescence apparent 1 to 2 minutes after fluorescein injection with persistent staining or leakage of dye in the overlying subretinal space by 10 minutes (Fig. 10.7). Fibrovascular PED differs from classic CNV in that the early hyperfluorescence

is not as discrete or as bright and the boundaries usually remain indeterminate. In addition, the smooth RPE elevation, uniform progressive hyperfluorescence, and late, well-demarcated pooling of a classic, serous PED should not be confused with fibrovascular PED.

Occult CNV with late-phase leakage of undetermined source lacks a discernible, well-demarcated area of leakage in the early frames of the FA. Speckled hyperfluorescence with no visible source becomes apparent 2 to 5 minutes after dye injection and later pools in the overlying subretinal

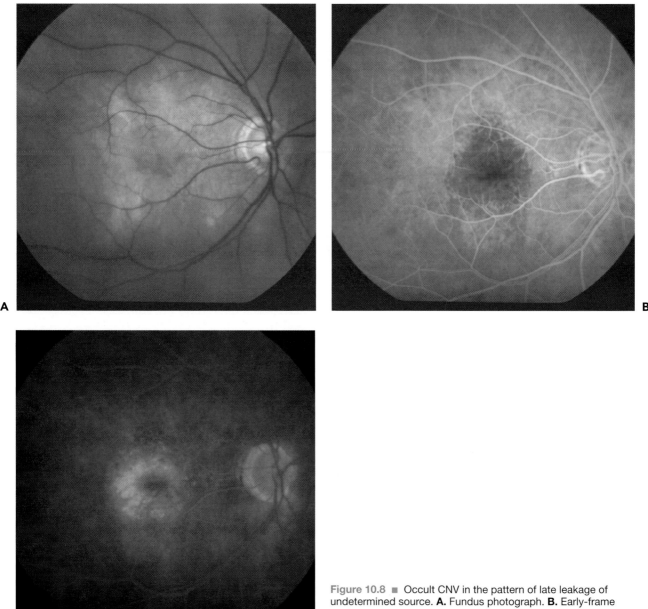

Figure 10.8 ■ Occult CNV in the pattern of late leakage of undetermined source. **A.** Fundus photograph. **B.** Early-frame angiograph demonstrating no apparent leakage source. **C.** Late frames reveal leakage into the subretinal space.

space (Fig. 10.8). This differs from the slow-filling variant of classic CNV in that the leakage source is never apparent.

Polypoidal choroidal vasculopathy (PCV) is a variant of occult neovascularization that has a predisposition for pigmented races (31). The reason PCV is more commonly seen in Asians and African Americans is that these individuals' eyes may have a more resilient RPE monolayer that is somewhat resistant to penetration by the underlying neovascular tissue. The individual "polyps" are found just below the RPE and typically represent only a small portion of a much larger type of occult neovascular lesion. Furthermore, this pattern appears to occur in eyes with long-standing CNV lesions better identified with ICG angiography.

Retinal angiomatous proliferation (RAP) has been described as a capillary proliferation within the retina that originates from the deep capillary plexus in the paramacular region (32,33). There has been considerable debate regarding whether this form of neovascularization originates from the retinal circulation, as Yannuzzi proposed and demonstrated in a histopathologic correlation by Lafaut et al. (28), or the choroidal circulation, as proposed by Gass. Despite this, Yannuzzi coined the term RAP that has predominated in the literature. He proposed that formation of RAP begins as IRN, which progresses to subretinal neovascularization (SRN) and finally an anastomosis to CNV (33) (Fig. 10.9).

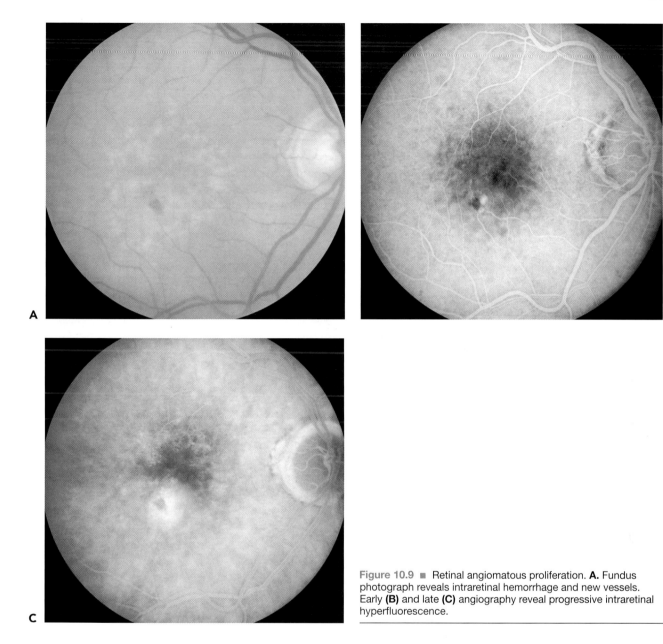

Figure 10.9 ■ Retinal angiomatous proliferation. **A.** Fundus photograph reveals intraretinal hemorrhage and new vessels. Early **(B)** and late **(C)** angiography reveal progressive intraretinal hyperfluorescence.

In angiographic studies, IRN usually reveals a focal area of intraretinal staining with indistinct borders and surrounding intraretinal edema (28). SRN occurs when the IRN extends posteriorly, beyond the photoreceptor layer of the retina into the subretinal space. Yannuzzi et al. demonstrated that the majority of these neovascularizations were categorized as occult CNV, mostly with a small component of classic CNV.

When the SRN reaches or fuses with RPE, a serous PED is seen in nearly all cases, which finally becomes vascularized. During the evolution of this vascularized process, an axonal communication between the retinal and choroidal circulation forms a retinal–choroidal anastomosis (RCA).

Angiographic examinations demonstrate the presence of CNV, sometimes associated with vascularized PED or a prediciform scar. In their series, the authors state that this form of neovascular AMD was found almost exclusively in whites, with a female to male ratio of 3:1. While the different stages

described were difficult to differentiate by examination and angiography, ICG was helpful in making the diagnosis.

Aside from drusenoid PED and the fibrovascular PED form of occult CNV discussed previously, other forms of PED exist in AMD, including serous and hemorrhagic PED. Serous PED may or may not be associated with CNV. Typically, serous PED is easily seen on fundus biomicroscopy as a round or oval translucent elevation of the RPE. Early arteriovenous phase of the angiogram reveals progressive, uniform hyperfluorescence with late, intense pooling of fluorescein. The progression of hyperfluorescence (often described as "turning up a rheostat") reflects the rapid movement of fluorescein across the Bruch's membrane into the sub-RPE space (7) (Fig. 10.3). A notch in the otherwise smooth border of a serous PED may be an indication of CNV. A hemorrhagic PED is easily differentiated from serous PED on clinical examination. The translucence of serous fluid is replaced by a dark, reddish-brown mass. While hemorrhagic PED can appear clinically similar to uveal melanoma, the blood blocks normal choroidal and CNV-associated fluorescence unlike the punctate hyper-fluorescence of the intrinsic circulation of melanoma. Furthermore, the standardized ultrasonographic patterns of the two lesions differ.

Lesion components associated with neovascular AMD that can obscure the boundaries of CNV include changes that block fluorescence, such as blood, fibrous tissue, RPE hyperplasia, or RPE redundancy (from an RPE tear). Alternatively, CNV can be obscured by greater fluorescence from staining fibrous tissue or a serous PED. When contiguous with CNV, such lesions can make it impossible to determine the exact boundary of the CNV and are referred to as components of the lesion. As such, they are included in the laser treatment plan unless otherwise indicated.

OTHER CNV PATTERNS IN AMD

Disciform scar represents the evolution of CNV and is comprised of variable amounts of active CNV as well as fibrovascular and cellular proliferation. The color varies from white to yellow to brown depending on the amount of fibrous tissue, RPE hyperplasia, blood, and lipid exudate present. Variable amounts of serous retinal detachment may be associated with disciform scar. Angiography, while not typically indicated at this stage of the disease, reveals blockage from RPE hyperplasia and blood, staining of the fibrous component, and leakage of the active CNV component, if present (Fig. 10.10). Like

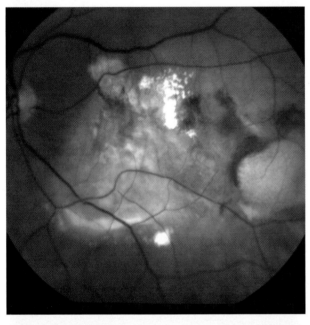

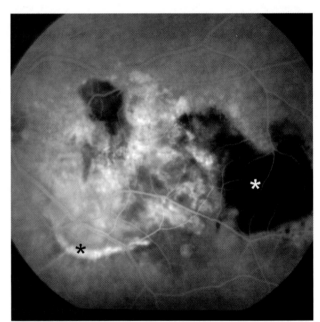

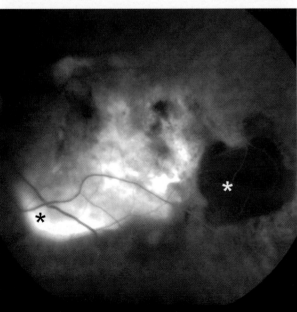

Figure 10.10 ■ Disciform scar. **A.** Fundus photograph. **B,C.** Angiographs with blockage from retinal pigment epithelial hyperplasia and blood (*white asterisk*) and staining of the fibrous component (*black asterisk*).

hemorrhagic PED, FA is helpful in differentiating an atypical, dark disciform scar from a uveal melanoma. A common vascular change that occurs during the disciform scar process is an RCA, in which CNV communicates with the retinal circulation (24).

In neovascular AMD, a tear in the RPE can occur spontaneously, as a result of thermal laser photocoagulation or after verteporfin PDT (34,35). Gass (36) has hypothesized that serous PED adjacent to fibrovascular PED tears at a point opposite the fibrovascular change and retracts toward the fibrovascular mound. His theory explains the uneven hyperfluorescence and distribution of drusen (not evident in the serous PED portion of the lesion) noted prior to RPE rip. The unique angiographic appearance after RPE rip includes early hyperfluorescence with late staining in the area of absent pigmented RPE and hypofluorescence with stippled hyperfluorescent staining in the area of redundant RPE and fibrovascular tissue (Fig. 10.11). Gass

explains that the reason the denuded Bruch's membrane does not leak fluorescein into the subretinal space is due to the growth of hypopigmented metaplastic RPE shortly after the tear occurs (36).

FA AFTER LASER TREATMENT

Thermal Laser Photocoagulation

Immediate effects of laser photocoagulation of CNV may include changes leading to hypofluorescence (retinal edema, temporary closure of retinal capillaries and choroidal vessels) and/or hyperfluorescence (thermal vasculitis of retinal and choroidal vessels). These immediate and variable changes usually stabilize by 2 to 4 weeks when the first postoperative FA is indicated. Features at the initial FA of a well-treated CNV membrane include early hypofluorescence in the area of treatment. Later frames may show areas of

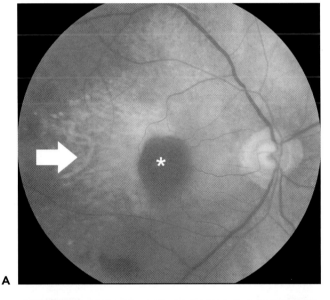
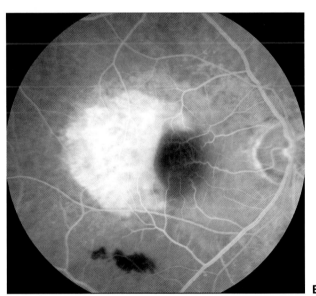
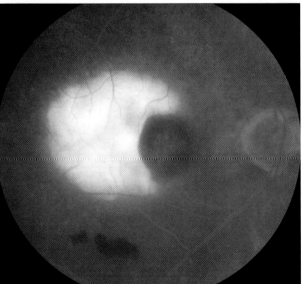

Figure 10.11 ■ Retinal pigment epithelial tear. **A.** Fundus photograph reveals a darkly pigmented mound (*asterisk*) with adjacent exposed choroidal pattern (*arrow*). **B,C.** Angiography reveals hyperfluorescence with late staining in the area of absent pigmented RPE and hypofluorescence in the area of redundant RPE and fibrovascular tissue.

staining or leakage within the area of treatment and uniform staining at the periphery of the lesion (37). Persistence of CNV is defined by the MPS as leakage at the periphery of the laser-treated area in the early (less than 6 weeks) post-operative FA and is considered inadequately treated original CNV tissue. CNV recurrence implies new fluorescein leakage contiguous to a previously treated lesion after initial FA showed no evidence of persistence. The leakage is present in the late frames of the study and is usually preceded by moderate hyperfluorescence in earlier frames (37) (Fig. 10.12).

In the MPS, a significant number of posttreatment angiograms could not be clearly interpreted as having recurrence or not (38). A category of questionable recurrence was defined as one of three angiographic patterns shown to carry a risk for developing recurrent CNV: (a) focal staining along the laser lesion edge, (b) new blocked fluorescence from hemorrhage, and (c) speckled hyperfluorescence beyond the edge of the laser lesion (38). Close follow-up is warranted if any of these patterns are present in the post-operative period.

A large choroidal vessel leading to the CNV may be visible on FA. Such feeder vessels may be seen in untreated neovascular AMD but are most commonly seen in recurrent CNV after thermal laser treatment. Feeder vessels are considered lesion components, which should be considered in the treatment plan (27).

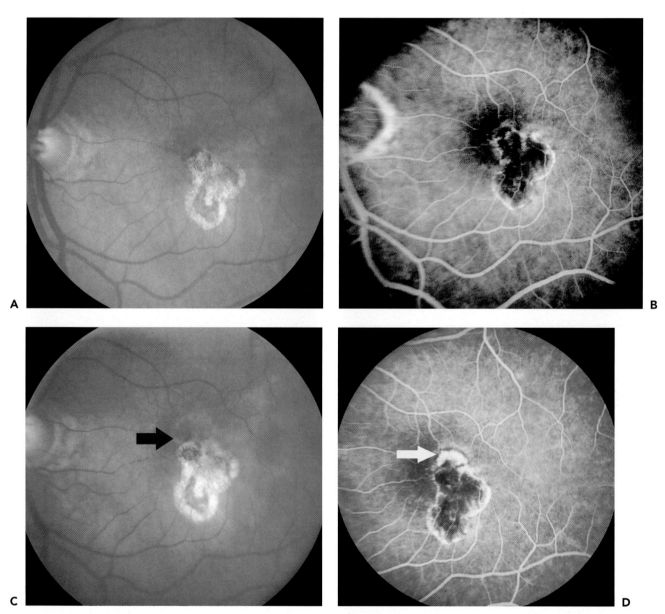

Figure 10.12 ■ Angiographic patterns after thermal laser treatment for CNV. Photograph **(A)** and midphase angiograph **(B)** of well-treated CNV. There is uniform staining at the periphery of the lesion. Two months later **(C)**, new subretinal fluid is present (*arrow*) with midphase angiograph **(D)** demonstrating progressive hyperfluorescence at the margin of CNV recurrence (*arrow*).

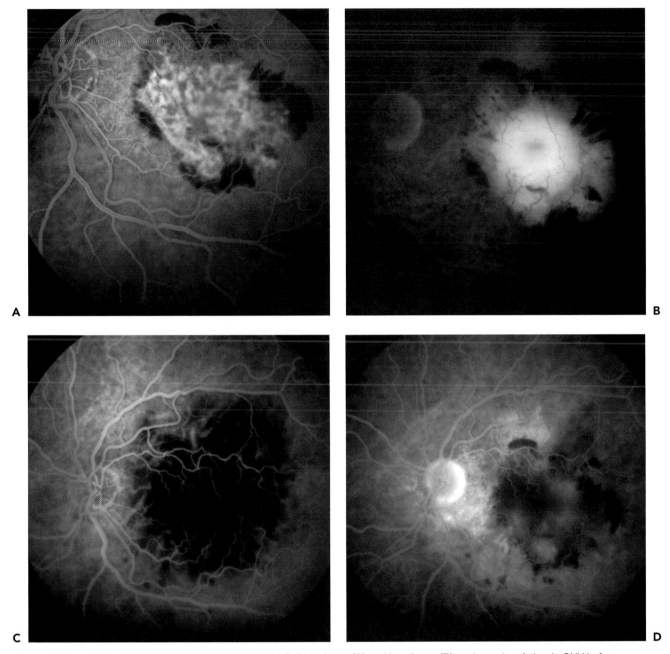

Figure 10.13 ■ Angiographic pattern after verteporfin PDT. Early-frame **(A)** and late-frame **(B)** angiographs of classic CNV before verteporfin PDT. One month after PDT, there is closure of the vessels in the early frames **(C)** with only mild staining within the original borders of the lesion in the late frames **(D)**.

Verteporfin PDT

In the TAP and VIP studies, follow-up angiograms were graded for evidence of leakage as (a) progression of leakage, CNV beyond the area of baseline CNV; (b) moderate leakage, area of active CNV occupying 50% of baseline CNV without progression; (c) minimal leakage, area of active CNV occupying less than 50% of baseline CNV; and (d) absence of leakage, no active CNV within baseline CNV and no progression (39). Lesions with leakage at follow-up visits were considered for retreatment at 3-month intervals (30). After treatment, the ability to differentiate classic from occult CNV became increasingly laborious (Fig. 10.13). Regardless, lesions with any leakage were considered for treatment. More importantly, the ability to differentiate leakage from staining of various lesion components becomes increasingly difficult after treatment (30–40).

CONCLUSIONS

AMD remains a challenging disease to evaluate and treat. The ideal imaging study for this disease would be (a) noninvasive, (b) rapid, (c) safe, (d) inexpensive, (e) able to detect neovascular changes under pigmented lesions or serous PED, (f) able to differentiate neovascular from nonneovascular disease, and (g) able to differentiate active from inactive CNV. FA falls short of ideal because it requires an intravenous injection, has known (albeit minimal) risks, and is limited in its ability to differentiate neovascular from other lesions and to detect CNV margins due to obscuring lesions. Regardless, FA remains the gold standard in the diagnosis and treatment of neovascular AMD. More importantly, FA has been crucial in our understanding of the pathophysiology of AMD.

Digital FA is replacing film angiography in clinical trials just as it largely has in practice. All new retinal imaging technologies must be compared to FA in efficacy and cost (41). A combination of FA with ICG facilitated the detection and demarcation of occult or poorly defined CNV, and providing a more detailed representation through RPE, blood, and exudative material also contributed more information, essentially in PCV and RAP.

A combination of FA with optical coherence tomography (OCT) in patients with CNV provides a quantitative measure of retinal thickness and subretinal fluid, but it does not provide a direct indication of the current amount of leakage. This information is provided by FA, which also demonstrates CNV lesion size, another outcome measure that cannot be assessed by OCT. Currently multimodal imaging technologies, including OCT, FA and ICG, aid in developing understanding of the underlying pathophysiology of the diseases we treat.

REFERENCES

1. Ehrlich P. Uber provicierte Fluoreszenzerscheinungen am Auge. Dtsch Med Wschr. 1882;8:8–21.

2. Novotny HR, Alvis DL. A method of photographing fluorescence in circulating blood in the human retina. Circulation. 1961;24:82–86.

3. Malamos P, Sacu S, Georgopoulos M, et al. Correlation of high-definition optical coherence tomography and fluorescein angiography imaging in neovascular macular degeneration. Invest Ophthalmol Vis Sci. 2009;50(10):4926–4933. Epub 2009 Jun 3.

4. Norton EW. Doyne memorial lecture, 1981. Fluorescein angiography. Twenty years later. Trans Ophthalmol Soc UK. 1981;101(Pt2):229–233.

5. Wolfe DR. Fluorescein angiography: basic science and engineering. Ophthalmology. 1986;93:1617–1620.

6. Yannuzzi LA, Rohrer KT, Tindel LJ, et al. Fluorescein angiography complication survey. Ophthalmology. 1986;93:611–617.

7. Johnson RN, Schatz H, McDonald HR, et al. Fluorescein angiography: basic principles and interpretation. In: Ryan SJ, Schachat AP, Eds. Retina. St. Louis, MO: Mosby. 2001:875–942.

8. Chamberlin JA, Bressler NM, Bressler SB, et al. The use of fundus photographs and fluorescein angiograms in the identification and treatment of choroidal neovascularization in the Macular Photocoagulation Study. The Macular Photocoagulation Study Group. Ophthalmology. 1989;96:1526–1534.

9. Chew EY, Benson WE, Boldt HC, et al. Preferred practice patterns: age-related macular degeneration. San Francisco, CA: American Academy of Ophthalmology; 2003.

10. Yannuzzi LA, Ober MD, Slakter JS, et al. Ophthalmic fundus imaging: today and beyond. Am J Ophthalmol. 2004;137(3):511–524.

11. Kwiterovich KA, Maguire MG, Murphy RP, et al. Frequency of adverse systemic reactions after fluorescein angiography. Results of a prospective study. Ophthalmology. 1991;98:1139–1142.

12. Rabb MF, Burton TC, Schatz H, et al. Fluorescein angiography of the fundus: a schematic approach to interpretation. Surv Ophthalmol. 1978;22:387–403.

13. Pieramici DJ, Bressler SB. Fluorescein angiography. In: Berger JW, Fine SL, Maguire MG, eds. Age-related macular degeneration. St. Louis, MO: Mosby. 1999:219–236.

14. Macular Photocoagulation Study Group. Laser photocoagulation of subfoveal neovascular lesions in age-related macular degeneration. Results of a randomized clinical trial. Arch Ophthalmol. 1991;109:1220–1231.

15. Macular Photocoagulation Study Group. Laser photocoagulation for juxtafoveal choroidal neovascularization. Five-year results from randomized clinical trials. Arch Ophthalmol. 1994;112:500–509.

16. Pieramici DJ, Bressler SB. Age-related macular degeneration and risk factors for the development of choroidal neovascularization in the fellow eye. Curr Opin Ophthalmol. 1998;9:38–46.

17. Wilkinson CP. The clinical examination. Limitation and over-utilization of angiographic services. Ophthalmology. 1986;93:401–404.

18. Sykes SO, Bressler NM, Maguire MG, et al. Detecting recurrent choroidal neovascularization. Comparison of clinical examination with and without fluorescein angiography. Arch Ophthalmol. 1994;112:1561–1566.

19. Bressler NM. Verteporfin therapy of subfoveal choroidal neovascularization in age-related macular degeneration: two-year results of a randomized clinical trial including lesions with occult with no classic choroidal neovascularization—verteporfin in photodynamic therapy report 2. Am J Ophthalmol. 2002;133:168–169.

20. Sarks SH. Council lecture. Drusen and their relationship to senile macular degeneration. Aust J Ophthalmol. 1980;8:117–130.

21. Green WR, Key SN III. Senile macular degeneration: a histopathologic study. Trans Am Ophthalmol Soc. 1977;75:180–254.

22. Bressler NM, Bressler SB, Fine SL. Age-related macular degeneration. Surv Ophthalmol. 1988;32:375–413.

23. Bressler NM, Silva JC, Bressler SB, et al. Clinicopathologic correlation of drusen and retinal pigment epithelial abnormalities in age-related macular degeneration. Retina. 1994;14:130–142.

24. Green WR, McDonnell PJ, Yeo JH. Pathologic features of senile macular degeneration. Ophthalmology. 1985;92:615–627.

25. Gass JD, Jallow S, Davis B. Adult vitelliform macular detachment occurring in patients with basal laminar drusen. Am J Ophthalmol. 1985;99:445–459.

26. Meredith TA, Braley RE, Aaberg TM. Natural history of serous detachments of the retinal pigment epithelium. Am J Ophthalmol. 1979;88:643–651.

27. Macular Photocoagulation Study Group. Subfoveal neovascular lesions in age-related macular degeneration. Guidelines for evaluation and treatment in the macular photocoagulation study. Arch Ophthalmol. 1991;109:1242–1257.

28. Lafaut BA, Aisenbrey S, van den Broecke C, et al. Polypoidal choroidal vasculopathy pattern in age-related macular degeneration. A clinicopathologic correlation. Retina. 2000;20:650–654.

29. Bressler NM, Bressler SB, Alexander J, et al. Loculated fluid. A previously undescribed fluorescein angiographic finding in choroidal neovascularization associated with macular degeneration. Macular Photocoagulation Study Reading Center. Arch Ophthalmol. 1991;109:211–215.

30. Barbazetto I, Burdan A, Bressler NM, et al. Photodynamic therapy of subfoveal choroidal neovascularization with verteporfin: fluorescein angiographic guidelines for evaluation and treatment—TAP and VIP report No. 2. Arch Ophthalmol. 2003;121:1:1253–1268.

31. Yannuzzi LA, Wong DW, Sforzolini BS, et al. Polypoidal choroidal vasculopathy and neovascularized age-related macular degeneration. Arch Ophthalmol. 1999;117(11):1503–1510.

32. Hartnett ME, Weiter JJ, Staurenghi G, et al. Deep retinal vascular anomalous complexes in advanced age-related macular degeneration. Ophthalmology. 1996;103:2042–2053.

33. Yannuzzi LA, Negrão S, Iida T, et al. Retinal angiomatous proliferation in age–related macular degeneration. Retina. 2012;32(Suppl 1):416–434.

34. Cantrill HL, Ramsay RC, Knobloch WH. Rips in the pigment epithelium. Arch Ophthalmol. 1983;101:1074–1079.

35. Gelisken F, Inhoffen W, Partsch M, et al. Retinal pigment epithelial tear after photodynamic therapy for choroidal neovascularization. Am J Ophthalmol. 2001;131:518–520.

36. Gass JD. Pathogenesis of tears of the retinal pigment epithelium. Br J Ophthalmol. 1984;68:513–519.

37. Macular Photocoagulation Study Group. Recurrent choroidal neovascularization after argon laser photocoagulation for neovascular maculopathy. Arch Ophthalmol. 1986;104:503–512.

38. Dyer DS, Brant AM, Schachat AP, et al. Angiographic features and outcome of questionable recurrent choroidal neovascularization. Am J Ophthalmol. 1995;120:497–505.

39. Treatment of Age-Related Macular Degeneration with Photodynamic Therapy (TAP) Study Group. Photodynamic therapy of subfoveal choroidal neovascularization in age-related macular degeneration with verteporfin: one-year results of 2 randomized clinical trials—TAP report 1. Arch Ophthalmol. 1999;117:1329–1345.

40. Kaiser RS, Berger JW, Williams GA, et al. Variability in fluorescein angiography interpretation for photodynamic therapy in age-related macular degeneration. Retina. 2002;22:683–690.

41. Bressler NM. Evaluating new retinal imaging techniques. Arch Ophthalmol. 1998;116:521–522.

11

INDOCYANINE GREEN ANGIOGRAPHY IN AGE-RELATED MACULAR DEGENERATION

IRENE A. BARBAZETTO • JASON S. SLAKTER

INTRODUCTION

Indocyanine green (ICG) angiography has evolved since the introduction of the technique and is used today to complement other imaging modalities such as spectral-domain optical coherence tomography (SD-OCT) and fluorescein angiography (FA). In neovascular age-related macular degeneration (AMD), ICG angiography is recommended for patients with serosanguineous macular detachments in the peripapillary area; serosanguineous macular detachments in the absence of drusen; large vascularized pigment epithelial detachments (PEDs), particularly with extensive lipid, blood, or minimal cystoid macular edema; hemorrhagic lesions in the peripheral retina; and lesions that are resistant or show suboptimal response to multiple anti–vascular endothelial growth factor (VEGF) indications and is based on the patients' ethnicity (1).

HISTORIC BACKGROUND

ICG was introduced into medicine by Fox et al. (2) in 1957 as part of an indicator dilution technique for measuring cardiac output (3). Shortly thereafter, clinical applications were expanded, and ICG was utilized to quantify hepatic blood flow

and assess liver function (4,5). It was the unique optical property of ICG that allowed for visualization of the dye through overlying melanin and xanthophyll (6) that made it interesting for ophthalmic imaging. Kogure and Choromokos were the first to image the choroid by injecting ICG dye into the carotid artery of monkeys. They were able to image choroidal veins but could not identify choroidal arteries or capillaries (7). In 1972, Flower and Hochheimer (8) were successful in imaging the choroidal circulation using ICG absorption angiography. One year later, technology evolved, and ICG fluorescence was imaged using ICG angiography, which allowed imaging of the choroidal arteries on a regular basis (9). The initial utility of ICG angiography was limited by the low fluorescence of the dye and recording techniques available, making imaging of the choriocapillaris difficult, if not impossible (10). The earliest studies using ICG angiography for AMD were done on film-based systems. Given the low fluence of the ICG dye, the detection of choroidal abnormalities was difficult. Patz et al. (10) were the first to describe the use of ICG angiography for choroidal neovascularization (CNV). They were able to identify choroidal lesions in only 2 of 25 patients. Other publications reported a similar low yield in regard to CNV detection (11–13). However, choroidal filling abnormalities were described in a significant subset of patients with advanced AMD (11). It took 20 years and major advances in technology for this technique to become a standard diagnostic tool (14–16). Today, clinical images are recorded using digital angiography with a highly weighted camera in the near-infrared and high-speed imaging capacity (1,17) or scanning laser ophthalmoscope (SLO)–based technology (18–20). Together with FA, it has become a standard clinical tool for imaging choroidal pathologies such as AMD, central serous chorioretinopathy (CSC), uveitis, and choroidal tumors.

CHEMICAL AND OPTICAL PROPERTIES OF INDOCYANINE GREEN

ICG ($C_{43}H_{47}N_2NaO_6S_2$) is a tricarbocyanine dye that has a complex molecular structure with amphiphilic properties, meaning it has both hydrophilic and lipophilic characteristics. It appears to be rapidly and almost completely (98%) bound to plasma protein following its intravenous administration (5). Initially, it was thought that serum albumin was the main binding protein (5), but studies later suggested that 80% of ICG molecules actually bind to globulins such as alpha-1 lipoprotein (21–23). A recent study by Yoneya et al. (24) not only confirmed this finding but showed that ICG intensely binds to high-density lipoprotein (HDL) and moderately to low-density lipoproteins (LDLs). These lipoproteins have a large molecular size and may explain the limited vascular and tissue permeability of the dye (24).

The absorption and emission spectra of ICG are within the near-infrared range (21). ICG absorbs light between 790 and 805 nm and fluoresces between 770 and 880 nm, with a peak absorption or fluorescence at around 805 nm in plasma. The absorption spectrum is dependent on the solvent (saline solution vs. plasma and proteins) and the dye concentration, which tends to promote aggregate formation in higher concentrations and in the absence of protein binding (21,25). Clinically, the retinal pigment epithelium (RPE) and choroid absorb about 21% to 38% of the near-infrared light (800 nm) used in ICG angiography. By comparison, this is less than half of the amount of light absorbed during FA (500 nm) (6), thereby allowing for better visualization of choroidal pathologies. ICG fluence, however, reaches only 4% of the effective efficiency of fluorescein in the eye (26).

For clinical use, ICG is diluted with sterile water prior to injection with the exception of iodine-free ICG, which is dissolved into a 5% glucose solution. Diluted ICG is stable for 4 hours in plasma. Conversely, ICG in distilled water alone shows considerable decrease of optical density, which can be significantly accelerated by exposure to light (25).

Safety and Toxicity of ICG Angiography

ICG dye is well tolerated, and the rates of adverse reactions rank below those reported for FA. Severe adverse reactions were estimated at 0.05%, and the death rate following ICG angiography is approximately 1:333,333 (27).

Most commercially available ICG dyes contain about 5% sodium iodide. Therefore, the use of ICG is usually considered contraindicated in patients with iodine or shellfish allergies. Other relative contraindications include liver disease, uremia (11), and pregnancy (category C).

PHOTOGRAPHIC TECHNIQUE AND SYSTEM REQUIREMENTS

The introduction of digitized imaging in the 1990s allowed for bypassing some of the exposure problems experienced during the early experiments with ICG angiography due to the weak fluorescence emitted by the dye. Imaging systems used today are either modified fundus camera systems or laser scanning ophthalmoscopes. Regardless of the camera used, the basic technique remains the same: Prior to injection, infrared images are obtained. Twenty-five to fifty mg of ICG diluted in 2 mL aqueous solvent is injected intravenously followed by a 5-mL saline flush. Eight to ten seconds following the injection, rapid sequential photographs (1 per second) are acquired. When using videoangiography or SLO-based systems, short video segments (with a frame rate up to 30 images per second) can be recorded immediately after injection. It is important to start imaging prior to the dye appearance in the fundus in order to capture the earliest choroidal filling phase. Thereafter, images are obtained at 3- to 5-minute intervals for a total duration of 30 to 50 minutes. ICG angiography can be performed before, after, or simultaneously with FA.

ICG ANGIOGRAPHY FOR AGE-RELATED MACULAR DEGENERATION

ICG Angiography: Nonneovascular AMD

ICG angiography is not routinely used or recommended in nonneovascular AMD. Some studies, however, indicated that choroidal abnormalities in conjunction with drusen could be predictive of future progression to advanced AMD (28,29). Hanutsaha et al. (28) showed that in patients with unilateral CNV, the presence of focal hot spots or hyperintense plaques on ICG angiography in the fellow eye was associated with a significantly higher risk of progression to neovascularization (27% vs. 10% over an average of 22 months of follow-up). Pauleikhoff et al. (29) reported a study where a prolonged choroidal filling phase on ICG angiography increased the risk of geographic atrophy.

Drusen

While angiography is not routinely indicated in the diagnosis of drusen, ICG studies have provided interesting details and thus enhanced our understanding of this pathology. Drusen fluorescence on ICG angiography varies with drusen size, location, and age. While hard drusen are hyper- or isofluorescent, soft drusen usually remain hypofluorescent throughout the study (30,31). In younger patients who are more likely to have basal laminar drusen or malattia leventinese, drusen seem to be hyperfluorescent in the early and late phases of the ICG angiography (31). The exception are the large, aggregated drusen in the later stages of malattia leventinese, which are hypofluorescent in the early phases of ICG and present as hyperfluorescent spots surrounded by halos of hypofluorescence in the late phases (32).

Basal Laminar Drusen

Basal laminar drusen appear as minimally hyperfluorescent spots on early-phase ICG angiography. With time, they increase in fluorescence and become more confluent. However, a small subset of basal laminar drusen are described as being hypofluorescent in the late phase (33).

Reticular Drusen/Pseudodrusen/Subretinal Drusenoid Deposits

Reticular pseudodrusen, also referred to as subretinal drusenoid deposits, first described by Mimoun and associates in 1990, have been of interest because of their associated risk for developing advanced AMD (34–36). Querques et al. (37) described reticular pseudodrusen as hypofluorescent dots and dot pattern on ICG angiography, confirming observations reported by Arnold et al. (30) in an earlier publication. These patterns seemed to project on the choroidal stroma and follow but not overlay larger choroidal vessels.

ICG Angiography: Choroidal Neovascularization

Because of its specific properties, ICG angiography has been found to be especially useful in imaging CNV. ICG allows for imaging the near-infrared end of the spectrum, thereby enhancing the visualization of structures through the RPE, melanin, xanthophyll, blood, and serous fluid. As a proof of principle, histopathology of a patient with occult CNV confirmed that a late-staining, well-circumscribed, hyperfluorescent "plaque" seen on ICG imaging correlated precisely with a thin layer of fibrovascular tissue beneath the pigment epithelium (38).

Initially in the 1990s, ICG angiography was intended to expand the spectrum of lesions amenable to laser photocoagulation in patients with occult CNV. By using videoangiography, Yannuzzi et al. (17) were able to identify well-demarcated areas of CNV in 39% of patients previously classified as purely "occult" or type 1 neovascularization. Today, with the advent of anti-VEGF therapy, laser therapy has only a marginal role in managing AMD. The main purpose of ICG angiography in AMD has become to identify and monitor subgroups such as polypoidal choroidal vasculopathy (PCV) and retinal angiomatous proliferations (RAPs) or conditions that may mimic AMD like CSC.

Occult or Type 1 Choroidal Neovascularization

Guyer, Yannuzzi, and coworkers were the first to classify ill-defined CNV (occult or type 1 CNV) into subgroups based on their ICG angiographic appearance (27,39). The first group consists of patients presenting with a solitary, focal, and well-delineated area of hyperfluorescent CNV (*hot spot*). By definition, hot spots are less than 1 disk diameter in size. They represent hyperpermeable, active parts of the neovascular lesions and also include polyps in PCV and type 3 neovascularization in RAP and its final stage of chorioretinal anastomosis.

The second group is comprised of patients with continuous, fluorescent areas (*plaques*) of CNV larger than 1 disk diameter with either sharp or indistinct margins (Fig. 11.1). Frequently, these plaques are formed by late-staining vessels and may represent less active parts of the neovascularization.

The third group combined both hot spots and plaques in one lesion.

ICG angiography has proven to be particularly useful in detecting neovascular components in PEDs. Unlike on FA, serous PEDs appear comparatively hypofluorescent on ICG angiography because only minimal ICG leakage occurs beneath the serous detachment (27). Vascularized components of a PED, on the other hand, are hyperfluorescent. Patients with vascularized PEDs are further classified by the location of the CNV as seen on ICG. Small areas of hyperfluorescent CNV at the margin or outside and indenting the PED are termed *notch* (Fig. 11.2) (40). Intraretinal proliferations (INRs) associated with PEDs are suggestive of RAP lesions or type 3 lesions, which may advance to chorioretinal anastomosis (41).

Using the above classification system, Guyer et al. (42) found that out of 680 patients with occult CNV, 22% had localized lesions, previously undetected by FA and potentially amenable to laser therapy, the treatment of choice at that time. Still, about 1% of patients with occult CNV on FA did not show any changes on ICG angiography (39).

Polypoidal Choroidal Vasculopathy

Currently, the most common indication for the use of ICG angiography in AMD is the detection of PCV. Although PCV is most common in Asian populations where it has been described in as many as 50% of AMD patients (43–45), it can be found in all ethnic groups (43,46,47). Missing the diagnosis potentially leads to treatment failures given the less robust response of these lesions to anti-VEGF therapy (48). Active PCV presents as an inner choroidal vascular network ending in aneurysmal bulges. At times, these bulges can be seen as red-orange, spheroid-like structures with indirect ophthalmoscopy. More frequently, they are obscured by hemorrhages and/or the overlying retina and RPE. ICG can be used to identify and characterize the vascular abnormality with high sensitivity and specificity (1,46,49–57). In the early phase

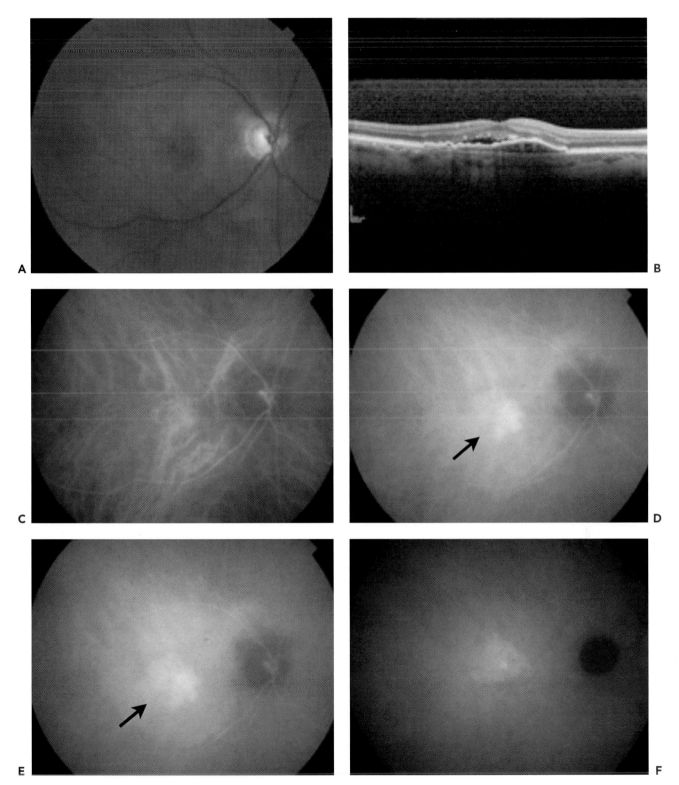

Figure 11.1 ■ Type 1 CNV in a 72-year-old patient with AMD **(A)**. OCT imaging sub-RPE neovascularization with subretinal fluid **(B)**. ICG angiography shows a hyperfluorescent "plaque" of neovascularization (*black arrow*) **(C–F)**.

of the ICG angiogram, PCV appears as a distinct, branching vascular network. Soon after the lesion is first visible on ICG angiography, small hyperfluorescent "polyps" emerge within the lesion actively leaking into the surrounding hypofluorescent area and creating increasing hyperfluorescence. In the late phases of the ICG angiogram, the dye disappears from the polypoidal vascular structure ("washout") (Fig. 11.3).

Wide-field angiography, which currently combines SLO-based imaging devices with a handheld wide-angle viewing

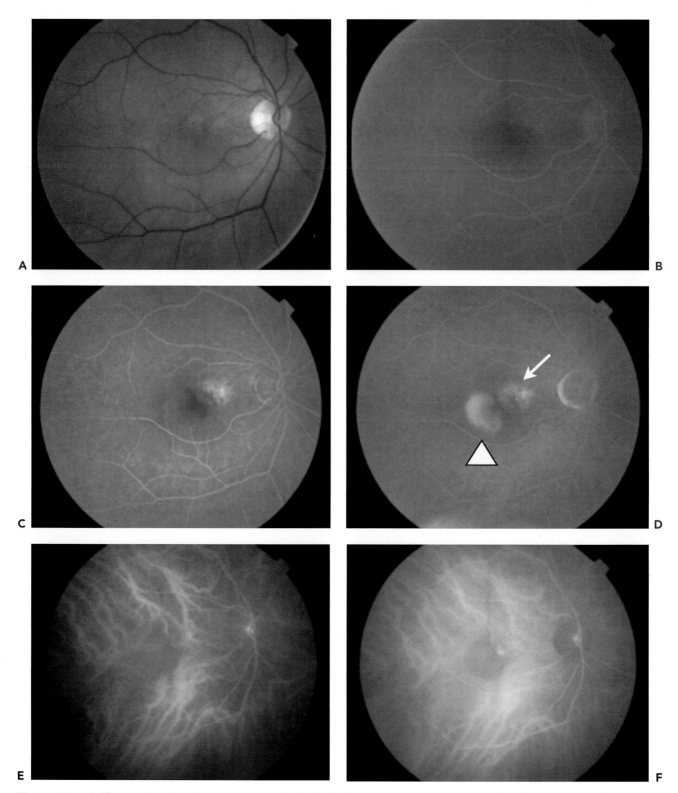

Figure 11.2 ■ A 79-year-old patient with type 1 neovascular AMD. FA shows a vascularized pigment epithelial detachment (*white arrowhead*) with a neighboring serous retinal PED (*white arrow*) **(A–D)**. ICG angiography shows hypofluorescence of the serous PED (*black arrowhead*) with a small area of hyperfluorescent CNV ("notch," *black arrow*) **(E–H)**.

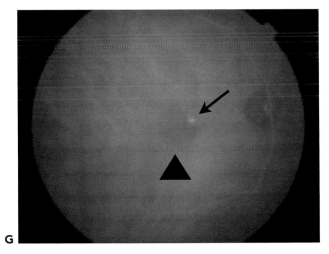

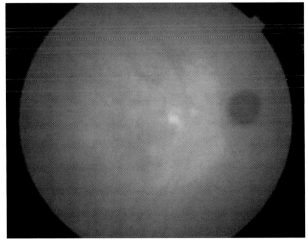

Figure 11.2 ■ *(Continued)*

lens system (e.g., Staurenghi 230 SLO retina lens), allows detection of choroidal abnormalities in the outer periphery. Using this new technique, Mantel and coworkers found that two-thirds of patients with peripheral exudative hemorrhagic chorioretinopathy have polyp-like structures and share many features with PCV.

Classic or Type 2 Choroidal Neovascularization

Classic (type 2) CNV has variable appearance on ICG imaging, with most lesions showing at both the early and late phases or, less commonly, only at the late phase as well-defined, hyperfluorescent structures. However, there is a subset of patients that present with ill-defined

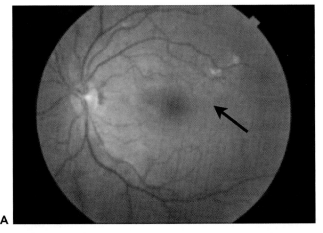

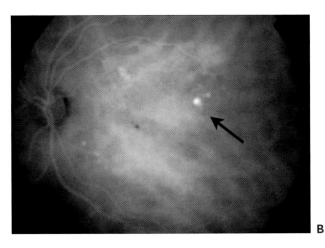

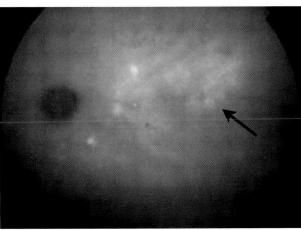

Figure 11.3 ■ Color photography of a patient with AMD: The typical orange polypoidal lesions are almost undetectable *(arrow)* **(A)**. Midphase ICG angiography reveals hyperfluorescent "hot spots" representing individual polyps, the hallmark of PCV *(arrow)* **(B)**. The polyps leak into the surrounding hypofluorescent area, creating patterns of increasing hyperfluorescence. A "washout" effect is seen as the dye disappears from the polypoidal vascular structure in the late phases of the ICG angiogram *(arrow)* **(C)**.

or no detectable hyperfluorescence, confirming FA as the method of choice for imaging this type of lesion (58–60). Most authors have found that ICG angiography is the most valuable form of imaging in studying details of occult (type 1) (17,39,58,61,62) and RAP (type 3) lesions (1,41,63–66).

Retinal Angiomatous Proliferation

RAP, also known as type 3 neovascularization, is a distinct subgroup of neovascular AMD lesions in which intraretinal vascular proliferations are the characteristic manifestation. The neovascularization, which extends into the outer retina and subretinal space, is typically accompanied by dilated retinal vessels, hemorrhages (preretinal, intraretinal, and subretinal), and exudates. One or more of the related compensatory retinal vessels may perfuse and drain the neovascularization, forming a retinal–retinal anastomosis (RRA) in more advanced stages. On FA, RAP lesions show the same indistinct staining as seen in occult CNV; therefore, most cases require the use of ICG angiography to make the diagnosis (41). RAP lesions reveal a focal area of early and intense hyperfluorescence ("hot spot") on ICG.

In the later phases of the ICG study, the leakage originating from the intraretinal neovascularization extends within the deep layers of the retina. Koizumi et al. (67) were able to show that the majority of patients with early-stage RAP also present with abnormal choroidal filling. In later stages of RAP, ICG angiography allows differentiation between the serous PED and the neovascular complex connecting the INR with the choroidal vasculature (Fig. 11.4) (68,69).

Although standard ICG angiography is excellent in detecting RAP lesions, detection rates may be even higher when using high-speed or dynamic ICG videoangiography provided by SLO-based technology imaging systems (66). This technique allows for visualization of the blood flow from the retinal artery to the intraretinal complex to the retinal venule in real time.

ICG: THERAPEUTIC APPLICATIONS

When ICG angiography was first adapted for diagnosing retinal and choroidal pathologies, clinicians and scientists focused on expanding the spectrum of neovascular lesions amendable to thermal laser photocoagulation. Over time, diagnostic and therapeutic indications evolved, using ICG-guided and ICG-enhanced feeder-vessel photocoagulation as well as ICG-mediated photodynamic therapy (PDT). Most recently, Flower et al. (70) pioneered a technique injecting ICG-loaded erythrocyte ghost cells to visualize retinal capillary and choriocapillaris hemodynamics.

ICG-Guided and ICG-Enhanced Feeder-Vessel Photocoagulation

In some cases of CNV, distinct vessels within the choroid that seem to form the basic source of blood flow to the neovascular lesion, the so-called feeder vessels (FVs), can be identified in the early phase of the angiographic study, especially using video sequences with an SLO-based imaging system. Analysis of the images permits identification of the FVs, based on the dye-filling pattern of the choroidal blood vessels in the vicinity of the CNV (71,72). Selective treatment of the FVs is applied by either using an argon laser (72) or using an ICG bolus injection with a diode laser at 810 nm ("ICG enhanced") (73). The underlying principle is that successful closure of the FV(s) can shut down the perfusion of the entire neovascular network and thereby indirectly obliterate the CNV. While initially success rates of 40% to 70% were reported (72,74,75), most clinicians have stopped investigating "feeder-vessel" treatment. Today, thermal laser photocoagulation is largely reserved to treat singular eccentric polypoidal CNV lesions that are not responsive to conventional medical therapy (1).

ICG-Mediated Photodynamic Therapy

ICG has photochemical properties, which allow for it to be used as a photosensitizer. Activated in the near-infrared spectrum, it was thought to be of special use for choroidal and sub-RPE lesions, which can be imaged with the same dye used for treatment. First described by Reichel, "indocyanine green dye-enhanced diode laser photocoagulation" showed variable results, from successful obliteration of CNV to significant vision loss post treatment (76). Due to increasing interest in PDT for AMD in the late 1990s and early 2000s, clinicians explored again the use of ICG as a more affordable substitute for the photosensitizer verteporfin (Visudyne™, QLT Inc., Vancouver, Canada) (77–83). Although some of the reported results seemed promising, the treatment never gained wider popularity due to lack of sufficient dosimetry data, the concerns of additional thermal damage, and the introduction of anti-VEGF therapy.

ICG Angiography and Anti-VEGF Therapy

Since the advent of anti-VEGF therapy for neovascular AMD, the use of ICG angiography has shifted, focusing on identifying lesion subtypes, which may show a less favorable or no response to anti-VEGF therapy. This group is mostly comprised of PCV lesions either mimicking other AMD subtypes or as a sign of vascular maturation seen mainly in ill-defined CNV lesions (48).

Chronic central serous chorioretinopathy is another important differential diagnosis to make with the help ICG angiography (1). Especially with more advanced age, the

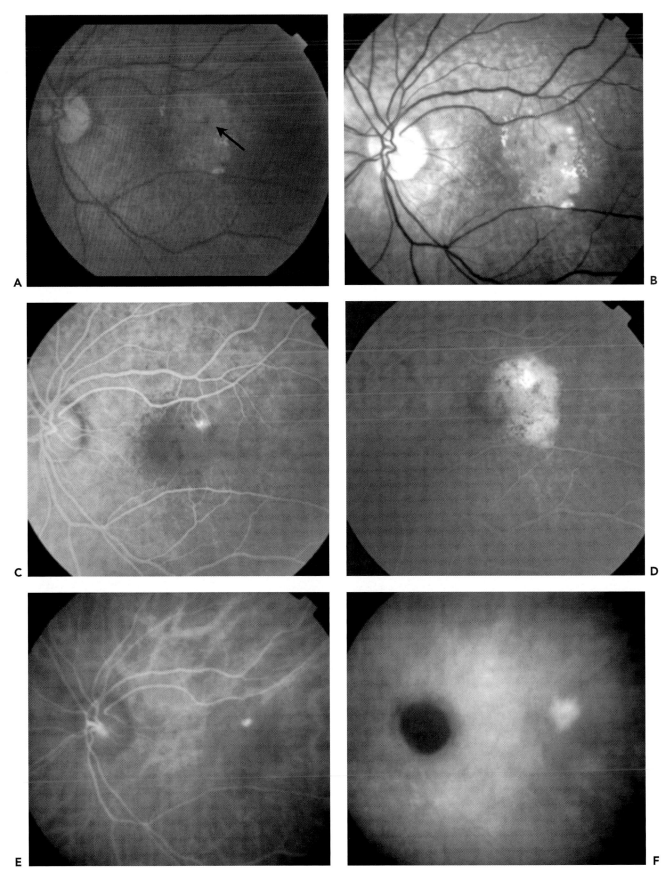

Figure 11.4 ■ Color photograph **(A)** and red-free photograph **(B)** of a patient with RAP: Note the small hemorrhage indicating the area of INR (*arrow*). FA shows a small area of hyperfluorescent proliferation **(C)** with late leakage **(D)**. ICG angiography shows a focal INR **(E)** with increasing hyperfluorescence in the late phase **(F)**.

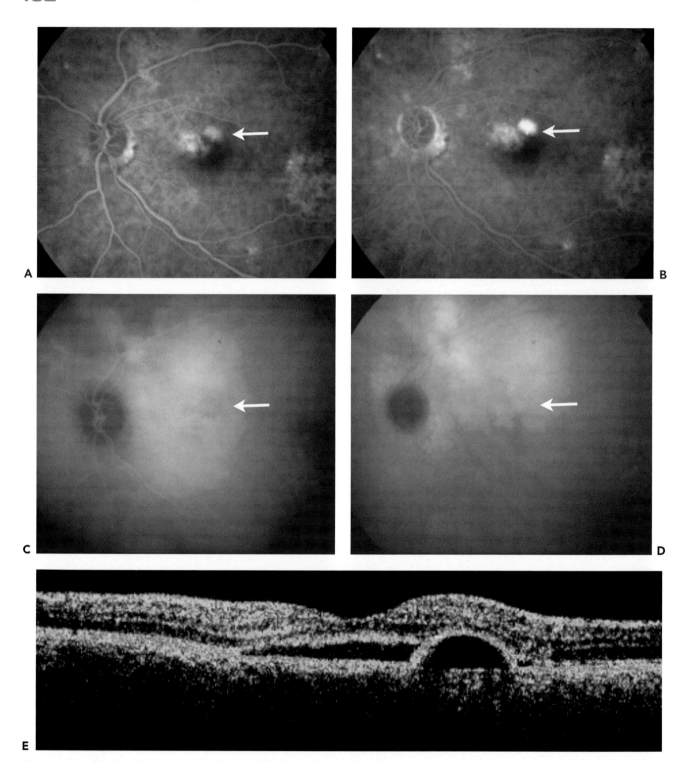

Figure 11.5 ■ FA of a patient with chronic central serous chorioretinopathy: Note the pooling in the small PED (*arrow*) as well as the multiple window defects due to RPE atrophy **(A,B)**. ICG angiography shows areas of increased fluorescence delineating choroidal hyperpermeability. The PED presents as early hypo- and later hyperfluorescence (*arrow*) **(C,D)**. OCT imaging shows a PED with subretinal fluid **(E)**.

typical funduscopic changes of CSC appear more similar to AMD. ICG angiography permits visualization of the characteristic choroidal hyperpermeability presenting as multifocal areas of patchy hyperfluorescence (84) (Fig. 11.5). When approaching a treatment strategy beyond anti-VEGF drugs, these areas can be targeted with standard or reduced fluence

PDT. ICG angiography–guided PDT has been shown to be very successful and frequently yields better results than standard anti-VEGF therapy in this subset of patients (85). It is also important to note that the success of PDT correlates directly with the degree of vascular hyperpermeability/hyperfluorescence seen on ICG (86).

SUMMARY

Although less utilized than before the advent of anti-VEGF therapy, ICG angiography continues to play a crucial role in diagnosing specific subtypes of age-related macular degeneration such as RAP and PCV lesions as well as identifying unsuspected underlying conditions such as CSC. In these forms of AMD, the combined use of ICG angiography in conjunction with SD-OCT is the best way to understand the exact composition of the neovascular lesion and to guide appropriate treatment.

REFERENCES

1. Yannuzzi LA. Indocyanine green angiography: a perspective on use in the clinical setting. Am J Ophthalmol. 2011;151(5):745–751, e741.

2. Fox IJ, Brooker LG, Heseltine DW, et al. A tricarbocyanine dye for continuous recording of dilution curves in whole blood independent of variations in blood oxygen saturation. Proc Staff Meet Mayo Clin. 1957;32(18):478–484.

3. Fox IJ, Wood EH. Applications of dilution curves recorded from the right side of the heart or venous circulation with the aid of a new indicator dye. Proc Staff Meet Mayo Clin. 1957;32(19):541–550.

4. Cherrick GR, Pothier L, Dufour JJ, et al. Immunologic response to tetanus toxoid inoculation in patients with hepatic cirrhosis. N Engl J Med. 1959; 261(7):340–342.

5. Cherrick GR, Stein SW, Leevy CM, et al. Indocyanine green: observations on its physical properties, plasma decay, and hepatic extraction. J Clin Invest. 1960;39:592–600.

6. Geeraets WJ, Berry ER. Ocular spectral characteristics as related to hazards from lasers and other light sources. Am J Ophthalmol. 1968;66(1):15–20.

7. Kogure K, David NJ, Yamanouchi U, et al. Infrared absorption angiography of the fundus circulation. Arch Ophthalmol. 1970;83(2):209–214.

8. Flower RW, Hochheimer BF. Clinical infrared absorption angiography of the choroid. Am J Ophthalmol. 1972;73(3):458–459.

9. Flower RW, Hochheimer BF. A clinical technique and apparatus for simultaneous angiography of the separate retinal and choroidal circulations. Invest Ophthalmol. 1973;12(4):248–261.

10. Patz A, Flower RW, Klein ML, et al. Clinical applications of indocyanine green angiography. Doc Ophthalmol Proc Series. 1976;9:245–251.

11. Bischoff PM, Flower RW. Ten years experience with choroidal angiography using indocyanine green dye: a new routine examination or an epilogue? Doc Ophthalmol. 1985;60(3):235–291.

12. Archer DB, Krill AE, Ernest JT. Choroidal vascular aspects of degenerations of the retinal pigment epithelium. Trans Ophthalmol Soc U K. 1972;92:187–207.

13. Hyvarinen L, Maumenee AE, George T, et al. Fluorescein angiography of the choriocapillaris. Am J Ophthalmol. 1969;67(5):653–666.

14. Hayashi K, de Laey JJ. Indocyanine green angiography of choroidal neovascular membranes. Ophthalmologica. 1985;190(1):30–39.

15. Hyvarinen L, Flower RW. Indocyanine green fluorescence angiography. Acta Ophthalmol (Copenh). 1980;58(4):528–538.

16. Yannuzzi LA, Sorenson JA, Guyer DR, et al. Indocyanine green videoangiography: current status. Eur J Ophthalmol. 1994;4(2):69–81.

17. Yannuzzi LA, Slakter JS, Sorenson JA, et al. Digital indocyanine green videoangiography and choroidal neovascularization. Retina. 1992;12(3):191–223.

18. Scheider A, Schroedel C. High resolution indocyanine green angiography with a scanning laser ophthalmoscope. Am J Ophthalmol. 1989;108(4):458–459.

19. Scheider A, Kaboth A, Neuhauser L. Detection of subretinal neovascular membranes with indocyanine green and an infrared scanning laser ophthalmoscope. Am J Ophthalmol. 1992;113(1):45–51.

20. Wolf S, Wald KJ, Elsner AE, et al. Indocyanine green choroidal videoangiography: a comparison of imaging analysis with the scanning laser ophthalmoscope and the fundus camera. Retina. 1993;13(3):266–269.

21. Baker K. Binding of sulfobromophthalein (BSP) sodium and indocyanine green (ICG) by plasma ?1-lipoproteins. Proc Soc Exp Biol Med. 1966; 122:957–963.

22. Janecki J, Krawcynski J. Labeling with indocyanine green of serum protein from normal persons and patients with acute viral hepatitis. Clin Chem. 1970;16(12):1008–1011.

23. Kamisaka K, Yatsuji Y, Yamada H, et al. The binding of indocyanine green and other organic anions to serum proteins in liver diseases. Clin Chim Acta. 1974;53(2):255–264.

24. Yoneya S, Saito T, Komatsu Y, et al. Binding properties of indocyanine green in human blood. Invest Ophthalmol Vis Sci. 1998;39(7):1286–1290.

25. Landsman ML, Kwant G, Mook GA, et al. Light-absorbing properties, stability, and spectral stabilization of indocyanine green. J Appl Physiol. 1976; 40(4):575–583.

26. Hochheimer BF, D'Anna SA. Angiography with new dyes. Exp Eye Res. 1978;27(1):1–16.

27. Yannuzzi LA, Flower RW, Slakter JS. Indocyanine green angiography. St. Louis, MO: Mosby; 1997.

28. Hanutsaha P, Guyer DR, Yannuzzi LA, et al. Indocyanine-green videoangiography of drusen as a possible predictive indicator of exudative maculopathy. Ophthalmology. 1998;105(9):1632–1636.

29. Pauleikhoff D, Spital G, Radermacher M, et al. A fluorescein and indocyanine green angiographic study of choriocapillaris in age-related macular disease. Arch Ophthalmol. 1999;117(10):1353–1358.

30. Arnold JJ, Quaranta M, Soubrane G, et al. Indocyanine green angiography of drusen. Am J Ophthalmol. 1997;124(3):344–356.

31. Chang AA, Guyer DR, Orlock DR, et al. Age-dependent variations in the drusen fluorescence on indocyanine green angiography. Clin Experiment Ophthalmol. 2003;31(4):300–304.

32. Souied EH, Leveziel N, Querques G, et al. Indocyanine green angiography features of Malattia leventinese. Br J Ophthalmol. 2006;90(3):296–300.

33. Guigui B, Leveziel N, Martinet V, et al. Angiography features of early onset drusen. Br J Ophthalmol. 2011;95(2):238–244.

34. Arnold JJ, Sarks SH, Killingsworth MC, et al. Reticular pseudodrusen. A risk factor in age-related maculopathy. Retina. 1995;15(3):183–191.

35. Zweifel SA, Imamura Y, Spaide TC, et al. Prevalence and significance of subretinal drusenoid deposits (reticular pseudodrusen) in age-related macular degeneration. Ophthalmology. 2010;117(9):1775–1781.

36. Klein R, Meuer SM, Knudtson MD, et al. The epidemiology of retinal reticular drusen. Am J Ophthalmol. 2008;145(2):317–326.

37. Querques G, Querques L, Forte R, et al. Choroidal changes associated with reticular pseudodrusen. Invest Ophthalmol Vis Sci. 2012;53(3):1258–1263.

38. Chang AA, Morse LS, Handa JT, et al. Histologic localization of indocyanine green dye in aging primate and human ocular tissues with clinical angiographic correlation. Ophthalmology. 1998;105(6):1060–1068.

39. Guyer DR, Yannuzzi LA, Slakter JS, et al. Classification of choroidal neovascularization by digital indocyanine green videoangiography. Ophthalmology. 1996;103(12):2054–2060.

40. Gass JD. Serous retinal pigment epithelial detachment with a notch. A sign of occult choroidal neovascularization. Retina. 1984;4(4):205–220.

41. Yannuzzi LA, Negrao S, Iida T, et al. Retinal angiomatous proliferation in age-related macular degeneration. Retina. 2001;21(5):416–434.

42. Guyer DR, Yannuzzi LA, Slakter JS, et al. Digital indocyanine-green videoangiography of occult choroidal neovascularization. Ophthalmology. 1994;101(10):1727–1735; discussion 1735–1727.

43. Yannuzzi LA, Wong DW, Sforzolini BS, et al. Polypoidal choroidal vasculopathy and neovascularized age-related macular degeneration. Arch Ophthalmol. 1999;117(11):1503–1510.

44. Maruko I, Iida T, Saito M, et al. Combined cases of polypoidal choroidal vasculopathy and typical age-related macular degeneration. Graefes Arch Clin Exp Ophthalmol. 2010;248(3):361–368.

45. Wen F, Chen C, Wu D, et al. Polypoidal choroidal vasculopathy in elderly Chinese patients. Graefes Arch Clin Exp Ophthalmol. 2004;242(8):625–629.

46. Lafaut BA, Leys AM, Snyers B, et al. Polypoidal choroidal vasculopathy in Caucasians. Graefes Arch Clin Exp Ophthalmol. 2000;238(9):752–759.

47. Imamura Y, Engelbert M, Iida T, et al. Polypoidal choroidal vasculopathy: a review. Surv Ophthalmol. 2010;55(6):501–515.

48. Cho M, Barbazetto IA, Freund KB. Refractory neovascular age-related macular degeneration secondary to polypoidal choroidal vasculopathy. Am J Ophthalmol. 2009;148(1):70–78, e71.

49. Kwok AK, Lai TY, Chan CW, et al. Polypoidal choroidal vasculopathy in Chinese patients. Br J Ophthalmol. 2002;86(8):892–897.

50. Schneider U, Gelisken F, Inhoffen W. Clinical characteristics of idiopathic polypoidal choroid vasculopathy. Ophthalmologe. 2001;98(12):1186–1191.

51. Smith RE, Wise K, Kingsley RM. Idiopathic polypoidal choroidal vasculopathy and sickle cell retinopathy. Am J Ophthalmol. 2000;129(4):544–546.

52. Scassellati-Sforzolini B, Mariotti C, Bryan R, et al. Polypoidal choroidal vasculopathy in Italy. Retina. 2001;21(2):121–125.

53. Tateiwa H, Kuroiwa S, Gaun S, et al. Polypoidal choroidal vasculopathy with large vascular network. Graefes Arch Clin Exp Ophthalmol. 2002;240(5):354–361.

54. Lafaut BA, Aisenbrey S, Van den Broecke C, et al. Polypoidal choroidal vasculopathy pattern in age-related macular degeneration: a clinicopathologic correlation. Retina. 2000;20(6):650–654.

55. Lip PL, Hope-Ross MW, Gibson JM. Idiopathic polypoidal choroidal vasculopathy: a disease with diverse clinical spectrum and systemic associations. Eye (Lond). 2000;14 Pt 5:695–700.

56. Lois N. Idiopathic polypoidal choroidal vasculopathy in a patient with atrophic age related macular degeneration. Br J Ophthalmol. 2001;85(8):1011–1012.

57. Ross RD, Gitter KA, Cohen G, et al. Idiopathic polypoidal choroidal vasculopathy associated with retinal arterial macroaneurysm and hypertensive retinopathy. Retina. 1996;16(2):105–111.

58. Watzke RC, Klein ML, Hiner CJ, et al. A comparison of stereoscopic fluorescein angiography with indocyanine green videoangiography in age-related macular degeneration. Ophthalmology. 2000;107(8):1601–1606.

59. Gelisken F, Inhoffen W, Schneider U, et al. Indocyanine green angiography in classic choroidal neovascularization. Jpn J Ophthalmol. 1998;42(4):300–303.

60. Avvad FK, Duker JS, Reichel E, et al. The digital indocyanine green videoangiography characteristics of well-defined choroidal neovascularization. Ophthalmology. 1995;102(3):401–405.

61. Destro M, Puliafito CA. Indocyanine green videoangiography of choroidal neovascularization. Ophthalmology. 1989;96(6):846–853.

62. Regillo CD, Benson WE, Maguire JI, et al. Indocyanine green angiography and occult choroidal neovascularization. Ophthalmology. 1994;101(2):280–288.

63. Iranmanesh R, Eandi CM, Peiretti E, et al. The nature and frequency of neovascular age-related macular degeneration. Eur J Ophthalmol. 2007;17(1):75–83.

64. Cohen SY, Creuzot-Garcher C, Darmon J, et al. Types of choroidal neovascularisation in newly diagnosed exudative age-related macular degeneration. Br J Ophthalmol. 2007;91(9):1173–1176.

65. Viola F, Massacesi A, Orzalesi N, et al. Retinal angiomatous proliferation: natural history and progression of visual loss. Retina. 2009;29(6):732–739.

66. Massacesi AL, Sacchi L, Bergamini F, et al. The prevalence of retinal angiomatous proliferation in age-related macular degeneration with occult choroidal neovascularization. Graefes Arch Clin Exp Ophthalmol. 2008;246(1):89–92.

67. Koizumi H, Iida T, Saito M, et al. Choroidal circulatory disturbances associated with retinal angiomatous proliferation on indocyanine green angiography. Graefes Arch Clin Exp Ophthalmol. 2008;246(4):515–520.

68. Bottoni F, Massacesi A, Cigada M, et al. Treatment of retinal angiomatous proliferation in age-related macular degeneration: a series of 104 cases of retinal angiomatous proliferation. Arch Ophthalmol. 2005;123(12):1644–1650.

69. Bottoni F, Romano M, Massacesi A, et al. Remodeling of the vascular channels in retinal angiomatous proliferations treated with intravitreal triamcinolone acetonide and photodynamic therapy. Graefes Arch Clin Exp Ophthalmol. 2006;244(11):1528–1533.

70. Flower R, Peiretti E, Magnani M, et al. Observation of erythrocyte dynamics in the retinal capillaries and choriocapillaris using ICG-loaded erythrocyte ghost cells. Invest Ophthalmol Vis Sci. 2008;49(12):5510–5516.

71. Staurenghi G, Flower RW. Clinical observations supporting a theoretical model of choriocapillaris blood flow in treatment of choroidal neovascularization associated with age-related macular degeneration. Am J Ophthalmol. 2002;133(6):801–808.

72. Staurenghi G, Orzalesi N, La Capria A, et al. Laser treatment of feeder vessels in subfoveal choroidal neovascular membranes: a revisitation using dynamic indocyanine green angiography. Ophthalmology. 1998;105(12):2297–2305.

73. Flower RW. Optimizing treatment of choroidal neovascularization feeder vessels associated with age-related macular degeneration. Am J Ophthalmol. 2002;134(2):228–239.

74. Shiraga F, Ojima Y, Matsuo T, et al. Feeder vessel photocoagulation of subfoveal choroidal neovascularization secondary to age-related macular degeneration. Ophthalmology. 1998;105(4):662–669.

75. Stanga PE, Lim JI, Hamilton P. Indocyanine green angiography in chorioretinal diseases: indications and interpretation: an evidence-based update. Ophthalmology. 2003;110(1):15–21; quiz 22–13.

76. Reichel E, Puliafito CA, Duker JS, et al. Indocyanine green dye-enhanced diode laser photocoagulation of poorly defined subfoveal choroidal neovascularization. Ophthalmic Surg. 1994;25(3):195–201.

77. Costa RA. Severe retinal thermal injury after indocyanine green-mediated photothrombosis for central serous chorioretinopathy. Am J Ophthalmol. 2007;144(3):480–481.

78. Costa RA, Calucci D, Cardillo JA, et al. Selective occlusion of subfoveal choroidal neovascularization in angioid streaks by using a new technique of ingrowth site treatment. Ophthalmology. 2003;110(6):1192–1203.

79. Costa RA, Farah ME, Cardillo JA, et al Photodynamic therapy with indocyanine green for occult subfoveal choroidal neovascularization caused by age-related macular degeneration. Curr Eye Res. 2001;23(4):271–275.

80. Costa RA, Rocha KM, Calucci D, et al. Neovascular ingrowth site photothrombosis in choroidal neovascularization associated with retinal pigment epithelial detachment. Graefes Arch Clin Exp Ophthalmol. 2003;241(3):245–250.

81. Costa RA, Scapucin L, Moraes NS, et al. Indocyanine green-mediated photothrombosis as a new technique of treatment for persistent central serous chorioretinopathy. Curr Eye Res. 2002;25(5):287–297.

82. Cardillo JA, Jorge R, Costa RA, et al. Experimental selective choriocapillaris photothrombosis using a modified indocyanine green formulation. Br J Ophthalmol. 2008;92(2):276–280.

83. Farah ME, Cardillo JA, Luzardo AC, et al. Indocyanine green mediated photothrombosis for the management of predominantly classic choroidal neovascularisation caused by age related macular degeneration. Br J Ophthalmol. 2004;88(8):1055–1059.

84. Guyer DR, Yannuzzi LA, Slakter JS, et al. Digital indocyanine green videoangiography of central serous chorioretinopathy. Arch Ophthalmol. 1994;112(8):1057–1062.

85. Yannuzzi LA, Slakter JS, Gross NE, et al. Indocyanine green angiography-guided photodynamic therapy for treatment of chronic central serous chorioretinopathy: a pilot study. Retina. 2003;23(3):288–298.

86. Inoue R, Sawa M, Tsujikawa M, Gomi F. Association between the efficacy of photodynamic therapy and indocyanine green angiography findings for central serous chorioretinopathy. Am J Ophthalmol. 2010;149(3):441–446, e1–e6.

12

FUNDUS AUTOFLUORESCENCE IMAGING IN AGE-RELATED MACULAR DEGENERATION

MONICA RODRIGUEZ FONTAL • CRAIG M. GREVEN
D. VIRGIL ALFARO III • ERIC P. JABLON

■ INTRODUCTION

More than 9 million Americans and 60 million individuals worldwide exhibit some form of age-related macular degeneration (AMD). Most of these patients are affected by the early changes of the disease. Close to 20% of AMD patients will progress to a more severe and blinding form of the disease: geographic atrophy (GA) and neovascular AMD.

GA is the advanced form of dry AMD. It accounts for up to one-third of the cases of late AMD and is responsible for 20% of cases of severe visual loss due to the disease. The traditional method for documenting and quantifying GA is with color fundus photographs. However, it can be difficult to distinguish between absence of retinal pigment epithelium (RPE) or real GA and the presence of depigmented normal-function RPE. In addition, the predictive sensitivity of color photos is poor and is capable of identifying only 5% to 7% of eyes that progress to late stages of AMD.

Autofluorescence is an intrinsic property of certain materials that is characterized by the transient emission of light when the substance is illuminated by an exogenous source. Many tissues and structures in the eye, such as the RPE, are composed of biologic molecules that have autofluorescent properties. Fundus autofluorescence (FAF) is an imaging technology that measures the autofluorescence

properties of the retina. FAF is a new tool that seems promising in measuring and predicting GA. GA currently lacks effective treatment, but there has been a renewed interest in this condition as suggested by the exponential growth in the number of therapies under investigation that have emerged in recent years. By evaluating risk for disease progression, FAF imaging could help differentiate eyes that progress slowly from those that progress rapidly, and thus enable smaller clinical trials with shorter duration and enhanced power.

■ RETINAL PIGMENT EPITHELIUM AND LIPOFUSCIN

The RPE is a monolayer of hexagonal cells between the neurosensory retina and the vascular choroid. The RPE has multiple functions: It is responsible for the transport of metabolic wastes from the retina into the choroid, it is part of the photoreceptor renewal, and it is in charge of absorbing light (through melanin within the RPE cells) that has not been captured by photoreceptors conferring protection to the retina from photo-oxidative stress. Given the multiple functions of the RPE, it is not surprising that its dysfunction has been implicated in a variety of blinding retinal disorders (1,2).

135

Photoreceptor renewal is one of RPE's most important roles. RPE is in charge of phagocytosis of the oldest disks at the distal end of the outer segments; meanwhile, new outer segment disks are continually added proximal to the base. As a result of this process of membrane renewal (the entire photoreceptor outer segment is turned over every 10–14 days), lipofuscin granules are deposited in the cytoplasm of the RPE cells (3). Accumulation of lipofuscin is a hallmark of aging in metabolically active postmitotic RPE cells.

Ultrastructural analysis of RPE cells reveals the presence of inclusions that have morphologic features of both phagocytized outer segments and lipofuscin granules (4). Delori et al. (5,6) demonstrated with spectrophotometric investigations that lipofuscin granules in the RPE contain the main fluorophores responsible for FAF.

The lysosomal bodies in which RPE lipofuscin is housed have revealed amino acid content and bisretinoid compounds (7–9). The bisretinoid compounds (A2E is one of the most prominent ones) are the fluorescent constituents of the RPE's lipofuscin. They are formed in the membranes of photoreceptor outer segments before the segments are phagocytized by the RPE. The formation of these bisretinoid fluorophores is light dependent. Bisretinoid compounds are formed in the photoreceptor from random inadvertent reactions of vitamin A aldehyde.

The autofluorescent properties of lipofuscin's compounds allow visualization of lipofuscin accumulation in the RPE cell. Lipofuscin has a broad-range excitation; it goes from 300 to 600 nm, so visible light can be used to elicit its fluorescence in vivo. The emission spectrum is broad (480–800 nm) and maximal in the 600- to 640-nm region of the spectrum, shifting slightly toward deep red with increasing excitation wavelength. The excitation used for imaging with a confocal scanning laser ophthalmoscope (cSLO) is typically 488 nm; for imaging by fundus camera, 535 to 580 nm; and for spectrofluorometry, 550 nm (6,10). The fluorescence emission of FAF is broad and centered at approximately 610 nm.

FUNDUS AUTOFLUORESCENCE IMAGING

FAF imaging is a photographic technique that measures emitted fluorescent light from the retina after excitation with 488- to 580-nm light. Several devices can be used to capture the emitted fluorescent light: fundus camera with special filters, fundus spectrophotometer, or cSLO.

The fundus spectrophotometer, developed by Delori in 1994, was designed to measure the excitation and emission spectra of the autofluorescence from small retinal areas of the fundus. The spectrophotometer incorporates an image-intensifier diode array as a detector and beam separation in the pupil to minimize the contribution of autofluorescence from the lens; this device allowed absolute measurements of FAF (Fig. 12.1).

A *fundus camera* with a bandpass filter from 535 to 580 nm for excitation and a bandpass filter from 615 to 715 nm as a barrier can be used to capture FAF. This camera uses a single flash to get an image of the entire retina at the same time (Fig. 12.2). The detected fluorescence signal derives from all tissue levels, in the light beam, with fluorescent properties. The filters allow long wavelengths to pass and filter short wavelengths. Filtering short wavelength reduces interference from fluorophores in the lens (which mainly emit in the range between 510 and 670 nm) especially in presence of nuclear sclerosis.

Confocal scanning laser ophthalmoscopy, originally developed by Webb et al. (11), has a focused low-power laser beam that sweeps across the fundus in a raster pattern and then captures the reflected light through a small aperture (a confocal pinhole). The confocal pinhole suppresses light reflected or scattered from outside of the focal plane (Fig. 12.3). Light originating in the light beam, but out of the focal plane, is suppressed, reducing the autofluorescence from sources anterior to the retina (12). In contrast to the small field of the fundus spectrophotometer, cSLO allows imaging FAF over larger retinal areas and achieves high-contrast images of the posterior segment.

Three different cSLOs have been used for obtaining FAF images: the Heidelberg Retina Angiograph (HRA), the Rodenstock cSLO (RcSLO, Rodenstock, Weco, Düsseldorf, Germany), and the Zeiss prototype SM 30 4024 (ZcSLO, Zeiss, Oberkochen, Germany). The three cameras use an excitation wavelength of 488 nm. Emitted light is detected above 500 nm for the HRA, above 515 nm for the RcSLO, and above 521 nm for the ZcSLO (barrier filter). Bellmann et al. compared the three cameras taking in account image contrast, image brightness, and background noise. Their study showed that both image contrast and image brightness were significantly higher with the Zeiss prototype and the HRA than the RcSLO. Using a model eye to measure the background noise, they found that the highest background noise was measured with the ZcSLO and lowest with the HRA classic (13).

The Heidelberg Retinal Angiograph (the HRA classic, HRA 2, and Spectralis HRA; Heidelberg Engineering, Heidelberg, Germany HRA) is the currently commercially available cSLO equipped with excitation 488-nm solid-state laser and Heidelberg image analysis software (Fig. 12.4). The HRA can register and average multiple FAF images (typically from 9 to 15 single images) in order to amplify the FAF signal. With the signal amplification, the background noise is reduced and the image contrast is enhanced.

The differing wavelengths used by cSLO and fundus camera systems suggest that each system may record fluorescence from a different complement of fluorophores. To compare two FAF images from different cameras, it is useful to identify pathognomonic fundus changes undetectable by only either FAF equipment (14). An example of this situation is the difference in the hypoautofluorescence

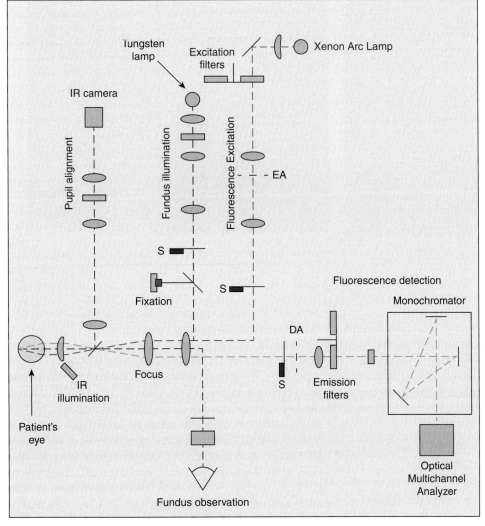

Figure 12.1 ■ Optical diagram of the fundus spectrophotometer. EA, confocal excitation; DA, detection apertures; S, shutters; IR, infrared.

of macula with no pathology; normal macula with cSLO appears darker than with the fundus camera.

FUNDUS AUTOFLUORESCENCE IN RETINAL DISEASES

The FAF image shows the spatial distribution of the intensity of the signal for each pixel in gray values. These are arbitrary values from 0 to 255. Low pixel values (dark or hypoautofluorescence) shows low intensities. High pixel values (bright or hyperautofluorescence) shows high intensities.

Normal Fundus

The topographical distribution of an FAF in normal retina shows a consistent pattern (12). Retinal vessels are associated with a reduced FAF signal because of the absorption

of the signal by blood. The optic nerve head appears hypoautofluorescent due to the absence of the RPE (no lipofuscin). The posterior pole shows a diffused autofluorescence signal. In the macula area, the FAF signal shows high degree of interindividual variability; in general, the signal is reduced at the fovea due to absorption of the signal by the luteal pigment. The signal in the parafoveal area is higher than in the fovea but still exhibits a relatively decreased intensity compared with the background signal. It has been speculated that this observation is caused by increased melanin deposition and lower density of lipofuscin granules in central RPE cells (5).

Abnormal autofluorescence signals can be derived either from a change in the amount or composition of lipofuscin in the RPE cell or from the presence of absorbing material (blood, lens opacity) anterior to the RPE. The identification of abnormalities in the FAF image is dependent on the quality of the recorded image (Fig. 12.5). Vitreous opacities, cataract or lens changes, and cornea abnormalities may

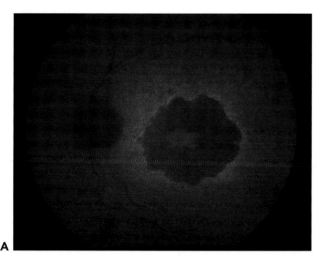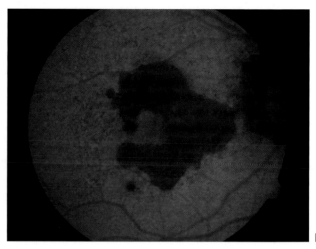

Figure 12.2 ■ Fundus autofluorescence image with fundus camera and filters. **A.** Topcom camera. **B.** Zeiss camera.

affect the autofluorescence signal at the level of the RPE (Table 12.1).

There are qualitative descriptions of localized FAF changes that are widely used. The FAF signal over a certain retinal location is categorized as decreased (hypoautofluorescence), normal, or increased intensities (hyperautofluorescence) in comparison to the background signal of the same image (Fig. 12.6).

Fundus Autofluorescence Image for Dry Age-Related Macular Degeneration

Early Manifestation of Age-Related Macular Degeneration

Early manifestations of AMD include focal hypopigmentation and hyperpigmentation at the RPE level and drusen with extracellular material accumulating in the inner

aspects of the Bruch's membrane. Postmortem analyses demonstrate that some molecular species in drusen material possess autofluorescent properties.

The FAF image for early changes in AMD has been described by several investigators using both cSLO device and fundus camera–based systems. Drusen visible by fundus photography are not necessarily correlated with notable FAF changes; areas of hyperautofluorescence may or may not correspond with areas of hyperpigmentation or drusen (Fig. 12.7). In general, larger drusen are associated with more pronounced FAF abnormalities than smaller ones (15); there are two exceptions for this observation: the basal laminar drusen, which have a prominent appearance, and the crystalline drusen, which have a decreased FAF signal.

FAF (especially with fundus camera–based system) may show a pattern of ring distribution associated with drusen.

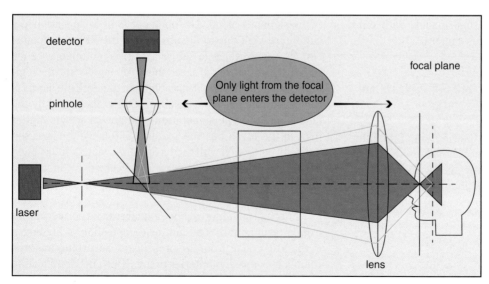

Figure 12.3 ■ Confocal scanning laser ophthalmoscopy. The confocal pinhole suppresses light reflected or scattered from outside of the focal plane.

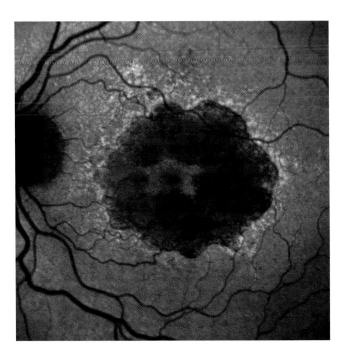

Figure 12.4 ■ Fundus autofluorescence image with cSLO.

This pattern consists of hypoautofluorescence in the center of the drusen surrounded by an annulus of hyperautofluorescence (16). It has been speculated that this appearance is caused by a peripheral displacement of the overlying RPE cytoplasm and/or lipofuscin granules. Confluent drusen and large foveal soft drusen topographically correspond with mildly increased FAF. Coalescence of several small, hard, or soft drusen shows irregular areas of FAF. Focal areas of hyperpigmentation (areas with increased melano-lipofuscin) on fundus photographs may show as increased FAF intensity (Fig. 12.8). Areas of hypopigmentation (areas with absence of RPE cells) on fundus photographs tend to be associated with a corresponding decreased FAF signal (Fig. 12.8). Reticular drusen are identified as a peculiar

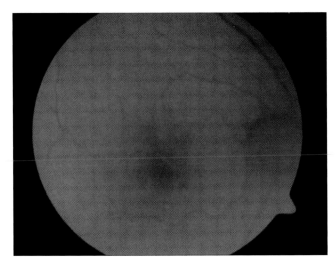

Figure 12.5 ■ FAF in a patient with cataract.

pattern on FAF images (especially with cSLO). Reticular drusen present with multiple, relatively uniform, roundish, or elongated spots with decreased intensities that are surrounded by an interlacing network of normal-appearing FAF signals.

To describe various abnormal FAF patterns in early AMD and to develop an FAF classification system, a workshop was organized by the Fundus Autofluorescence in Age-Related Macular Degeneration Group (FAM study group) in Germany on July 2003. The International FAM study group (17) has identified eight patterns: minimal change, focal increase, lacelike, reticular, speckled, patchy, linear, and plaque-like patterns (Fig. 12.9):

Minimal change: Eyes with minimal variations form the normal homogenous background; FAF without an obvious topographic pattern.

Focal increased pattern: Presence of at least one spot (less than 200 μm diameter) of markedly increased FAF much brighter than the surrounding backgrounds. The borders are well defined, with no gradual decrease of FAF observed between the background and the area with focal increased FAF. Some areas of focal increased FAF may be surrounded by a darker-appearing halo. These areas may or may not correspond to visible alterations (like drusen or focal hyperpigmentation).

Patchy pattern: Presence of at least one larger area (greater than 200 μm diameter) of markedly increased FAF. These areas are brighter than the surrounding background fluorescence. The borders of the areas are typically less well defined than the previous patterns. These areas may or may not correspond to visible alterations.

Linear pattern: Defined by the presence of at least one linear area of markedly increased FAF. The borders of the areas are typically well demarcated with no gradual decrease in FAF observed between the background and the linear structure. These linear structures of increased FAF correspond to hyperpigmented lines on color fundus photographs.

Lacelike pattern: Shows multiple-branching linear structures of increased FAF (lacelike pattern). This pattern may or may not correspond to hyperpigmentation on color fundus photos.

Reticular pattern: Multiple small areas of decreased FAF (less than 200 μm diameter). This pattern is found in the macula and in a superotemporal location. It may be associated with numerous small drusen or areas with pigmentary changes.

Speckled pattern: Characterized by simultaneous presence of a variety of FAF abnormalities in a large area and may cover the entire posterior fundus. The corresponding abnormalities on color fundus photographs include hyper- or hypopigmentation and multiple confluent drusen.

The FAM study group demonstrated with these observations that it is a poor correlation between the visible alterations on fundus photographs and the changes in the FAF. The findings of the FAF may indicate more widespread

Table 12.1	CATEGORIES FOR INCREASED OR REDUCED FAF SIGNALS

Causes for a reduced FAF signal
 Absence or reduction in RPE lipofuscin density
 RPE loss or atrophy (e.g., GA)
 Hereditary retinal dystrophies (e.g., RPE65 mutations)
 Increased RPE melanin content (e.g., RPE hypertrophy)
 Absorption from extracellular material, cells, or fluid anterior to the RPE
 Intraretinal fluid (e.g., macular edema)
 Migrated melanin-containing cells
 Intraretinal and subretinal lipid
 Fresh intraretinal and subretinal hemorrhages
 Fibrosis, scar tissue, or borders of laser scars
 Retinal vessels
 Luteal pigment (lutein and zeaxanthin)
 Media opacities (vitreous, lens, anterior chamber, or cornea)

Causes for an increased FAF signal
 Excessive RPE lipofuscin accumulation
 Stargardt's disease, Best's disease, and adult vitelliform macular dystrophy
 AMD (e.g., RPE in the junctional zone preceding enlargement of occurrence of GA)
 Intraretinal fluid, (e.g., macula edema[a])
 Subretinal fluid leading to separation of the outer segments of the photoreceptors from the underlying RPE, which leads to improper outer segment turnover
 Macrophages containing lipofuscin in the subretinal space (choroidal tumors such as nevi and melanomas)
 Drusen in the subpigment epithelial space
 Migrated RPE cells or macrophages containing lipofuscin or melanolipofuscin (seen as pigment clumping or hyperpigmentation by funduscopy)
 Older intraretinal and subretinal hemorrhages
 Choroidal vessel in the presence of RPE and choriocapillaris atrophy (e.g., in the center of laser scars or within patches of RPE atrophy)
 Lack of absorbing material
 Depletion of luteal pigment (e.g., in idiopathic macular telangiectasia type 2)
 Displacement of luteal pigment (e.g., cystoid macular edema)
 Optic nerve head drusen

Artifacts

[a]Diabetic macular edema can have either increased or decreased autofluorescence.
Data from Schmitz-Valckenberg S, Holz FG, Bird AC, et al. Fundus autofluorescence imaging: review and perspectives. Retina. 2008;28(3):385–409.

damage and may precede the visible lesions. This group also identified a few patients with very early dry AMD and a normal homogenous background at the FAF; the absence of abnormal alterations at the FAF, even in the presence of drusen at the fovea, was explained by the masking effects of the luteal pigment.

The progression in the fundus appearance, marked by changes in the drusen size, does not necessarily correlate with intensity changes in the FAF and vice versa (15). A longitudinal analysis within the FAM study included 125 eyes with soft drusen and no history of laser treatment (18). During the follow-up (mean 18 months), severe visual loss occurred in 11 patients, whereas two developed GA and nine exudative advanced AMD. The two GA eyes were classified as having the focal FAF pattern and the focal plaque-like pattern at baseline. The GA in these eyes developed following the collapse and flattening of large drusenoid RPE detachment. The patchy FAF pattern was found to be the most

frequent in the eyes with progression to exudative AMD. A total of 35 eyes were classified to exhibit patchy pattern at baseline, and six of them developed exudative AMD over the review period. This finding strongly suggests that the patchy FAF pattern in early AMD may represent indeed a high-risk marker for progression to advanced AMD.

Geographic Atrophy

GA represents the late manifestation of dry AMD. It is characterized by the development of atrophic patches that initially occur in the parafoveal area. During the natural course of the disease, atrophy slowly enlarges over time, and the fovea itself is typically not involved until later. Histopathologic studies have shown that clinically visible areas of atrophy are confined to areas with absence of photoreceptor cells, RPE atrophy, and atrophy at the collateral tissue layers. With the disappearance of RPE, lipofuscin is also absent resulting in a corresponding marked decrease

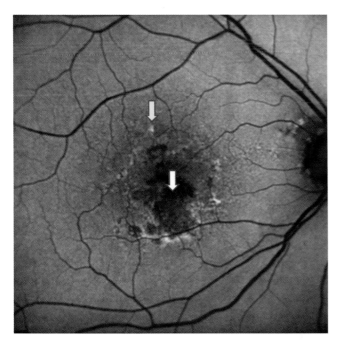

Figure 12.6 ■ FAF showing areas of hyperautofluorescence (*yellow arrow*) and areas of hypoautofluorescence (*white arrow*).

in FAF intensity over atrophic areas. The areas surrounding the atrophy (junctional zone) show high-intensity FAF levels. This junctional zone may appear to be slightly darker than the adjacent RPE by biomicroscopy and may appear to subtly block the background choroidal fluorescence during fluorescein angiography.

The photoreceptors and the RPE function in the junctional zone are impaired. The hyperautofluorescence of this area is indicative of exceptional levels of lipofuscin. The accumulation of lipofuscin occurs before cell loss and predisposes to atrophy expansion. Photoreceptor function is dependent on normal RPE function. Several compounds

in the lipofuscin are toxic for the RPE and interfere with its normal work. An impaired RPE, loaded with lipofuscin, is not able to phagocytize the photoreceptor's outer segments leading to photoreceptor damage. Furthermore, there is some evidence that the ongoing photoreceptor cell dysfunction and degeneration could also be responsible for the hyperautofluorescence in the junctional zone (19).

Natural history of advance atrophic AMD demonstrated a high variability in the progression of the atrophy. Using color fundus photos, the mean progression rate is 2.6 mm²/year; with FAF, the mean progression rate is 1.74 mm²/year (20,21). The variability in the progression rate between patients cannot be explained by the baseline atrophy or any demographic factor (e.g., smoking, lens status, family history) (22,23). Furthermore, there is a linear growth of atrophy over time, and the best predictor of future atrophy would be the growth rate in the previous year. The progression of GA is best studied in the junctional zone at the margin of intact and atrophic RPE, where increased FAF signal may be noted in varying levels. The diversity patterns of abnormal FAF in the junctional zone have a high degree of intraindividual symmetry between the eyes (24). FAF has shown that the extension of areas of hyperautofluorescence surrounding atrophy patches correlates with atrophy progression over time.

The FAM study introduced a classification of the FAF pattern for eyes with GA (25). This classification consists of five main patterns (none, focal, banded, diffuse, and patchy), and the "diffuse" pattern is further subdivided into five subtypes (Table 12.2) (21). A recent analysis of atrophy progression rates over time and FAF pattern at baseline revealed that variation in GA growth rates is dependent on the specific phenotype of abnormal FAF pattern at baseline (21). The progression rates in eyes with the "banded" (median 1.81 mm²/year) and the "diffuse" FAF patterns (1.77 mm²/year) were significantly higher compared with

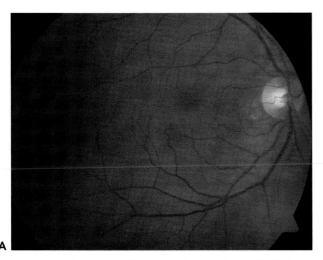
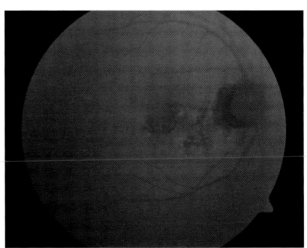

Figure 12.7 ■ **A.** Color fundus photo showing drusen. **B.** FAF of the same eye showing areas of hypo- and hyperautofluorescence that do not correspond with drusen at the color fundus photo.

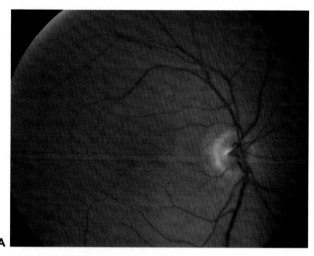
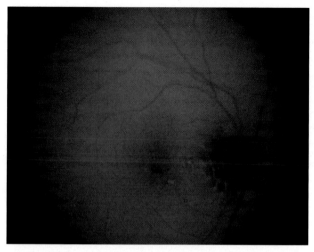

Figure 12.8 ■ **A.** Color fundus photo shows hyperpigmented area secondary to RPE clumping and hypopigmented area secondary to RPE loss. **B.** FAF of the same eye shows hyperautofluorescence area corresponding with RPE clumping and hypoautofluorescence area corresponding with RPE loss.

eyes without FAF abnormalities (0.38 mm²/year) and "focal" FAF patterns (0.81 mm²/year). Within the group of the "diffuse" pattern, eyes with a "diffuse trickling" pattern were identified that exhibited an even higher spread rate (median 3.02 mm²/year) compared to the other diffuse types (1.67 mm²/year) (Fig. 12.10).

Recently, Bearelly et al. (27) proposed a simplified classification scheme using the measure of the rim area focal hyperautofluorescence (RAFH) to group eyes with GA and predict progression rate. The authors measure the area of RAFH in the 500-μm perimeter bordering the GA. The rationale for using a 500-μm rim was to select a measure that allows adequate assessment of increased autofluorescence in the margin around the GA without resulting in much overlap between adjacent areas of GA. They identified three categories (Fig. 12.11):

Category 1: Eyes with RAFH less than or equal to 33% of the 500-μm margin surrounding the GA

Category 2: Eyes with RAFH greater than 33% but less than 67% of the 500-μm margin surrounding the GA

Category 3: Eyes with RAFH greater or equal to 67% of the 500-μm margin surrounding the GA

In this classification, eyes with a larger area of initial RAFH (Categories 2 and 3) had a faster increase in size of GA during the follow-up interval compared to eyes with a smaller amount of baseline rim hyperautofluorescence (Category 1).

Pigmented Epithelium Detachment Secondary to AMD

Pigmented epithelium detachments (PEDs) usually present with a corresponding hyperautofluorescence evenly distributed over the lesion, surrounded by a well-defined and less autofluorescent halo (28,29). There are PEDs with intermediate or decreased FAF signal over the lesion that may not correspond to areas of RPE loss or atrophy. A less common presentation is an increase in autofluorescence in a radial pattern; the radial lines are hyperpigmented streaks also seen by optical coherence tomography. These variations may reflect different stages of evolutions in the PEDs.

A new PED usually shows a mild, diffuse increase in the FAF signal. The fluorescence material inside the PED may derive from RPE lipofuscin and/or degraded photoreceptors. Over time, the FAF signal of the PEDs tends to decrease. Finally, the flattening of the PED or development of RPE tear, GA, or fibrovascular scarring is associated with marked decrease of the signal in the area.

Choroidal Neovascularization in AMD

The FAF signal intensity in choroidal neovascularization (CNV) is irregular. In early CNV, patches of continuous or normal autofluorescence are seen in the corresponding areas of hyperfluorescence on fluorescein angiography. In eyes with long-standing CNV, areas of decreased FAF intensity are typically detected (30,31). Several possible reasons were proposed to explain these observations. In general, it is believed that in early CNV, the photoreceptors and the RPE are less affected than in the long-standing CNV.

Hemorrhages and intraretinal exudates, in contrast to subretinal fluid, show a decrease of the FAF signal because of absorption phenomena. The presence of blood or exudates blocks the underlying retina details, and other image studies are important to differentiate them from RPE atrophy.

Retinal Pigment Epithelium Tears

Areas with RPE tears are characterized by very low signal in the FAF. This lack of autofluorescence is sharply

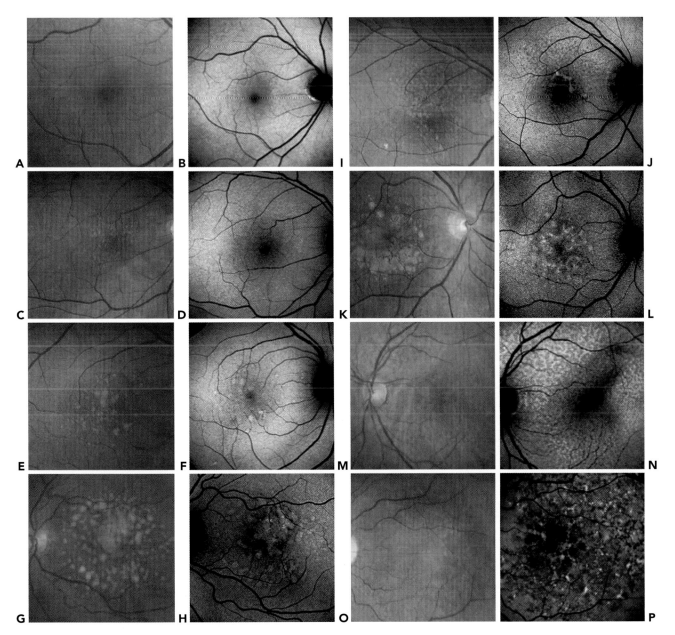

Figure 12.9 ■ The International FAM study group has identified eight patterns: minimal change, focal increase, lace-like, reticular, speckled, patchy, linear, and plaque-like patterns. **A,B.** Normal. **C,D.** Minimal change: minimal variations from normal background FAF. **E,F.** Focal: several well-defined spots with markedly increased FAF. Fundus photograph of the same eye with multiple hard and soft drusen. **G,H.** Patchy: multiple large areas of increased FAF corresponding to large or soft drusen and/or hyperpigmentation on the fundus photograph. **I,J.** Linear: characterized by the presence of at least one linear area with markedly increased FAF. A corresponding hyperpigmented line is visible in the fundus photograph. **K,L.** Lace-like: multiple branching linear structures of increased FAF. This pattern may correspond to hyperpigmentation on the fundus photograph or to no visible abnormalities. **M,N.** Reticular: multiple, specific small areas of decreased FAF with brighter lines in between. The reticular pattern not only occurs in the macular area but also is found more typically in a superotemporal location. There may be visible reticular drusen in the corresponding fundus photograph. **O,P.** Speckled: variety of FAF abnormalities in a larger area of the FAF image. There seem to be fewer pathologic areas in the corresponding fundus. (Reprinted from Bindewald A, Bird AC, Dandekar SS, et al. Classification of fundus autofluorescence patterns in early age-related macular disease. Invest Ophthalmol Vis Sci. 2005;46(9):3309–3314, with permission.)

demarcated, and it is secondary to the loss of lipofuscin. The adjacent area with enrolled RPE is characterized by heterogenous signal of distinct increased FAF. With FAF, it is possible to recognize the exact location of the tear in most cases.

Disciform Scars

Areas with scarring and fibrosis show decrease in FAF signal. Some scar areas have a rim of increased signal surrounding them. This rim is secondary to a multilayered RPE area around the scar (28).

Table 12.2	ABNORMAL PATTERN OF FAF IN THE JUNCTIONAL ZONE OF GA

None: no increase in FAF intensity

Focal increased autofluorescence: single or multiple small spots of markedly focal increased FAF at the margin of the atrophic patch

Band of increased autofluorescence: a continuous stippled band of increased FAF surrounding the entire atrophic area

Patchy increased autofluorescence: large areas of patchy increased FAF outside the area of GA

Diffuse increase of autofluorescence: FAF changes show a larger spread at the posterior pole. These diffuse changes showed interindividual differences that were classified into four subtypes.
  Reticular: various lines of increased FAF with a preferred radial orientation
  Trickling: Atrophy is grayish, with high intensity at the margin, seeping toward the periphery.
  Branching: diffuse increased FAF with a fine branching pattern of an increased FAF signal
  Fine granular: large area of increased FAF with a granular-like appearance surrounding the GA
  Fine granular with peripheral punctate spots: In a diffuse FAF change surrounding the atrophic area, there were elongated small lesions with increased FAF signal.

Data from Holz FG, Bindewald-Wittich A, Fleckenstein M, et al. Progression of geographic atrophy and impact of fundus autofluorescence patterns in age-related macular degeneration. Am J Ophthalmol. 2007;143(3):463–472.

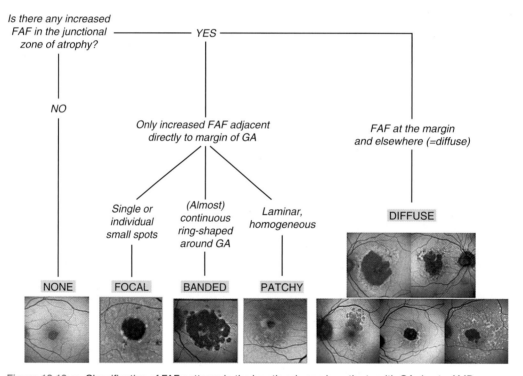

Figure 12.10 ■ Classification of FAF patterns in the junctional zone in patients with GA due to AMD (26). Eyes with no increased FAF intensity at all are graded as "NONE" (slow progressor). The eyes with increased FAF are divided into two groups depending on the configuration of increased FAF surrounding atrophy. Eyes showing areas with increased FAF only at the margin of the GA (focal, banded, and patchy), and eyes showing areas with increased FAF directly adjacent to the margin of the atrophic patch(es) and elsewhere are diffuse (rapid progressors). The diffuse pattern is subdivided in five groups. From left to right: (**Top row**) fine granular, branching, (**bottom row**) trickling, reticular, and fine granular with punctated spots. (Reprinted from Schmitz-Valckenberg S, Fleckenstein M, Scholl HP, et al. Fundus autofluorescence and progression of age-related macular degeneration. Surv Ophthalmol. 2009;54(1):96–117. Review., with permission.)

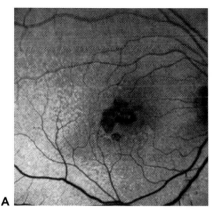 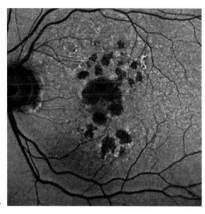 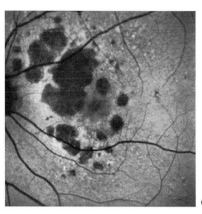

A   B   C

Figure 12.11 ■ Categories of rim area with FAF. Category 1: ≤1/3 of the 500-μm zone bordering the GA with increased autofluorescence. Category 2: between 1/3 and 2/3 of the 500-μm zone bordering the GA with increased autofluorescence. Category 3: ≥2/3 of the 500-μm zone bordering the GA with increased autofluorescence. (Reprinted from Bearelly S, Khanifar AA, Lederer DE, et al. Use of fundus autofluorescence images to predict geographic atrophy progression. Retina. 2011;31(1):81–86, with permission.)

REFERENCES

1. Schraermeyer U, Heimann K. Current understanding on the role of retinal pigment epithelium and its pigmentation. Pigment Cell Res. 1999;12:219–236.

2. Boulton M, Dayhaw-Barker P. The role of the retinal pigment epithelium: topographical variation and ageing changes. Eye (Lond). 2001;15:384–389.

3. Terman A, Brunk UT. Oxidative stress, accumulation of biological 'garbage', and aging. Antioxid Redox Signal. 2006;8(1–2):197–204.

4. Katz ML, Parker KR, Handelman GJ, et al. Effects of antioxidant nutrient deficiency on the retina and retinal pigment epithelium of albino rats: a light and electron microscopic study. Exp Eye Res. 1982;34:339–369.

5. Delori FC, Dorey CK, Staurenghi G, et al. In vivo fluorescence of the ocular fundus exhibits retinal pigment epithelium lipofuscin characteristics. Invest Ophthalmol Vis Sci. 1995;36(3):718–729.

6. Delori FC, Goger DG, Dorey CK. Age-related accumulation and spatial distribution of lipofuscin in the RPE of normal subjects. Invest Ophthalmol Vis Sci. 2001;42(8):1855–1866.

7. Ng KP, Gugiu BG, Renganathan K, et al. Retinal pigment epithelium lipofuscin proteomics. Mol Cell Proteomics. 2008;7:1397–1405.

8. Kim SR, Jang YP, Jockusch S, et al. The all-trans-retinal dimer series of lipofuscin pigments in retinal pigment epithelial cells in a recessive Stargardt disease model. Proc Natl Acad Sci U S A. 2007;104:19273–19278.

9. Wu Y, Fishkin NE, Pande A, et al. Novel lipofuscin bisretinoids prominent in human retina and in a model of recessive Stargardt disease. J Biol Chem. 2009;284:20155–20166

10. Spaide RF. Autofluorescence imaging with the fundus camera. In: Holz FG, Schmitz-Valckenberg S, Spaide RF, et al, eds. Atlas of fundus autofluorescence imaging. Berlin-Heidelberg, Germany: Springer-Verlag; 2007:49–54.

11. Webb RH, Hughes GW, Delori FC. Confocal scanning laser ophthalmoscope. Appl Opt. 1987;26(8):1492–1499.

12. Von Ruckmann A, Fitzke FW, Bird AC. Distribution of fundus autofluorescence with a scanning laser ophthalmoscope. Br J Ophthalmol. 1995;79:407–412.

13. Bellmann C, Rubin GS, Kabanarou SA, et al. Fundus autofluorescence imaging compared with different confocal scanning laser ophthalmoscopes. Br J Ophthalmol. 2003;87(11):1381–1386.

14. Yamamoto M, Kohno T, Shiraki K. Comparison of fundus autofluorescence of age-related macular degeneration between a fundus camera and a confocal scanning laser ophthalmoscope. Osaka City Med J. 2009;55(1):19–27.

15. Lois N, Owens SL, Coco R, et al. Fundus autofluorescence in patients with age-related macular degeneration and high risk of visual loss. Am J Ophthalmol. 2002;133(3):341–349.

16. Delori FC, Fleckner MR, Goger DG, et al. Autofluorescence distribution associated with drusen in age-related macular degeneration. Invest Ophthalmol Vis Sci. 2000;41(2):496–504.

17. Bindewald A, Bird AC, Dandekar SS, et al. Classification of fundus autofluorescence patterns in early age-related macular disease. Invest Ophthalmol Vis Sci. 2005;46(9):3309–3314.

18. Einbock W, Moessner A, Schnurrbusch UE, et al. Changes in fundus autofluorescence in patients with age-related maculopathy. Correlation to visual function: a prospective study. Graefes Arch Clin Exp Ophthalmol. 2005;243(4):300–305.

19. Sparrow JR, Yoon KD, Wu Y, et al. Interpretations of fundus autofluorescence from studies of the bisretinoids of the retina. Invest Ophthalmol Vis Sci. 2010;51(9):4351–4357.

20. Sunness JS, Margalit E, Srikumaran D, et al. The long-term natural history of geographic atrophy from age-related macular degeneration: enlargement of atrophy and implications for interventional trials. Ophthalmology. 2007;114(2):271–277.

21. Holz FG, Bindewald-Wittich A, Fleckenstein M, et al. Progression of geographic atrophy and impact of fundus autofluorescence patterns in age-related macular degeneration. Am J Ophthalmol. 2007;143(3):463–472.

22. Sunness JS, Gonzalez-Baron J, Applegate CA, et al. Enlargement of atrophy and visual acuity loss in the geographic atrophy form of age-related macular degeneration. Ophthalmology. 1999;106(9):1768–1779.

23. Schatz H, McDonald HR. Atrophic macular degeneration. Rate of spread of geographic atrophy and visual loss. Ophthalmology. 1989;96(10):1541–1551.

24. Bellmann C, Jorzik J, Spital G, et al. Symmetry of bilateral lesions in geographic atrophy in patients with age-related macular degeneration. Arch Ophthalmol. 2002;120(5):579–584.

25. Bindewald A, Schmitz-Valckenberg S, Jorzik JJ, et al. Classification of abnormal fundus autofluorescence patterns in the junctional zone of geographic atrophy in patients with age related macular degeneration. Br J Ophthalmol. 2005;89(7):874–878.

26. Schmitz-Valckenberg S, Fleckenstein M, Scholl HP, et al. Fundus autofluorescence and progression of age-related macular degeneration. Surv Ophthalmol. 2009;54(1):96–117. Review.

27. Bearelly S, Khanifar AA, Lederer DE, et al. Use of fundus autofluorescence images to predict geographic atrophy progression. Retina. 2011;31(1):81–86.

28. von Ruckmann A, Fitzke FW, Bird AC. Fundus autofluorescence in age-related macular disease imaged with a laser scanning ophthalmoscope. Invest Ophthalmol Vis Sci. 1997;38(2):478–486.

29. Karadimas P, Bouzas EA. Fundus autofluorescence imaging in serous and drusenoid pigment epithelial detachments associated with age-related macular degeneration. Am J Ophthalmol. 2005;140(6):1163–1165.

30. Dandekar SS, Jenkins SA, Peto T, et al. Autofluorescence imaging of choroidal neovascularization due to age-related macular degeneration. Arch Ophthalmol. 2005;123:1507–1513.

31. von Ruckmann A, Schmidt KG, Fitzke FW, et al. [Dynamics of accumulation and degradation of lipofuscin in retinal pigment epithelium in senile macular degeneration]. Klin Monatsbl Augenheilkd. 1998;213(1):32–37.

13

OPTICAL COHERENCE TOMOGRAPHY

CAIO V. REGATIERI • ROBIN A. VORA • JAY S. DUKER

■ INTRODUCTION

Age-related macular degeneration (AMD) is the leading cause of severe visual loss in adults older than 60 years (1,2). It is estimated that approximately 30% of adults older than 75 years have some sign of AMD and around 10% develop advanced stages of the disease. More than 1.6 million people in the United States currently have one or both eyes affected by an advanced stage of AMD, and it is estimated that there are another 7 million individuals "at risk" (1). Due to rapid aging of the population in many developed countries, this number is expected to double by the year of 2020 (1,3). Although neovascular AMD only accounts for about 10% to 20% of the overall AMD incidence, this subtype is responsible for 90% of cases of severe vision loss (20/200 or worse) (4,5).

Until recently, fluorescein angiography (FA) was the primary imaging modality used to detect choroidal neovascularization (CNV) presence and activity. Although FA is useful for determining presence of leakage in neovascular AMD, this technique does not provide any three-dimensional anatomic information about retinal layers, the retinal pigment epithelium (RPE), or the choroid. The development of optical coherence tomography (OCT) makes it possible to have cross-sectional images of the macula or optic nerve head analogous to ultrasonography.

Instead of sound, OCT uses light waves to obtain a reflectivity profile of the tissue under investigation (6). Light from a broadband light source is divided into a reference beam traveling a delay path and a sample beam that is directed onto the subject's retina. Light backscattered by retinal structures interferes with light from the reference beam. The interference of echoes is detected to create a measurement of light echoes versus depth. The first commercially available OCT systems such as the Stratus OCT (Carl Zeiss Meditec, Inc., Dublin, CA) used time-domain (TD) detection, in which the reference mirror position and delay are mechanically scanned to produce axial scans (A-scans) of light echoes versus depth. Scan rates of 400 A-scans per second with an axial resolution of 8 to 10 μm in the eye are achieved with the Stratus OCT (7). In cases with active neovascular AMD, OCT can be used to detect signs of activity and to establish a baseline retinal thickness, volume, and fluid involvement. Additionally, OCT is particularly helpful in identifying the location and level of CNV (intraretinal, subretinal, sub-RPE) and other lesion components (blood, fluid, pigment, and fibrosis) (8). In cases suspicious for exudative changes, OCT can be extremely helpful in detecting suspected intraretinal, subretinal, or sub-RPE fluid, especially when angiographic interpretation is equivocal, inconvenient, or not readily accessible (9,10).

Spectral domain (SD), a type of Fourier domain detection, uses a high-speed spectrometer to measure light echoes from all time delays simultaneously enhancing OCT capabilities. The reference mirror does not require mechanical scanning. Improved sensitivity enables dramatic improvements in sampling speed and signal-to-noise ratio (11,12). SD detection, coupled with improvements in light sources, achieves axial scanning speeds of greater than 20,000 A-scans per second with an axial resolution of 3 to 7 μm in the eye (Fig. 13.1). At present, at least nine commercial spectral/Fourier domain OCT systems are available worldwide. SD-OCT has emerged as the ancillary examination of choice to assist the diagnosis and management of neovascular AMD. SD-OCT has the advantage of detecting small changes in the morphology of the retinal layers and subretinal space, allowing for precise anatomic detection of structural changes that may correspond to progression or regression of the neovascular lesions (13,14).

Several types of treatment directed at CNV have been developed to prevent the severe visual loss in neovascular AMD patients. These include laser photocoagulation (15), photodynamic therapy (PDT) (16), and the combination of PDT with intraocular injections of triamcinolone acetonide. Despite anatomical success in some cases, there is a low chance for visual improvement when these treatments are used. In recent years, research has provided new insights into the pathogenesis of macular disease. Today, less destructive treatments directly targeting the leakage produced by CNV and its pathogenic cascade have become available (17,18). Antibodies against vascular endothelial growth factor (VEGF) uniquely offer a significant chance to improve visual acuity in patients affected by neovascular AMD. Anti-VEGF therapy can provide long-term vision maintenance in over 90% and substantial visual improvement in 25% to 40% of patients (19,20).

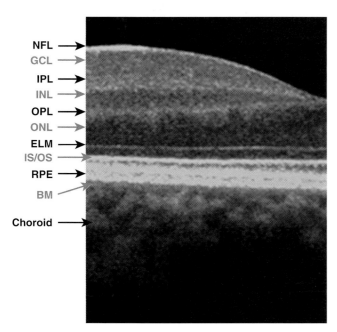

Figure 13.1 ■ Spectral-domain OCT image demonstrating location of retinal layers in a healthy subject. Note *black arrows* denoting nerve fiber layer, inner plexiform layer, outer plexiform layer, external limiting membrane, RPE, and choroid. Note *green arrows* denoting the ganglion cell layer, inner nuclear layer, outer nuclear layer, photoreceptor inner segment/outer segment junction, and Bruch's membrane.

Monitoring response to therapy is one of the most important clinical uses of OCT. OCT can be used to quantify changes in central retinal thickness, macular volume, and subretinal fluid. These parameters, in combination with visual acuity, are used to analyze the response to therapy in several diseases including neovascular AMD. Fung et al. (21) used OCT to guide the treatment of neovascular AMD and demonstrated that OCT could detect the earliest signs of recurrent fluid in the macula after the ranibizumab injections were stopped.

This chapter discusses the OCT findings in neovascular and dry AMD, the importance of the OCT on AMD management, and the choroidal changes observed with OCT.

OCT FINDINGS IN NEOVASCULAR AMD

FA remains the gold standard for initial diagnosis of CNV, the defining characteristic of neovascular AMD. Correlation between OCT findings and leakage and staining on FA has been demonstrated using both TD-OCT and SD-OCT systems (10,14). Small changes in the structure of the retinal layers and subretinal space can readily be noted allowing the detection of morphologic changes that may signal progression or regression of the lesions. As such, SD-OCT is a useful tool in diagnosing and monitoring anatomical changes associated with neovascular AMD.

Classic CNV on OCT can be seen as a highly reflective fibrovascular tissue with irregular yet defined borders between the RPE and Bruch's membrane or above the RPE (22). Likewise, CNV may also appear as a localized fusiform serous or fibrovascular pigmented epithelial detachment (PED) (23). CNV not well defined by FA, or occult CNV, may present as an RPE elevation from the underlying choroidal plane and may be composed of either serous or fibrovascular tissue (23,24).

CNV, when active, is associated with presence of fluid, which appears on OCT as well-circumscribed hyporeflective spaces that distort the surrounding retinal architecture. The fluid can accumulate in the subretinal space, sub-RPE space, or between all layers of the inner retina, and it can be quantitatively evaluated with OCT (Fig. 13.2) (24,25). Recent studies show that SD-OCT is superior to TD-OCT in detecting subretinal, sub-RPE, and intraretinal fluid making it better for evaluation of CNV activity (26).

Freund et al. (27) proposed a more refined classification of CNV that is based on information from a variety of imaging techniques, such as combined FA/SD-OCT, high-speed SD-OCT, and indocyanine green (ICG) angiography, when necessary. This new classification system divides the neovascularization into three types with the goal of honing treatment strategies and providing better prognostic information.

Type 1 neovascularization is characterized by vessels proliferating under the RPE. With FA, it appears as occult or poorly defined CNV. With ICG angiography, it

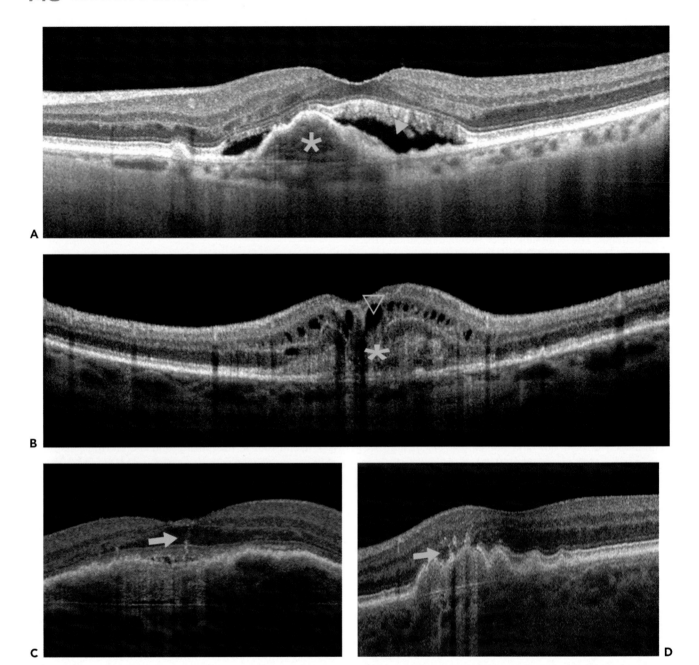

Figure 13.2 ■ Cross-sectional OCT images showing different types of CNV. **A.** Cross-sectional image (Spectralis; Heidelberg Engineering, Heidelberg, Germany) showing a fibrovascular PED, type 1 neovascularization (*green asterisk*), and the presence of subretinal fluid (*green arrowhead*). **B.** Cross-sectional image (RTVue; Optovue, Inc., Fremont, CA) showing a classic CNV, type 2 neovascularization, delineated as a nonuniform moderately hyperreflective formation above the RPE (*green asterisk*) and the presence of intraretinal cysts (*green arrowhead*). **C,D.** Cross-sectional images (Cirrus OCT; Carl Zeiss Meditec, Dublin, CA) of type 3 neovascularization (RAP). *Green arrow* (C) illustrates a retinal vessel transversing the retina toward the choroid. There is a small amount of visible subretinal fluid. In a different patient (D), infiltrating choroidal neovascular tissue (*green arrow*) can be appreciated overlying an irregular PED.

presents as a low-intensity hyperfluorescence. On OCT, it appears as localized fusiform serous or fibrovascular PED (Fig. 13.2A). Type 1 neovascularization usually presents as a fairly mature neovascular tissue that may incompletely respond to anti-VEGF therapy (27). Polypoidal choroidal vasculopathy (PCV) is included in this classification as a variant of the type 1 neovascularization.

Type 2 neovascularization is characterized by proliferation of neovascular tissue above the RPE, in the subretinal space. With FA, such CNV is described as classic. Using ICG angiography, it is usually more difficult to identify type 2 neovascularization due to the hyperfluorescence of the background choroidal circulation. SD-OCT localizes the vessels in between the RPE and the photoreceptor outer segments (Fig. 13.2B). Disruption of the inner/outer photoreceptor junction and intraretinal cystic spaces is often observed. Type 2 vessels may show a complete anatomic response to anti-VEGF therapy (27).

Type 3 neovascularization, commonly referred to as retinal angiomatous proliferation (RAP), is characterized by intraretinal neovascularization and has a distinct appearance on OCT. Imaging characteristics include sub-RPE CNV with intraretinal angiomatous change along with subretinal neovascularization and cystic change within the retina. These changes correlate with clinical and angiographic findings and are hypothesized to be caused by aberrant retinal–choroidal anastomosis (Fig. 13.2C and D) (28). Type 3 neovascularization appears to be sensitive to anti-VEGF therapy, if detected very early in its evolution (27).

Additional features of neovascular AMD are RPE tears or rips. They are known to occur in the setting of an RPE detachment both spontaneously as a feature of the disease and as the result of therapy. On OCT, a tear in the RPE is characterized by a focal defect in the RPE with scrolling at the borders along with pleating of the adjacent continuous RPE (Fig. 13.3). RPE rips are associated with the presence of a dome-shaped PED (29).

Additionally, end-stage AMD can be visualized as a disciform scar made up of hyperreflective tissue in the same location as the inciting CNV accompanied by retinal atrophy (24).

ANATOMIC ASSESSMENT OF THERAPEUTIC RESPONSE IN NEOVASCULAR AMD

Currently, inhibition of VEGF-A is the first-choice therapy for neovascular AMD. Such therapy often stabilizes the vision but can result in significant visual acuity improvement in about 1/3 of treated eyes. Two of the most effective preparations, bevacizumab (Avastin, Genentech Inc. South San Francisco, CA) and ranibizumab (Lucentis, Genentech Inc.), are recombinant monoclonal antibodies (Fab) that neutralize all biologically active forms of VEGF (18). One other highly effective therapy, VEGF trap (Eylea, Regeneron, Tarrytown, NY), is a fully human fusion protein, consisting of portions of VEGF receptors 1 and 2, that binds all forms of VEGF-A along with the related placental growth factor (PlGF) (30). A fourth anti-VEGF therapy, pegaptanib sodium (Macugen, Eyetech Inc.), is available but not widely used due to its less robust clinical effectiveness (31). Two phase III clinical trials (MARINA and ANCHOR) used ranibizumab for the treatment of CNV associated with neovascular AMD (19,20). In both of these studies, ranibizumab was administered every 4 weeks (fixed schedule) for up

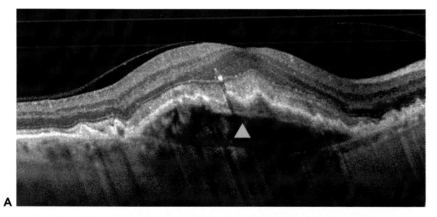

A

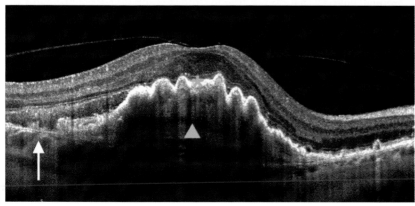

B

Figure 13.3 ■ Cross-sectional Cirrus HD-OCT image of a fibrovascular PED before and after RPE rip. A. Cross-sectional image before rip. Note dome-shaped PED (*green closed arrowhead*) and intact RPE layer. B. Cross-sectional image after rip. Arrow denotes discontinuity of the RPE layer. Note RPE scrolling at the edge of the RPE defect and pleating RPE over the PED (*green closed arrowhead*). (Reprinted from Regatieri CV, Branchini L, Duker JS. The role of spectral domain OCT in the diagnosis and management of neovascular age-related macular degeneration. Ophthalmic Surg Lasers Imaging. 2011;42 Suppl:S56–66, with permission.)

to 2 years without monthly imaging. Both trials demonstrated prevention of substantial vision loss (lost less than 15 letters) in more than 90% of subjects. Additionally, approximately 30% to 40% of the subjects experienced substantial visual acuity gain (gain greater than 15 letters). Though these dramatic results have revolutionized the treatment of neovascular AMD, the monthly treatment schedule used in the clinical trials has a number of drawbacks including the high number of injections and the challenge of determining an end point to treatment.

Consequently, in order to evaluate the effectiveness of less frequent ranibizumab treatment schedules on neovascular AMD, the PIER study (32) evaluated a reduced-frequency treatment schedule that consisted of intravitreal injection of ranibizumab once a month for the first 3 months followed by injections once every 3 months. A reduced chance of substantial vision loss was observed. However, the treatment schedule tested failed to demonstrate an increased chance of substantial vision gain compared with sham.

As such, the best criteria for retreatment are uncertain. The strategies for treatment indication and particularly follow-up have to be adapted to new treatment modalities. Previously, when considering retreatment in neovascular AMD, FA commonly was used as an indicator of CNV activity; however, several reports have indicated inability to differentiate between leakage and staining and poor agreement in interpretation of FA in neovascular AMD between doctors, especially after treatment (10,33). Further, FA is an invasive modality rendering it not ideal for a monthly follow-up. Visual acuity alone depends on many factors such as cataract progression. It is a psychophysical measurement with limited reliability. By contrast, OCT offers many advantages: It is noninvasive and provides an objective measurement of retinal thickening and extravasated fluid. Further, OCT has been validated against FA, the gold standard, in the evaluation of retinal vascular leakage (10,13,14). OCT detects abnormalities, such as interstitial fluid, retinal cystoid abnormalities, and subretinal fluid, when fluorescein leakage from CNV is present. SD-OCT also seems to detect abnormalities frequently in the absence of fluorescein leakage from CNV. Khurana et al. (14) confirmed that the abnormalities more frequently detected on SD-OCT seemed to correspond to 90% of cases with fluorescein leakage from CNV. Additionally, studies have shown a correlation between retinal morphology on SD-OCT and visual function. For example, reduction in thickness of the neurosensory retina at the foveal center correlates with improvement in visual acuity (34). Likewise, reduction of the size of subretinal tissue on OCT has been correlated with amelioration of contrast sensitivity (35). Furthermore, disruption of the inner segment/outer segment junction (IS/OS) on SD-OCT, which is an important indicator of photoreceptor integrity, has been correlated with irreversible reduction in visual function (13,36).

In contrast with previous clinical trials, PrONTO study (Prospective OCT Imaging of Patients with Neovascular AMD Treated with Intraocular Lucentis) included macular TD-OCT features as part of the retreatment criteria (21). In this OCT-guided study, visual outcomes were similar to the results from MARINA and ANCHOR clinical trial regimen; however, the patients in the PrONTO study received an average of 9.9 injections over 24 months. In analysis of the study data after completion of the clinical trial, it was demonstrated that OCT findings predicted the need for retreatment based upon features, such as appearance of macular cysts or subretinal fluid, and these signs were thought to represent the earliest manifestations of recurrent CNV. Other OCT-guided studies using ranibizumab (37,38) or bevacizumab (39) confirmed the visual outcomes reported by PrONTO using similar numbers of intravitreous injections.

These OCT-guided studies used TD-OCT that has an axial resolution of less than 10 μm, with a relatively slow data acquisition speed (400 A-scans/second). Recently, developed SD-OCT devices offer improved image resolution of less than 3 to 7 μm with dramatically faster acquisition speeds (18,000 to 40,000 A-scan/second). Studies demonstrated that SD-OCT provides more detailed views of the intraretinal cysts, intraretinal fluid, subretinal fluid, and sub-RPE fluid, when compared with TD-OCT (13). There is a correlation between retinal morphology on OCT and visual function (34,35,40). For these reasons, SD-OCT devices have higher and earlier detection rates of CNV activity. For an average patient, earlier detection means a significant gain of vision, which may be equivalent to or better than the gain achieved with most CNV treatments (41).

The incorporation of SD-OCT into clinical practice has improved decision-making ability in the treatment of neovascular AMD (Fig. 13.4). However, these instruments have not yet been validated in the context of anti-VEGF therapy. The Comparison of Age-Related Macular Degeneration Treatments Trial (CATT) will identify the best approach to anti-VEGF therapy (bevacizumab and ranibizumab) to be used as the standard of comparison for subsequent clinical trials for neovascular AMD. This trial has four arms: two with fixed schedule for every 4 weeks and two with variable dosing schedule. On the variable dosing arm, patients are monthly evaluated using visual acuity and TD-OCT or SD-OCT images. The treatment in the follow-up will be driven by the presence or absence of fluid (subretinal, intraretinal fluid, or sub-RPE) on the OCT. This study will identify if there is any difference between anti-VEGF therapies and evaluate whether or not use of SD-OCT images can improve outcomes.

In future studies, photoreceptor anatomy may be more readily assessed and quantified by SD-OCT and could become an important prognostic factor for patients undergoing treatment for neovascular AMD (42). Three-dimensional rendering of retinal and intraretinal structures may enable more detailed assessment of CNV, facilitating the decision-making ability in the treatment of neovascular AMD.

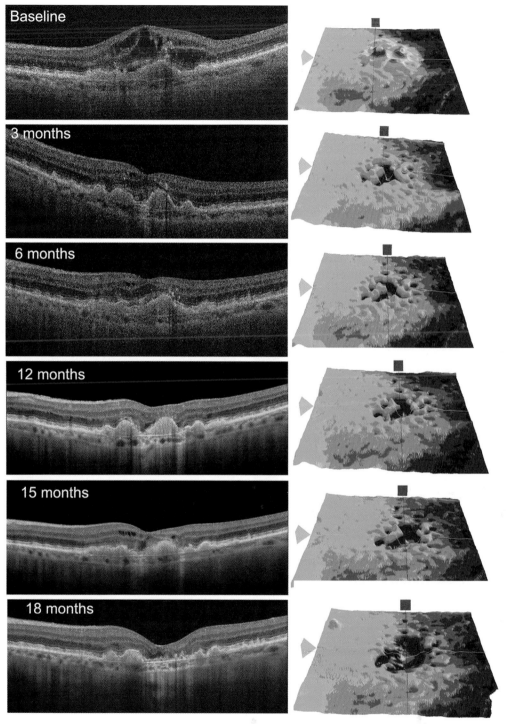

Figure 13.4 ■ Sequential spectral-domain OCT scans of a 75-year-old woman with subfoveal CNV. A baseline scan depicted an elevation of the RPE layer, a localized fusiform thickening and duplication of the highly reflective external band (RPE/choriocapillaris complex), and intraretinal fluid corresponding to CNV. The patient was treated with intravitreous injection of ranibizumab at baseline, month 1, and month 2. Three months after the first injection, the OCT scan demonstrated improvement of macular architecture with mild intraretinal fluid. Additionally, the thickness map showed a significant decrease in the retinal thickness at the macular region. Between 3 and 12 months after treatment, three injections were administered due to the presence of discrete intraretinal fluid. It is important to note the better resolution of the 12-month scan due to image oversampling. The improvement in the resolution leads to a better visualization of retinal layers, and it is possible to note the inner/outer segment junction interruption. At 15 months from the first injection, the patient presented with intraretinal fluid and was treated with intravitreous ranibizumab. At 18 months of follow-up, no fluid was detected in the macular area, but the thickness map showed a diffuse thinning. (Reprinted from Regatieri CV, Branchini L, Duker JS. The role of spectral-domain OCT in the diagnosis and management of neovascular age-related macular degeneration. Ophthalmic Surg Lasers Imaging. 2011;42 Suppl:S56–66, with permission.)

■ OCT FINDINGS IN DRY AMD

Drusen

The presence of drusen is a hallmark feature of dry macular degeneration. Conventional high-resolution fundus photography has been the traditional gold standard in the evaluation of patients with drusen and the imaging modality chosen by reading centers to follow patients in large longitudinal, epidemiologic studies (43). However, interpretation of color photographs is subject to considerable variation, and it is difficult to reproducibly outline indistinct drusen (44). Furthermore, stereoscopic images provide no direct information regarding drusen anatomy and their effect on surrounding retinal tissue and the RPE. Due to these limitations, OCT is gaining popularity in the evaluation of drusen (Fig. 13.5).

A descriptive study of drusen revealed 17 different types of OCT abnormalities (45). Interobserver and intraobserver reliability were high. The most common pattern revealed drusen as convex and homogenous with medium internal reflectivity. Also commonly noted are hyperreflective foci overlying drusen, which are felt to be either RPE migration or pigment (46). Of interest, it was nearly impossible to predict the ultrastructural characteristics of drusen based on their photographic appearance (45). Other possible qualitative changes on OCT include disruption of the inner segment/outer segment junction and a hyperreflective haze within the remaining outer nuclear layer, though this may simply be the unveiling of the Henle's layer (47,48).

The photoreceptor layer overlying drusen also has been shown to be significantly thinned, with the degree of thinning directly correlated with the height of the drusen (49). It is unclear whether the anatomical changes in the outer retina are primary and precede drusen formation and RPE loss or are secondary and form as a result of alterations in their microenvironment from drusen or RPE dysfunction (49). It is also feasible that the observed retinal thinning, in some

October 2010   **October 2011**

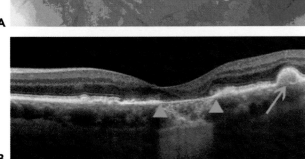
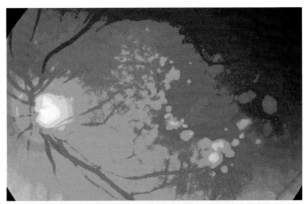
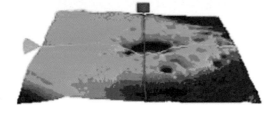
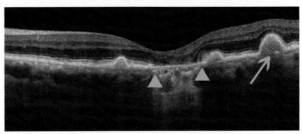
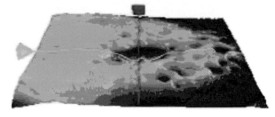

Figure 13.5 ■ Evolution of drusen in this patient with AMD. **A.** The color fundus photos show subtle changes in drusen morphology. **B.** The high-definition OCT image illustrates drusen as homogenous elevations of the RPE with medium internal reflectivity (Cirrus OCT; Carl Zeiss Meditec, Dublin, CA). There has been a slight increase in the volume and height of the larger drusen over the interval as seen on OCT B-scan image (*green arrow*) and the **(C)** OCT-generated elevation map. New, smaller drusen have also appeared. *Arrowheads* denote an area of geographic atrophy as illustrated by OCT. There is loss of the outer retina and RPE and increased transmission of light into the choroid.

cases, is solely due to mechanical compression and that if the compressive forces are relieved, outer retinal anatomy could normalize (50). This has been demonstrated in a recent study of the natural history of drusen. Using SD-OCT and a novel segmentation algorithm, it was shown that drusen evolve dynamically over time, growing and shrinking with an overall tendency to increase in volume and area over time (50,51).

Geographic Atrophy

Geographic atrophy is the principal cause of visual loss in 20% of patients with AMD (52). The gold standard in the assessment and evaluation of geographic atrophy has traditionally been conventional fundus photography. In the AREDS study, for example, high-resolution stereoscopic images were taken yearly and ultimately used to develop a severity scale to predict progression toward advanced AMD (53). There are limitations to this approach, however. For one, there is the nontrivial degree of intraobserver and interobserver variability in interpreting fundus photos (54). Standard photography also only renders a two-dimensional image of the retina, providing little direct information about the anatomy of the outer retina, RPE, and choroid.

Fundus autofluorescence (FAF) is another ancillary test useful in the evaluation of geographic atrophy. It relies on the fluorescent characteristics of the fluorophore lipofuscin, a toxic metabolite within the RPE. Areas of retinal pigment atrophy are devoid of lipofuscin and appear hypo-autofluorescent. A hyper-autofluorescent border may often be seen at the margins of the atrophic area. This is thought to represent swollen RPE cells filled with lipofuscin granules. These cells are at significant risk for necrosis, and this finding has been linked to progressive atrophy (55). Unfortunately, there are drawbacks to this imaging modality as well. FAF provides no direct information about the deeper retinal layers and choroid. Image quality degrades quickly in the presence of significant media opacity. The main disadvantage, however, is the poor discrimination of atrophy in the foveal and parafoveal area. Central macular pigments absorb the excitation light—necessarily making this area hypo-autofluorescent. Thus, there is not enough contrast to clearly discriminate geographic atrophy as it approaches the fovea.

Because of these limitations, OCT has taken an expanding role in the assessment of geographic atrophy. OCT systems offer several complementary imaging protocols to illustrate the extent of geographic atrophy. Patients with geographic atrophy show attenuation of the outer retina with loss of the external limiting membrane and inner segment/outer segment junction. The outer nuclear layer is thinned, and there is a posterior bowing of the outer plexiform layer (56). At the margins of atrophy, two patterns have been described: smooth and irregular (57). There is minimal outer retinal and RPE structural change in patients with the smooth margin pattern. These patients have corresponding normal autofluorescence signal at the border of atrophy. However, those patients with an irregular pattern have severe outer retinal abnormalities with significant RPE alterations at the margin. These patients have corresponding hyper-autofluorescent borders and are felt to be at risk for progressive atrophy.

Another key finding on OCT is the increased transmission of light through the retina and into the choroid. Atrophic pigment epithelium and choriocapillaris fail to scatter light, allowing deeper penetration of light into the choroid. This feature serves as the basis for the rendered OCT fundus image, which is an en face compilation of reflected light from each A-scan. Because more light is transmitted through, areas of geographic atrophy appear bright on the virtual image. Studies have shown that geographic atrophy can be measured reproducibly with these images and correlate well with measurements from FAF (58–60). Foveal sparing has been shown to be identified much more reliably and with more certainty than FAF (59). Based on OCT images, an enlargement rate (ER) of 1.2 mm²/year has been calculated (60).

The main advantage of OCT over other imaging modalities is that it provides both an en face two-dimensional view along with cross-sectional images that allow direct visualization of outer retinal anatomy. Given that visual acuity is a poor indicator of progression of geographic atrophy and that FAF does not discriminately image parafoveal atrophy, OCT will likely become the ancillary test of choice in clinical trials involving pharmaceuticals designed to delay the progression of geographic atrophy.

Geographic Atrophy Enlargement

Early attempts to determine the progression rate of GA relied mainly on serial fundus photography. In 1989, Schatz and McDonald (61) reported a mean ER of 139 μm/year in the horizontal direction. The Beaver Dam Eye Study also looked at total growth in GA over a 5-year period. They found that all

Jan - 2010   Nov - 2011

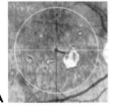
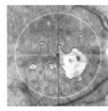

Sub RPE illumination		
	Jan-10	Nov-11
Area in 5 mm circle (mm²)	1.2	2.9
Closest distance from the fovea	0.5	0

A   **B**

Figure 13.6 ■ Geographic atrophy analysis. **A.** Sub-RPE illumination map shows an enlargement of the geographic atrophy area from January 2010 to November 2011. **B.** Table shows the analysis made by the Cirrus HD-OCT software regarding the atrophy area and distance from the fovea.

of their study eyes showed some progression of GA and that the mean overall increase was 2.5 disk areas or 6.4 mm² (61). The AREDS study similarly found an ER of 1.78 mm²/year and a mean change of 7.45 mm² (62). FAF has also been used to assess progression, and in a study by Holz et al., a median ER of 1.52 mm²/year was found. As discussed previously, OCT can also reliably measure the area of geographic atrophy, and, as such, it can be utilized to calculate an ER. Using OCT, Yehoshua et al. (60) found an ER of 1.2 mm²/year. This ER initially seemed to correlate with baseline lesion area, but after a square root transformation of lesion area was performed, the correlation no longer existed (Fig. 13.6). It is unclear why their growth rate as measured by OCT is slower than rates previously published, but it is possible that it is due to the more precise measurements of area as rendered by OCT.

CHOROIDAL IMAGING IN AMD

Choroidal structure is of particular interest in AMD since abnormalities of the choroidal circulation have been hypothesized to contribute to the development of AMD. However, there are only a few studies examining choroidal anatomy using SD-OCT in this disease.

Spaide described a distinct entity, termed age-related choroidal atrophy, which has some overlap with dry AMD. He described 28 eyes of 17 patients with a mean age 80.6 ± 7.3 years, with mean choroidal thickness less than 125 μm. The mean subfoveal choroidal thickness was 69.8 μm, and 35.7% (10 of 28 eyes) of the eyes presented with late-stage AMD. It suggests that choroidal thickness decrease with increasing age and the choroidal circulation might play a role in the pathophysiology of AMD (63).

Another study compared subfoveal choroidal thickness in eyes with neovascular AMD (21 eyes of 21 patients) versus PCV (23 eyes of 23 patients). This study demonstrated that eyes with PCV have a thicker subfoveal choroid (293 ± 72.3 μm) when compared with eyes featuring typical neovascular AMD (245 ± 73.1 μm), $P = 0.032$ (64). Additionally, it was found that eyes with a subfoveal choroidal thickness of 300 μm or greater are more than five times more likely to have PCV. Similar results were also observed in another study that compared the choroidal thickness among eyes with neovascular AMD, PCV, and CSC. It was demonstrated that the choroid was thicker in eyes with PCV and CSC than in normal subjects or those with neovascular AMD (65). The thicker choroid could be partially attributed to dilation of middle and large choroidal vessels or increase in the choroidal vascular permeability that is observed by ICG (64).

Both PCV and neovascular AMD feature abnormal vascular lesions arising from the choroid, which lead to recurrent serous exudation and hemorrhages. These same studies suggest that PCV lesions respond better to focal treatment with laser or PDT as compared to lesions from neovascular AMD. As it is often difficult to differentiate both diseases clinically, measurement of choroidal thickness may play a role in the differentiation of these diseases.

REFERENCES

1. Friedman DS, O'Colmain BJ, Munoz B, et al. Prevalence of age-related macular degeneration in the United States. Arch Ophthalmol. 2004;122(4):564–572.
2. Klein R, Klein BE, Linton KL. Prevalence of age-related maculopathy. The Beaver Dam Eye Study. Ophthalmology. 1992;99(6):933–943.
3. Thylefors B. A global initiative for the elimination of avoidable blindness. Indian J Ophthalmol. 1998;46(3):129–130.
4. Bressler NM, Bressler SB, Fine SL. Age-related macular degeneration. Surv Ophthalmol. 1988;32(6):375–413.
5. Votruba M, Gregor Z. Neovascular age-related macular degeneration: present and future treatment options. Eye (Lond). 2001;15(Pt 3):424–429.
6. Huang D, Swanson EA, Lin CP, et al. Optical coherence tomography. Science. 1991;254(5035):1178–1181.
7. Sull AC, Vuong LN, Price LL, et al. Comparison of spectral/Fourier domain optical coherence tomography instruments for assessment of normal macular thickness. Retina. 2010;30(2):235–245.
8. Hee MR, Baumal CR, Puliafito CA, et al. Optical coherence tomography of age-related macular degeneration and choroidal neovascularization. Ophthalmology. 1996;103(8):1260–1270.
9. Coscas F, Coscas G, Souied E, et al. Optical coherence tomography identification of occult choroidal neovascularization in age-related macular degeneration. Am J Ophthalmol. 2007;144(4):592–599.
10. Eter N, Spaide RF. Comparison of fluorescein angiography and optical coherence tomography for patients with choroidal neovascularization after photodynamic therapy. Retina. 2005;25(6):691–696.
11. de Boer JF, Cense B, Park BH, et al. Improved signal-to-noise ratio in spectral-domain compared with time-domain optical coherence tomography. Opt Lett. 2003;28(21):2067–2069.
12. Leitgeb R, Hitzenberger C, Fercher A. Performance of fourier domain vs. time domain optical coherence tomography. Opt Express. 2003;11(8):889–894.
13. Sayanagi K, Sharma S, Yamamoto T, et al. Comparison of spectral-domain versus time-domain optical coherence tomography in management of age-related macular degeneration with ranibizumab. Ophthalmology. 2009;116(5):947–955.
14. Khurana RN, Dupas B, Bressler NM. Agreement of time-domain and spectral-domain optical coherence tomography with fluorescein leakage from choroidal neovascularization. Ophthalmology. 2010;117(7):1376–1380.
15. Argon laser photocoagulation for neovascular maculopathy. Five-year results from randomized clinical trials. Macular Photocoagulation Study Group. Arch Ophthalmol. 1991;109(8):1109–1114.
16. Bressler NM, Arnold J, Benchaboune M, et al. Verteporfin therapy of subfoveal choroidal neovascularization in patients with age-related macular degeneration: additional information regarding baseline lesion composition's impact on vision outcomes-TAP report No. 3. Arch Ophthalmol. 2002;120(11):1443–1454.
17. Ferrara N, Gerber HP, LeCouter J. The biology of VEGF and its receptors. Nat Med. 2003;9(6):669–676.
18. Chen Y, Wiesmann C, Fuh G, et al. Selection and analysis of an optimized anti-VEGF antibody: crystal structure of an affinity-matured Fab in complex with antigen. J Mol Biol. 1999;293(4):865–881.
19. Rosenfeld PJ, Brown DM, Heier JS, et al. Ranibizumab for neovascular age-related macular degeneration. N Engl J Med. 2006;355(14):1419–1431.
20. Brown DM, Kaiser PK, Michels M, et al. Ranibizumab versus verteporfin for neovascular age-related macular degeneration. N Engl J Med. 2006;355(14):1432–1444.
21. Fung AE, Lalwani GA, Rosenfeld PJ, et al. An optical coherence tomography-guided, variable dosing regimen with intravitreal ranibizumab (Lucentis) for neovascular age-related macular degeneration. Am J Ophthalmol. 2007;143(4):566–583.
22. Giovannini A, Amato GP, Mariotti C, et al. OCT imaging of choroidal neovascularisation and its role in the determination of patients' eligibility for surgery. Br J Ophthalmol. 1999;83(4):438–442.
23. Ahlers C, Michels S, Beckendorf A, et al. Three-dimensional imaging of pigment epithelial detachment in age-related macular degeneration using optical coherence tomography, retinal thickness analysis and topographic angiography. Graefes Arch Clin Exp Ophthalmol. 2006;244(10):1233–1239.
24. Castro LC. Exudative age-related macular degeneration. In: Imaging the eye from front to back with RTVue Fourier-domain optical coherence tomography, 1st Ed. Thorofare, NJ: Slack Inc.; 2010.

25. Chen Y, Vuong LN, Liu J, et al. Three-dimensional ultrahigh resolution optical coherence tomography imaging of age-related macular degeneration. Opt Express. 2009;17(5):4046–4060.

26. Cukras C, Wang YD, Meyerle CB, et al. Optical coherence tomography-based decision making in exudative age-related macular degeneration: comparison of time- vs spectral-domain devices. Eye (Lond). 2010;24(5): 775–783.

27. Freund KB, Zweifel SA, Engelbert M. Do we need a new classification for choroidal neovascularization in age-related macular degeneration? Retina. 2010;30(9):1333–1349.

28. Truong SN, Alam S, Zawadzki RJ, et al. High resolution Fourier-domain optical coherence tomography of retinal angiomatous proliferation. Retina. 2007;27(7):915–925.

29. Chang LK, Flaxel CJ, Lauer AK, et al. RPE tears after pegaptanib treatment in age-related macular degeneration. Retina. 2007;27(7):857–863.

30. Heier JS, Boyer D, Nguyen QD, et al. The 1-year results of CLEAR-IT 2, a phase 2 study of vascular endothelial growth factor trap-eye dosed as-needed after 12-week fixed dosing. Ophthalmology. 2011;118(6):1098–1106.

31. Gragoudas ES, Adamis AP, Cunningham ET Jr, et al. Pegaptanib for neovascular age-related macular degeneration. N Engl J Med. 2004;351(27): 2805–2816.

32. Regillo CD, Brown DM, Abraham P, et al. Randomized, double-masked, sham-controlled trial of ranibizumab for neovascular age-related macular degeneration: PIER Study year 1. Am J Ophthalmol. 2008;145(2):239–248.

33. Friedman SM, Margo CE. Choroidal neovascular membranes: reproducibility of angiographic interpretation. Am J Ophthalmol. 2000;130(6):839–841.

34. Keane PA, Liakopoulos S, Chang KT, et al. Relationship between optical coherence tomography retinal parameters and visual acuity in neovascular age-related macular degeneration. Ophthalmology. 2008;115(12):2206–2214.

35. Keane PA, Patel PJ, Ouyang Y, et al. Effects of retinal morphology on contrast sensitivity and reading ability in neovascular age-related macular degeneration. Invest Ophthalmol Vis Sci. 2010;51(11):5431–5437.

36. Hayashi H, Yamashiro K, Tsujikawa A, et al. Association between foveal photoreceptor integrity and visual outcome in neovascular age-related macular degeneration. Am J Ophthalmol. 2009;148(1):83–89.e1.

37. Rothenbuehler SP, Waeber D, Brinkmann CK, et al. Effects of ranibizumab in patients with subfoveal choroidal neovascularization attributable to age-related macular degeneration. Am J Ophthalmol. 2009;147(5):831–837.

38. Querques G, Azrya S, Martinelli D, et al. Ranibizumab for exudative age-related macular degeneration: 24-month outcomes from a single-centre institutional setting. Br J Ophthalmol. 2010;94(3):292–296.

39. Leydolt C, Michels S, Prager F, et al. Effect of intravitreal bevacizumab (Avastin) in neovascular age-related macular degeneration using a treatment regimen based on optical coherence tomography: 6- and 12-month results. Acta Ophthalmol. 2010;88(5):594–600.

40. Regatieri CV, Branchini L, Duker JS. The role of spectral-domain OCT in the diagnosis and management of neovascular age-related macular degeneration. Ophthalmic Surg Lasers Imaging. 2011;42(Suppl):S56–S66.

41. Loewenstein A. The significance of early detection of age-related macular degeneration: Richard & Hinda Rosenthal Foundation lecture, The Macula Society 29th Annual Meeting. Retina. 2007;27(7):873–878.

42. Witkin AJ, Vuong LN, Srinivasan VJ, et al. High-speed ultrahigh resolution optical coherence tomography before and after ranibizumab for age-related macular degeneration. Ophthalmology. 2009;116(5):956–963.

43. Age-Related Eye Disease Study Research Group. The Age-Related Eye Disease Study system for classifying age-related macular degeneration from stereoscopic color fundus photographs: the Age-Related Eye Disease Study Report Number 6. Am J Ophthalmol. 2001;132(5):668–681.

44. Klein R, Davis MD, Magli YL, et al. The Wisconsin age-related maculopathy grading system. Ophthalmology. 1991;98(7):1128–1134.

45. Khanifar AA, Koreishi AF, Izatt JA, et al. Drusen ultrastructure imaging with spectral domain optical coherence tomography in age-related macular degeneration. Ophthalmology. 2008;115(11):1883–1890.

46. Pieroni CG, Witkin AJ, Ko TH, et al. Ultrahigh resolution optical coherence tomography in non-exudative age related macular degeneration. Br J Ophthalmol. 2006;90(2):191–197.

47. Lujan BJ, Roorda A, Knighton RW, et al. Revealing Henle's fiber layer using spectral domain optical coherence tomography. Invest Ophthalmol Vis Sci. 2011;52(3):1486–1492.

48. Zarbin MA. Current concepts in the pathogenesis of age-related macular degeneration. Arch Ophthalmol. 2004;122(4):598–614.

49. Schuman SG, Koreishi AF, Farsiu S, et al. Photoreceptor layer thinning over drusen in eyes with age-related macular degeneration imaged in vivo with spectral-domain optical coherence tomography. Ophthalmology. 2009;116(3):488–496 e2.

50. Gregori G, Wang F, Rosenfeld PJ, et al. Spectral domain optical coherence tomography imaging of drusen in nonexudative age-related macular degeneration. Ophthalmology. 2011;118(7):1373–1379.

51. Yehoshua Z, Wang F, Rosenfeld PJ, et al. Natural history of drusen morphology in age-related macular degeneration using spectral domain optical coherence tomography. Ophthalmology. 2011;118(12):2434–2441.

52. Ferris FL 3rd, Fine SL, Hyman L. Age-related macular degeneration and blindness due to neovascular maculopathy. Arch Ophthalmol. 1984;102(11):1640–1642.

53. Davis MD, Gangnon RE, Lee LY, et al. The Age-Related Eye Disease Study severity scale for age-related macular degeneration: AREDS Report No. 17. Arch Ophthalmol. 2005;123(11):1484–1498.

54. Scholl HP, Peto T, Dandekar S, et al. Inter- and intra-observer variability in grading lesions of age-related maculopathy and macular degeneration. Graefes Arch Clin Exp Ophthalmol. 2003;241(1):39–47.

55. Holz FG, Bindewald-Wittich A, Fleckenstein M, et al. Progression of geographic atrophy and impact of fundus autofluorescence patterns in age-related macular degeneration. Am J Ophthalmol. 2007;143(3):463–472.

56. Fleckenstein M, Schmitz-Valckenberg S, Adrion C, et al. Tracking progression with spectral-domain optical coherence tomography in geographic atrophy caused by age-related macular degeneration. Invest Ophthalmol Vis Sci. 2010;51(8):3846–3852.

57. Brar M, Kozak I, Cheng L, et al. Correlation between spectral-domain optical coherence tomography and fundus autofluorescence at the margins of geographic atrophy. Am J Ophthalmol. 2009;148(3):439–444.

58. Lujan BJ, Rosenfeld PJ, Gregori G, et al. Spectral domain optical coherence tomographic imaging of geographic atrophy. Ophthalmic Surg Lasers Imaging. 2009;40(2):96–101.

59. Sayegh RG, Simader C, Scheschy U, et al. A systematic comparison of spectral-domain optical coherence tomography and fundus autofluorescence in patients with geographic atrophy. Ophthalmology. 2011;118(9):1844–1851.

60. Yehoshua Z, Rosenfeld PJ, Gregori G, et al. Progression of geographic atrophy in age-related macular degeneration imaged with spectral domain optical coherence tomography. Ophthalmology. 2011;118(4):679–686.

61. Schatz H, McDonald HR. Atrophic macular degeneration. Rate of spread of geographic atrophy and visual loss. Ophthalmology. 1989;96(10):1541–1551.

62. Lindblad AS, Lloyd PC, Clemons TE, et al. Change in area of geographic atrophy in the Age-Related Eye Disease Study: AREDS report number 26. Arch Ophthalmol. 2009;127(9):1168–1174.

63. Spaide RF. Age-related choroidal atrophy. Am J Ophthalmol. 2009;147(5): 801–810.

64. Koizumi H, Yamagishi T, Yamazaki T, et al. Subfoveal choroidal thickness in typical age-related macular degeneration and polypoidal choroidal vasculopathy. Graefes Arch Clin Exp Ophthalmol. 2011;249(8):1123–1128.

65. Kim SW, Oh J, Kwon SS, et al. Comparison of choroidal thickness among patients with healthy eyes, early age-related maculopathy, neovascular age-related macular degeneration, central serous chorioretinopathy, and polypoidal choroidal vasculopathy. Retina. 2011;31(9):1904–1911.

14

ANTIOXIDANTS AND AGE-RELATED MACULAR DEGENERATION: CLINICAL ASSOCIATIONS AND BASIC MECHANISMS

YAN CHEN • PAUL STERNBERG JR.

◼ INTRODUCTION

Age-related macular degeneration (AMD), like many other chronic degenerative diseases, is a multifactorial disease involving environmental, genetic, and sometimes concomitant systemic disease. These risk factors impact a physiologic state of tissue and cells known as oxidative stress, which is defined as an imbalance of reactive oxygen species (ROS) and the protective antioxidant system. With aging, a decline in the retinal antioxidant defense and an increase in ROS production may shift the balance toward oxidative damage. The cellular and molecular mechanisms of retinal oxidative injury and protection, and their associations with chronic inflammation in AMD, have not yet been clearly defined. Nonetheless, there is a great body of evidence supporting the causative role of oxidative stress in the pathogenesis of AMD, and clinical studies of antioxidant supplementation have demonstrated beneficial effects in slowing the progression of AMD.

In this chapter, we review our current understanding of the role of oxidative stress in AMD based on the results of both patient-based and animal model studies. We address the experimental evidence supporting potential mechanisms of oxidative injury in the pathogenesis of AMD. We also discuss the use of antioxidants and other related novel therapeutic options in the prevention and treatment of AMD.

◼ OXIDATIVE STRESS IN THE PATHOGENESIS OF AMD

During the past few years, tremendous progress has been made in deciphering the etiology of AMD. Major genetic variations of AMD have been mapped to genes encoding complement factor proteins and chromosome region 10q26 (1–10). Single nucleotide polymorphisms in the complement factor H (CFH) gene have been detected in a high percentage of AMD cases (1–4). However, animal models with either CFH knockout or replacement with human risk alleles have only produced minor signs of accelerated aging in the outer retina (11,12). The discrepancy between the predominant effects of genetic variations predicted by the clinical association studies and the mild phenotypic expression in the animal models suggest that other undefined mechanisms are involved in the initiation process of macular degeneration. Considerable evidence implicates inflammatory processes as participants. Complement proteins and other proinflammatory factors may greatly amplify the initial lesions of AMD in the retinal pigment epithelium (RPE), Bruch's membrane, and choroid. Accumulating evidence suggests that oxidative stress can be an initiating factor in the pathogenesis of AMD.

The Retina Is Subjected to Oxidative Stress

As noted, oxidative stress occurs when the ROS exceeds the antioxidant capacity at the tissue and cellular level. ROS is divided into two groups based on the presence or absence of unpaired electrons: (a) Free radicals, such as superoxide anion (O_2^-) and hydroxyl radical ($OH\bullet$), have unpaired electrons, and (b) nonradicals, such as hydrogen peroxide (H_2O_2), have only paired electrons. Normal physiologic processes generate ROS as by-products. For example, mitochondria produce most of the energy required by the cell via oxidative phosphorylation. During this process, around 1% to 4% of electrons leak from the electron transport chain and form O_2^- (13). O_2^- quickly converts to H_2O_2, which can be further transformed into highly reactive OH^- in the presence of transition metals via the Fenton reaction (14,15).

Unquenched ROS readily reacts with macromolecules including proteins, lipids, and nucleic acids, which can lead to oxidative damage. To counteract the deleterious effects of ROS, cells use multilayered antioxidant systems to promptly neutralize reactive intermediates. Two types of antioxidant mechanisms serve the purpose: enzymatic detoxification systems and nonenzymatic compounds. Enzymatic antioxidants work in a coordinated manner to remove intracellular ROS. This is exemplified by the decomposition of superoxide anions (Fig. 14.1), which occurs in two sequential steps.

First, superoxide dismutase (SOD) facilitates the conversion of O_2^- to H_2O_2 (16). Second, three different enzymes, catalase, glutathione peroxidase (Gpx), and peroxiredoxin (Prx), catalyze the clearance of H_2O_2. Mammalian catalase degrades H_2O_2 to water via heme groups in its active center (17). Reduction of H_2O_2 by Gpx occurs in the expense of reduced glutathione (GSH). In the reaction, GSH provides electrons and is oxidized to form glutathione disulfide (GSSG), and GSSG is reduced back by glutathione reductase (GR), which uses NADPH as the ultimate electron donor (18,19). The Prx system consists of three enzymes: Prx, thioredoxin (Trx), and thioredoxin reductase (TR). Prx reduces peroxides and is regenerated by Trx in conjunction with TR (20,21). Given the synchronized manner by which antioxidant enzymes work, it is easy to understand why correcting a dysfunction in a single component would often be insufficient to achieve the optimal protective effects (22–24).

Nonenzymatic compounds are also key components of the antioxidant network. The tripeptide GSH is one of several highly important small compounds. It contains a free sulfhydryl (SH) group, which is highly reactive with ROS. In RPE cells, the intercellular concentration of GSH is in the millimolar range and provides a first-line buffer system against free radical attack. GSH also serves as a cofactor in the detoxification of ROS by antioxidant enzymes. Several other small molecule antioxidants, including vitamin C, vitamin E, and zinc, are also of particular importance in protecting the retina from oxidative stress. They are discussed in more detail later in the chapter.

The antioxidant systems in RPE cells are highly efficient and highly error resistant under normal physiologic conditions. However, the balance between the generation of ROS and their clearance by the antioxidant systems can be disturbed by exogenous factors, such as pollutants and tobacco use, or physiologic conditions, such as aging and concomitant systemic disease. The retina is prone

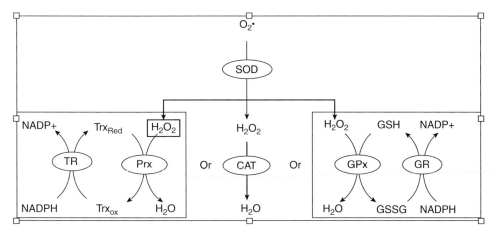

Figure 14.1 ■ Diagrammatic representation of detoxification of ROS superoxide anion. In the presence of SOD, superoxide anion is immediately transformed into hydrogen peroxide. Three enzymes catalyze decomposition of hydrogen peroxide: catalase (CAT), Gpx, and Prx. Reduced glutathione (GSH) and Trx (Trx$_{Red}$) provide electrons for Gpx and Prx, respectively. Using NADPH as the final electron donor, oxidized glutathione (GSSG) and Trx are reduced back by GR and TR.

to oxidative stress for several reasons. First, the rate of oxygen consumption in the retina is greater than in any other tissue of the human body (25). This high-energy utilization is necessarily accompanied by high ROS production. Second, the retina is continually subjected to intense focal light exposure. In the presence of photosensitizers or chromophores (visual pigments and lipofuscin), photo-oxidation occurs resulting in the production of ROS, which includes singlet oxygen, superoxide, hydrogen peroxide, and hydroxyl radicals (26). Third, RPE cells can function as phagocytes, phagocytizing and degrading shed photoreceptor outer segments (POS). The phagocytosis of POS stimulates respiratory burst (rapid release of ROS), which likely occurs by utilizing plasma membrane NADPH oxidase (27–29). Moreover, the outer segments are extremely abundant in polyunsaturated fatty acids (PUFAs), which readily undergo lipid peroxidation. The resultant oxidized intermediates are long-lived and covalently modify various kinds of molecules including proteins, thereby impairing the stability and functions of their targets. Thus, lipid peroxidation initiates a chain reaction, which amplifies the initial number of free radicals. Two major products of lipid peroxidation, carboxyethylpyrrole (CEP) and malondialdehyde (MDA), have been recently linked to AMD and are discussed in more detail later in the chapter.

As the retina ages, it becomes more susceptible to oxidative injury due partly to an age-related decline in the antioxidant capacity. For example, a reduction in catalase activity in aging RPE was demonstrated by both biochemical and immunohistochemical analyses of human donor eyes (30,31). Systemically, the plasma GSH pool has an age-dependent decrease in total level as well as an oxidation in the redox status (32,33). Meanwhile, age-related

increases in chromophores like lipofuscin cause increases in pro-oxidants that further stress and sometimes surpass the antioxidant system capacity.

Lipofuscin

Lipofuscin, also known as aging pigment, is an autofluorescent and electron-dense material that accumulates with age in postmitotic cells, including the RPE (34). It has a brown-yellow color and is enzymatically nondegradable. The rate of lipofuscin accumulation shows a negative correlation with longevity in animals. Thus, the accumulation of lipofuscin is considered a hallmark of aging (35,36). An age-dependent buildup of lipofuscin occurs in human RPE cells; at the age of 90, lipofuscin occupies about 19% of the RPE cell volume, whereas in the first 10 years of life, it occupies only 1% (37). The increased lipofuscin in the RPE causes an increase in autofluorescence of the fundus and precedes the development of geographic atrophy. Thus, high autofluorescence of the fundus can be a useful clinical biomarker that can assist in monitoring the progression of atrophic AMD (37–39) (Fig. 14.2).

The composition of lipofuscin is highly heterogeneous and includes oxidized proteins and lipids. Two degradation pathways, autophagy and phagocytosis, contribute to lipofuscin accumulation in the lysosomes. In the RPE, the role of phagocytosis has been well established by multilayered evidence. On the molecular level, the best-characterized fluorophore of the RPE lipofuscin, N-retinylidene-N-retinylethanolamine (A2E), derives from unique components of phagocytized POS (40,41). On the cellular level, long-term exposure of POS leads to formation of lipofuscin-like autofluorescent granules in cultured RPE cells (42). On the whole animal level, RCS

Figure 14.2 ■ Increased lipofuscin fluorescence in aging RPE from Nrf2-deficient mice. RPE/choroid flat mount was prepared from age-matched (14 M) wild-type (WT) and Nrf2 knockout (KO) mice. Autofluorescence (green) was monitored over a broad spectrum of excitation wavelengths (e.g., 488 and 555 nm). F-actin was stained with phalloidin (red) to delineate the boundaries of the RPE. Increased autofluorescence in Nrf2-deficient RPE is an indicator of lipofuscin accumulation. Scale bar: 20 μm.

rats (which have early photoreceptor degeneration) show less lipofuscin accumulation with age in the RPE (43). Compared to phagocytosis, the role of autophagy in RPE lipofuscin formation is less defined. However, results from both in vivo and in vitro studies indicate that RPE lipofuscin is not produced solely from phagocytosis. Studies with long-term cultured RPE cells show that autofluorescent inclusions resembling lipofuscin granules accumulate in the absence of outer segments or the A2E (44). Mice lacking alphaVbeta5 integrin are defective in phagocytosis of POS; nonetheless, lipofuscin accumulation with age is still apparent in the RPE of these mice (45). We recently developed a murine model of AMD using nuclear factor erythroid 2–related factor (Nrf2)–deficient mice. In this model, increased presence of autophagy intermediate structures was detected in the aging RPE, indicating dysregulated autophagy (46). Lipofuscin-associated fluorescence was more pronounced in aging RPE from knockout mice than in an age-matched wild-type control. More conclusively, components originating from autophagy have been identified in human RPE lipofuscin using proteomic approaches (47,48). Thus, like in other postmitotic tissues, autophagy appears to be involved in lipofuscinogenesis in the RPE (49).

Lipofuscin augments oxidative stress by increasing ROS generation and weakening antioxidant defense. Lipofuscin granules are photosensitizers that produce ROS in response to light exposure (50–53). It has recently been reported that photo-oxidation products of the major lipofuscin fluorophore A2E may contribute to drusen formation in human AMD (54). They may also directly damage the intracellular antioxidant defense. In fact, RPE cells fed with the aging pigment have decreased activity of SOD and catalase (55). Accumulated lipofuscin compromises cellular functions including lysosome-mediated degradative pathways, which are responsible for removal of damaged proteins and organelles (55–58). Altogether, lipofuscin causes considerable oxidative damage in aging RPE by increasing ROS production and impairing removal of ROS.

ASSOCIATION BETWEEN AMD AND OXIDATIVE STRESS: EVIDENCE BASED ON EPIDEMIOLOGIC AND CLINICAL ASSOCIATION STUDIES

Population-based studies have established a strong correlation between oxidative stress and AMD. Risk factors of AMD, such as aging, smoking, and sunlight exposure, are closely linked to oxidative stress (59–66). Markers of oxidative damage are detected both locally and systemically in patients with AMD. Moreover, antioxidant supplementation is an effective intervention in delaying the progression of AMD (67). Together, epidemiologic and clinical studies clearly demonstrate an association between oxidative stress and AMD.

Oxidation Markers in the AMD

Oxidative stress can be evaluated by various markers. In the past, we used plasma thiol/disulfide redox status and/or the concentration of thiol metabolites as a systemic indicator of oxidative stress. We showed that oxidation of plasma GSH and cysteine pools is associated with AMD risk factors including aging, smoking, and CFH polymorphism (32,62,68,69). Our recent studies further showed that plasma level of oxidized cysteine is sensitive to the supplements recommended by the Age-Related Eye Disease Study (AREDS). Dietary antioxidants and zinc indeed reverse the tendency of oxidation of the plasma cysteine in patients with AMD (70,71). Therefore, monitoring the redox status of plasma cysteine may provide a tool for predicting the effectiveness of antioxidant intervention in AMD patients.

The retina is rich in PUFA and susceptible to lipid peroxidation, and therefore, lipid peroxidation has been widely studied in the context of AMD. A relationship between dietary intake of PUFA and AMD is proposed by several published studies. In human eyes with AMD, an increased staining of oxidized phospholipids is prominent in the outer segments and the RPE (72). Presence of lipid modification in lipofuscin from human RPE is confirmed by proteomic analysis (48). Drusen, the earliest clinical manifestation of AMD, contains adducts of CEP and MDA, both of which are products of lipid peroxidation (73,74). The increased level of those two adducts is observed not only in the RPE/Bruch's membrane/choroid complex but also in the plasma of patients with AMD (74–76). Recent studies on those two lipid peroxidation markers have provided critical information in elucidating functional roles for oxidative stress in AMD.

CEP adducts are derived from oxidation of docosahexaenoic acid (DHA), a fatty acid component of the membrane. DHA is an essential PUFA with highest abundance in the retina and accounts for approximately 50% of the fatty acids in POS membrane (77). Oxidative cleavage of DHA gives rise to 4-hydroxy-7-oxohept-5-enoic acid, and the latter covalently modifies proteins to form CEP adducts (78). Immunocytochemical studies showed that in the eye, CEP adducts mainly locate in the POS and RPE (76). CEP modifications have been identified in drusen of human AMD eyes. In addition, human AMD eyes have more CEP adducts in RPE/Bruch's membrane/choroid complex than do age-matched controls (73). Systemically, AMD human plasma has increased levels of CEP adducts and anti-CEP autoantibodies compared with age-matched non-AMD control human plasma (76,79). CEP adducts are not only an oxidative damage marker associated with AMD. A recent study by Hollyfield et al. (80) showed that systemic administration of CEP adducts can initiate dry AMD-like phenotype in animal models. Thus, these studies convincingly suggest that the CEP adducts contribute to the AMD pathology of the outer retina.

MDA is a commonly used lipid peroxidation marker. In contrast to CEP (which is uniquely generated from DHA), MDA is the decomposition product from oxidation of PUFAs that contain more than two methylene-interrupted double bonds (81). Plasma samples from patients with AMD have higher levels of MDA than that of a control cohort (82,83). The negative regulator of the complement system, CFH, was recently found to specifically bind to the plasma MDA adducts, but not to the other oxidative modifications tested, such as CEP and 4-hydroxynonenal (74). CFH binds to MDA adducts via its two short consensus repeats (SCRs), SCR7 or SCR20, and neutralizes proinflammatory effects of MDA adducts. More strikingly, the AMD risk allele of CFH Y402H, which has an amino acid substitution in the region of SCR7, has impaired binding ability to MDA modifications and decreased protection. Together, using both clinical and experimental approaches, this elaborate study provides the first clue to solve the mystery on functional roles of the genetic risk factor CFH in AMD.

CAUSAL ROLES OF OXIDATIVE STRESS IN AMD: EVIDENCE FROM ANIMAL MODELS

Despite decades of efforts and the strong clinical association between oxidative stress and AMD, mechanisms of how oxidative injury leads to RPE degeneration and the link with chronic inflammation remain elusive. Severe oxidative stress induces apoptosis, but loss of RPE cells occurs mainly in the late stages of AMD. Cellular and molecular mechanisms of the early RPE degeneration remain largely unknown. In recent years, compelling evidence has been obtained from animal models, in which oxidative stress is introduced either by increasing exogenous pro-oxidant level, such as injection of CEP, or by compromising endogenous antioxidant systems such as deletion of the stress response gene Nrf2.

Superoxide Dismutase Knockout Mice

Mammals have three isoforms of SOD: the cytoplasmic Cu/Zn-SOD (SOD1), the mitochondrial MnSOD (SOD2), and the extracellular Cu/Zn-SOD (SOD3). All three require catalytic metals (Cu or Mn) for their activities (16). SODs play significant roles in oxidative defense, which is evident by increased oxidative damage in mice deficient of the cytoplasmic SOD1 or the mitochondrial SOD2. In fact, mice that completely lack the SOD1 have accelerated aging and shortened lifespan, and SOD2 knockout mice are lethal (84,85).

SODs are highly expressed in the retina (86), and manipulation of SODs in mice generates phenotypes related to human AMD. Mice deficient of the cytoplasmic SOD1 are the first animal model that demonstrated the causative roles of oxidative stress in pathogenesis of AMD (87). The SOD1 knockout mice showed AMD-like pathology in the outer retina (deposition of inflammatory proteins in the RPE/choroid complex, thickened Bruch's membrane, and sub-RPE deposition) and developed drusen after 9 months.

In young knockouts, constant light exposure at an intensity similar to outdoor sunlight caused drusen formation within a few weeks. After 10 months, about 10% of the mice developed choroidal neovascularization (CNV) and subretinal fluid leakage during fluorescein angiography. SOD2 is critical in defense against mitochondrial oxidative stress. Sod2-/- mice have dilated cardiomyopathy and die within weeks after birth (85). Retinal toxicity is evident even in these short-lived mutant mice, which show a progressive thinning of retina mainly involving the inner retinal and photoreceptor layers (88). RPE-specific knockdown of SOD2 leads to phenotypic changes related to AMD, but mainly in the RPE/Bruch's membrane. Those changes include accumulation of oxidized proteins in the RPE/choroid complex, vacuolization and degeneration of the RPE, thickening of Bruch's membrane, and increased levels of autofluorescence and A2E (89).

While the SOD models proved the concept that oxidative injury can lead to RPE degeneration and AMD-like pathology, they had certain limitations. SOD1 is a universal enzyme that directly scavenges superoxide anions and provides the first line of defense against oxidative stress. Lack of SOD1 resulted in severe damage to the neural retina with degeneration of the retina and the RPE occurring at almost the same time (90). Significant changes in the thickness of outer nuclear layer were noted as early as 30 weeks. This is in contrast to the clinical observation in AMD patients who typically retain their retinal function until late stages of the disease.

Mice Deficient of Nuclear Factor Erythroid 2–Related Factor

Nrf2 is a transcription factor controlling the cellular antioxidant and detoxification responses. Under basal conditions, Nrf2 is targeted for degradation by its inhibitor protein, Keap1, and remains at low to undetectable level in nontransformed cells (91,92). Upon conditions of oxidative stress or exposure to electrophilic compounds, Nrf2 dissociates from Keap1 and translocates into the nucleus in which it up-regulates genes containing a *cis*-acting antioxidant response element (ARE) in their promoter region (93). Genes under the transcriptional control of Nrf2 encode various enzymes, such as Trx1, Prx, glutamate–cysteine ligase, GSH S-transferase, heme oxygenase, NAD(P)H–quinone reductase, and glutamate–cysteine exchanger, which are essential for detoxification of xenobiotics and endogenous reactive intermediates (93,94).

Nrf2 knockout mice have normal embryonic development and comparable basal level of antioxidant status to the wild-type animals at young age (94,95). Accelerated aging is evident in Nrf2 null mice. The life expectancy is about 20 months, which is the life expectancy of only 60% of wild-type mice with the same genetic background (96). Nrf2 knockout mice have increased sensitivity to a variety of pharmacologic and environmental toxicants, and the manifestation depends on tissues and stimuli (94,97,98). Certain stimuli can induce ocular pathology in Nrf2-deficient mice. Hyperoxia results in more severe retinal vaso-obliteration in neonatal Nrf2 knockout mice compared with wild-type controls (99). Nrf2 null mice are more sensitive to ischemia/reperfusion-induced retinal toxicity. In response to ischemia/reperfusion, knockout mice have increased proinflammatory mediators, leukocyte infiltration, loss of ganglion cells, and retinal capillary degeneration (100). Chronic exposure to cigarette smoking induces more oxidative stress in Nrf2-deficient mice as evidenced by increased staining of 8-hydroxydeoxyguanosine in the RPE. Accordingly, Nrf2−/− mice displayed abnormal RPE basal infoldings and vacuoles and thickening of Bruch's membrane (98).

We recently reported that Nrf2−/− mice developed age-related RPE and choroidal degeneration resembling cardinal features of human AMD, including RPE degeneration, Bruch's membrane thickening, and spontaneous CNV (46). Between 8 and 11 months, drusen-like deposits emerged in fundus of Nrf2 KO knockout mice. With aging, atrophic RPE lesions occurred, and some of these lesions would eventually develop into sites of CNV. Knockout mice have moderate decrease in retinal function, as measured by ERG. Drusen formation, RPE atrophy, and CNV are also confirmed by histologic studies. Using histologic and electron microscopy, we further showed increased thickness of Bruch's membrane and RPE vacuolation. Basal laminar and basal linear deposits were found exclusively in Nrf2−/− mice. Accumulation of lipofuscin granules was detected by fluorescence and electron microscopy. Immunostaining of eye sections revealed increased deposition of proteins that related to innate immunity (i.e., C3d, vitronectin, and serum amyloid P) and a marker of oxidative injury (nitrotyrosine) between the RPE and Bruch's membrane in Nrf2−/− mice. The same proteins have been found in drusen and Bruch's membrane of human AMD eyes (73,101).

Dry AMD-Like Pathology in Mice Immunized with CEP-Conjugated Albumin

CEP adducts originate from lipid peroxidation and have increased levels in patients with AMD both locally and systemically. Mice immunized with CEP-modified mouse serum albumin (CEP-MSA) have some phenotypic changes resembling AMD (80). Pathologic changes are apparent in the RPE, including vacuolation, hyperpigmentation, hypopigmentation, and atrophy. Effects of CEP-MSA immunization are long-lasting and progressive. Twelve months after the immunization, changes in the RPE persist and further extend to Bruch's membrane. Sub-RPE elevation and basal laminar deposits occur, and there is significant increase in thickness of Bruch's membrane. Deposition of complement-related proteins on Bruch's membrane is also evident although no spontaneous CNV develops in the whole time frame. Thus, CEP-immunized mice provide a model of the atrophic form of AMD.

Findings from the CEP model suggest that a systemic challenge with immunogens can cause localized responses in the outer retina, and highlight the contributions of systemic factors such as complement protein and humoral or cell-mediated immunity to AMD. This is consistent with our previous findings that showed a more oxidized environment in plasma of AMD patients. These data support the use of antioxidant compounds to alleviate oxidative stress throughout the entire body.

Retinal and RPE Degeneration in Mouse Models of Iron Overload

Iron overload is clinically associated with AMD. Compared to normal donors, human AMD eyes have increased iron within the RPE (60,102). Although iron acts as essential cofactor of enzymes, ferrous iron is a potent source of ROS through the Fenton reaction. To mimic the condition of iron overload, Dunaief et al. generated double knockout mice (DKO) with both Cp and Heph deficiency (103). Cp and Heph are both multicopper ferroxidases that facilitate iron export from cells. Consequently, reduced activity of Cp and Heph in the DKO results in an age-dependent iron accumulation in the retina with the highest level in the RPE/choroid (104). The mice eventually develop retinal degeneration, which shares many features with AMD including photoreceptor degeneration, lipofuscin accumulation, RPE hyperplasia, RPE atrophy, sub-RPE deposits, and CNV (103,104). Infiltration of macrophages and deposition of complement components are also evident in the mice. Since iron overload has definite clinical associations with AMD, iron-chelating compounds may have a role in the development of novel therapeutic agents (105).

HOW OXIDATIVE STRESS CONTRIBUTES TO AMD: POTENTIAL MECHANISMS

Although clinical and laboratory studies indicate functional roles of oxidative stress in AMD, underlying mechanisms remain undefined. Available data suggested that oxidative stress could contribute to the pathophysiology of AMD in multiple ways, both locally and systemically.

Interaction Between Oxidative Stress and Inflammation in AMD

AMD involves inflammation, which is supported by the presence of complement proteins in drusen (73,106), association of multiple complement gene polymorphisms with AMD (1–4), and accumulation of inflammatory and immune response proteins in the Bruch's membrane/choroid complex of AMD eyes (107). Available evidence suggests that oxidative stress may favor a proinflammatory environment and serve either as an initiating insult or as an amplifying adjuvant of the inflammatory responses in the pathogenesis of AMD. Oxidative stress and inflammation can also be involved in feed-forward loops to greatly accelerate the disease progression. Similar to observations in many other chronic human diseases, the interactive roles of oxidative stress and inflammation have been clearly demonstrated in the pathogenesis of AMD (108–111).

Oxidatively modified molecules may serve as an initial signal for innate immunity. Studies from recent years have shown that oxidized phospholipids modify endogenous molecules and generate immunogenic and proinflammatory oxidation-specific epitopes (OSE). The pathophysiologic significance of OSE has been established in several chronic diseases (112). CEP and MDA adducts are major OSE associated with AMD. The proinflammatory and immunogenic features of those epitopes are demonstrated by the following: (a) Intravitreal injections of MDA-BSA in mice trigger IL-8 production in the RPE (74), and (b) mice immunized with CEP-BSA have C3 deposition in the RPE/Bruch's membrane and develop some AMD-resembling phenotypes (80). Interestingly, proteins encoded from normal and risk alleles of CFH show different reactivity to MDA adducts. Plasma CFH can bind to MDA-related OSE and inhibit their proinflammatory effects, while the AMD risk allele of CFH (Y402H) has impaired ability of binding MDA adducts and decreased efficiency in neutralizing their proinflammatory effects (74).

Oxidative stress may foster a proinflammatory environment in the eye by other means as well. Transcription factors responsible for up-regulating the inflammatory response, such as nuclear factor kappa B (NFκB), can be activated by oxidative stress (113–115). RPE cells are known to produce chemokines and cytokines and are involved in local immune responses. Oxidative stress can change the profile of cytokines and chemokines secreted by the RPE. Phagocytosis of oxidized POS induces IL-8 and MCP-1 production and decreases CFH production from RPE cells (116,117). In the presence of complement sufficient medium, hydrogen peroxide can reduce the surface expression of complement inhibitors DAF and CD59, decrease the surface inhibition mediated by CFH, and lead to complement activation on the surface of RPE cells (118). Oxidative damage induced by bisretinoid pigments of RPE lipofuscin has similar effects on complement activation, as evidenced by the accumulation of C3 split product iC3b (119,120). A direct molecular link between oxidative stress and CFH expression in the RPE has been demonstrated by Wu et al. (121). They identified an FOXO3 binding site in the promoter region of CFH and showed that the binding of the repressor FOXO3 to CFH promoter is subject to regulation by oxidative stress.

Oxidative Stress and Choroidal Neovascularization

Oxidative stress may generate a proangiogenic environment in the retina and contribute to the development of exudative AMD. In vitro cell culture studies have shown that oxidative stress stimulates VEGF production from the RPE (122,123). Furthermore, CEP adducts induce VEGF secretion and promote angiogenesis in vivo (124,125). About 10% of Sod1 knockout mice develop spontaneous CNV (126). Sod1 knockout mice crossed with transgenic mice expressing VEGF under the rhodopsin promoter developed significantly increased neovascularization in the subretinal space. Sod1 null mice also showed increased retinal neovascularization when subjected to oxygen-induced ischemia (127,128). These results suggest that when choroidal and retinal neovascularization begin to develop, oxidative stress potentiates VEGF production (from the RPE and other types of cells), thereby promoting the proliferation of the neovascularization.

Other Mechanisms

Oxidative stress may be involved in AMD pathology independent of inflammation. For example, DICER1 is a ribonuclease required for maturation of small interference RNA and microRNA (129). Recently, it has been attributed to the pathology of atrophic AMD (130,131). Expression of DICER1 is susceptible to oxidants, and therefore, direct down-regulation of DICER1 can be one possible mechanism mediating the contribution of oxidative stress to AMD. A common feature shared by mouse models of AMD involving oxidative stress is RPE pathology, including atrophy. Oxidative stress may induce RPE cell death and lead to atrophic AMD.

Intervention Targeting Oxidative Stress

Currently, antioxidant and zinc supplementation is the only treatment proven effective to impede the development and progression of AMD except for antiangiogenic pharmacotherapy that solely targets the exudative form of AMD. The therapeutic potential of antioxidant supplementation was supported by several clinical studies including the AREDS I. The multicentered, randomized AREDS I showed that high intake of the supplemental antioxidants (vitamin C, vitamin E, and beta-carotene) and zinc decreased the risk of progression from intermediate AMD to advanced AMD by 25% (132). Modifying antioxidant status can actually reduce the genetic risk as indicated by the Rotterdam Study (133). However, protection achieved by dietary antioxidant supplementation is modest, and the effectiveness remains controversial. The controversy may result from the lack of sufficient statistical power in detecting the phenotypic changes of the chronic disease and low potency of the current antioxidant regimen. More potent antioxidants with less long-term toxicities prove to be more effective. Furthermore, nonenzymatic antioxidants act in a synergistic fashion as is seen among vitamin C, vitamin E, and GSH, which greatly complicates the task of formulating an antioxidant supplement balanced to achieve optimal efficacy. Alternatively, reagents boosting the endogenous antioxidant network may offer a new direction to improve therapeutic outcomes.

Vitamin C (Ascorbate)

Vitamin C, the most effective water-soluble antioxidant found in the blood, may be essential for protection against diseases that involve oxidative stress (134). Vitamin C exists at high levels in the retina and is very efficient in removing hydrogen peroxide (135). Pretreatment with vitamin C protects against light toxicity in rats (67). AREDS I showed that vitamin C, together with vitamin E, beta-carotene, and zinc, reduced the risk for progression of AMD. However, vitamin C alone does not appear sufficient to provide adequate protection against oxidative stress (136).

Vitamin E

Vitamin E comprises a class of tocopherol compounds of which alpha-tocopherol is the most common and potent form (25). They are lipid-soluble and membrane-bound antioxidants considered as a primary nonenzymatic defense against lipid peroxidation. The RPE and the outer segments of the rods in the retina are rich in vitamin E, which is important in protecting the retina from oxidative injury (137,138). Typically, vitamin E acts as a chain-breaking antioxidant, which prevents the propagation of free radical damage to lipids in biologic membranes. To achieve maximum efficiency, vitamin E requires the presence of ascorbate and GSH (139). Deficiency of vitamin E causes retinal degeneration in monkeys (140,141). Supplementation of vitamin E protects outer segments from oxidative damage (67,132,142,143). Similar to vitamin C, there is no strong evidence that supports the efficacy of vitamin E when used alone, but it is included in the AREDS supplement formula, which has been proven effective (142,144).

Carotenoids

Carotenoids are tetraterpenoid organic pigments naturally occurring in photosynthetic organisms especially plants. They can be divided into two classes: non–oxygen-containing carotenes, such as beta-carotene, and oxygen-containing xanthophylls, such as lutein and zeaxanthin. Dietary analyses by the Eye Disease Case–Control Study (EDCCS) group suggest carotenoids have protective effects in AMD (145,146). In this study, an inverse relationship between carotenoid supplementation and risk for exudative AMD was demonstrated. Lutein, zeaxanthin, and beta-carotene were the major species (of those examined) that accounted for the protective effect of the carotenoids against oxidative stress.

Beta-carotene is a precursor to vitamin A. It is highly abundant in the blood but normally is present only in trace amounts in the retina (67). Beta-carotene acts as general scavenger to a broad spectrum of ROS, including superoxide radicals, lipid peroxidation intermediates, and Fenton-generated radicals. However, the role of beta-carotene in AMD is inconsistent. The AREDS supplementation regimen contained 15 mg of beta-carotene and resulted in the aforementioned 25% risk reduction in progression to advanced

AMD (147). The risk reduction effect is confirmed by the Rotterdam Study (148), but challenged by the Blue Mountain Eye Study, in which an increased risk of developing neovascular AMD was associated with increased intake of beta-carotene (146,149).

The xanthophyll carotenoids, lutein and zeaxanthin, are the major components of macular pigment (150). These membrane-localized carotenoids function as lipid antioxidants by two means: (a) as light filters and (b) as ROS quenchers. Lutein and zeaxanthin efficiently absorb blue light that passes through the anterior segment and decrease the short-wavelength light exposure of the macula (151,152). The high content of double bonds in the tetraterpenoid backbone enables these carotenoids to easily supply electrons to quench ROS and prevent further damage to lipids. Thus, they prevent lipid peroxidation and stabilize the membrane.

As discussed above, carotenoid intake from food was negatively associated with the risk of exudative AMD in the EDCCS. Several other clinical studies have evaluated the effects of the macular carotenoids. However, the results are still controversial due to the limited sample size, the relatively short lengths of follow-up, and outcome measures concerns (137). There currently is a large-scale longitudinal clinical trial, AREDS 2, that is designed to evaluate the effects of supplemental lutein, zeaxanthin, and omega-3 on the progression to advanced AMD (http://clinicaltrials.gov/ct2/show/NCT00345176) that will be invaluable in answering the question about the benefit of carotenoids in the treatment of AMD.

Glutathione

GSH is a major component of the endogenous antioxidant system that protects cells from oxidative stress. As briefly mentioned above, the nonenzymatic antioxidants vitamin C and vitamin E require GSH for maximal activity. Vitamin C (ascorbate) scavenges hydrogen peroxide forming oxidized dehydroascorbate whose reduction depends on GSH. Vitamin C further supports antioxidant function of vitamin E by reducing the radical form of vitamin E (138). Thus, by fulfilling the redox cycle of vitamin C and vitamin E, GSH plays a critical role in the maintenance of the eye mediated by these antioxidants (153,154). In addition, GSH serves both as a direct antioxidant and as an important substrate for the enzymatic antioxidant systems such as GSH peroxidase (155,156). Deficiency of GSH leads to tissue damage in animals and even early mortality in newborn rats and guinea pigs (157). In the context of the eye, GSH protects photoreceptor cell membranes from lipid peroxidation (158,159). Furthermore, compounds inducing GSH synthesis protect against oxidative injury in cultured RPE (160).

Zinc

Zinc is a trace element present in high concentrations in eye tissues, particularly the retina and choroid (161,162).

It participates in the antioxidant defense in both direct and indirect ways (163–165). Zinc protects susceptible protein SH groups from oxidative modification by binding directly to these groups; by binding to adjacent sites, thus creating steric hindrance to the SHs; and by binding to distant sites and causing a conformational change in the protein's tertiary structure to sequester the SHs. Zinc can also antagonize redox-active transition metal catalysts in the Fenton reaction such as copper and iron, thereby inhibiting the production of ROS. Zinc is indispensable for activity of Cu/Zn-SOD, the first-line enzymatic antioxidant defense. Moreover, zinc can induce enzymes that are critical for the antioxidant network, such as catalase, metallothioneins (MTs), and Nrf2 (67,148). Zinc deficiency results in increased lipid peroxidation in subcellular membranes of the liver.

The beneficial effects of zinc with regard to the progression of AMD have been demonstrated by both large-scale randomized controlled clinical trials and population-based studies (67). In AREDS, zinc, either alone or with antioxidants, significantly reduced the risk of progression from an intermediate stage to an advanced stage of AMD (164). Of particular note was the observation that both zinc alone and zinc with antioxidant supplementation had much greater efficacy than was found with supplementation of the three antioxidants, vitamin C, vitamin E, and beta-carotene. The potency of zinc may be attributed to effects other than directly scavenging ROS. Our study using in vitro cultured RPE cells showed that zinc activates the Nrf2-dependent antioxidant system in the RPE, which is the major activation site in the eye. We also found that feeding mice a high-zinc diet increased Nrf2 activity (unpublished data) (46). Increasing cellular GSH synthesis is one of the downstream events of Nrf2. Accordingly, higher levels of GSH were found in the retina and RPE from the mice fed a high-zinc diet than were found in tissues from the mice fed a normal diet. Nrf2 is a master regulator of cellular antioxidant and detoxification systems. Mice deficient of Nrf2 have ocular pathology resembling human AMD, and enhancing transcriptional activity of Nrf2 can protect against oxidative injury to the RPE in this model (166). Thus, our data from both in vitro and in vivo studies indicate that Nrf2 is a potential node that mediates the protective effect of zinc in AMD.

Nrf2 Inducers

Besides zinc, several structurally different Nrf2 inducers have been tested for their protective effects against oxidative retinal injury. The majority of these inducers are naturally occurring compounds, such as sulforaphane and curcumin, or from compounds biochemically derived from them, such as triterpenoid analogs. Sulforaphane [(-)-1-isothiocyanato-(4R)-(methylsulfinyl)butane] is a potent Nrf2 inducer existing in vegetables such as broccoli and Brussels sprouts (167,168). It activates an array of detoxification responses dependent on Nrf2. Protection against oxidative and proto-oxidative damage is evident in RPE cells

pretreated with sulforaphane (169). In vivo study in rodent models of retinal injury has also confirmed the protection conferred by sulforaphane. Using a light damage model, Yodoi et al. showed that sulforaphane is effective in protecting photoreceptors and the RPE from oxidative injury and the protective signals emanating from Nrf2-mediated pathways (170). Sulforaphane delayed photoreceptor cell death in tubby mouse, a model of Usher syndrome, which exhibits progressive photoreceptor degeneration shortly after birth (171). Compared to vehicle-treated animals, sulforaphane-treated tub/tub mice showed increased thickness of outer nuclear layer and improved visual function as detected by ERG recording.

A new class of Nrf2 inducers, triterpenoid derivatives, has been investigated recently. These compounds have strong potencies, capable of inducing phase 2 enzymes and protecting against oxidative stress at subnanomolar concentrations (172). One of the most potent synthetic triterpenoid analogs, 2-cyano-3,12-dioxooleanan-1,9(11)-dien-28-oci acid (CDDO) (172,173) and its relatives, confer cytoprotection against light-induced retinal damage in vivo (100). Another type of retinal injury can be induced in an ischemia–reperfusion model, which involves loss of ganglion cell layer and degeneration of retinal capillaries. CDDO-methyl ester was effective in diminishing the retinal damage caused in this model by inhibiting neutrophil infiltration and retinal capillary degeneration in an Nrf2-dependent way (133). The CDDO compounds are currently under clinical trials for treating solid tumors, leukemia, chronic kidney disease, and type 2 diabetes. Their potential usefulness in treating dry AMD will likely be explored in human studies in the near future.

SUMMARY, CONCLUSION, AND FUTURE DIRECTIONS

The involvement of oxidative stress in AMD is based on a compelling theoretical rationale and is supported by a variety of population-based studies. Recent studies using multiple animal models have confirmed the contributing roles of oxidative stress. Mechanisms underlying the participation of oxidative stress in AMD pathology are under further investigation. The interrelationship between oxidative stress and inflammation suggested by numerous studies will require further mechanistic studies to elucidate their complementary roles in the pathogenesis of AMD. Fortunately, the increased number of available animal models of AMD has made these complex studies feasible.

Antioxidant supplementation is one of the few effective ways in delaying the progression of AMD. Modifying antioxidant status can actually reduce the genetic risk. However, the effectiveness of current antioxidant regimen is modest. Exploring new approaches to boosting endogenous antioxidant system may provide a new direction for the development of more efficacious treatments for this disease.

REFERENCES

1. Haines JL, Hauser MA, Schmidt S, et al. Complement factor H variant increases the risk of age-related macular degeneration. Science. 2005;308:419–421.

2. Klein RJ, Zeiss C, Chew EY, et al. Complement factor H polymorphism in age-related macular degeneration. Science. 2005;308:385–389.

3. Edwards AO, Ritter R III, Abel KJ, et al. Complement factor H polymorphism and age-related macular degeneration. Science. 2005;308:421–424.

4. Hageman GS, Anderson DH, Johnson LV, et al. A common haplotype in the complement regulatory gene factor H (HF1/CFH) predisposes individuals to age-related macular degeneration. Proc Natl Acad Sci U S A. 2005;102:7227–7232.

5. Yates JR, Sepp T, Matharu BK, et al. Complement C3 variant and the risk of age-related macular degeneration. N Engl J Med. 2007;357:553–561.

6. Maller JB, Fagerness JA, Reynolds RC, et al. Variation in complement factor 3 is associated with risk of age-related macular degeneration. Nat Genet. 2007;39:1200–1201.

7. Rivera A, Fisher SA, Fritsche LG, et al. Hypothetical LOC387715 is a second major susceptibility gene for age-related macular degeneration, contributing independently of complement factor H to disease risk. Hum Mol Genet. 2005;14:3227–3236.

8. Fritsche LG, Loenhardt T, Janssen A, et al. Age-related macular degeneration is associated with an unstable ARMS2 (LOC387715) mRNA. Nat Genet. 2008;40:892–896.

9. Gold B, Merriam JE, Zernant J, et al. Variation in factor B (BF) and complement component 2 (C2) genes is associated with age-related macular degeneration. Nat Genet. 2006;38:458–462.

10. Spencer KL, Hauser MA, Olson LM, et al. Protective effect of complement factor B and complement component 2 variants in age-related macular degeneration. Hum Mol Genet. 2007;16:1986–1992.

11. Coffey PJ, Gias C, McDermott CJ, et al. Complement factor H deficiency in aged mice causes retinal abnormalities and visual dysfunction. Proc Natl Acad Sci U S A. 2007;104:16651–16656.

12. Zeiss CJ. Animals as models of age-related macular degeneration: an imperfect measure of the truth. Vet Pathol. 2010;47:396–413.

13. Richter C. Do mitochondrial DNA fragments promote cancer and aging? FEBS Lett. 1988;241:1–5.

14. Loschen G, Azzi A, Flohe L. Mitochondrial H_2O_2 formation: relationship with energy conservation. FEBS Lett. 1973;33:84–87.

15. Turrens JF, Boveris A. Generation of superoxide anion by the NADH dehydrogenase of bovine heart mitochondria. Biochem J. 1980;191:421–427.

16. Fridovich I. Superoxide radical and superoxide dismutases. Annu Rev Biochem. 1995;64:97–112.

17. Nicholls P, Fita I, Loewen PC. Enzymology and structure of catalases. Adv Inorg Chem. 2000;51:51–106.

18. Epp O, Ladenstein R, Wendel A. The refined structure of the selenoenzyme glutathione peroxidase at 0.2-nm resolution. Eur J Biochem. 1983;133:51–69.

19. Esworthy RS, Ho YS, Chu FF. The Gpx1 gene encodes mitochondrial glutathione peroxidase in the mouse liver. Arch Biochem Biophys. 1997;340:59–63.

20. Chen Y, Cai J, Murphy TJ, et al. Overexpressed human mitochondrial thioredoxin confers resistance to oxidant-induced apoptosis in human osteosarcoma cells. J Biol Chem. 2002;277:33242–33248.

21. Miranda-Vizuete A, Damdimopoulos AE, Pedrajas JR, et al. Human mitochondrial thioredoxin reductase cDNA cloning, expression and genomic organization. Eur J Biochem. 1999;261:405–412.

22. Elroy-Stein O, Bernstein Y, Groner Y. Overproduction of human Cu/Zn-superoxide dismutase in transfected cells: extenuation of paraquat-mediated cytotoxicity and enhancement of lipid peroxidation. EMBO J. 1986;5:615–622.

23. Jaarsma D, Haasdijk ED, Grashorn JA, et al. Human Cu/Zn superoxide dismutase (SOD1) overexpression in mice causes mitochondrial vacuolization, axonal degeneration, and premature motoneuron death and accelerates motoneuron disease in mice expressing a familial amyotrophic lateral sclerosis mutant SOD1. Neurobiol Dis. 2000;7:623–643.

24. Lu L, Oveson BC, Jo YJ, et al. Increased expression of glutathione peroxidase 4 strongly protects retina from oxidative damage. Antioxid Redox Signal. 2009;11:715–724.

25. Handelman GJ, Dratz EA. The role of antioxidants in the retina and retinal pigment epithelium and the nature of prooxidant-induced damage. Adv Free Radic Biol Med. 1986;2:1–89.

26. Margrain TH, Boulton M, Marshall J, et al. Do blue light filters confer protection against age-related macular degeneration? Prog Retin Eye Res. 2004;23:523–531.

27. Dorey CK, Khouri GG, Syniuta LA, et al. Superoxide production by porcine retinal pigment epithelium in vitro. Invest Ophthalmol Vis Sci. 1989;30:1047–1054.

28. Miceli MV, Liles MR, Newsome DA. Evaluation of oxidative processes in human pigment epithelial cells associated with retinal outer segment phagocytosis. Exp Cell Res. 1994;214:242–249.

29. Kindzelskii AL, Elner VM, Elner SG, et al. Toll-like receptor 4 (TLR4) of retinal pigment epithelial cells participates in transmembrane signaling in response to photoreceptor outer segments. J Gen Physiol. 2004;124:139–149.

30. Liles MR, Newsome DA, Oliver PD. Antioxidant enzymes in the aging human retinal pigment epithelium. Arch Ophthalmol. 1991;109:1285–1288.

31. Frank RN, Amin RH, Puklin JE. Antioxidant enzymes in the macular retinal pigment epithelium of eyes with neovascular age-related macular degeneration. Am J Ophthalmol. 1999;127:694–709.

32. Jones DP, Mody VC Jr, Carlson JL, et al. Redox analysis of human plasma allows separation of pro-oxidant events of aging from decline in antioxidant defenses. Free Radic Biol Med. 2002;33:1290–1300.

33. Samiec PS, Drews-Botsch C, Flagg EW, et al. Glutathione in human plasma: decline in association with aging, age-related macular degeneration, and diabetes. Free Radic Biol Med. 1998;24:699–704.

34. Brunk UT, Terman A. Lipofuscin: mechanisms of age-related accumulation and influence on cell function. Free Radic Biol Med. 2002;33:611–619.

35. Nakano M, Oenzil F, Mizuno T, et al. Age-related changes in the lipofuscin accumulation of brain and heart. Gerontology. 1995;41(Suppl 2):69–79.

36. Sohal RS, Marzabadi MR, Galaris D, et al. Effect of ambient oxygen concentration on lipofuscin accumulation in cultured rat heart myocytes—a novel in vitro model of lipofuscinogenesis. Free Radic Biol Med. 1989;6:23–30.

37. Feeney-Burns L, Hilderbrand ES, Eldridge S. Aging human RPE: morphometric analysis of macular, equatorial, and peripheral cells. Invest Ophthalmol Vis Sci. 1984;25:195–200.

38. Holz FG, Bellmann C, Margaritidis M., et al. Patterns of increased in vivo fundus autofluorescence in the junctional zone of geographic atrophy of the retinal pigment epithelium associated with age-related macular degeneration. Graefes Arch Clin Exp Ophthalmol. 1999;237:145–152.

39. Holz FG, Bellman C, Staudt S, et al. Fundus autofluorescence and development of geographic atrophy in age-related macular degeneration. Invest Ophthalmol Vis Sci. 2001;42:1051–1056.

40. Katz ML, Gao CL, Rice LM. Formation of lipofuscin-like fluorophores by reaction of retinal with photoreceptor outer segments and liposomes. Mech Ageing Dev. 1996;92:159–174.

41. Liu J, Itagaki Y, Ben-Shabat S, et al. The biosynthesis of A2E, a fluorophore of aging retina, involves the formation of the precursor, A2-PE, in the photoreceptor outer segment membrane. J Biol Chem. 2000;275:29354–29360.

42. Boulton M, McKechnie NM, Breda J, et al. The formation of autofluorescent granules in cultured human RPE. Invest Ophthalmol Vis Sci. 1989;30:82–89.

43. Katz ML, Drea CM, Eldred GE, et al. Influence of early photoreceptor degeneration on lipofuscin in the retinal pigment epithelium. Exp Eye Res. 1986;43:561–573.

44. Burke JM, Skumatz CM. Autofluorescent inclusions in long-term postconfluent cultures of retinal pigment epithelium. Invest Ophthalmol Vis Sci. 1998;39:1478–1486.

45. Nandrot EF, Kim Y, Brodie SE, et al. Loss of synchronized retinal phagocytosis and age-related blindness in mice lacking alphavbeta5 integrin. J Exp Med. 2004;200:1539–1545.

46. Zhao Z, Chen Y, Wang J, et al. Age-related retinopathy in NRF2-deficient mice. PLoS One. 2011;6:e19456.

47. Schutt F, Ueberle B, Schnolzer M, et al. Proteome analysis of lipofuscin in human retinal pigment epithelial cells. FEBS Lett. 2002;528:217–221.

48. Schutt F, Bergmann M, Holz FG, et al. Proteins modified by malondialdehyde, 4-hydroxynonenal, or advanced glycation end products in lipofuscin of human retinal pigment epithelium. Invest Ophthalmol Vis Sci. 2003;44:3663–3668.

49. Terman A, Brunk UT. Lipofuscin. Int J Biochem Cell Biol. 2004;36:1400–1404.

50. Boulton M, Dontsov A, Jarvis-Evans J, et al. Lipofuscin is a photoinducible free radical generator. J Photochem Photobiol B. 1993;19:201–204.

51. Gaillard ER, Atherton SJ, Eldred G., et al. Photophysical studies on human retinal lipofuscin. Photochem Photobiol. 1995;61:448–453.

52. Rozanowska M, Jarvis-Evans J, Korytowski W, et al. Blue light-induced reactivity of retinal age pigment. In vitro generation of oxygen-reactive species. J Biol Chem. 1995;270:18825–18830.

53. Davies S, Elliott MH, Floor E, et al. Photocytotoxicity of lipofuscin in human retinal pigment epithelial cells. Free Radic Biol Med. 2001;31:256–265.

54. Wu Y, Yanase E, Feng X, et al. Structural characterization of bisretinoid A2E photocleavage products and implications for age-related macular degeneration. Proc Natl Acad Sci U S A. 2010;107:7275–7280.

55. Shamsi FA, Boulton M. Inhibition of RPE lysosomal and antioxidant activity by the age pigment lipofuscin. Invest Ophthalmol Vis Sci. 2001;42:3041–3046.

56. Sundelin S, Wihlmark U, Nilsson SE, et al. Lipofuscin accumulation in cultured retinal pigment epithelial cells reduces their phagocytic capacity. Curr Eye Res. 1998;17:851–857.

57. Terman A, Dalen H, Brunk UT. Ceroid/lipofuscin-loaded human fibroblasts show decreased survival time and diminished autophagocytosis during amino acid starvation. Exp Gerontol. 1999;34:943–957.

58. Sitte N, Huber M, Grune T, et al. Proteasome inhibition by lipofuscin/ceroid during postmitotic aging of fibroblasts. FASEB J. 2000;14:1490–1498.

59. Pryor WA, Prier DG, Church DF. Electron-spin resonance study of mainstream and sidestream cigarette smoke: nature of the free radicals in gas-phase smoke and in cigarette tar. Environ Health Perspect. 1983;47:345–355.

60. Smith W, Assink J, Klein R, et al. Risk factors for age-related macular degeneration: pooled findings from three continents. Ophthalmology. 2001;108:697–704.

61. Mitchell P, Wang JJ, Smith W, et al. Smoking and the 5-year incidence of age-related maculopathy: the Blue Mountains Eye Study. Arch Ophthalmol. 2002;120:1357–1363.

62. Moriarty SE, Shah JH, Lynn M, et al. Oxidation of glutathione and cysteine in human plasma associated with smoking. Free Radic Biol Med. 2003;35:1582–1588.

63. Young RW. Solar radiation and age-related macular degeneration. Surv Ophthalmol. 1988;32:252–269.

64. Cruickshanks KJ, Klein R, Klein BE. Sunlight and age-related macular degeneration. The Beaver Dam Eye Study. Arch Ophthalmol. 1993;111:514–518.

65. Vingerling JR, Hofman A, Grobbee DE, et al. Age-related macular degeneration and smoking. The Rotterdam Study. Arch Ophthalmol. 1996;114:1193–1196.

66. Tomany SC, Cruickshanks KJ, Klein R, et al. Sunlight and the 10-year incidence of age-related maculopathy: the Beaver Dam Eye Study. Arch Ophthalmol. 2004;122:750–757.

67. A randomized, placebo-controlled, clinical trial of high-dose supplementation with vitamins C and E, beta carotene, and zinc for age-related macular degeneration and vision loss: AREDS report no. 8. Arch Ophthalmol. 2001;119:1417–1436.

68. Moriarty-Craige SE, Adkison J, Lynn M, et al. Antioxidant supplements prevent oxidation of cysteine/cystine redox in patients with age-related macular degeneration. Am J Ophthalmol. 2005;140:1020–1026.

69. Brantley MA Jr, Osborn MP, Sanders BJ, et al. Plasma biomarkers of oxidative stress and genetic variants in age-related macular degeneration. Am J Ophthalmol. 2012;153:460.e1–467.e1.

70. Moriarty-Craige SE, Ha KN, Sternberg P Jr, et al. Effects of long-term zinc supplementation on plasma thiol metabolites and redox status in patients with age-related macular degeneration. Am J Ophthalmol. 2007;143:206–211.

71. Brantley MA Jr, Osborn MP, Sanders BJ, et al. The short-term effects of antioxidant and zinc supplements on oxidative stress biomarker levels in plasma: a pilot investigation. Am J Ophthalmol. 2012;153:1104.e2–1109.e2.

72. Suzuki M, Kamei M, Itabe H, et al. Oxidized phospholipids in the macula increase with age and in eyes with age-related macular degeneration. Mol Vis. 2007;13:772–778.

73. Crabb JW, Miyagi M, Gu X, et al. Drusen proteome analysis: an approach to the etiology of age-related macular degeneration. Proc Natl Acad Sci U S A. 2002;99:14682–14687.

74. Weismann D, Hartvigsen K, Lauer N, et al. Complement factor H binds malondialdehyde epitopes and protects from oxidative stress. Nature. 2011;478:76–81.

75. Nowak M, Swietochowska E, Wielkoszynski T, et al. Changes in blood antioxidants and several lipid peroxidation products in women with age-related macular degeneration. Eur J Ophthalmol. 2003;13:281–286.

76. Gu X, Meer SG, Miyagi M, et al. Carboxyethylpyrrole protein adducts and autoantibodies, biomarkers for age-related macular degeneration. J Biol Chem. 2003;278:42027–42035.

77. Fliesler SJ, Anderson RE. Chemistry and metabolism of lipids in the vertebrate retina. Prog Lipid Res. 1983;22:79–131.

78. Gu X, Sun M, Gugiu B, et al. Oxidatively truncated docosahexaenoate phospholipids: total synthesis, generation, and peptide adduction chemistry. J Org Chem. 2003;68:3749–3761.

79. Gu J, Pauer GJ, Yue X, et al. Assessing susceptibility to age-related macular degeneration with proteomic and genomic biomarkers. Mol Cell Proteomics. 2009;8:1338–1349.

80. Hollyfield JG, Bonilha VL, Rayborn ME, et al. Oxidative damage-induced inflammation initiates age-related macular degeneration. Nat Med. 2008;14:194–198.

81. Esterbauer H, Schaur RJ, Zollner H. Chemistry and biochemistry of 4-hydroxynonenal, malonaldehyde and related aldehydes. Free Radic Biol Med. 1991;11:81–128.

82. Totan Y, Cekic O, Borazan M, et al. Plasma malondialdehyde and nitric oxide levels in age related macular degeneration. Br J Ophthalmol. 2001;85:1426–1428.

83. Evereklioglu C, Er, H, Doganay S, et al. Nitric oxide and lipid peroxidation are increased and associated with decreased antioxidant enzyme activities in patients with age-related macular degeneration. Doc Ophthalmol. 2003;106:129–136.

84. Elchuri S, Oberley TD, Qi W, et al. CuZnSOD deficiency leads to persistent and widespread oxidative damage and hepatocarcinogenesis later in life. Oncogene. 2005;24:367–380.

85. Li Y, Huang TT, Carlson EJ, et al. Dilated cardiomyopathy and neonatal lethality in mutant mice lacking manganese superoxide dismutase. Nat Genet. 1995;11:376–381.

86. Rao NA, Thaete LG, Delmage JM, et al. Superoxide dismutase in ocular structures. Invest Ophthalmol Vis Sci. 1985;26:1778–1781.

87. Imamura Y, Noda S, Hashizume K, et al. Drusen, choroidal neovascularization, and retinal pigment epithelium dysfunction in SOD1-deficient mice: a model of age-related macular degeneration. Proc Natl Acad Sci U S A. 2006;103:11282–11287.

88. Sandbach JM, Coscun PE, Grossniklaus HE, et al. Ocular pathology in mitochondrial superoxide dismutase (Sod2)-deficient mice. Invest Ophthalmol Vis Sci. 2001;42:2173–2178.

89. Justilien V, Pang JJ, Renganathan K, et al. SOD2 knockdown mouse model of early AMD. Invest Ophthalmol Vis Sci. 2007;48:4407–4420.

90. Hashizume K, Hirasawa M, Imamura Y, et al. Retinal dysfunction and progressive retinal cell death in SOD1-deficient mice. Am J Pathol. 2008;172:1325–1331.

91. Cullinan SB, Gordan JD, Jin J, et al. The Keap1-BTB protein is an adaptor that bridges Nrf2 to a Cul3-based E3 ligase: oxidative stress sensing by a Cul3-Keap1 ligase. Mol Cell Biol. 2004;24:8477–8486.

92. Kobayashi A, Kang MI, Okawa H, et al. Oxidative stress sensor Keap1 functions as an adaptor for Cul3-based E3 ligase to regulate proteasomal degradation of Nrf2. Mol Cell Biol. 2004;24:7130–7139.

93. Wakabayashi N, Slocum SL, Skoko JJ, et al. When NRF2 talks, who's listening? Antioxid Redox Signal. 2010;13:1649–1663.

94. Kensler TW, Wakabayashi N, Biswal S. Cell survival responses to environmental stresses via the Keap1-Nrf2-ARE pathway. Annu Rev Pharmacol Toxicol. 2007;47:89–116.

95. Chan K, Lu R, Chang JC, et al. NRF2, a member of the NFE2 family of transcription factors, is not essential for murine erythropoiesis, growth, and development. Proc Natl Acad Sci U S A. 1996;93:13943–13948.

96. Pearson KJ, Lewis KN, Price NL, et al. Nrf2 mediates cancer protection but not prolongevity induced by caloric restriction. Proc Natl Acad Sci U S A. 2008;105:2325–2330.

97. Osburn WO, Kensler TW. Nrf2 signaling: an adaptive response pathway for protection against environmental toxic insults. Mutat Res. 2008;659:31–39.

98. Cano M, Thimmalappula R, Fujihara M, et al. Cigarette smoking, oxidative stress, the anti-oxidant response through Nrf2 signaling, and age-related macular degeneration. Vision Res. 2010;50:652–664.

99. Uno K, Prow TW, Bhutto IA, et al. Role of Nrf2 in retinal vascular development and the vaso-obliterative phase of oxygen-induced retinopathy. Exp Eye Res. 2010;90:493–500.

100. Wei Y, Gong J, Yoshida T, et al. Nrf2 has a protective role against neuronal and capillary degeneration in retinal ischemia-reperfusion injury. Free Radic Biol Med. 2011;51:216–224.

101. Mullins RF, Russell SR, Anderson DH, et al. Drusen associated with aging and age-related macular degeneration contain proteins common to extracellular deposits associated with atherosclerosis, elastosis, amyloidosis, and dense deposit disease. FASEB J. 2000;14:835–846.

102. Hahn P, Milam AH, Dunaief JL. Maculas affected by age-related macular degeneration contain increased chelatable iron in the retinal pigment epithelium and Bruch's membrane. Arch Ophthalmol. 2003;121:1099–1105.

103. Hahn P, Qian Y, Dentchev T, et al. Disruption of ceruloplasmin and hephaestin in mice causes retinal iron overload and retinal degeneration with features of age-related macular degeneration. Proc Natl Acad Sci U S A. 2004;101:13850–13855.

104. Hadziahmetovic M, Dentchev T, Song Y, et al. Ceruloplasmin/hephaestin knockout mice model morphologic and molecular features of AMD. Invest Ophthalmol Vis Sci. 2008;49:2728–2736.

105. Dunaief JL. Iron induced oxidative damage as a potential factor in age-related macular degeneration: the Cogan Lecture. Invest Ophthalmol Vis Sci. 2006;47:4660–4664.

106. Hageman GS, Luthert PJ, Victor Chong NH, et al. An integrated hypothesis that considers drusen as biomarkers of immune-mediated processes at the RPE-Bruch's membrane interface in aging and age-related macular degeneration. Prog Retin Eye Res. 2001;20:705–732.

107. Yuan X, Gu X, Crabb JS, et al. Quantitative proteomics: comparison of the macular Bruch membrane/choroid complex from age-related macular degeneration and normal eyes. Mol Cell Proteomics. 2010;9:1031–1046.

108. McGeer PL, McGeer EG. Inflammation and the degenerative diseases of aging. Ann N Y Acad Sci. 2004;1035:104–116.

109. Jofre-Monseny L, Minihane AM, Rimbach G. Impact of apoE genotype on oxidative stress, inflammation and disease risk. Mol Nutr Food Res. 2008;52:131–145.

110. Vaziri ND, Rodriguez-Iturbe B. Mechanisms of disease: oxidative stress and inflammation in the pathogenesis of hypertension. Nat Clin Pract Nephrol. 2006;2:582–593.

111. Singh U, Devaraj S, Jialal I. Vitamin E, oxidative stress, and inflammation. Annu Rev Nutr. 2005;25:151–174.

112. Chou MY, Hartvigsen K, Hansen LF, et al. Oxidation-specific epitopes are important targets of innate immunity. J Intern Med. 2008;263:479–488.

113. Richmond A. Nf-kappa B, chemokine gene transcription and tumour growth. Nat Rev Immunol. 2002;2:664–674.

114. Ziegler-Heitbrock HW, Sternsdorf T, Liese J, et al. Pyrrolidine dithiocarbamate inhibits NF-kappa B mobilization and TNF production in human monocytes. J Immunol. 1993;151:6986–6993.

115. Brennan P, O'Neill LA. Inhibition of NF kappa B activity by oxidative processes in intact cells mechanism of action of pyrrolidine dithiocarbamate and diamide. Biochem Soc Trans. 1996;24:3S.

116. Higgins GT, Wang JH, Dockery P, et al. Induction of angiogenic cytokine expression in cultured RPE by ingestion of oxidized photoreceptor outer segments. Invest Ophthalmol Vis Sci. 2003;44:1775–1782.

117. Chen M, Forrester JV, Xu H. Synthesis of complement factor H by retinal pigment epithelial cells is down-regulated by oxidized photoreceptor outer segments. Exp Eye Res. 2007;84:635–645.

118. Thurman JM, Renner B, Kunchithapautham K, et al. Oxidative stress renders retinal pigment epithelial cells susceptible to complement-mediated injury. J Biol Chem. 2009;284:16939–16947.

119. Zhou J, Jang YP, Kim SR, et al. Complement activation by photooxidation products of A2E, a lipofuscin constituent of the retinal pigment epithelium. Proc Natl Acad Sci U S A. 2006;103:16182–16187.

120. Zhou J, Kim SR, Westlund BS, et al. Complement activation by bisretinoid constituents of RPE lipofuscin. Invest Ophthalmol Vis Sci. 2009;50:1392–1399.

121. Wu Z, Lauer TW, Sick A, et al. Oxidative stress modulates complement factor H expression in retinal pigmented epithelial cells by acetylation of FOXO3. J Biol Chem. 2007;282:22414–22425.

122. Sreekumar PG, Kannan R, de Silva AT, et al. Thiol regulation of vascular endothelial growth factor-A and its receptors in human retinal pigment epithelial cells. Biochem Biophys Res Commun. 2006;346:1200–1206.

123. Kannan R, Zhang N, Sreekumar PG, et al. Stimulation of apical and basolateral VEGF-A and VEGF-C secretion by oxidative stress in polarized retinal pigment epithelial cells. Mol Vis. 2006;12:1649–1659.

124. Ebrahem Q, Renganathan K, Sears J, et al. Carboxyethylpyrrole oxidative protein modifications stimulate neovascularization: implications for age-related macular degeneration. Proc Natl Acad Sci U S A. 2006;103:13480–13484.

125. West XZ, Malinin NL, Merkulova AA, et al. Oxidative stress induces angiogenesis by activating TLR2 with novel endogenous ligands. Nature. 2010;467:972–976.

126. Dong A, Xie B, Shen J, et al. Oxidative stress promotes ocular neovascularization. J Cell Physiol. 2009;219:544–552.

127. Bernstein E, Caudy AA, Hammond SM, et al. Role for a bidentate ribonuclease in the initiation step of RNA interference. Nature. 2001;409:363–366.

128. Lee Y, Jeon K, Lee JT, et al. MicroRNA maturation: stepwise processing and subcellular localization. EMBO J. 2002;21:4663–4670.

129. Kaneko H, Dridi S, Tarallo V, et al. DICER1 deficit induces Alu RNA toxicity in age-related macular degeneration. Nature. 2011;471:325–330.

130. Frei B, England L, Ames BN. Ascorbate is an outstanding antioxidant in human blood plasma. Proc Natl Acad Sci U S A. 1989;86:6377–6381.

131. Harman D. The aging process. Proc Natl Acad Sci U S A. 1981;78:7124–7128.

132. VandenLangenberg GM, Mares-Perlman JA, Klein R, et al. Associations between antioxidant and zinc intake and the 5-year incidence of early age-related maculopathy in the Beaver Dam Eye Study. Am J Epidemiol. 1998;148:204–214.

133. Ho L, van Leeuwen R, Witteman JC, et al. Reducing the genetic risk of age-related macular degeneration with dietary antioxidants, zinc, and omega-3 fatty acids: the Rotterdam study. Arch Ophthalmol. 2011;129:758–766.

134. Varma SD, Chand D, Sharma YR, et al. Oxidative stress on lens and cataract formation: role of light and oxygen. Curr Eye Res. 1984;3:35–57.

135. Organisciak DT, Wang HM, Li ZY, et al. The protective effect of ascorbate in retinal light damage of rats. Invest Ophthalmol Vis Sci. 1985;26:1580–1588.

136. Drevon CA. Absorption, transport and metabolism of vitamin E. Free Radic Res Commun. 1991;14:229–246.

137. Palozza P, Krinsky NI. beta-Carotene and alpha-tocopherol are synergistic antioxidants. Arch Biochem Biophys. 1992;297:184–187.

138. Meister A. Glutathione-ascorbic acid antioxidant system in animals. J Biol Chem. 1994;269:9397–9400.

139. Hayes KC. Retinal degeneration in monkeys induced by deficiencies of vitamin E or A. Invest Ophthalmol. 1974;13:499–510.

140. Penn JS, Naash MI, Anderson RE. Effect of light history on retinal antioxidants and light damage susceptibility in the rat. Exp Eye Res. 1987;44:779–788.

141. Farnsworth CC, Dratz EA. Oxidative damage of retinal rod outer segment membranes and the role of vitamin E. Biochim Biophys Acta. 1976;443:556–570.

142. Seddon JM, Ajani UA, Sperduto RD, et al. Dietary carotenoids, vitamins A, C, and E, and advanced age-related macular degeneration. Eye Disease Case-Control Study Group. JAMA. 1994;272:1413–1420.

143. Taylor HR, Tikellis G, Robman LD, et al. Vitamin E supplementation and macular degeneration: randomised controlled trial. BMJ. 2002;325:11.

144. Antioxidant status and neovascular age-related macular degeneration. Eye Disease Case-Control Study Group. Arch Ophthalmol. 1993;111:104–109.

145. Krinsky NI, Russett MD, Handelman GJ, et al. Structural and geometrical isomers of carotenoids in human plasma. J Nutr. 1990;120:1654–1662.

146. Handelman GJ, Dratz EA, Reay CC, et al. Carotenoids in the human macula and whole retina. Invest Ophthalmol Vis Sci. 1988;29:850–855.

147. van Leeuwen R, Boekhoorn S, Vingerling JR, et al. Dietary intake of antioxidants and risk of age-related macular degeneration. JAMA. 2005;294:3101–3107.

148. Tan JS, Wang JJ, Flood V, et al. Dietary antioxidants and the long-term incidence of age-related macular degeneration: the Blue Mountains Eye Study. Ophthalmology. 2008;115:334–341.

149. Bone RA, Landrum JT, Tarsis SL. Preliminary identification of the human macular pigment. Vision Res. 1985;25:1531–1535.

150. Landrum JT, Bone RA. Lutein, zeaxanthin, and the macular pigment. Arch Biochem Biophys. 2001;385:28–40.

151. Sabour-Pickett S, Nolan JM, Loughman J, et al. A review of the evidence germane to the putative protective role of the macular carotenoids for age-related macular degeneration. Mol Nutr Food Res. 2012;56:270–286.

152. Krishnadev N, Meleth AD, Chew EY. Nutritional supplements for age-related macular degeneration. Curr Opin Ophthalmol. 2010;21:184–189.

153. Jones DP, Brown LA, Sternberg P. Variability in glutathione-dependent detoxification in vivo and its relevance to detoxification of chemical mixtures. Toxicology. 1995;105:267–274.

154. Reed DJ. Glutathione: toxicological implications. Annu Rev Pharmacol Toxicol. 1990;30:603–631.

155. Martensson J, Jain A, Stole E, et al. Inhibition of glutathione synthesis in the newborn rat: a model for endogenously produced oxidative stress. Proc Natl Acad Sci U S A. 1991;88:9360–9364.

156. Martensson J, Meister A. Glutathione deficiency decreases tissue ascorbate levels in newborn rats: ascorbate spares glutathione and protects. Proc Natl Acad Sci U S A. 1991;88:4656–4660.

157. Keys SA, Zimmerman WF. Antioxidant activity of retinol, glutathione, and taurine in bovine photoreceptor cell membranes. Exp Eye Res. 1999;68:693–702.

158. Nelson KC, Armstrong JS, Moriarty S, et al. Protection of retinal pigment epithelial cells from oxidative damage by oltipraz, a cancer chemopreventive agent. Invest Ophthalmol Vis Sci. 2002;43:3550–3554.

159. Nelson KC, Carlson JL, Newman ML, et al. Effect of dietary inducer dimethylfumarate on glutathione in cultured human retinal pigment epithelial cells. Invest Ophthalmol Vis Sci. 1999;40:1927–1935.

160. Karcioglu ZA. Zinc in the eye. Surv Ophthalmol. 1982;27:114–122.

161. Bray TM, Bettger WJ. The physiological role of zinc as an antioxidant. Free Radic Biol Med. 1990;8:281–291.

162. Powell SR. The antioxidant properties of zinc. J Nutr. 2000;130:1447S–1454S.

163. Tate DJ Jr, Miceli MV, Newsome DA. Zinc induces catalase expression in cultured fetal human retinal pigment epithelial cells. Curr Eye Res. 1997;16:1017–1023.

164. Ha KN, Chen Y, Cai J, et al. Increased glutathione synthesis through an ARE-Nrf2-dependent pathway by zinc in the RPE: implication for protection against oxidative stress. Invest Ophthalmol Vis Sci. 2006;47:2709–2715.

165. McCormick CC, Menard MP, Cousins RJ. Induction of hepatic metallothionein by feeding zinc to rats of depleted zinc status. Am J Physiol. 1981;240:E414–E421.

166. Zhang Y, Talalay P, Cho CG, et al. A major inducer of anticarcinogenic protective enzymes from broccoli: isolation and elucidation of structure. Proc Natl Acad Sci U S A. 1992;89:2399–2403.

167. Gao X, Talalay P. Induction of phase 2 genes by sulforaphane protects retinal pigment epithelial cells against photooxidative damage. Proc Natl Acad Sci U S A. 2004;101:10446–10451.

168. Wang L, Chen Y, Sternberg P, et al. Essential roles of the PI3 kinase/Akt pathway in regulating Nrf2-dependent antioxidant functions in the RPE. Invest Ophthalmol Vis Sci. 2008;49:1671–1678.

169. Tanito M, Masutani H, Kim YC, et al. Sulforaphane induces thioredoxin through the antioxidant-responsive element and attenuates retinal light damage in mice. Invest Ophthalmol Vis Sci. 2005;46:979–987.

170. Kong L, Tanito M, Huang Z, et al. Delay of photoreceptor degeneration in tubby mouse by sulforaphane. J Neurochem. 2007;101:1041–1052.

171. Dinkova-Kostova AT, Liby KT, Stephenson KK, et al. Extremely potent triterpenoid inducers of the phase 2 response: correlations of protection against oxidant and inflammatory stress. Proc Natl Acad Sci U S A. 2005;102:4584–4589.

172. Liby K, Hock T, Yore MM, et al. The synthetic triterpenoids, CDDO and CDDO-imidazolide, are potent inducers of heme oxygenase-1 and Nrf2/ARE signaling. Cancer Res. 2005;65:4789–4798.

173. Pitha-Rowe I, Liby K, Royce D, et al. Synthetic triterpenoids attenuate cytotoxic retinal injury: cross-talk between Nrf2 and PI3K/AKT signaling through inhibition of the lipid phosphatase PTEN. Invest Ophthalmol Vis Sci. 2009;50:5339–5347.

15

PRE–ANTI-VEGF ERA

REINALDO A. GARCIA • VERONICA ORIA
LUIS M. SUÁREZ TATA • MARIANA MATA-PLATHY

INTRODUCTION

The purpose of this chapter is to discuss the different treatment modalities that were available in clinical practice before the use of anti–vascular endothelial growth factors (anti-VEGF), according to their date of appearance and their clinical significance. At present, many of these techniques have been abandoned, as the reader will conclude, given their efficacy compared to the modern anti-VEGF treatments available. However, we are still far from having an ideal treatment for wet age-related macular degeneration (AMD), and in some circumstances, history has shown that retaking old treatment strategies and combining them with newer modalities, or rethinking previously used principles, can lead science toward new steps in managing these disorders, thus offering novel treatment strategies and improving visual outcomes.

In this chapter, the reader will find a brief review of the different treatment modalities available for AMD previous to the introduction of anti-VEGF in clinical practice. In each treatment option mentioned, we summarized an introduction, the most relevant multicenter studies, their principle and results, and their current use. In those treatments where no randomized, double-blind, placebo-controlled study data were available, we included those obtained from small case series that had significant results and relevance that lead to their application in different disorders.

PHOTOCOAGULATION FOR CHOROIDAL NEOVASCULARIZATION

Between 1979 and 1994, the Macular Photocoagulation Study Group (MPS) conducted three sets of randomized clinical trials (1–21). The purpose of these studies was to determine if laser photocoagulation was of benefit in preventing or delaying large losses of visual acuity (VA) in comparison with observation without treatment. The Argon and Krypton studies included patients with choroidal neovascularization (CNV) secondary to AMD, presumed ocular histoplasmosis (POH), and idiopathic choroidal neovascularizations (ICNV). The Argon study studied the effectiveness of photocoagulation with argon blue-green laser in eyes with extrafoveal CNV (200–2,500 μm from the center of the foveal avascular zone [FAZ]). The Krypton study examined CNV lesions with the posterior border 1 to 199 μm from the center of the FAZ, and the Foveal study was carried out in patients with new (never treated) or recurrent (previously treated with laser photocoagulation) subfoveal CNV (CNV with blood or blocked fluorescence within 200 μm of the foveal center).

PRINCIPLES OF TREATMENT

Ocular photocoagulation uses heat produced through the absorption of light by ocular pigments. Absorption of light can take place either in the tissue to be photocoagulated or in a neighboring tissue, where heat is then transferred to the tissue of interest by thermal conduction. Therefore, photocoagulation is used to obliterate single blood vessels and neovascular networks such as subretinal neovascularization. The most common light sources used for this type of surgery were argon ion (488 and 514 µm) and krypton ion (568 and 647 µm) (20).

SUMMARIZED MPS RESULTS OF TREATMENT BY LESION LOCATION

Extrafoveal Choroidal Neovascularization

In 1982, the MPS group reported that covering the entire extent of the extrafoveal CNV and contiguous blood reduced the risk of additional severe VA loss when compared with the natural course of the disease (1). The benefits were greatest during the first posttreatment year and persisted over 5 years of follow-up; at that time, 64% of untreated eyes versus 46% of treated eyes progressed to severe visual loss. After 5 years, untreated eyes lost a mean of 7.1 lines of VA, while laser-treated eyes lost 5.2 lines. Unfortunately, persistent or recurrent CNV was observed in 54% of treated eyes, usually on the foveal (posterior) side of the treated lesion (3,4,7,21).

Juxtafoveal Choroidal Neovascularization

The 5-year results for juxtafoveal lesions in AMD were published in 1994. They also demonstrated the benefit of treatment over observation. As compared to no treatment, laser photocoagulation reduced the risk of severe visual loss by approximately 10%. The baseline level of VA was maintained in 25% of the treated eyes, compared to 15% of the untreated eyes over the study period. In addition, more than twice as many treated patients as untreated patients retained VA of 20/40 or better. Unfortunately, by the 5-year follow-up examination, 78% of those treated had either persistent or recurrent CNV involving the foveal center (5,6,15,18,21).

Subfoveal Choroidal Neovascularization

In 1991, the MPS reported that laser treatment of new subfoveal CNV (i.e., no prior laser treatment) was better than observation alone in preventing large losses of VA for eligible lesions. Overall, eyes receiving direct laser treatment to the fovea for new CNV immediately lost more VA than did observed eyes. However, the amount of VA loss in observed eyes increased to the level of loss in treated eyes at 12 months and exceeded the level thereafter. By 24 months, VA still had decreased by six or more lines in 20% of laser-treated eyes compared to 37% of untreated eyes (8–10). Additional follow-up at 4 years continued to show this same trend, despite both treated and untreated eyes losing additional lines of VA (12,21). Eyes with smaller lesions and worse initial VA had greater and earlier

benefits of laser treatment (13). Eyes with large subfoveal neovascular lesions and good initial VA were not good candidates for focal laser photocoagulation. In all probability, the wavelength specificity for laser photocoagulation of the CNV was not as critical as the completeness of treatment (16).

UTILITY IN CURRENT CLINICAL PRACTICE

Although photocoagulation treatment could change the natural history of the disease, it would not restore vision, and unfortunately with the appropriate follow-up, persistent or recurrent CNV would be observed in all kinds of extrafoveal, juxtafoveal, and subfoveal CNVs. Therefore, thermal coagulation produces a scar that goes through all layers of the retina and that manifests itself clinically as a visual field defect.

In light of recent findings on anti-VEGF therapy, it seems like at present photocoagulation for CNV should only be applied for small extrafoveal lesions, which accounts for 5% of all patients. There is no doubt that laser photocoagulation is still useful for peripapillary CNV. However, some ophthalmologists are hesitant to treat peripapillary CNV with photocoagulation, fearing that the procedure may lead to thermal damage of the nerve fiber layer in the papillomacular bundle. Others are hesitant because they believe that the natural course of peripapillary lesions might be more benign than the treatment (21). The MPS reported that in those eyes with peripapillary CNV lesions nasal to the fovea and below the papillomacular bundle, 44% of treated eyes versus 29% of untreated eyes would achieve VA of 20/40 or better at 3-year follow-up. In addition, only 9% of treated eyes compared to 54% of untreated eyes lost six or more lines of VA. The MPS group reported that severe VA loss was noted after treatment only when recurrent CNV extended through the center of the fovea (17–21). This finding suggests that severe visual loss only from nerve fiber layer damage after this treatment approach, in the absence of subfoveal recurrence, must be a rare complication.

In order to avoid thermal necrosis of disc tissue and following the MPS photocoagulation technique, one should consider refraining from treatment within 100 to 200 µm of the optic nerve and consider treatment only when at least 1 ½ clock hours of papillomacular bundle on the temporal side of the disc is uninvolved with CNV so that at least 1 ½ clock hours of papillomacular bundle can be spared of treatment (17).

Subretinal Surgery

In 1988, De Juan and Machemer (22) described a vitrectomy technique with a large flap retinotomy for the removal of blood and disciform scars in four end-stage cases of AMD.

Although three of their patients improved their vision, two of them developed severe proliferative vitreoretinopathy (PVR). Subsequent surgeons reported discouraging results in terms of VA (23). As a result of these experiences, large flap retinotomy was not widely employed. Investigators speculated that the postsurgical absence of retinal pigment epithelium (RPE) was the cause of poor vision, and thus, they attempted to replace subfoveal RPE with autologous or homologous RPE. However, the surgical transplantation of RPE failed to improve vision (23). In January 1991, Thomas and Kaplan (24) reported in two patients an alternative approach to subfoveal neovascularization in POHS, with dramatic improvements in VA from 20/400 to 20/20 and 20/400 to 20/40, respectively. Instead of a large flap retinotomy, their technique employed a small retinal hole through which instruments were introduced into the subretinal space (23,24).

PRINCIPLES OF TREATMENT

The surgery for CNV is appealing because it offers the promise of removing abnormal tissue without causing as much damage to normal tissue (neurosensory retina) as occurs with laser photocoagulation (23). However, it has also been realized that the numerous pre-RPE and sub-RPE attachments of the neovascular complex in AMD (in contrast to the neovascular complex in ocular histoplasmosis that lie predominantly anterior to the RPE and have eccentric ingrowth sites), carry an increased risk of damage to the underlying RPE thereby resulting in poorer visual outcome.

SUMMARIZED MULTICENTER, RANDOMIZED, AND DOUBLE-BLIND CLINICAL TRIAL RESULTS IN SUBMACULAR SURGERY

The Submacular Surgery Trials (SST) was initiated in 1997, prior to the advent of photodynamic therapy (PDT) (25). They were designed to compare the outcome of surgical treatment versus observation in three categories: (a) (SST-N): New subfoveal CNV (without prior laser) secondary to AMD, (b) (SST-H): CNV secondary to POHS or idiopathic etiology, and (c) (SST-B): Thick submacular blood or hematomas associated with AMD. In the three arms, a successful outcome was defined to be either improvement of best-corrected visual acuity or visual acuity no more than 1 line worse at 24-month follow-up. However, none of the three arms showed a benefit over the observation group at the end of the study period (25–28), according to the following results:

SST-N: Forty-four percent of observed eyes and 41% of eyes assigned to surgery had a successful outcome as defined in the study. Median VA loss at 24 months was 2.1

lines in observed eyes and 2.0 lines in eyes assigned to surgery. Median VA declined from 20/100 to 20/400 at 2 years in both groups (26).

SST-H: Forty-six percent of eyes in the observation arm and 55% of those in the surgery arm had a successful outcome as defined in the study. Median VA at 24 months was 20/250 among eyes in the observation group and 20/160 in the surgery group. A subgroup of eyes with VA worse than 20/100 at baseline had more success with surgery; 76% in the surgery arm versus 50% in the observation arm. However, recurrent CNV developed in 54% of surgically treated eyes at 24 months (27).

SST-B: Forty-one percent of observed eyes and 44% of eyes assigned to surgery achieved a successful outcome as defined in the study (28).

UTILITY IN CURRENT CLINICAL PRACTICE

Vitrectomy surgery for removal of subretinal CNV, whether subfoveal or nonsubfoveal, has not been shown to be more beneficial over laser photocoagulation, PDT, or observation in any prospective clinical trial. However, massive subretinal hemorrhage is a medically untreatable entity that will remain in the domain of surgical treatment.

Intravitreal Triamcinolone

The use of intravitreal triamcinolone was largely overlooked until 2002 when Jonas et al. (29–31) published their findings on the beneficial effects of the triamcinolone on macular edema, on ocular neovascularization, and during difficult surgical cases. Subsequently, several animal studies showed the benefits of triamcinolone acetonide in the treatment of experimental CNV (32,33). Ciulla et al. (33) noted that the rodents failed to develop iatrogenic created krypton laser CNV if laser photocoagulation was followed by an intravitreal injection of triamcinolone. In contrast, nearly 70% of eyes that received intravitreal saline after laser photocoagulation developed CNV.

Rationale

Triamcinolone acetonide exerts an anti-inflammatory effect due to the induction of the phospholipase A2 inhibitory proteins. These proteins control the biosynthesis of prostaglandins and leukotrienes by inhibiting the release of arachidonic acid, which is released from membrane phospholipids by phospholipase A2 (34).

Results

In 1994, Dominguez-Collazo (35) detailed the safety and efficacy of intravitreal triamcinolone in the treatment of subfoveal CNV secondary to AMD. One year later,

Penfold et al. (36) published the first results from a large series of patients. In the long-term follow-up, intravitreal triamcinolone acetonide (IVTA) as monotherapy had no effect on the risk of severe VA loss, despite a significant antiangiogenic effect found 3 months after the treatment. The first randomized, double-blind, placebo-controlled study in a relatively large study population was reported by Gillies et al. (37) in 2003. They treated patients with a single dose of intravitreal triamcinolone, and after 1 year of follow-up, they found a 35% risk of severe visual loss in both groups (treatment vs. observation). Further studies with conventional (4 mg) and higher doses (20–25 mg) did not show any other beneficial effects (38,39).

UTILITY IN CURRENT CLINICAL PRACTICE

Although an important number of publications were written, several issues remained unsolved regarding the type of CNV that responded best to intravitreal triamcinolone, the dose (from 4 to 25 mg depending on the study), and the frequency of injection (34). The intravitreal administration of steroids alone can no longer be recommended, in view of the results of new VEGF inhibitor treatments and the high rate of complications such as cataract, glaucoma, vitreous hemorrhage, and pseudoendophthalmitis (34). Nowadays, IVTA has been tested as a part of the triple combined treatment (see combined treatment).

Photodynamic Therapy

Until 1999, no treatment other than laser photocoagulation had been shown to reduce the risk of vision loss in patients with CNV from AMD in large-scale, randomized clinical trials (40). The first experience with the use of PDT in ophthalmology was reported in 1994 treating intraocular tumors and subretinal neovascularization (41,42). The propitious results obtained in the treatment of choroidal melanomas initiated the study of PDT in animal models of CNV (43). In 1998, Schmidt-Erfurth et al. (44) reported the results of 61 patients with subfoveal CNV secondary to AMD treated with PDT in whom a temporary closing of the CNV was observed, and stabilization of VA was achieved. Based on this experiment, phase III randomized clinical trials were designed and developed (45).

Rationale

PDT involves the use of a photoactivatable compound (photosensitizer: Benzoporphyrin derivate [BPD-verteporfin; Ciba Vision AG, Balateh, Switzerland & QLT Phototherapeutics, Vancouver, Canada]), which accumulates in, and is retained by, proliferating tissues. When injected intravenously and complexed with low-density lipoprotein (LDL), verteporfin may be taken up selectively by rapidly proliferating endothelial cells that have an increased number of LDL receptors active in their plasma membranes. When this molecule is activated by light of appropriate wavelength (laser light of low power to avoid thermal damage), active forms of oxygen and free radicals are generated, causing a photochemical reaction that appears to result in direct cellular injury, including damage to vascular endothelial cells and vessel thrombosis (46).

SUMMARIZED MULTICENTER, RANDOMIZED, AND DOUBLE-BLIND CLINICAL TRIAL RESULTS IN PHOTODYNAMIC THERAPY

TTAP Results

The treatment of AMD with photodynamic therapy (TAP) study was carried out in 22 centers in Europe and the United States with 609 patients recruited between December 1996 and October 1997 and randomized in a proportion of two to one (verteporfin to placebo). Cases enrolled were to have subfoveal CNV with a component of classic CNV and a greatest linear dimension ≤5,400 μm. Results at 1 year showed that verteporfin therapy significantly reduced the risk of moderate and severe visual loss compared to placebo (47). At 12-month follow-up examination for primary outcome, 39% of 402 verteporfin-treated patients compared with 54% of 207 placebo-treated patients had three or more lines of VA loss ($P < 0.001$). Subgroup analysis showed that the treatment benefit was judged to be quite clinically relevant in eyes with predominantly classic CNV (where the classic CNV was ≥50% of the area of the lesion), especially when no occult CNV was present. No VA benefit was noted for cases with classic CNV in which the area of classic CNV was greater than 0 but less than 50% of the area of the lesion. At 24-month follow-up, moderate visual loss was observed in 47% of the patients in the verteporfin group and 62% in the placebo group ($P < 0.001$) (48). An extension to 36 months demonstrated that the visual results of patients with predominantly classic lesions treated with verteporfin remained stable (49).

VIP Results

The Verteporfin in Photodynamic Therapy (VIP) Study began in 1998 and included 459 patients (120 patients with CNV secondary to myopia and 339 patients with occult CNV secondary to AMD) recruited in 28 centers in Europe and the United States. Results at 1 year showed that 51% of the group treated with verteporfin suffered from moderate visual loss compared to 55% in the placebo group; in other words, verteporfin did not perform any better than letting the disease run its natural course (45). However, at 2 years, the results showed that a smaller percentage of the group treated with verteporfin suffered from moderate visual loss (55% vs. 68%, $P = 0.023$). Analyzing the group with occult active CNV secondary to AMD, the results showed a benefit when the patient had small lesions (less than 4 MPS disc diameters) with independence of the VA or VA less than 20/50, regardless of the size of the lesion (50).

In those patients with CNV secondary to myopia, the VIP results showed that at 1 year, 72% of the patients treated with verteporfin lost less than 1.5 lines of vision compared with 44% of the patients in the placebo group ($P = 0.003$) (51). At the conclusion of the 2nd year, 39% of the patients treated with verteporfin versus 13% in the placebo group gained at least one line of VA (52).

VIM Results

The Visudyne in Minimally Classic CNV (VIM) trial was developed because in a retrospective analysis, the group of patients with minimally classic CNV secondary to AMD (with lesions measuring less than 4 MPS disc diameters and visual acuities less than 20/50) lost less vision when they were treated with verteporfin compared to patients who did not receive PDT (42% vs. 63% in the placebo group). Previous studies suggested that diminishing the light fluence could maximize the photodynamic effects of verteporfin. For this reason, a phase II study was designed to compare the application of verteporfin using standard-fluence PDT (600 mW/cm^2) compared to low-fluence PDT (300 mW/cm^2) (45). After 12 months, it was observed that the group treated with verteporfin had better visual acuities than did the control group (low-fluence PDT compared to placebo $P = 0.02$; standard-fluence PDT compared to placebo $P = 0.08$; PDT with verteporfin group compared to placebo $P = 0.01$) (53).

Other PDT Studies

The Verteporfin in Ocular Histoplasmosis (VOH) Study was developed to evaluate the response of PDT treatment in 26 patients with CNV secondary to ocular histoplasmosis. At 12 months, a mean of seven lines of improvement was observed (54).

The Visudyne with Altered (delayed) Light in Occult CNV Trial (VALIO) was designed to determine if delayed laser application (30 minutes) had a positive impact on the visual and angiographic results of patients with occult CNV. The results at 6 months did not show any difference (55).

The Visudyne Early Retreatment (VER) Trial was to determine if earlier retreatments reduced the risk of moderate visual loss in patients with subfoveal predominantly classic CNV secondary to AMD. Re-treating the patients every 6 weeks during the first 6 months and later every 3 months until 2 years did not show any difference after 12 months of follow-up when comparing the results with the control group (45).

UTILITY IN CURRENT CLINICAL PRACTICE

After the introduction of PDT, the location of lesions to be treated (extrafoveal, juxtafoveal, or subfoveal) became irrelevant. Instead, the composition of the lesion was more important (classic or occult). In other words, when PDT with verteporfin was initiated, a reduction of the risk of moderate and severe visual loss in patients with classic CNV and some occult CNVs was achieved, regardless of the localization of the CNV. However, later studies showed that PDT with verteporfin could cause choroidal ischemia with the subsequent stimulation of VEGF expression (56). For this reason and as a result of newer modalities like anti-VEGF therapy, the PDT treatment of CNV secondary to AMD patients evolved to double (PDT + verterporfin + intravitreal steroids) or triple (PDT + verterporfin + intravitreal steroids + anti-VEGF) combination therapies. At present, PDT with verteporfin alone is particularly useful in choroidal hemangioma and central serous chorioretinopathy among other disorders.

Transpupillary Thermotherapy

The first experience with the use of transpupillary thermotherapy (TTT) in ophthalmology was reported by Journee-de Kover and Oosterhuis (57) in 1992 for the treatment of choroidal melanomas. The beneficial results obtained in the treatment of choroidal melanomas initiated the study of TTT in CNV secondary to AMD (58–62). It was particularly indicated in patients with purely occult CNV where PDT + verteporfin treatment had not shown any advantage over untreated patients according to the 1-year follow-up VIP results.

Rationale

TTT is a low irradiance (810 nm), large spot size (3 mm), long pulse (60 seconds in a continuous mode), infrared diode laser photocoagulation technique that is poorly absorbed by hemoglobin and xanthophylls, allowing transmission through preretinal and subretinal hemorrhage, and reducing nerve fiber layer damage. Melanin in the RPE and choroid converts laser radiation into heat energy, which increases the temperature of the treated tissue. Vascular damage most likely occurs by heat conversion from the pigmented targets of the irradiation, including the RPE cells and choroidal melanocytes.

Summarized Multicenter, Randomized, and Double-Blind Clinical Trial Results in TTT

The preliminary results of a multicenter, randomized, double-blind clinical trial were presented at the American Academy of Ophthalmology (AAO) Annual Meeting in 2004. The TTT4CNV compared TTT to sham for subfoveal occult CNV caused by AMD. In its preliminary results in 303 patients enrolled, TTT, as applied in this trial, did not result in a significantly advantageous effect relative to sham. However, a subgroup analysis of eyes with poorer baseline VA (20/100 or worse) indicated a statistically significant treatment benefit. Improvement in VA (by two or more lines) was significantly greater ($P = 0.03$) in TTT-treated eyes at 12 months (19% vs. 0%) and at 18 months (17% vs. 0%). The best results occurred in TTT-treated eyes that were not re-treated (63).

Indocyanine Green–Enhanced Diode Laser Transpupillary Thermotherapy (i-TTT)

The first experience with the use of i-TTT for the treatment of CNV secondary to AMD was reported by Puliafito et al. (64,65).

Rationale

i-TTT is a technique that requires intravenous injection of a photosensitizing agent (ICG dye) that accumulates in neovascular tissue. This photosensitized tissue is then irradiated by light at the absorption peak of the dye (805 nm), which is close to the peak emission (810 nm) of the conventional diode laser. ICG is an anionic tricarbocyanine dye with a large protein-bound component that provides a selective intravascular retention advantage in the large choroidal vessels (with a great concentration of ICG) compared to retinal vessels. In exudative AMD, there is less melanin pigment in the proliferative pigment epithelium that covers the CNV, and this less-pigmented RPE absorbs little laser light. However, the therapy is still effective because ICG becomes a new chromophore and absorbs the infrared light, which leads to vascular toxicity.

■ SUMMARIZED RESULTS

i-TTT results are quite similar to TTT alone (66). A possible explanation for this might include differences between adjustments in ICG concentration during i-TTT, laser power, and/or the timing of laser application following ICG infusion (67).

Utility in Current Clinical Practice

Like PDT + verteporfin, the TTT and i-TTT therapies evolved into combined treatment modalities with intravitreal steroids or anti-VEGF therapy. TTT and i-TTT are still popular methods for the treatment of small and medium-sized choroidal melanomas.

Combined Therapy

Combination therapy for wet AMD started after V-PDT was approved for use in 2000. The first dual combinations involved V-PDT plus intravitreal triamcinolone (68).

When the anti-VEGF agent pegaptanib became the first agent in its class approved for use, studies of combination therapies of this drug plus V-PDT followed (69,70). Subsequent availability of the anti-VEGF agent ranibizumab generated considerable excitement because it demonstrated meaningful vision benefit for the first time in patients with wet AMD. Combination therapy with ranibizumab or the similar agent bevacizumab and a steroid, V-PDT, or both, followed.

Rationale

Combining various treatment modalities for exudative AMD targets multiple components of CNV. The intent is to provide different and complementary mechanisms of action to decrease inflammation, destroy existing CNV, prevent the formation of new CNV, and inhibit further VEGF production. This approach has the potential for improving efficacy and reducing treatment frequency.

Summarized Results in Combination Therapies

This chapter is focused on treatments available previous to the introduction of the new anti-VEGF agents, so it is beyond the scope of this review to analyze each of these modalities. However, the double therapy of PDT + verteporfin plus intravitreal triamcinolone is included here because it was done before the appearance of anti-VEGF therapies.

Double Therapy with PDT + Verteporfin Plus Intravitreal Triamcinolone

A large number of publications confirmed the positive synergic role of combining TA and PDT therapies for the treatment of all types of CNV (71,72). However, the advantages registered with the use of IVTA plus PDT compared to PDT alone were partially limited by the side effects, such as the rapid evolution of cataract. Furthermore, in large, randomized, clinical trials on combination therapy of TA and standard and low-fluence PDT, VA failed to show an improvement, even though the lesion size and subretinal fluid had decreased, compared to controls treated with PDT alone (73–76).

■ UTILITY IN CURRENT CLINICAL PRACTICE

The treatment options have expanded considerably over the past decade. Currently, combination therapies including ranibizumab or bevacizumab plus V-PDT (verteporfin photodynamic therapy) with and without steroids are being exhaustively investigated. The overall goal is to produce vision benefits comparable to those produced with ranibizumab monotherapy but with a reduced need for re-treatment. Dual combination trials comparing V-PDT plus ranibizumab with either V-PDT or ranibizumab monotherapy include FOCUS, PROTECT, MONT BLANC, and DENALI. Triple combinations with V-PDT, an anti-VEGF agent, and a steroid represent the next logical step in treating wet AMD. The RADICAL is a triple combination trial comparing V-PDT plus ranibizumab plus or minus dexamethasone with ranibizumab monotherapy.

Choroidal Feeder Vessel Photocoagulation Therapy

Feeder vessel photocoagulation therapy (FVT) is not a new technique in ophthalmology and has existed for more than 30 years (77). In fact, it was recommended in the guideline for MPS treatment published in 1991 (10). However, its use had been limited by difficulties in identifying the actual feeder vessel. The development of high-speed dynamic video indocyanine green angiography (HSICGA) allows identification of these feeder vessels as the afferent or arteriolar arm of the CNV complex in up to 90% of eyes regardless of the type of leakage (78).

Rationale

The concept of treating feeder vessels is based upon the concept that a single vessel often controls the majority of blood flow to an area of neovascularization within the choroid. The attenuation of the feeder vessel induces remodeling and maturation of the CNV complex resulting in resolution of exudative manifestations such as subretinal fluid, subretinal hemorrhage, and retinal edema (79,80). By treating only the afferent vessel, rather than the entire lesion, trauma to surrounding tissue is minimized.

Results

FVT has been successfully used in patients with classic, occult CNV and in several situations where a subfoveal CNV exists, since the feeder vessel itself is usually extrafoveal (79,81,82). Although there are no multicenter, double-blind, and randomized studies in large populations that would result in clinically relevant conclusions, in small series, application of FVT in classic CNV has shown improvements of more than two lines varying from 38% to 50% with recurrences between 13% and 19% of eyes according to a few available studies (81,82). In occult CNV, Roh and Glaser (83) reported improvements greater than three lines in 24.3% of 37 eyes included for analysis. Other successful results with regression of subretinal fluid and retinal edema have also been reported in pigment epithelial detachments, recurrent CNV, retinal–choroidal anastomosis, polypoidal choroidal vasculopathy, and retinal angiomatous proliferation (80,84–87).

UTILITY IN CURRENT CLINICAL PRACTICE

FVT requires a certain amount of experience in order to successfully identify the feeder vessel. Initially, argon green was used to achieve feeder vessel closure and subsequently yellow dye lasers were applied, thus creating a hemoglobin-absorbing wavelength to damage feeder vessels. However, recurrences were still an issue, and complications such as full-thickness retinal damage needed to be considered. Furthermore, the ICG dye–enhanced diode laser was studied because of its ability to penetrate tissue and potentially spare the overlying retina (88). With this wavelength, vascular closure was difficult because the laser is poorly absorbed by hemoglobin, and coupling the laser with ICG as a desirable photosensitising agent was suggested to make this modality more effective (89). As a result, a combination of standard or high-dose PDT and subsequent FVT laser coagulation using standard photocoagulation wavelengths were used in the treatment of CNV in AMD (89). Although the treatment is less expensive than is anti-VEGF therapy, the preliminary results in small series of patients could not be comparable with the benefits of vision achieved with the latter. However, FVT alone or in combination with other modality treatments could still be considered as an option in patients who do not respond to other therapies.

Radiation Therapy

Early ophthalmology studies investigated external beam radiation to treat wet AMD. These used high-energy radiation to penetrate the ocular and periocular tissue, targeting the macula. While some studies showed results better than the natural history of the disease, the results do not compare favorably to those in the anti-VEGF era (90–92). This may be because of collateral damage to ocular tissue and difficulty targeting macular lesions using technology that was designed for lesions that are usually several orders of magnitude larger. Another factor could have been the time-delay before radiation has an effect. In the era before anti-VEGF therapy, this meant the disease progressed before the benefit of radiation occurred. A disadvantage of early external beam therapy was that linear accelerators were used to generate the energy. These accelerators produce extremely high levels of energy that are tightly regulated and need special precautions to prevent escape of the radiation: usually lead-lined concrete walls, large power supplies, and cooling measures (93,94).

Rationale

Radiation therapy has been proposed as an alternative treatment for exudative AMD because of the known radiosensitivity of vascular endothelial cells. Ionizing radiation is used in neoplasias to inhibit cellular proliferation and is particularly lethal for rapidly dividing cells (95). In vitro studies have indicated that proliferating endothelium is particularly radiosensitive. In vivo experiments in rats have shown that with a single large dose of 15 to 20 Gy, there is capillary closure (96,97). Animal models have also demonstrated choriocapillary occlusion with sparing of larger choroidal vessels (98).

Clinical Experience

While it is beyond the scope of this chapter to review each of these modalities, there are several nonrandomized (99–104) and a few randomized (105,106) clinical trials studying the treatment of classic, occult, or mixed subfoveal CNVs, showing both beneficial (99–102,105) and no beneficial (101–103,106) effects. A multicenter randomized controlled clinical trial is necessary to determine if a therapeutic window exists.

■ UTILITY IN CURRENT CLINICAL PRACTICE

It is clear that so far, published data are not conclusive enough to currently recommend radiotherapy in AMD aside from experimental treatment protocols (107). However, there are two radiation therapy approaches in the treatment of neovascular AMD that are being investigated: epimacular brachytherapy (VIDION; NeoVista Inc., Fremont, CA) and stereotactic radiosurgery (IRay system; Oraya Therapeutics Inc., Newark, CA). Ongoing multicenter, randomized, controlled clinical trials on epimacular brachytherapy include the MERITAGE, CABERNET, and MERLOT studies. The CLH002 and CLH003 are multicenter randomized controlled clinical trials evaluating the efficacy of stereotactic radiosurgery.

Macular Rotation Surgery

In 1993, Machemer and Steinhorst (108) suggested macular translocation detaching the retina by transscleral subretinal injection of fluid, followed by a 360-degree peripheral retinotomy (translocation with 360-degree retinotomy). The retina was then rotated around the optic disc under silicone oil by 10 to 45 degrees. Wolf et al. (109,110) used intraoperative perfluorinated and semifluorinated liquid fluorocarbons to facilitate the procedure. Eckardt et al. (111) supplemented retinal translocation with counter rotation of the whole eye by extraocular muscle surgery. Nimoniya et al. (112) confined the retinal translocation to a temporal retinal flap, thereby reducing the extent of retinotomy to 180 degrees (translocation with partial retinotomy). De Juan et al. (113) and later Lewis et al. (114) replaced retinotomy with scleral shortening (limited macular translocation). In their technique, the temporal half of the retina is detached by transretinal injection of balanced salt solution

(BSS) into the subretinal space using a 39-gauge flexible needle. The superior temporal sclera is then shortened either by means of preplaced mattress sutures (de Juan) or by special clips (Lewis). The retina is then reattached by gas tamponade from superior to inferior. Later, Fujikado et al. (115) recommend removal of the CNV at the time of limited macular translocation.

Rationale

Macular translocation was proposed to improve vision in cases with subfoveal CNV by relocation of the fovea away from the CNV to an adjacent area of intact RPE and choriocapillaris where nourishment from healthier tissues could be received. Therefore, moving the fovea away from the CNV allows laser photocoagulation of the neovascular tissue with minimal risk of foveal damage.

■ RESULTS

Each technique has advantages and disadvantages regarding effectiveness and complications. Postoperative recovery is gradual, and usually, it takes 6 to 12 months to reach the maximum VA. In general, vision improves more than two lines in one-third of eyes, decreases by more than two lines in another one-third of eyes, and vision gets stabilized in the remaining patients (111,112). Functional prognosis seems to be independent of the type of translocation but appears to depend on the initial VA.

Complications vary according to the procedure, but it is important to briefly comment on the following three: (a) Tilted image. The angle of translocation may be as little as 10 to 15 degrees following limited translocation, but cyclotropia can occur up to 50 degrees or more after 360-degree retinotomy. The small angle of limited macular translocation is likely to be compensated spontaneously; but the tilted vision from higher angles of rotation regresses over 3 to 6 months (116). (b) PVR. Besides the long operating time of 2 to 4 hours, the rate of PVR in procedures with large retinotomies was as high as 30% in the earlier series of Wolf et al. (110) and Eckardt et al. (111). Limited translocation avoided retinotomy all together and showed a rate of PVR around 4% (+10% incidence of retinal detachment) (114). (c) Recurrence of subfoveal CNV. The rate of CNV recurrence is reported in up to 10% of eyes (110,111) following the Machemer type of translocation. CNV recurrence following "limited rotation" is equally common. However, recurrence of CNV after surgical removal or laser photocoagulation after limited macular translocation surgery occurred in 14% to 63% of patients. Postoperative enlargement of the CNV in cases that did not receive any direct treatment during the limited macular translocation surgery occurred in 59% of patients. This high rate of recurrence argues against limited translocation, because recurrent CNV being nearly always subfoveal compromises surgical success.

Eckardt et al. (111) recommend rotation of the retina to an extent that the fovea is overlapped by at least one disc diameter of intact RPE at its new location. This safety margin leaves sufficient space for eventual laser photocoagulation.

UTILITY IN CURRENT CLINICAL PRACTICE

Macular rotation surgery requires a considerable learning curve for each of the described procedures. The high rate of complications related with surgical techniques and visual results that unfortunately do not compare to those obtained with the new anti-VEGF therapies explain why these procedures do not offer success rates that would prove to be more beneficial than current treatment options.

REFERENCES

1. Macular Photocoagulation Study Group. Argon laser photocoagulation for senile macular degeneration: results of a randomized clinical trial. Arch Ophthalmol. 1982;100:912–918.

2. Macular Photocoagulation Study Group. Argon laser photocoagulation for ocular histoplasmosis syndrome: results of a randomized clinical trial. Arch Ophthalmol. 1983;101:1347–1357.

3. Macular Photocoagulation Study Group. Recurrent choroidal neovascularization after argon laser photocoagulation for neovascular maculopathy. Arch Ophthalmol. 1986;104:503–512.

4. Macular Photocoagulation Study Group. Recurrent choroidal neovascularization after argon laser photocoagulation for neovascular maculopathy: 3-year results from randomized clinical trials. Arch Ophthalmol. 1986;104:694–701.

5. Macular Photocoagulation Study Group. Krypton laser photocoagulation for neovascular lesions of ocular histoplasmosis: results of a randomized clinical trial. Arch Ophthalmol. 1987;105:1499–1507.

6. Macular Photocoagulation Study Group. Persistent and recurrent neovascularization after Krypton laser photocoagulation for neovascular lesions of age-related macular degeneration. Arch Ophthalmol. 1990;108:825–833.

7. Macular Photocoagulation Study Group. Argon laser photocoagulation for neovascular maculopathy after 5 years: results from randomized clinical trials. Arch Ophthalmol. 1991;109:1109–1114.

8. Macular Photocoagulation Study Group. Laser photocoagulation of subfoveal neovascular lesions in age-related macular degeneration: results of a randomized clinical trial. Arch Ophthalmol. 1991;109:1220–1231.

9. Macular Photocoagulation Study Group. Subfoveal neovascular lesions in age-related macular degeneration: results of a randomized clinical trial. Arch Ophthalmol. 1991;109:1232–1241.

10. Macular Photocoagulation Study Group. Subfoveal neovascular lesions in age-related macular degeneration: guidelines for evaluation and treatment in the Macular Photocoagulation Study. Arch Ophthalmol. 1991;109:1242–1257.

11. Macular Photocoagulation Study Group. Five-year follow-up of fellow eyes of patients with age-related macular degeneration and unilateral extrafoveal choroidal neovascularization. Arch Ophthalmol. 1993;111:1189–1199.

12. Macular Photocoagulation Study Group. Laser photocoagulation of subfoveal neovascular lesions of age-related macular degeneration: updated findings from two clinical trials. Arch Ophthalmol. 1993;111:1200–1209.

13. Macular Photocoagulation Study Group. Visual outcome after laser photocoagulation for subfoveal choroidal neovascularization secondary to age-related macular degeneration: the influence of initial lesion size and initial visual acuity. Arch Ophthalmol. 1994;112:480–488.

14. Macular Photocoagulation Study Group. Persistent and recurrent choroidal neovascularization after argon laser photocoagulation for subfoveal choroidal neovascularization of age-related macular degeneration. Arch Ophthalmol. 1994;112:489–499.

15. Macular Photocoagulation Study Group. Laser photocoagulation of juxtafoveal choroidal neovascularization: 5-year results from randomized clinical trials. Arch Ophthalmol. 1994;111:500–509.

16. Macular Photocoagulation Study Group. Evaluation of green versus red laser for photocoagulation of subfoveal choroidal neovascularization in the Macular Photocoagulation Study. Arch Ophthalmol. 1994;112:1176–1184.

17. Macular Photocoagulation Study Group. Laser photocoagulation for neovascular lesions nasal to the fovea associated with ocular histoplasmosis or idiopathic causes. Arch Ophthalmol. 1995;113:56–61.

18. Macular Photocoagulation Study Group. The influence of treatment coverage on the visual acuity of eyes treated with Krypton laser for juxtafoveal choroidal neovascularization. Arch Ophthalmol. 1995;113:190–194.

19. Macular Photocoagulation Study Group. Occult choroidal neovascularization: influence on visual outcome in patients with age-related macular degeneration. Arch Ophthalmol. 1996;114:400–412.

20. Weiter JJ. Retinal laser surgery: principles and techniques. In: Ryan SJ, Schachat AP, eds. Retina, 3rd ed. Medical retina. St. Louis, MO: Mosby; 2001:1025–1031.

21. Weisz JM, O'Conell SR. Choroidal neovascularization and the macular photocoagulation study. In: Alfaro V, et al., eds. Age-related macular degeneration: a comprehensive textbook, 1st ed. Philadelphia, PA: Lippincott Williams & Wilkins; 2006:189–199.

22. De Juan E, Machemer R. Vitreous surgery for hemorrhagic and fibrous complications of age-related macular degeneration. Am J Ophthalmol. 1988;105:25–29.

23. Joseph DP, Thomas MA. Surgical removal of subretinal choroidal neovascular membranes. In: Ryan SJ, Schachat AP, eds. Retina, 3rd ed. Surgical retina. St. Louis, MO: Mosby; 2001:2562–2572.

24. Thomas MA, Kaplan HJ. Surgical removal of subfoveal neovascularization in the presumed ocular histoplasmosis syndrome. Am J Ophthalmol. 1991;111:1–7.

25. Holekamp NM, Thomas MA. Submacular surgery and the submacular surgery trials. In: Alfaro V, et al., eds. Age-related macular degeneration: a comprehensive textbook, 1st ed. Philadelphia, PA: Lippincott Williams & Wilkins; 2006:254–263.

26. Hawkins BS, Bressler NM, Miskala PH, et al. Submacular Surgery Trials (SST) Research Group. Surgery for subfoveal choroidal neovascularization in age-related macular degeneration: ophthalmic findings: SST report no. 11. [Clinical Trial. Journal Article. Multicenter Study. Randomized Controlled Trial] Ophthalmology. 2004;111:1967–1980.

27. Hawkins BS, Bressler NM, Bressler SB, et al. Submacular Surgery Trials Research Group. Surgical removal vs observation for subfoveal choroidal neovascularization, either associated with the ocular histoplasmosis syndrome or idiopathic. I. Ophthalmic findings from a randomized clinical trial: Submacular Surgery Trials (SST) Group H Trial: SST Report No. 9 [see comment] [erratum appears in Arch Ophthalmol. 2005;123:28. [Clinical Trial. Journal Article. Multicenter Study. Randomized Controlled Trial] Arch Ophthalmol. 2004;122:1597–1611.

28. Bressler NM, Bressler SB, Childs AL, et al. Submacular Surgery Trials (SST) Research Group. Surgery for hemorrhagic choroidal neovascular lesions of age-related macular degeneration: ophthalmic findings: SST report no. 13. [Clinical Trial. Journal Article. Multicenter Study. Randomized Controlled Trial] Ophthalmology. 2004;111:1993–2006.

29. Jonas JB, Degenring R. Intravitreal injection of crystalline triamcinolone acetonide in the treatment of diffuse diabetic macular oedema. Klin Monatsbi Augenheilkd. 2002;219:429–432.

30. Jonas JB, Sofker A. Intravitreal triamcinolone for cataract surgery with iris neovascularization. J Cataract Refract Surg. 2002;28:2040–2041.

31. Jonas JB, Sofker A, Degenring R. Intravitreal triamcinolone acetonide as an additional tool in pars plana vitrectomy for proliferative diabetic retinopathy. Eur J Ophthalmol. 2003;13:468–473.

32. Ishibashi T, Miki K, Sorgente N, et al. Effects of intravitreal administration of steroids on experimental subretinal neovascularization in the subhuman primate. Arch Ophthalmol. 1985;103:708–711.

33. Ciulla TA, Criswell MH, Danis RP, et al. Intravitreal triamcinolone acetonide inhibits choroidal neovascularization in a laser-treated rat model. Arch Ophthalmol. 2001;119:399–404.

34. Alfaro V, Rodriguez-Fontal M, Rodriguez E, et al. Intravitreal triamcinolone for choroidal neovascularization. In: Alfaro V, et al., eds. Age-related macular degeneration: a comprehensive textbook, 1st ed. Philadelphia, PA: Lippincott Williams & Wilkins; 2006:295–299.

35. Dominguez Collazo A. Devices and drugs introduced intraocularly for the treatment of eye diseases "in the office." An R Acad Nac Med (Madr). 1994;111:377–385.

36. Penfold PL, Gyory JF, Hunyor AB, et al. Exudative macular degeneration and intravitreal triamcinolone. A pilot study. Aust NZJ Ophthalmol. 1995;23:293–298.

37. Gillies MC, Simpson JM, Luo W, et al. A randomized clinical trial of a single dose of intravitreal triamcinolone acetonide for neovascular age-related macular degeneration: one year results. Arch Ophthalmol. 2003;121:667–673.

38. Lee J, Freeman WR, Azen SP, et al. Prospective, randomized clinical trial of intravitreal triamcinolone treatment of neovascular age-related macular degeneration: one-year results. Retina. 2007;27:1205–1213.

39. Jonas JB. Intravitreal triamcinolone acetonide for treatment of intraocular oedematous and neovascular diseases. Acta Ophthalmol Scand. 2005;83:645–663.

40. Bressler NM, Bressler SB, Fine SL. Neovascular (exudative) age-related macular degeneration. In: Ryan SJ, Schachat AP, eds. Retina, 3rd ed. Medical retina. St. Louis, MO: Mosby; 2001:1100–1135.

41. Schmidt-Erfurth U, Hasan T, Flotte T. Photodynamic therapy of experimental intraocular tumors with benzoporphyrin-lipoprotein. Ophthalmology. 1994;91:348–356.

42. Schmidt-Erfurth U, Hasan T, Gragoudas ES, et al. Vascular targeting in photodynamic occlusion of subretinal vessels. Ophthalmology. 1994;101:1953–1961.

43. Organisciak DT, Darrow RM, Barsalou L, et al. Light history and age-related changes in retinal light damage. Invest Ophthalmol Vis Sci. 1998;39:1107–1116.

44. Schmidt-Erfurth U, Miller J, Sickenberg M, et al. Photodynamic therapy of subfoveal choroidal neovascularization: clinical and angiographic examples. Graefes Arch Clin Exp Ophthalmol. 1998;236:365–374.

45. Barquet LA, Mones JM, Lavaque AJ, et al. Photodynamic therapy for choroidal neovascularization and age-related macular degeneration. In: Alfaro V, et al., eds. Age-related macular degeneration: a comprehensive textbook, 1st ed. Philadelphia, PA: Lippincott Williams & Wilkins; 2006:200–213.

46. Hussain D, Gragoudas ES, Miller J. Photodynamic therapy. In Berger JQ, Fine SL, Maguire MG, eds. Age-related macular degeneration. St. Louis, MO: Mosby; 1999:297–307.

47. Treatment of Age-Related Macular Degeneration with Photodynamic Therapy (TAP) Study Group (prepared by Bressler, NM). Verteporfin (Visudyne) therapy of subfoveal choroidal neovascularization in age-related macular degeneration: 1-year results of two randomized clinical trials, TAP report no. 1. Arch Ophthalmol. 1999;117:1329–1345.

48. Treatment of Age-Related Macular Degeneration with Photodynamic Therapy (TAP) Study Group. Photodynamic therapy of subfoveal choroidal neovascularization in age-related macular degeneration with verteporfin. Two-year results of 2 randomized clinical trials-TAP report 2. Arch Ophthalmol. 2001;119:198–207.

49. Treatment of Age-Related Macular Degeneration with Photodynamic Therapy (TAP) Study Group. Verteporfin therapy of subfoveal choroidal neovascularization in age-related macular degeneration. Three-year results of an open label extension of 2 randomized clinical trials-TAP report no. 5. Arch Ophthalmol. 2002;120:1307–1313.

50. Verteporfin in Photodynamic Therapy (VIP) Study Group. Verteporfin therapy of subfoveal choroidal neovascularization in age-related macular degeneration: 2-year results of a randomized clinical trial including lesions with occult with no classic choroidal neovascularization-VIP report 2. Am J Ophthalmol. 2001;131:541–560.

51. Verteporfin in Photodynamic Therapy (VIP) Study Group. Photodynamic therapy of subfoveal choroidal neovascularization in pathologic myopia with verteporfin: 1-year results of a randomized clinical trial-VIP report 1. Ophthalmology. 2001;108:841–853.

52. Verteporfin in Photodynamic Therapy (VIP) Study Group. Verteporfin therapy of subfoveal choroidal neovascularization in pathologic myopia: two-year results of a randomized clinical trial-VIP report 3. Ophthalmology. 2003;110:667–873.

53. Rosenfeld PJ for TAP Study Group. Visual outcomes in patients with minimally classic choroidal neovascularization (CNV): rationale for the Visudyne in Minimally Classic CNV (VIM) Trial. Invest Ophthalmol Vis Sci. 2001;42:S512.

54. Bressler NM. New photodynamic therapy investigations. Presented at the annual meeting of the American Academy of Ophthalmology. New Orleans, LA: 2001.

55. Kaiser PK. Photodynamic therapy update: update on verteporfin ocular photodynamic therapy clinical trials. Presented at the Annual Meeting of the American Academy of Ophthalmology, Anaheim, CA: 2003.

56. Isola V, Pece A, Parodi MB. Choroidal ischemia after photodynamic therapy with verteporfin for choroidal neovascularization. Am J Ophthalmol. 2006;142:680–683.

57. Journee-de Kover JG, Oosterhuis JA, Kakebeeke-Kemme HM, et al. Transpupillary thermotherapy (TTT) by infrared irradiation of choroidal melanoma. Doc Ophthalmol. 1992;82:185–191.

58. Reichel E, Berrocal AM, Ip M, et al. Transpupillary thermotherapy of occult subfoveal choroidal neovascularization in patients with age-related macular degeneration. Ophthalmology. 1999;106:1908–1914.

59. Ip M, Kroll A, Reichel E. Transpupillary thermotherapy. Semin Ophthalmol. 1999;14:11–18.

60. Hooper CY, Guymer RH. New treatments in age-related macular degeneration. Clin Exp Ophthalmol. 2003;3:376–391.

61. Algvere PV, Seregard S. Age-related maculopathy: pathogenic features and new treatment modalities. Acta Ophthalmol Scand. 2002;80:136–143.

62. Algvere PV, Libert C, Lindgarde G, et al. Transpupillary thermotherapy of predominantly occult choroidal neovascularization in age-related macular degeneration with 12 months follow-up. Acta Ophthalmol Scand. 2003;81:110–117.

63. Reichel E, Musch DC, Blodi BA. TTT4CNV Study Group. Results from the TTT4CNV Clinical Trial. Invest Ophthalmol Vis Sci. 2005;46:E-Abstract 2311.

64. Puliafito CA, Destro M, To K, et al. Dye-enhanced photocoagulation of choroidal neovascularization. Invest Ophthalmol Vis Sci. 1998;29:414.

65. Puliafito CA, Guyer DR, Mones JM, et al. Indocyanine green digital angiography and dye-enhanced diode laser photocoagulation of choroidal neovascularization. Invest Ophthalmol Vis Sci. 1991;32:712.

66. Kim JE, Shah KB, Han DP, et al. Transpupillary thermotherapy with indocyanine green dye enhancement for the treatment of occult subfoveal choroidal neovascularization in age-related macular degeneration. Ophthalmic Surg Lasers Imaging. 2006;37:272–277.

67. Ligget PE, Lavaque AJ, Jablon EP, et al. Transpupillary thermotherapy for the treatment of choroidal neovascularization associated with age-related macular degeneration. In: Alfaro V, et al., eds. Age-related macular degeneration: a comprehensive textbook, 1st ed. Philadelphia, PA: Lippincott Williams & Wilkins; 2006:214–230.

68. Spaide RF, Sorenson J, Maranan L. Combined photodynamic therapy with verteporfin and intravitreal triamcinolone acetonide for choroidal neovascularization. Ophthalmology. 2003;110:1517–1525.

69. Eter N, Krohne TU, Holz FG. New pharmacologic approaches to therapy for age-related macular degeneration. BioDrugs. 2006;20:167–179.

70. Kaiser PK. Verteporfin photodynamic therapy and anti-angiogenic drugs: potential for combination therapy in exudative age-related macular degeneration. Curr Med Res Opin. 2007;23:477–487.

71. Chan WM, Lai TY, Wong AL, et al. Combined photodynamic therapy and intravitreal triamcinolone injection for the treatment of subfoveal choroidal neovascularisation in age related macular degeneration: a comparative study. Br J Ophthalmol. 2006;90:337–341.

72. Arias L, Garcia-Arumi J, Ramon JM, et al. Photodynamic therapy with intravitreal triamcinolone in predominantly classic choroidal neovascularization: one-year results of a randomized study. Ophthalmology. 2006;113:2243–2250.

73. Becerra EM, Morescalchi F, Gandolfo F, et al. Clinical evidence of intravitreal triamcinolone acetonide in the management of age-related macular degeneration. Curr Drug Targets. 2011;12:149–172.

74. Maberley D. Canadian Retinal Trials Group. Photodynamic therapy and intravitreal triamcinolone for neovascular age-related macular degeneration: a randomized clinical trial. Ophthalmology. 2009;116:2149–2157.

75. Dunavoelgyi R, Sacu S, Simader C, et al. Changes in macular sensitivity after reduced fluence photodynamic therapy combined with intravitreal triamcinolone. Acta Ophthalmol. 2011;89:166–171.

76. Piermarocchi S, Sartore M, Lo Giudice G, et al. Source Combination of photodynamic therapy and intraocular triamcinolone for exudative age-related macular degeneration and long-term chorioretinal macular atrophy. Arch Ophthalmol. 2008;126:1367–1374.

77. Little HL, Zweng HC, Jack RL, et al. Techniques of argon laser photocoagulation of diabetic disk new vessels. Am J Ophthalmol. 1976;82:675–683.

78. Glaser B, Johnson TM. Choroidal feeder vessel photocoagulation therapy. In: Alfaro V, et al., eds. Age-related macular degeneration: a comprehensive textbook, 1st ed. Philadelphia, PA: Lippincott Williams & Wilkins; 2006:231–241.

79. Glaser BM, Murphy R, Lakhanpal R, et al. Identification and treatment of modulating choroidal vessels associated with occult choroidal neovascularization. [ARVO Meeting Abstracts]. Invest Opthalmol Vis Sci. 2000;41:S320.

80. Coscas F, Stanescu D, Coscas G, et al. Feeder vessel treatment of choroidal neovascularization in age-related macular degeneration. J Fr Ophtalmol. 2003;26:602–608.

81. Staurenghi G, Orzalesi N, La Capria A, et al. Laser treatment of feeder vessels in subfoveal choroidal neovascular membranes: a revisitation using dynamic indocyanine green angiography. Ophthalmology. 1998;105:2297–2305.

82. Shiraga F, Ojima Y, Matsuo T, et al. Feeder vessel photocoagulation of subfoveal choroidal neovascularization secondary to age-related macular degeneration. Ophthalmology. 1998;105:662–669.

83. Roh ML, Glaser BM. Feeder vessel treatment of occult with no classic choroidal neovascularization in age-related macular degeneration. ARVO Meeting Abstracts. 2003;44:1776.

84. Luu J, Baudo T, Glaser B. Feeder vessel treatment of recurrent choroidal neovascularization (CNV). ARVO Meeting Abstracts. 2002;43:2510.

85. Johnson TM, Glaser BM. High speed ICG guided focal laser treatment of retinal angiomatous proliferations. ARVO Meeting Abstracts. 2003;44:5034.

86. Johnson TM, Luu J, Glaser BM. Micropulse laser modulation of retinal choroidal anastomoses in exudative macular degeneration. ARVO Meeting Abstracts. 2002;43:2506.

87. Somaiya M, Glaser B. High-speed phi-motion ICG characteristics and feeder vessel treatment of polypoidal choroidal vasculopathy in age-related macular degeneration. ARVO Meeting Abstracts. 2002;43:2509.

88. Flower RW. Optimizing treatment of choroidal neovascularization feeder vessels associated with age-related macular degeneration. Am J Ophthalmol. 2002;134:228–239.

89. Staurenghi G, Massacesi A, Musicco I, et al. Combining photodynamic therapy and feeder vessel photocoagulation: a pilot study. Semin Ophthalmol. 2001;16:233–236.

90. Chakravarthy U, MacKenzie G. External beam radiotherapy in exudative age-related macular degeneration: a pooled analysis of phase I data. Br J Radiol. 2000;73:305–313.

91. Jaakkola A, Heikkonen J, Tommila P, et al. Strontium plaque brachytherapy for exudative age-related macular degeneration: three-year results of a randomized study. Ophthalmology. 2005;112:567–573.

92. Evans JR, Sivagnanavel V, Chong V. Radiotherapy for neovascular age-related macular degeneration. Cochrane Database Syst Rev. 2010;(5):CD004004.

93. Rokni SH, Fassò A, Liu JC. Operational radiation protection in high-energy physics accelerators. Radiat Prot Dosimetry. 2009;137:3–17.

94. Petrarca R, Jackson TL. Radiation therapy for neovascular age-related macular degeneration. Clin Ophthalmol. 2011;5:57–63.

95. Arlett CF, Harcourt SA. Survey of radiosensitivity in a variety of human cell strains. Cancer Res. 1980;40:926–932.

96. Amoaku WM, Frew L, Mahon GJ, et al. Early ultrastructural changes after low dose X-irradiation in the retina of the rat. Eye (Lond). 1989;3:638–646.

97. Archer DB, Amoaku WM, Gardiner TA. Radiation retinopathy- clinical, histological, ultrastructural and experimental correlation. Eye (Lond). 1991;5:239–251.

98. Irvine AR, Wood IS. Radiation retinopathy as an experimental model for ischemic proliferative retinopathy and rubeosis iridis. Am J Ophthalmol. 1987;103:790–797.

99. Sherr DL, Finger PT. Radiation therapy for age-related macular degeneration. Semin Ophthalmol. 1997;12:26–33.

100. Chakrabarthy U, Houston RF, Archer DB. Treatment of age-related subfoveal neovascular membrane by tele therapy: a pilot study. Br J Ophthalmol. 1993;77:265–273.

101. Donati G, Soubrane D, Quaranta M, et al. Radiotherapy for isolated occult subfoveal neovascularisation in age-related macular degeneration: a pilot study. Br J Ophthalmol. 1999;83:646–651.

102. Stalmans P, Leys A, van Limbergen E. External beam radiotherapy (20 gy, 2 gy fractions) fails to control the growth of choroid neovascularization in age-related macular degeneration: a review of 111 cases. Retina. 1997;17:481–492.

103. Spaide RF, Guyer DR, McCormick B, et al. External beam radiation therapy for choroidal neovascularization. Ophthalmology. 1998;105:24–30.

104. Tholen AM, Meisher A, Bernasconi PP, et al. Radiotherapy for choroidal neovascularization in age-related macular degeneration. A pilot study using low- versus high dose proton beam radiation in age-related related macular degeneration. Ophthalmology. 1998;95:691–698.

105. Bergink GJ, Hoyng CB, Vander Maazen RW, et al. A randomized controlled clinical trial on the efficacy of radiation therapy in the control of subfoveal choroidal neovascularization in age-related macular degeneration: radiation versus observation. Graefes Arch Clin Exp Ophihalmol. 1998;236:321–325.

106. Holz FR, Eugenhart-Cabillic R, Unnebrink KK, et al. A prospective, randomized, double-blind trial on radiation therapy for neovascular age-related macular degeneration (RAD study). Ophthalmology. 1999;106:2239–2247.

107. Verma L, Das T, Binder S, et al. New approaches in the management of choroidal neovascular membrane in age-related macular degeneration. Indian J Ophthalmol. 2000;48:263–278.

108. Machemer R, Steinhorst UH. Retinal separation, retinotomy, and macular relocation: II. A surgical approach for age-related macular degeneration. Graefes Arch Clin Exp Ophthalmol. 1993;231:635–641.

109. Wolf S, Lapas A, Weinberger A, et al. Erste Erfahrungen mit makularer translocation zur behnadlung subfovealer choroidaler neovascularisationen. Klin Monatsble Augenheilkd. 1997;210:5.

110. Wolf S, Lappas A, Weinberger AW, et al. Macular translocation for surgical management of subfoveal choroidal neovascularizations in patients with AMD: First results. Graefes Arch Clin Exp Ophthalmol. 1999;237:51–57.

111. Eckardt C, Eckardt U, Conrad HG. Macular rotation with and without counter-rotation of the globe in patients with age-related macular degeneration. Graefes Arch Clin Exp Ophthalmol. 1999;237:313–325.

112. Nimoniya Y, Lewis JM, Hasegawa T, et al. Retinotomy and foveal translocation for surgical management of subfoveal choroidal neovascular membranes. Am J Ophthalmol. 1996;122:613–621.

113. de Juan E Jr, Lowenstein AL, Bressler NM, et al. Translocation of the retina for management of subfoveal choroidal neovascularization. II: a preliminary report in humans. Am J Ophthalmol. 1998;125:635–646.

114. Lewis H, Kaiser PK, Lewis S, et al. Macular translocation for subfoveal choroidal neovascularization in age-related macular degeneration: a prospective study. Am J Ophthalmol. 1999;128:135–146.

115. Fujikado T, Ohji M, Hayashi A. Anatomic and functional recovery of the fovea after foveal translocation surgery without large retinotomy and simultaneous excision of neovascular membrane. Am J Ophthalmol. 1998;126:839–842.

116. Fricke J, Neugebauer A, Kirsch A, et al. Muskelchirurgische gegenrotation des bulbus bei makulatranslokation. Jahrestagung der DOG Ophthalmoge. 1999;96:S3.

16

MACUGEN FOR AGE-RELATED MACULAR DEGENERATION

PABLO CARNOTA MÉNDEZ • CARLOS MÉNDEZ VÁZQUEZ

■ INTRODUCTION

Pegaptanib sodium for injection (Macugen, Eyetech Pharmaceuticals Inc., and Pfizer Inc.,) was the first pharmacologic agent for age-related macular degeneration (AMD) since the introduction of verteporfin photodynamic therapy (PDT) in the late 1990s. It was approved by the FDA in December 2004 for the treatment of neovascular AMD, becoming the first anti–vascular endothelial growth factor (anti-VEGF) molecule used for the treatment of ocular disease. Most patients with neovascular AMD have choroidal neovascularization (CNV) characterized as occult or minimally classic as determined by fluorescein angiography (1), whereas a minority of patients have predominantly classic CNV (2).

Before the appearance of pegaptanib sodium, there was no FDA-approved treatment for the majority of patients with neovascular AMD. PDT was only approved for patients with subfoveal membranes with the predominantly classic subtype of CNV (3,4). Later, this indication was extended to cases with minimally classic or occult subtype of CNV, but only if they were less than four disk areas in size and were associated with progression of the disease. Extra- and juxtafoveal CNV had traditionally been treated with thermal laser photocoagulation, and prior to the advent of PDT, subfoveal lesions had been treated with laser as well (5). These traditional treatment approaches to neovascular AMD (i.e., PDT and thermal laser photocoagulation) were destructive therapies that led to retinal tissue scarring. Pegaptanib sodium emerged as a nondestructive therapy and showed efficacy for the treatment of most subtypes of neovascular AMD.

■ MECHANISM OF ACTION

Pegaptanib sodium is a pegylated aptamer with high affinity for VEGF (6,7). An aptamer is a synthetic short strand of RNA oligonucleotide that adopts a specific three-dimensional conformation (8), joining to its target molecule (Fig. 16.1). Because aptamers have high affinity for their target molecules, the aptamer–target interaction is very similar to that of an antibody and antigen.

Aptamers are created using a process known as the systematic evolution of ligands of exponential (SELEX) enrichment process (9). Through this process, 10^{14} aptamers are produced in a test tube and then screened for their ability to bind or interfere with various target molecules (9). Using $VEGF_{165}$ as the target, SELEX methodology was performed in three separate approaches at NeXstar Pharmaceuticals, ultimately producing the aptamer that became pegaptanib. Aptamers that blocked the actions of VEGF in vitro were first described in 1994 (10) followed by the use of amino-substituted nucleotides to improve the resistance of anti-VEGF aptamers to nuclease attack in 1995 (11) and, subsequently, the use of additional substitutions to further improve stability and affinity in 1998 (12). In the latter work, three stable, high-affinity candidate anti-VEGF aptamers were characterized, one of which was selected for development as pegaptanib. In a process called pegylation, the addition of a 40-kDa polyethylene glycol (PEG) moiety to the 5′ end of the aptamer improved bioavailability (12). Pegylation is the process of covalent attachment of PEG polymer chains to another molecule, normally a drug or therapeutic protein (13).

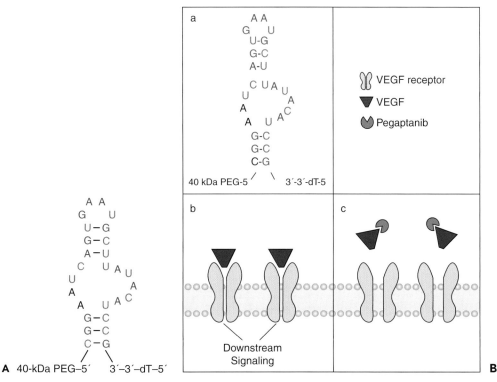

Figure 16.1 ■ Pegaptanib structure and target binding. **A.** Sequence and predicted secondary structure of pegaptanib. 2′-O-methylated purines are shown in red, 2′-fluorine-modified pyrimidines are shown in blue, and unmodified ribonucleotides are shown in black. The site of attachment of a 40-kDa PEG moiety is shown. **B.** Interaction between the 55-amino-acid heparin-binding domain of VEGF$_{165}$ and pegaptanib. (From Ng EW, Shima DT, Calias P, et al. Pegaptanib, a targeted anti-VEGF aptamer for ocular vascular disease. Nat Rev Drug Discov. 2006;5(2):123–132.)

This covalent attachment can "mask" the agent from the host's immune system (reducing immunogenicity and antigenicity) and increase the hydrodynamic size (size in solution) of the agent, which prolongs its terminal half-life by reducing clearance from the eye (14).

The selectivity of pegaptanib derives from its interaction with cysteine-137, an amino acid that is contained within the 55 amino acid heparin-binding domain of VEGF, which is not present in VEGF$_{121}$ (15); the interaction between pegaptanib and this domain is shown in Figure 16.1B (16).

CHEMICAL STRUCTURE

The molecular formula for pegaptanib sodium is C$_{294}$H$_{342}$F$_{13}$N$_{107}$Na$_{28}$O$_{188}$P$_{28}$[C$_2$H$_4$O]n (where n is approximately 900), and the molecular weight is 49 kDa (17). The chemical structure of pegaptanib sodium is depicted in Figure 16.2.

RATIONALE FOR CLINICAL USE

The VEGF family is a group of secreted proteins that include VEGF-A, -B, -C, -D, and placental growth factor (PlGF). These factors selectively bind and activate receptors located primarily on the surface of vascular endothelial cells.

Among these, it is well known that VEGF-A acts as a key regulator of pathologic vessel growth and vascular permeability in ocular neovascular disease such as AMD (18,19). VEGF is produced by many cells types in the retina (20,21), but the underlying causes for its elevation during ocular neovascularization are not known. It has been suggested that VEGF can be up-regulated by plasminogen activator (22), endothelial nitric oxide synthase (23), and, most of all, hypoxia (24), which further contributes to the pathogenesis of ocular vascular disease. Several biologically active isoforms have been identified depending on the site of splicing of the VEGF gene: VEGF$_{121-165-189}$, and $_{-206}$. The isoform VEGF$_{165}$ is thought to be the most associated with pathologic ocular neovascularisation (25). Of the other isoforms, VEGF$_{189}$ and VEGF$_{206}$ are highly basic, are heparin binding, and exist primarily as matrix-bound forms. VEGF$_{121}$, lacking the heparin-binding domain, is freely secreted (22). Pegaptanib sodium was developed to selectively inhibit the isoform VEGF$_{165}$. In this way, the choice of aptamer was based on the characteristic of having high affinity and specificity for VEGF$_{165}$. In fact, preclinical studies in mouse models of pathologic ocular neovascularisation demonstrate the effectiveness of pegaptanib sodium at inhibiting the activity of VEGF$_{164}$ (the murine homologue to the human isoform VEGF$_{165}$) (26,27). However, one of the main concerns during drug development was whether or not the inhibition of

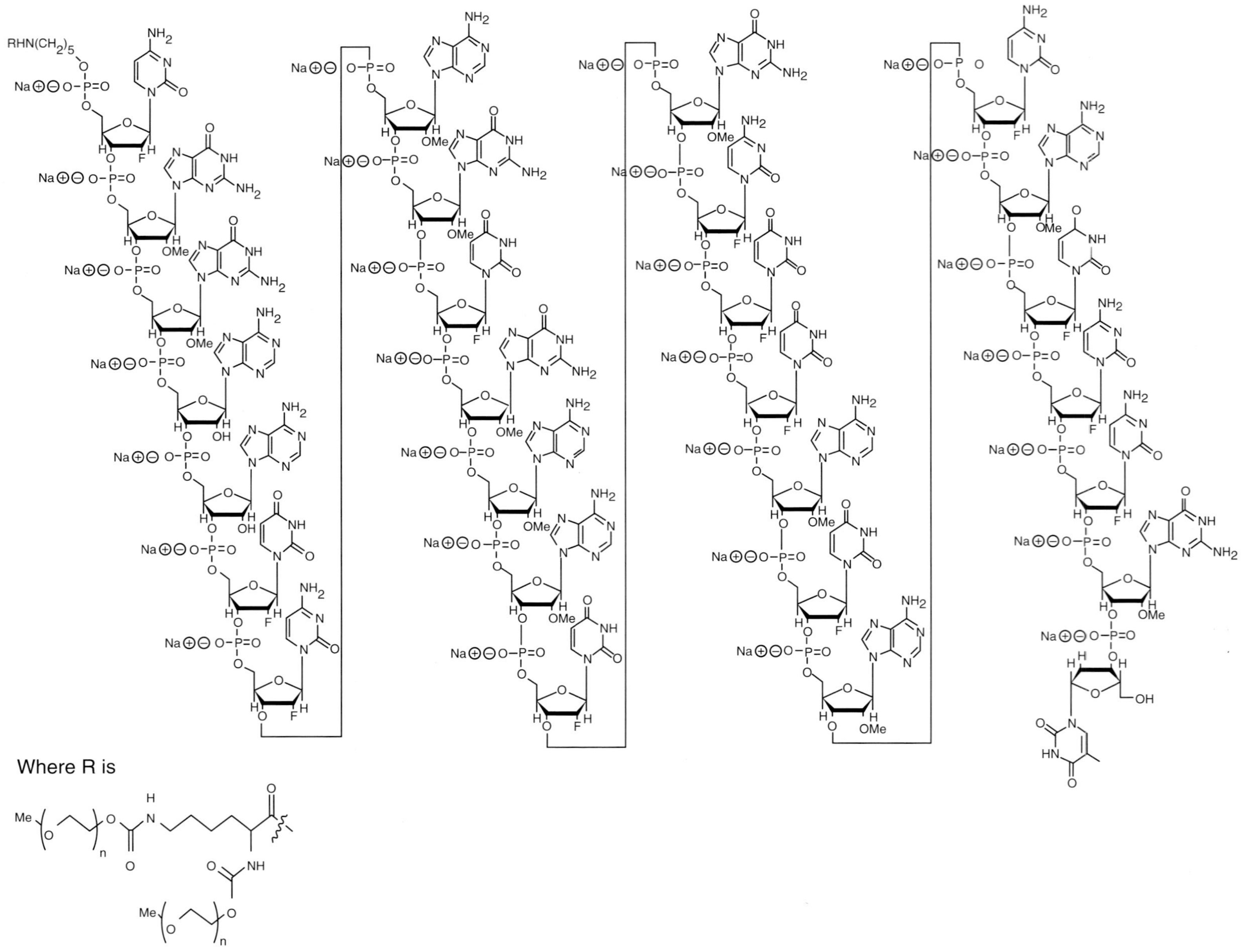

Figure 16.2 ■ Schematic depicting chemical structure of pegaptanib sodium. (From Eyetech/Pfizer: Pegaptanib sodium injection in the treatment of neovascular AMD. Briefing Document for the FDA Dermatologic and Ophthalmic Drugs Advisory Committee. Rockville, MD, 2004.)

VEGF$_{165}$ could inhibit not only pathologic neovascularisation but physiologic vasculogenesis and vascular homeostasis. The studies mentioned above showed that VEGF$_{164}$ was selectively increased in pathologic neovascularisation, and blocking it results in inhibition of pathologic angiogenesis and vascular permeability without damage to normal vasculature (26,27).

The rationale behind this approach is that eliminating the stimulus for the formation of abnormal blood vessels, one can eliminate the unwanted effects of the abnormal blood vessels (i.e., intraretinal, subretinal, and sub–retinal pigment epithelium [RPE] fluid accumulation and hemorrhage) without the "collateral" damage induced by thermal laser photocoagulation or PDT. One of the main advantages of anti-VEGF treatment over thermal laser or PDT is that normal retina, RPE, and choroid are spared from damage (28).

CLINICAL PHARMACOLOGY

Pharmacokinetics

Absorption

In animals, pegaptanib is slowly absorbed into the systemic circulation from the eye after intravitreous administration. The rate of absorption from the eye is the rate-limiting step in the disposition of pegaptanib in animals and is likely to be the rate-limiting step in humans, too (17). Vitreous levels appear to follow an apparent first-order elimination process. Preclinical studies determined the terminal half-life in the vitreous to be 83 hours in a rabbit model (6) and 94 hours (29) in a rhesus monkey model. The estimated plasma terminal half-life was 84 hours, and plasma concentration of the drug diminished via an apparent first-order elimination process as well. In humans, a mean maximum plasma concentration of about 80 ng/mL occurs within 1 to 4 days after a 3-mg monocular dose (10 times the recommended dose) (17). At doses less than 0.3 mg per eye, pegaptanib sodium plasma concentrations are not likely to exceed 10 ng/mL, which is more than 100 times less than the concentration observed in the nonclinical toxicology studies at the "no observed adverse effect level" doses (17). Circulating levels of pegaptanib sodium seen 4 to 6 weeks after an intravitreous 0.3-mg dose were below the lower limits of quantification (8 ng/mL) of the assay (17).

Metabolism

Based on preclinical data, pegaptanib is metabolized by endo- and exonucleases (17).

Excretion

After intravitreous and intravenous administration of radiolabeled pegaptanib to rabbits, the highest concentrations of radioactivity were obtained in the kidney. In rabbits, the component nucleotide 2′-fluorouridine is found in plasma and urine after single radiolabeled pegaptanib intravenous and intravitreous doses (17). However, dose adjustment for patients with renal impairment is not needed when administering the 0.3-mg dose (17).

Pharmacodynamics

Preclinical studies established that pegaptanib inhibited VEGF binding and VEGF-mediated cell signaling in cultured endothelial cells and that pretreatment of cells with pegaptanib inhibited proliferative responses only to VEGF$_{165}$, but not to VEGF$_{121}$ (30). In addition, pegaptanib dramatically inhibited VEGF$_{165}$-induced vascular permeability (6,12).

DRUG DELIVERY AND DOSING

Pegaptanib sodium is available in a single-use, pre-filled 1-mL glass syringe. Pegaptanib sodium (3.47 mg/mL solution) in a volume of 90 µL is delivered intravitreally via the pars plana for a total intraocular dose of 0.3 mg (17,31,32). The drug is packaged free of preservative, although pH buffers are a component of the clear, colorless solution (17).

PIVOTAL TRIALS OF CLINICAL EFFICACY

After phase I and phase II clinical trials demonstrated that pegaptanib was a safe drug (6,7), the hypothesis that pegaptanib would be effective in all types of CNV secondary to AMD was evaluated in two (EOP1003 and EOP1004) identically designed, concurrent, prospective, multicenter, randomized, double-masked, sham-controlled, dose-ranging pivotal trials: the VEGF Inhibition Study in Ocular Neovascularization (VISION) trials. The results were published by the VISION Clinical Trial Group in 2004 (31).

Study Design

Patients with subfoveal CNV due to neovascular AMD were treated every 6 weeks for 48 weeks with either a sham intravitreal injection or intravitreal pegaptanib sodium injection at doses of 0.3, 1, or 3 mg. Pharmacokinetic studies indicated that in order to maintain the intravitreal angiogenesis inhibitory concentration at therapeutic levels, pegaptanib doses ≥0.3 mg would need to be administered at least every 6 weeks (Fig. 16.3). The prespecified study end point was 54 weeks (6 weeks following the last study injection). The use of verteporfin PDT was allowed, in either sham injection groups or pegaptanib injection groups, at the treating physician's discretion if the FDA labeling indications for verteporfin treatment were met throughout the study.

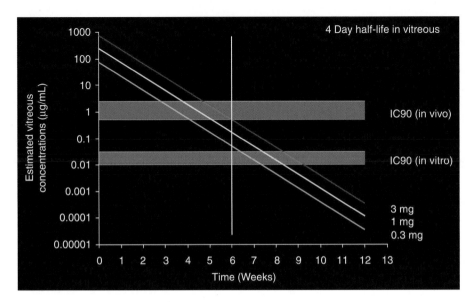

Figure 16.3 ■ A graph representing the in vivo and in vitro IC$_{90}$ of pegaptanib sodium (0.3, 1 or 3 mg) at varying time points following intravitreal injection. To maintain adequate inhibitory concentrations, reinjection is recommended every 6 weeks for doses of 0.3 mg. IC$_{90}$: concentration required to inhibit viral replication by 90%. (From Eyetech/Pfizer: Pegaptanib sodium injection (Macugen). Dermatologic and Ophthalmic Drugs Advisory Committee Meeting, August 27, 2004. Food and Drug Administration, Rockville, MD; 2004.)

At the end of 54 weeks, patients originally randomized to receive pegaptanib were rerandomized (1:1) to continue pegaptanib for an additional 48 weeks or to discontinue treatment; patients originally randomized to the sham group were rerandomized (1:1:1:1:1) to either continue in the sham group, to discontinue sham, or to be treated with one of the three pegaptanib doses. The purpose of rerandomization during the 2nd year of the study was to determine whether chronic treatment beyond 1 year was necessary and to identify any additional safety concerns of chronic treatment. The inclusion and exclusion criteria of the study are summarized in Table 16.1.

Table 16.1 INCLUSION AND EXCLUSION CRITERIA IN THE VISION TRIALS

Inclusion criteria	Exclusion criteria
■ Visual acuity between 20/40 and 20/320	■ Prior subfoveal thermal laser photocoagulation
■ Subfoveal location	■ >1 prior PDT treatment
■ Size ≤12 disk areas	■ ≥25% of CNV lesion with subfoveal fibrosis or atrophy
■ ≥50% of lesion consisting of active CNV	
■ Patients with occult or minimally classic lesions had to demonstrate recent disease progression (subretinal hemorrhage, subretinal lipid, or at least a three-line loss of visual acuity in the preceding 12 weeks)	

Data from Gragoudas ES, Adamis AP, Cunningham ET Jr, et al. Pegaptanib for neovascular age-related macular degeneration. N Engl J Med. 2004;351(27):2805–2816.

Outcome Measures

The prespecified efficacy end point was the proportion of patients who lost less than 15 Early Treatment Diabetic Retinopathy Study (ETDRS) letters from baseline to 54 weeks. This represents a doubling of the visual angle, which most ophthalmologists and patients consider as a meaningful change in vision. Secondary outcomes were the proportion of patients gaining ≥15 ETDRS letters from baseline to 54 weeks, the proportion of patients who experienced maintenance or gain of ≥0 letters from baseline to 54 weeks, and the change in mean visual acuity at 6, 12, and 54 weeks.

Clinical Efficacy Data

A total of 1,208 patients were randomly assigned in the two trials, of which 1,186 patients received at least one treatment and were included in 1-year efficacy analyses (622 patients included in EOP1003 and 586 patients included in EOP1004). During year one, 7,545 intravitreal injections of pegaptanib and 2,557 sham injections were administered. An average of 8.5 injections per patient was administered, and approximately 90% of patients in each group completed year 1 of the study.

The individual and combined data from the two clinical trials demonstrated that pegaptanib sodium provided a clear treatment benefit for doses of 0.3 or 1 mg when given intravitreally every 6 weeks for 54 weeks (data presented are from the combined analysis of the individual EOP1003 and EOP1004 trials). The greatest treatment benefit was seen with the lowest studied dose, 0.3 mg (17,31,32). The 0.3-mg dose demonstrated a significantly greater proportion (70%, combined analysis, $P < 0.0001$) of patients achieving the primary efficacy end point of a loss of less than 15 ETDRS letters of visual acuity at the end of 54 weeks compared with the sham injection group (55%). So far, there is no explanation for this phenomenon that the lowest dose

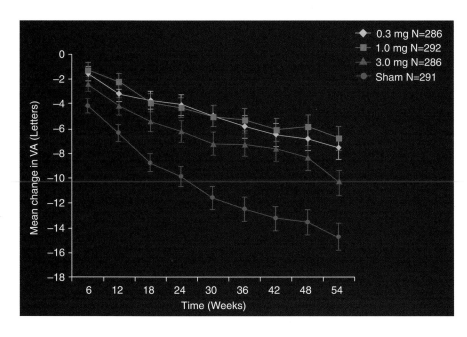

Figure 16.4 ■ Graph demonstrating the proportion of responders (those with less than 15 letters of visual acuity loss) at each study visit through 54 weeks for each treatment arm. The 0.3-mg dose of pegaptanib sodium in the VISION trials was associated with a 70% responder rate at 54 weeks compared with the sham group, which had a 55% responder rate ($P < 0.0001$). (From Eyetech/Pfizer: Pegaptanib sodium injection (Macugen™). Dermatologic and Ophthalmic Drugs Advisory Committee Meeting, August 27, 2004. Food and Drug Administration, Rockville, MD; 2004.)

was the most efficient. Figure 16.4 summarizes the results regarding the primary end point.

With regard to mean visual acuity loss, pegaptanib was significantly of benefit compared with sham from as early as the first study visit at 6 weeks. This early benefit was sustained at every visit through the 54-week follow-up (Fig. 16.5) and continued during the 2nd year of the trial (33). Moreover, pegaptanib has shown efficacy as maintenance therapy after any other treatments for neovascular AMD (34).

Maintenance or gain of visual acuity was seen in 33% of the 0.3-mg pegaptanib group compared with 23% in the sham group at the study end point ($P = 0.0032$). Six percent of patients in the 0.3-mg pegaptanib group gained three lines of vision or more compared to 2% in the sham group ($P = 0.0401$). On the other hand, 22% of patients in the sham group had a severe vision loss (≥ 30 ETDRS letters)

compared to 10% of patients in the 0.3-mg pegaptanib group ($P < 0.0001$) (Fig. 16.6).

In a posterior exploratory analysis, the good outcomes achieved with pegaptanib were validated also for the subgroup of patients with early subfoveal neovascular AMD (35). Early neovascular AMD was defined as lesions with less than 2 disk areas with baseline visual acuity of ≥ 54 letters, or as occult lesions with no classic CNV with an absence of lipid and worse visual acuity in the study eye versus the fellow eye.

■ SAFETY

There are several potential safety concerns for a treatment inhibiting VEGF, particularly in the context of prolonged treatment regimens (36). However, as discussed above, we know that isoform 165 of VEGF is involved in pathologic

Figure 16.5 ■ Graph representing the mean visual acuity change from baseline at each study visit for each treatment arm in the VISION trials for pegaptanib sodium. (From Eyetech/Pfizer: Pegaptanib sodium injection in the treatment of neovascular age-related macular degeneration. Briefing Document for the FDA Dermatologic and Ophthalmic Drugs Advisory Committee. Rockville, MD; 2004.)

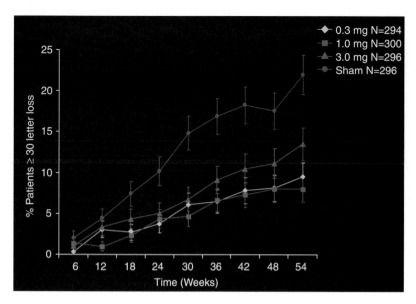

Figure 16.6 ■ Graph representing the proportion of patients with severe visual loss at each study visit for each treatment arm in the VISION trials for pegaptanib sodium. Patients in the sham group were more than twice as likely to develop severe vision loss than were those in the 0.3-mg pegaptanib sodium group ($P < 0.0001$). (From Eyetech/Pfizer: Pegaptanib sodium injection (Macugen™). Dermatologic and Ophthalmic Drugs Advisory Committee Meeting, August 27, 2004. Food and Drug Administration, Rockville, MD; 2004.)

neovascularization, not in physiologic vasculogenesis. The systemic risks of nonselective VEGF inhibition have been illustrated with the use of bevacizumab in the treatment of metastatic colorectal and non–small cell lung cancer. Thromboembolic events, potentially life-threatening bleeding complications, hypertension, and proteinuria are a few of the adverse events reported with its use systemically (37). In these terms, no evidence of systemic safety concerns, including hypertension and proteinuria, has been found related to the use of pegaptanib (38). Moreover, in the VISION trials, there was no difference in the mortality rate between the pegaptanib sodium and sham groups.

Pegaptanib has never been studied in pregnant women, so the potential risk to humans in this setting is unknown. However, the pregnancy classification for pegaptanib is category B in that no maternal toxicity, evidence of teratogenicity, or fetal mortality had been observed in mice given 7,000 times the recommended human intravitreous dose (39).

The main serious ocular adverse events related to intravitreal injections of pegaptanib sodium are endophthalmitis, traumatic cataract, and rhegmatogenous retinal detachment. The rates of these complications in the years 1, 2, and 3 of the VISION trials are summarized in Table 16.2 (31,40,41). These appear to be procedure-related adverse events rather than drug-related adverse events and are similar to those observed with other substances delivered with an intravitreous injection (42–44).

PEGAPTANIB FOR NEOVASCULAR AMD: NEW HORIZONS

Pegaptanib is the first anti-VEGF agent to be approved for the treatment of neovascular AMD. It has been shown to be efficacious in all angiographic subtypes of CNV lesions and has a 5-year safety record that differentiates it from other anti-VEGF drugs. Ranibizumab and bevacizumab,

two nonselective VEGF inhibitors approved for neovascular AMD, have been the first treatments to provide improvement in visual acuity for AMD patients (45–47). However, the implications for safety of nonselective VEGF inhibition remain unclear. Even though intravitreous administration requires low doses of drug, safety is of concern as these agents ultimately enter the systemic circulation. As mentioned previously, the $VEGF_{121}$ isoform is mostly involved in physiologic vasculogenesis and vascular homeostasis. As VEGF acts to up-regulate the synthesis of tissue factor, the initiator of the coagulation cascade, inhibition of VEGF could theoretically have antithrombotic consequences. In addition, VEGF up-regulates nitric oxide synthase and ultimately the production of nitric oxide, a potent anticoagulant. However, several other mechanisms are likely to promote thromboses in this setting (48). VEGF is an endothelial cell survival factor so its inhibition could favor apoptosis of endothelial cells, leading to their becoming

Table 16.2 SERIOUS OCULAR ADVERSE EVENTS, RATES (% PER INJECTION)

Event	Year 1	Year 2	Year 3
Endophthalmitis	0.16	0.10	0.06
Traumatic cataract	0.07	0.02	0
Retinal detachment	0.08	0.17	0.03

Data from Gragoudas ES, Adamis AP, Cunningham ET Jr, et al. Pegaptanib for neovascular age-related macular degeneration. N Engl J Med. 2004;351(27):2805–2816; D'Amico, DJ, Masonson, HN, Patel, M, et al. Pegaptanib sodium for age-related macular degeneration: two-year safety results of the two prospective, multicenter, controlled clinical trials. Ophthalmology. 113(6):992–1001, 2006; Singerman LJ, Masonson H, Patel M, et al. Pegaptanib sodium for age-related macular degeneration: third-year safety results of the VEGF Inhibition Study in Ocular Neovascularization (VISION) trial. Br J Ophthalmol. 2008;92:1606–1611.

procoagulant (49). Finally, VEGF has also been reported to destabilize cholesterol plaques, possibly through the inhibition of immature blood vessels forming in them (50). These findings could explain why an increased incidence of nonocular hemorrhage, cerebrovascular accidents, and stroke related to the use of nonselective anti-VEGF agents compared to control subjects has been reported (51–54).

Several strategies have been designed to try to minimize these potential systemic adverse events. One is to minimize the number of injections. Two-year data of the PrONTO study have indicated that increases in visual acuity can be attained with fewer injections than one every 6 weeks (55). Another approach is to combine the good safety profile of pegaptanib with the good visual outcome profile of nonselective agents. In two studies with relatively small numbers of patients, bevacizumab was employed as an initial inductive agent, followed by maintenance doses of pegaptanib, with encouraging results (56,57). A prospective, multicenter, uncontrolled, open-label study using pegaptanib as a maintenance anti-VEGF agent following an induction phase (with any combination of pegaptanib, bevacizumab, ranibizumab, or PDT) showed that pegaptanib maintained the visual acuity improvement achieved during the induction phase for at least 1 year (34). This strategy may have special relevance for patients with cardiovascular comorbidities who require anti-VEGF drugs to manage their neovascular AMD.

CONCLUSION

The development and application of pegaptanib, the first aptamer approved for clinical use, have fostered the study of the underlying molecular basis of ocular vascular diseases as a means of rationally developing new therapies. These studies have established the central role of VEGF in ocular neovascularization. In particular, they have highlighted the role of VEGF$_{165}$ isoform in mediating the inflammatory processes that are key to the development of both pathologic neovascularization and the vascular permeability abnormalities that lead to vision loss. Moreover, these VEGF-induced pathologic changes have been found to be associated not only with neovascular AMD but diabetic macular edema, diabetic retinopathy, and retinal vein occlusion. Therefore, pegaptanib has become a useful drug for neovascular AMD and other vascular ocular diseases, with an excellent safety record. This may be a capital advantage over other anti-VEGF agents given the cardiovascular risk profile of most of the patients suffering from these pathologies.

REFERENCES

1. Freund KB, Yannuzzi LA, Sorenson JA. Age-related macular degeneration and choroidal neovascularisation. Am J Ophthalmol. 1993;115(6):786–791.

2. Friedman DS, O'Colmain BJ, Munoz B, et al. Eye Diseases Prevalence Research Group. Prevalence of age-related macular degeneration in the United States. Arch Ophthalmol. 2004;122(4):564–572. Erratum in. Arch Ophthalmol. 2011;129(9):1188.

3. Photodynamic therapy of subfoveal choroidal neovascularization in age-related macular degeneration with verteporfin: one-year results of 2 randomized clinical trials-TAP report. Treatment of age-related macular degeneration with photodynamic therapy (TAP) Study Group. Arch Ophthalmol. 1999;117(10):1329–1345.

4. Bressler NM. Photodynamic therapy of subfoveal choroidal neovascularization in age-related macular degeneration with verteporfin: two-year results of 2 randomized clinical trials-TAP report 2. Arch Ophthalmol. 2001;119(2):198–207.

5. Laser photocoagulation of subfoveal neovascular lesions in age-related macular degeneration. Results of a randomized clinical trial. Macular Photocoagulation Study Group. Arch Ophthalmol. 1991;109(9):1220–1231.

6. The Eyetech Study Group. Preclinical and phase IA clinical evaluation of an anti-VEGF pegylated aptamer (EYE001) for the treatment of exudative age-related macular degeneration. Retina. 2002;22(2):143–152.

7. The Eyetech Study Group. Anti-vascular endothelial growth factor therapy for subfoveal choroidal neovascularization secondary to age-related macular degeneration: phase II study results. Ophthalmology. 2003;110(5):979–986.

8. Nimjee SM, Rusconi CP, Sullenger BA. Aptamers: an emerging class of therapeutics. Annu Rev Med. 2005;56:555–583.

9. Tuerk C, Gold L. Systematic evolution of ligands by exponential enrichment: RNA ligands to bacteriophage T4 DNA polymerase. Science. 1990;249(4968):505–510.

10. Jellinek D, Green LS, Bell C, et al. Inhibition of receptor binding by high-affinity RNA ligands to vascular endothelial growth factor. Biochemistry. 1994;33(34):10450–10456.

11. Green LS, Jellinek D, Bell C, et al. Nuclease-resistant nucleic acid ligands to vascular permeability factor/vascular endothelial growth factor. Chem Biol. 1995;2(10):683–695.

12. Ruckman J, Green LS, Beeson J, et al. 2-Fluoropyrimidine RNA-based aptamers to the 165-amino acid form of vascular endothelial growth factor (VEGF165). Inhibition of receptor binding and VEGF-induced vascular permeability through interactions requiring exon 7-encoded domain. J Biol Chem. 1998;273(32):20556–20567.

13. Davis FF. The origin of pegnology. Adv Drug Del Rev. 2002;54(4):457–458.

14. Hofman P, Blaauwgeers HG, Tolentino MJ, et al. VEGF-A induced hyperpermeability of blood-retinal barrier endothelium in vivo is predominantly associated with pinocytotic vesicular transport and not with formation of fenestrations. Curr Eye Res. 2000;21(2):637–645.

15. Lee JH, Canny MD, De Erkenez A, et al. A therapeutic aptamer inhibits angiogenesis by specifically targeting the heparin binding domain of VEGF165. Proc Natl Acad Sci U S A. 2005;102(52):18902–18907.

16. Ng EW, Shima DT, Calias P, et al. Pegaptanib, a targeted anti-VEGF aptamer for ocular vascular disease. Nat Rev Drug Discov. 2006;5(2):123–132.

17. Eyetech/Pfizer: Pegaptanib sodium injection in the treatment of neovascular age-related macular degeneration. Briefing Document for the FDA Dermatologic and Ophthalmic Drugs Advisory Committee. Rockville, MD; 2004.

18. Ambati J, Ambati BK, Yoo SH, et al. Age-related macular degeneration: etiology, pathogenesis, and therapeutic strategies. Surv Ophthalmol. 2003;48(3):257–293.

19. Ferrara N. Vascular endothelial growth factor: basic science and clinical progress. Endocr Rev. 2004;25(4):581–611.

20. Adamis AP, Shima DT, Yeo KT, et al. Synthesis and secretion of vascular permeability factor/vascular endothelial growth factor by human retina pigment epithelial cells. Biochem Biophys Res Commun. 1993;193(2):631–638.

21. Famiglietti EV, Stopa EG, McGookin ED, et al. Immunocytochemical localization of vascular endothelial growth factor in neurons and glial cells of human retina. Brain Res. 2003;969(1–2):195–204.

22. Park JE, Keller GA, Ferrara N. The vascular endothelial growth factor (VEGF) isoforms: differential deposition into the subepithelial extracellular matrix and bioactivity of extracellular matrix-bound VEGF. Mol Biol Cell. 1993;4:1317–1326.

23. Papapetropoulos A, García-Cardeña G, Madri JA, et al. Nitric oxide production contributes to the angiogenic properties of vascular endothelial growth factor in human endothelial cells. J Clin Invest. 1997;100:3131–3139.

24. Aiello LP, Northrup JM, Keyt BA, et al. Hypoxic regulation of vascular endothelial growth factor in retinal cells. Arch Ophthalmol. 1995;113(12):1538–1544.

25. Ferrara N, Hillan KJ, Gerer HP, et al. Discovery and development of bevacizumab, an anti-VEGF antibody for treating cancer. Nat Rev Drug Discov. 2004;3(5):391–400.

26. Usui T, Ishida S, Yamashiro K, et al. VEGF164(165) as the pathological isoform: differential leukocyte and endothelial responses through VEGFR1 and VEGFR2. Invest Ophthalmol Vis Sci. 2004;45(2):368–374.

27. Ishida S, Usui T, Yamashiro K, et al. VEGF164-mediated inflammation is required for pathological, but not physiological, ischemia-induced retinal neovascularization. J Exp Med. 2003;198(3):483–489.

28. Moshfeghi AA, Puliafito CA. Pegaptanib sodium for the treatment of neovascular age-related macular degeneration. Expert Opin Investig Drugs. 2005;14(5):671–682.

29. Drolet DW, Nelson J, Tucker CE, et al. Pharmacokinetics and safety of an anti-vascular endothelial growth factor aptamer (NX1838) following injection into the vitreous humor of rhesus monkeys. Pharm Res. 2000;17(12):1503–1510.

30. Bell C, Lynam E, Landfair DJ, et al. Oligonucleotide NX1838 inhibits VEGF165-mediated cellular responses in vitro. In Vitro Cell Dev Biol Anim. 1999;35(9):533–542.

31. Gragoudas ES, Adamis AP, Cunningham ET Jr, et al. Pegaptanib for neovascular age-related macular degeneration. N Engl J Med. 2004;351(27):2805–2816.

32. Eyetech/Pfizer: Pegaptanib sodium injection (Macugen™). Dermatologic and Ophthalmic Drugs Advisory Committee Meeting, August 27 2004. Food and Drug Administration. Rockville, MD; 2004.

33. Chakravarthy U, Adamis AP, Cunningham ET Jr, et al. Year 2 efficacy results of 2 randomized controlled clinical trials of pegaptanib for neovascular age-related macular degeneration. Ophthalmology. 2006;113(9):1508, e1501–e1525.

34. Friberg TR, Tolentino M. for the LEVEL Study Group: Pegaptanib sodium as maintenance therapy in neovascular age-related macular degeneration: the LEVEL study. Br J Ophthalmol. 2010;94:1611–1617.

35. The VEGF Inhibition Study in Ocular Neovascularization (VISION) Clinical Trial Group: Enhanced efficacy associated with early treatment of neovascular age-related macular degeneration with pegaptanib sodium: an exploratory analysis. Retina. 2005;25:815–827.

36. Apte RS. Pegaptanib sodium for the treatment of age-related macular degeneration. Expert Opin Pharmacother. 2008;9(3):499–508.

37. Genentech website (2011). Available from: http://www.gene.com/gene/products/information/oncology/avastin/insert.jsp#warnings

38. Apte RS, Modi M, Masonson H, et al. Pegaptanib 1-year systemic safety results from a safety-pharmacokinetic trial in patients with neovascular age-related macular degeneration. Ophthalmology. 2007;114(9):1702–1712.

39. Available from: www.agingeye.net/mainnews/macugenlabel.pdf

40. D'Amico DJ, Masonson HN, Patel M, et al. Pegaptanib sodium for age-related macular degeneration: two-year safety results of the two prospective, multicenter, controlled clinical trials. Ophthalmology. 2006;113(6):992–1001.

41. Singerman LJ, Masonson H, Patel M, et al. Pegaptanib sodium for age-related macular degeneration: third-year safety results of the VEGF Inhibition Study in Ocular Neovascularization (VISION) trial. Br J Ophthalmol. 2008;92:1606–1611.

42. Cavalcante LL, Cavalcante ML, Murray TG, et al. Intravitreal injection analysis at the Bascom Palmer Eye Institute: evaluation of clinical indications for the treatment and incidence rates of endophthalmitis. Clin Ophthalmol. 2010;25:519–524.

43. Moshfeghi AA. Rate of endophthalmitis after anti-VEGF intravitreal injection. Retina Today. 2008;2:75–76.

44. Pilli S, Kotsolis A, Spaide RF, et al. Endophthalmitis associated with intravitreal anti-vascular endothelial growth factor therapy injections in an office setting. Am J Ophthalmol. 2008;145:879–882.

45. Brown DM, Kaiser PK, Michels M, et al.; ANCHOR Study Group. Ranibizumab versus verteporfin for neovascular age-related macular degeneration. N Engl J Med. 2006;355(14):1432–1444.

46. Rosenfeld PJ, Brown DM, Heier JS, et al.; MARINA Study Group. Ranibizumab for neovascular age-related macular degeneration. N Engl J Med. 2006;355(14):1419–1431.

47. Martin DF, Maguire MG, Ying GS, et al.; CATT Research Group. Ranibizumab and bevacizumab for neovascular age-related macular degeneration. N Engl J Med. 2011;364(20):1897–1908.

48. Verheul HM, Pinedo HM. Possible molecular mechanisms involved in the toxicity of angiogenesis inhibition. Nat Rev Cancer. 2007;7:475–485.

49. Bombeli T, Karsan A, Tait JF, et al. Apoptotic vascular endothelial cells become procoagulant. Blood. 1997;89:2429–2442.

50. Russell DA, Abbott CR, Gough MJ. Vascular endothelial growth factor is associated with histological instability of carotid plaques. Br J Surg. 2008;95:576–581.

51. Van Wijngaarden P, Coster DJ, Williams KA. Inhibitors of ocular neovascularization: promises and potential problems. JAMA. 2005;293(12):1509–1513.

52. Gilles MC, Wong TY. Ranibizumab for neovascular age-related macular degeneration. N Engl J Med. 2007;356:748–749.

53. Ueta T, Yanagi Y, Tamaki Y, et al. Cerebrovascular accidents in ranibizumab. Ophthalmology. 2009;116:1731–1739.

54. Genentech website (2007). Available from: http://www.gene.com/gene/products/information/pdf/healthcare-provider-letter.pdf

55. Lalwani GA, Rosenfeld PJ, Fung AE, et al. A variable-dosing regimen with intravitreal ranibizumab for neovascular age-related macular degeneration: year 2 of the PrONTO Study. Am J Ophthalmol. 2009;148(1):43–58.

56. Hughes MS, Sang DN. Safety and efficacy of intravitreal bevacizumab followed by pegaptanib maintenance as a treatment regimen for age-related macular degeneration. Ophthalmic Surg Lasers Imaging. 2006;37(6):446–454.

57. Farah SE. Treatment of age-related macular degeneration with pegaptanib and boosting with bevacizumab or ranibizumab as needed. Ophthalmic Surg Lasers Imaging. 2008;39:294–298.

17

LUCENTIS (RANIBIZUMAB)

JOANNA L. GOULAH • D. VIRGIL ALFARO III • CARLOS E. ORTIZ

■ INTRODUCTION

Ranibizumab is marketed as LUCENTIS (ranibizumab injection) and was approved by the U.S. Food and Drug Administration (FDA) in June 2006 for the treatment of neovascular (wet) age-related macular degeneration (AMD). Ranibizumab has also received regulatory approval for the treatment of neovascular AMD in more than 100 countries worldwide. Ranibizumab binds to the receptor binding site of active forms of vascular endothelium growth factor-A (VEGF-A), including the biologically active, cleaved form of this molecule, VEGF110.

VEGF is a secreted homodimeric protein that is a potent vascular endothelial cell mitogen (1). VEGF stimulates vascular endothelial cell growth, functions as a survival factor for newly formed vessels, and induces vascular permeability. VEGF expression is up-regulated by hypoxia as well as by a number of other stimuli. Although other angiogenic factors have been identified, VEGF is perhaps the most potent and specific, with a well-defined role in normal and pathologic angiogenesis. Inappropriate overexpression of VEGF has been hypothesized as playing a key role in the growth of solid tumors and in vascular retinopathies such as AMD (Fig. 17.1).

VEGF-A has been shown to cause neovascularization and leakage in models of ocular angiogenesis and is thought to contribute to the progression of AMD. Inhibition of inappropriate VEGF activity is a so-called antiangiogenic approach to the treatment of these diseases. The binding of ranibizumab to VEGF-A prevents the interaction of VEGF-A with its receptors (VEGFR1 and VEGFR2) on the surface of endothelial cells, reducing endothelial cell proliferation, vascular leakage, and new blood vessel formation.

Ranibizumab, an anti–human VEGF, affinity-matured Fab, has been developed by Genentech as a therapeutic agent for treating ocular vascular disease by intravitreal (ITV) injection.

■ RANIBIZUMAB

Drug Biochemistry and Formulation

Affinity-matured ranibizumab is produced by standard recombinant technology methods in an *Escherichia coli* expression vector and bacterial fermentation. Ranibizumab is not glycosylated and has a molecular mass of approximately 48,000 Da.

The lyophilized form of the drug is produced from a freeze-drying process. The solid cake seen in each vial consists of protein and the excipient components that are stabilizing agents for the protein. The lyophilized form of ranibizumab requires reconstitution with Sterile Water for Injection (SWI), USP. After reconstitution with SWI, the highly concentrated protein solution is further diluted with vehicle prior to ITV administration. This presentation was useful in early clinical dose-ranging studies and was used in early phase I/phase II studies.

The liquid formulation is the commercial form. This presentation provides excellent stability and eliminates the need for reconstitution and further dilution. Liquid ranibizumab is formulated as a sterile solution aseptically filled in a sterile, 2-mL glass vial. Each vial is designed to deliver 0.05 mL of 10 mg/mL of ranibizumab aqueous solution with 10 mM histidine HCI, 10% α,α-trehalose dehydrate, and 0.01% polysorbate 20 (pH 5.5). The vial contains no preservative

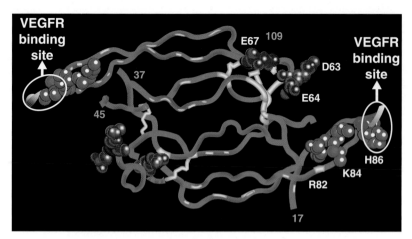

Figure 17.1 ■ Vascular endothelial growth factor (VEGF) is a homodimeric glycoprotein that is secreted in response to hypoxia and ischemia. VEGF induces angiogenesis and vascular permeability. *Arrows* show the binding site VEGFR. (Reprinted with permission from Quiroz-Mercado H, Kerrison JB, Alfaro DV, et al. Macular surgery, 2nd ed. Philadelphia, PA: Lippincott Williams & Wilkins; 2011.)

and is suitable for single use only. Vials should be protected from light. The liquid formulation was assayed for purity and identity as described for the lyophilized form. The assay for potency is a biologically relevant, cell-based assay in which the ability to inhibit VEGF-dependent growth in vitro with a cell line requiring VEGF for growth is quantified.

VEGF THE TARGET

Human VEGF exists as at least six isoforms (VEGF121, VEGF145, VEGF165, VEGF183, VEGF189, and VEGF206) that evolve from alternative splicing of mRNA of a single gene (1). VEGF165, the most abundant isoform, is a basic, heparin binding, dimeric glycoprotein with a molecular mass of approximately 45,000 Da (1). Two VEGF receptor tyrosine kinases, VEGFR1 and VEGFR2, have been identified (2–7). VEGFR1 has the highest affinity for VEGF, with a Kd of approximately 10 to 20 pM (8), and VEGFR2 has a somewhat lower affinity for VEGF with a Kd of approximately 75 to 125 pM (9–11).

VEGF has numerous biologic functions, including regulation of VEGF gene expression under hypoxic conditions (1), mitogenic activity for micro- and macrovascular endothelial cells (4–7,12–14), and induction of expression of plasminogen activators and collagenase (15). Of particular significance to wet AMD are the angiogenic properties of VEGF, which have been demonstrated in a variety of in vivo models, including the chick chorioallantoic membrane (15,16), rabbit cornea (17), and rabbit bone (17). VEGF also functions as a survival factor for newly formed endothelial cells (16,18). Consistent with prosurvival activity, VEGF stimulates expression of the antiapoptotic proteins Bcl-2 and A1 in human endothelial cells (19). VEGF has been shown to induce vascular leakage in guinea pig skin (19). Dvorak et al. (20,21) suggested that an increase in microvascular

permeability is a crucial step in angiogenesis associated with tumors and wound healing. According to this hypothesis, a core function of VEGF in the angiogenic process is the induction of plasma protein leakage. This outcome would result in the formation of an extravascular fibrin gel, which serves as a substrate for endothelial cells. This proposal may have substantial bearing for AMD as it is well known that permeability of the choroidal neovascularization (CNV) membrane results in the transduction of serum components beneath and into the retina, creating serous macular detachment, macular edema, and vision loss.

VEGF is expressed in an assortment of cells in the normal human retina. Colocalization of VEGF mRNA and protein is detected in the ganglion cell, inner nuclear and outer plexiform layers, the walls of the blood vessels, and photoreceptors (22). Retinal pigment epithelium (RPE), Müller cells, pericytes, vascular endothelium, and ganglion cells all manufacture VEGF (23,24).

Studies have documented the immunohistochemical localization of VEGF in surgically resected CNV membranes from AMD patients. Kvanta et al. (20) demonstrated the presence of VEGF mRNA and protein in RPE cells and fibroblast-like cells. Lopez et al. (19) noted that the RPE cells that were strongly immunoreactive for VEGF were present primarily in the highly vascularized regions of CNV membranes, whereas the RPE cells found in fibrotic regions of CNV membranes showed little VEGF reactivity. Kliffen et al. (25) also demonstrated increased VEGF expression in RPE cells and choroidal blood vessels in maculae from patients with wet AMD compared with controls.

An increase in VEGF expression has been noted in experimental models of CNV in rats and in nonhuman primates (26). In addition, transgenic mice with increased VEGF expression in photoreceptors (27) or RPE (28) developed neovascularization reminiscent of CNV seen in

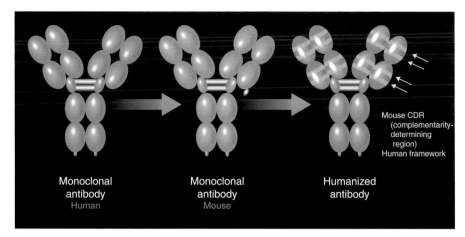

Figure 17.2 ■ The humanization of muMAb VEGF A.4.6.1 involved the transfer of six complimentary-determining regions (CDR) from muMAb VEGF A.4.6.1 to a human framework by site-directed mutagenesis. The final antibody is a rhuMAb (recombinant, humanized, monoclonal antibody). (Reprinted with permission from Quiroz-Mercado H, Kerrison JB, Alfaro DV, et al. Macular surgery, 2nd ed. Philadelphia, PA: Lippincott Williams & Wilkins; 2011.)

humans with neovascular AMD. This further supports the participation of VEGF in ocular neovascularization. These lines of evidence suggest that VEGF is a practical target for therapeutic intervention in neovascular AMD.

Inhibition of VEGF Activity by Ranibizumab

In Vitro Evaluation of Ranibizumab

A number of antibodies that can bind VEGF or inhibit VEGF activity were considered in vitro and in vivo for molecule selection. muMAb VEGF A.4.6.1 is a full-length murine monoclonal antibody of the IgG1 isotype that continuously and potently defuses the biologic activities of VEGF, including the endothelial cell mitogenic activity, vascular permeability–enhancing activity, and angiogenic properties in the chick chorioallantoic membrane (29). This antibody also inhibits growth of various human tumor types in animal models1, recognizes all isoforms of VEGF, binds to VEGF with a Kd of approximately 8×10^{-10} M, and neglects to recognize other peptide growth factors. Bevacizumab (rhuMAb VEGF) is a humanized version of muMAb VEGF A.4.6.1 that was produced by site-directed mutagenesis (30) (Figs. 17.2 and 17.3).

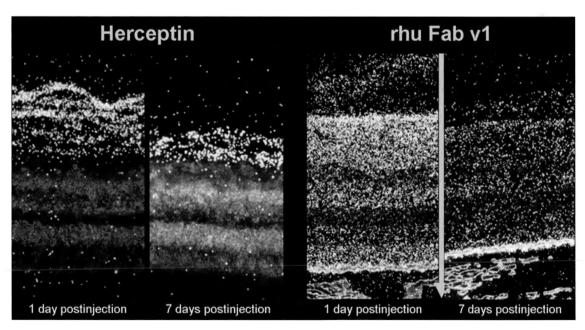

Figure 17.3 ■ Histoautoradiograph of ^{125}I-rhuMab VEGF Fab V1, the humanized Fab antibody (Column B), and ^{125}Iodine (I)-rhuMab HER2, the full-length humanized antibody (Column A) following bilateral intravitreal injections in rhesus monkeys. The Fab fragment penetrated all of the layers of the retina evenly extending as far back as the RPE while the full-length antibody failed to penetrate farther than the ILM at any point during the study. (Reprinted with permission from Quiroz-Mercado H, Kerrison JB, Alfaro DV, et al. Macular surgery, 2nd ed. Philadelphia, PA: Lippincott Williams & Wilkins; 2011.)

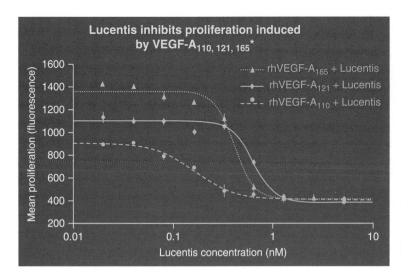

Figure 17.4 ■ HUVEC proliferation assay. rhuFab V2 Lucentis is capable of binding all three VEGF isoforms and thereby inhibits VEGF isoforms–induced endothelial cell proliferation. (Reprinted with permission from Quiroz-Mercado H, Kerrison JB, Alfaro DV, et al. Macular surgery, 2nd ed. Philadelphia, PA: Lippincott Williams & Wilkins; 2011.)

Ranibizumab is a recombinant humanized antibody Fab fragment that neutralizes VEGF. Ranibizumab shows high affinity for binding VEGF (Fig. 17.4). In addition, ranibizumab potently inhibits survival of human umbilical vein endothelial cells (HUVEC) stimulated with 5 ng/mL of recombinant human VEGF. Ranibizumab also inhibits VEGF-mediated vascular permeability in the Miles assay (Fig. 17.5).

Animal Models

Nonclinical pharmacology studies to measure the safety of ITV administration of ranibizumab during and following laser-induced CNV in cynomolgus monkeys were conducted. Study 99-166-1757 evaluated single-agent ranibizumab treatment, while study 00-580-1757 assessed ranibizumab in combination with verteporfin photodynamic therapy (PDT). The findings of these studies point out that ITV administration of ranibizumab during laser induction of a choroidal neovascular membrane and during its subsequent formation do not exhibit any irregular toxicity. Moreover, treatment with ranibizumab in the cynomolgus monkey model prevents membrane formation and attenuates permeability from already-formed choroidal neovascular membranes (31) (Figs. 17.6 and 17.7).

Following ITV administration in normal rabbits and cynomolgus monkeys, ranibizumab was cleared from the vitreous humor with a half-life of approximately 3 days and was distributed to all layers of the retina and cells where VEGF is expressed. In rabbits, a fraction of ranibizumab was cleared from the vitreous humor and through the choroidal capillaries. Concentrations of aqueous humor declined in parallel with those in the vitreous

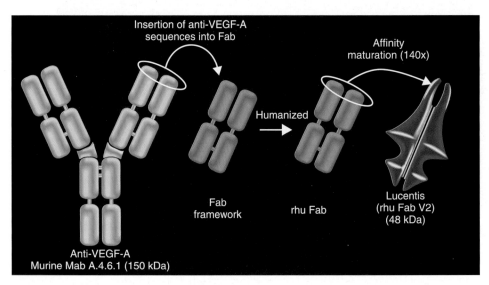

Figure 17.5 ■ RhuMAb VEGF was fragmented and affinity matured through complementarity-determining region (CDR) mutation and affinity selection by monovalent phage display. (Reprinted with permission from Quiroz-Mercado H, Kerrison JB, Alfaro DV, et al. Macular surgery, 2nd ed. Philadelphia, PA: Lippincott Williams & Wilkins; 2011.)

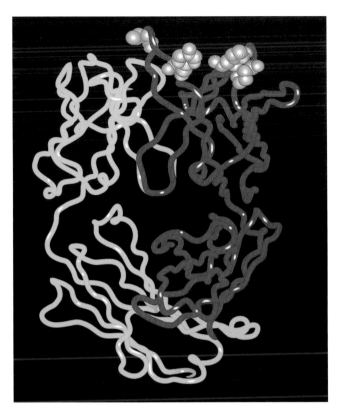

Figure 17.6 ■ The VEGF and the affinity-matured Fab fragment complex. Locally, it was possible to improve the contact between the antibody and the antigen through two mutations that improved the hydrogen bonding and van der Waals contact. (Reprinted with permission from Quiroz-Mercado H, Kerrison JB, Alfaro DV, et al. Macular surgery, 2nd ed. Philadelphia, PA: Lippincott Williams & Wilkins; 2011.)

beyond Day 7 (after IV administration, the mean terminal half-life of ranibizumab was 3.1 hours). The systemic bioavailability of ranibizumab following ITV administration was estimated to be approximately 67%, suggesting that intraocular metabolism is not the predominant mechanism for clearance of ranibizumab from the vitreous humor. As expected with administration of a human protein into rabbits, antibodies to ranibizumab were detected in the vitreous humor by Day 7 but did not seem to affect the decline of ranibizumab concentrations in this compartment. Day 14 also detected antibodies to ranibizumab in serum. In cynomolgus monkeys, there did not appear to be dose-related differences for vitreous humor clearance and steady-state volume. Dose-normalized areas under the curves (AUCs) were also similar and suggested no dose-related differences in ranibizumab vitreous humor pharmacokinetics. In aqueous humor and retina, the half-life of ranibizumab was similar to that in vitreous humor, while the AUC was approximately two- to threefold lower. The apparent elimination half-life of ranibizumab in serum was similar to that in vitreous humor, while after IV administration, it was approximately 15 hours. Ranibizumab concentrations in serum increased proportionally with dose and were 400 to 1,500 fold lower than those in vitreous humor. The systemic bioavailability of ranibizumab after bilateral ITV administration of 0.5 mg and 2 mg per eye was estimated to be 60% and 50%, respectively. Regardless of dose, antibodies against ranibizumab were detected in the serum of some of the animals following the second dose; the incidence of antibodies tended to increase with increasing dose. Consistent with the estimates of half-life in vitreous and serum, ranibizumab did not appear to accumulate in the serum of antibody-negative animals when it was administered every 14 days in rabbits (Fig. 17.8).

humor but were approximately 17 times lower. Serum ranibizumab concentrations were approximately 1/1,000 of vitreous concentrations and could not be quantified

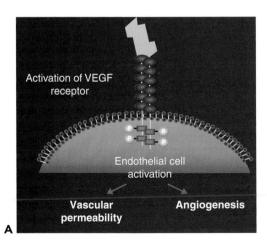
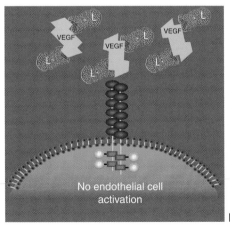

Figure 17.7 ■ **A.** Activation of the VEGF receptor (VEGFR1 and VEGFR2) of the endothelial cell by the VEGF generates an endothelial cell activation that increases the vascular permeability and induces angiogenesis. **B.** Lucentis binds to the receptor binding site of active forms of VEGF-A, avoid the interaction of VEGF-A with its receptors, on the surface of endothelial cells, reducing endothelial cell proliferation, vascular leakage, and new blood vessel formation. (Reprinted with permission from Quiroz-Mercado H, Kerrison JB, Alfaro DV, et al. Macular surgery, 2nd ed. Philadelphia, PA: Lippincott Williams & Wilkins; 2011.)

Nonclinical single and multidose toxicology studies were conducted to support the clinical use of ranibizumab administered up to once every 2 weeks by ITV. Based on flare and cell responses, 0.5 mg ranibizumab per eye were considered to be the maximum tolerated dose for a single dose in cynomolgus monkeys. In summary, the available data have shown that ranibizumab is successful in suppressing CNV in nonhuman primates.

In summary, ITV administered ranibizumab was shown to diffuse to sites of VEGF expression in the retina of rabbits and monkeys. Ranibizumab was cleared relatively slowly, with a half-life of approximately 3 days from the vitreous humor of both species. Combined the in vitro data, the in vivo ocular pharmacokinetics in animals, and the extrapolation to humans (adapting for ocular size and using the mean pharmacokinetic parameters obtained in monkeys) strongly recommend that concentrations capable of inhibiting neovascularization in the retina can be attained in humans following ITV ranibizumab doses of 0.3 to 0.5 mg per eye.

CLINICAL TRIALS

Ranibizumab in Humans: Phase I/II Studies

Three studies were designed to investigate the doses of ranibizumab that would be appropriate for the treatment of neovascular AMD in large, multicenter, randomized phase I/II clinical trials. The first, FVF 1770g, a phase I dose-escalating study with patients with neovascular AMD (32); the second, a larger, phase I/II clinical study, investigated the tolerability and efficacy of multiple monthly ITV injections of ranibizumab at doses of 0.3 mg or 0.5 mg in patients with neovascular AMD (33); and the third trial, a phase I clinical study, investigated doses of ranibizumab above 0.5 mg to determine if doses higher than the maximum tolerated single dose could be well accepted when injected in an escalating stepwise fashion every 2 or 4 weeks (34). From the data analysis of these three clinical trials, the study team concludes that dose-limiting toxicity resulting in ocular inflammation was reached at 1,000 µg per eye. A dose of 500 µg per eye was determined to be the maximum tolerated dose; ITV injections of ranibizumab at escalating doses ranging from 0.3 to 2.0 mg were well tolerated; no serum antibodies against ranibizumab were observed (no antimouse immunoresponse that might decrease ranibizumab's efficacy); the drug had a good safety profile with an improved VA and decreased leakage from CNV in subjects with neovascular AMD (Fig. 17.9).

Based on these results, Genentech initiated another phase I/II study: the FOCUS Study. This trial was a single-masked, multicenter study evaluating the safety, tolerability, and efficacy of multiple-dose ITV injections of ranibizumab used in combinations with PDT in patients with predominantly classic AMD. After 2 years, the study showed a clear visual acuity benefit of adding ranibizumab to PDT treatment (35) (Fig. 17.10).

The EXTENSION Study (FVF2508g) was a study to evaluate the long-term safety and tolerability of ranibizumab given as multiple ITV injections in subjects with primary or recurrent subfoveal CNV secondary to AMD who had completed the treatment phase of a Genentech-sponsored phase I or phase I/II ranibizumab study. The subjects were followed for treatment duration of up to 1,345 days, and subjects received up to 44 ITV injections. When the extension study concluded, at the time it represented the longest period of study of ranibizumab. The safety findings supported the further study of ranibizumab for long-term administration in subjects with neovascular AMD. Repeated ITV injection of ranibizumab was associated with a low rate

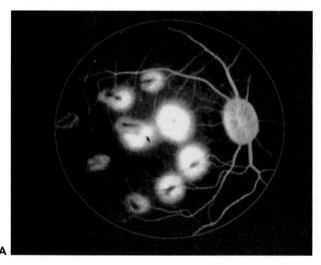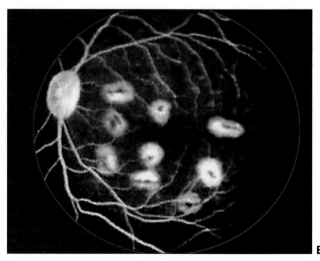

Figure 17.8 ■ Krzystolik assay. Cynomolgus monkeys, model of choroidal neovascularization. **A.** Pre-rhuFab injection. **B.** After rhuFab injection. (Reprinted with permission from Quiroz-Mercado H, Kerrison JB, Alfaro DV, et al. Macular surgery, 2nd ed. Philadelphia, PA: Lippincott Williams & Wilkins; 2011.)

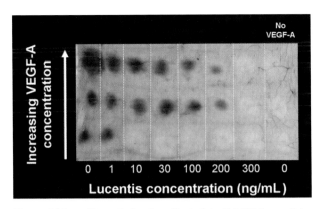

Figure 17.9 ■ Characterize the effect of rhuFab V2 (Lucentis) inhibition on VEGF-induced permeability in guinea pigs (Miles assay). (From Gaudreault J, Reich M, Arata A, et al. Ocular pharmacokinetics and antipermeability effect of rhuFab V2 in animals. Invest Ophthalmol Vis Sci. 2003;44(4):3942–3943.)

of serious ocular adverse events, and it commonly induced mild intraocular inflammation. Ranibizumab was well tolerated systemically after multiple ITV injections. There was a low incidence of serum immunoreactivity to the study drug. Positive serum immunoreactivity did not appear to be associated with adverse events such as intraocular inflammation or marked decrease in visual acuity; however, the number of patients with positive antitherapeutic antibodies was small. Although the study was not designed to assess efficacy in terms of visual acuity, most subjects treated in the extension study experienced improved or preserved visual function.

There have been several phase III/IV clinical trials developed by Genentech in the United States during the past 9 years to prove the efficacy and safety of ranibizumab: MARINA, ANCHOR, HARBOR, PIER, SAILOR, and PrONTO.

MARINA Study (FVF 2598g)

The MARINA study was the first phase III clinical trial designed. It was a multicenter, randomized, double-masked, sham injection–controlled study of the efficacy and safety of ranibizumab in subjects with minimally classic or occult subfoveal neovascular AMD (36). Subjects were randomized in a 1:1:1 ratio to receive 0.5-mg ranibizumab, 0.3-mg ranibizumab, or a sham injection administered monthly (30 ± 7 days) for up to a maximum of 24 injections during the 2-year study period. Approximately 3 months prior to the study's completion, subjects in the sham injection group who still remained on treatment were offered the opportunity to cross over to receive 0.5-mg ranibizumab for the remainder of the treatment period. The study met its primary end point, with nearly 95% of ranibizumab-treated subjects maintaining or improving vision at 12 months, compared with 62% of sham-treated subjects. The benefit of ranibizumab treatment over sham injections increased further through 24 months (Fig. 17.11). Ranibizumab administered as monthly ITV injections of 0.3 mg or 0.5 mg over 24 months was safe and well tolerated by subjects with minimally classic or occult subfoveal neovascular AMD.

ANCHOR Study (FVF2587g)

The ANCHOR study was a 2-year, phase III, multicenter, randomized, double-masked, active treatment–controlled study of the efficacy and safety of ranibizumab compared with PDT in subjects with predominantly classic subfoveal neovascular AMD (37). Subjects were randomized in a 1:1:1 ratio to receive 0.3 mg ranibizumab and sham PDT with saline infusion, 0.5-mg ranibizumab and sham PDT with saline infusion,

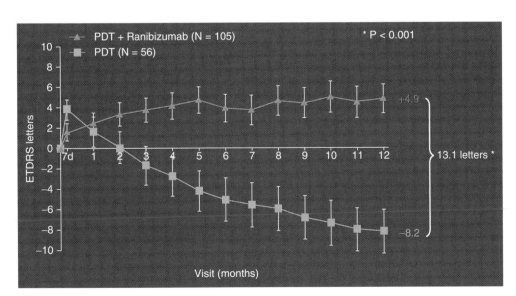

Figure 17.10 ■ Mean change in visual acuity in FOCUS study. (Reprinted with permission from Quiroz-Mercado H, Kerrison JB, Alfaro DV, et al. Macular surgery, 2nd ed. Philadelphia, PA: Lippincott Williams & Wilkins; 2011.)

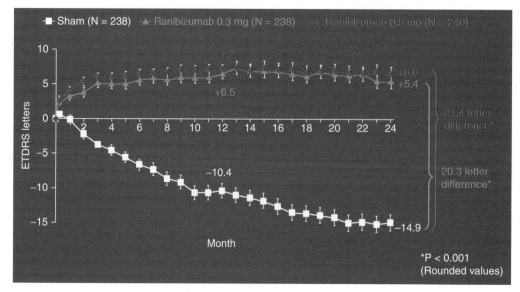

Figure 17.11 ■ Mean change in visual acuity in MARINA study. (Reprinted with permission from Quiroz-Mercado H, Kerrison JB, Alfaro DV, et al. Macular surgery, 2nd ed. Philadelphia, PA: Lippincott Williams & Wilkins; 2011.)

or sham injection of ranibizumab and active PDT. Subjects received a ranibizumab or sham injection monthly (30 ± 7 days) for 23 months of treatment (24 injections) and active (verteporfin) or sham (saline) PDT on Day 0 and every 3 months if needed (as determined by the assessment of FA by the evaluating physician) for 21 months of treatment. After review of the 12-month data of this study, the protocol was amended to allow subjects in the active verteporfin PDT study arm who still remained in the study the opportunity to receive treatment with 0.3-mg ranibizumab. The study met its primary efficacy objective, with approximately 94% of subjects treated with 0.3-mg ranibizumab and 96% of subjects treated with 0.5-mg ranibizumab maintaining or improving vision at Month 12 compared with approximately 64% of verteporfin PDT–treated subjects ($P < 0.0001$ for superiority for each of the ranibizumab groups vs. the verteporfin PDT group). At Month 12, approximately 36% of subjects in the 0.3-mg group and 40% of subjects in the 0.5-mg group gained ≥15 letters from baseline compared with approximately 6% of

subjects receiving verteporfin PDT ($P < 0.0001$ for treatment comparisons vs. verteporfin PDT). VA improved by an average of approximately 9 letters from baseline in the 0.3-mg group and 11 letters in the 0.5-mg group at Month 12 compared with a decline by an average of approximately 10 letters in the verteporfin PDT group ($P < 0.0001$ for treatment comparisons vs. verteporfin PDT) (Fig. 17.12).

PIER Study (FVF3192g)

The PIER study was a 2-year, phase IIIb, multicenter, randomized, double-masked, sham injection–controlled study of the efficacy and safety of ranibizumab in subjects with CNV with or without classic CNV secondary to AMD. This study assessed the efficacy and safety of ITV injections of ranibizumab administered monthly, for three doses, followed by doses every 3 months compared with sham injections. The PIER study met its primary end point, with an estimated benefit from baseline to 24 months in best-corrected

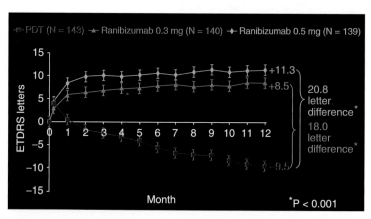

Figure 17.12 ■ Mean change in visual acuity in ANCHOR study.

visual acuity (BCVA) score compared with sham of 18.1 letters for the 0.3-mg group and 17.3 letters for the 0.5-mg group. Across the secondary end points, a statistically significant benefit was observed for the percentage of subjects losing less than 15 letters at 12 months compared with baseline, as well as for each of the secondary angiography and anatomic end points. The 2-year results demonstrated a statistically significant beneficial effect of ranibizumab on visual acuity and retinal anatomy. Within each of the ranibizumab dose groups, the outcomes of the primary end point and all secondary end points at 12 months were maintained at 24 months; in contrast, the outcomes continued to decline in subjects in the sham injection group. As a result, the estimated treatment benefit of each ranibizumab dose over the sham control was somewhat greater at 24 months than that at 12 months for the primary end point and most of the secondary efficacy end points and exploratory efficacy end points. Visual acuity decreased by an average of approximately two letters from baseline at 24 months in both ranibizumab groups compared with a decline by an average of approximately 21 letters in the sham injection group ($P < 0.0001$ for treatment comparisons vs. sham). At 24 months, 78.3% of subjects in the 0.3-mg group and 82.0% of subjects in the 0.5-mg group lost fewer than 15 letters from baseline compared with 41.3% of subjects given sham injections ($P < 0.0001$ for each ranibizumab dose group vs. sham).

A beneficial effect of ranibizumab on lesion anatomy was also observed based on optical coherence tomography (OCT) assessments in the first treatment year (no OCT assessment in the 2nd year). At Month 12, a statistically significant ($P < 0.007$) within-group reduction from baseline in retinal thickness and total retinal volume of the study eye was seen as early as Month 1 in ranibizumab-treated subjects. At 12 months, the mean change from baseline in foveal retinal thickness was approximately –123 to –126 µm for the ranibizumab groups; in the sham injection group, foveal retinal thickness decreased by an average of 28.5 µm ($P < 0.01$ for each ranibizumab dose group vs. sham). A beneficial effect of ranibizumab on lesion anatomy was observed based on fluorescein angiography assessments. At 24 months, the area of CNV increased, on average, by approximately 0.3 to 0.6 DA in

the ranibizumab groups; in the sham injection group, the area of CNV increased by an average of 1.9 DA ($P \leq 0.002$ for each ranibizumab dose group vs. sham). At 24 months, the area of leakage plus RPE staining decreased by an average of approximately 1.2 to 1.5 DA in the ranibizumab groups, while decreasing by an average of approximately 0.78 DA in the sham injection group. At Month 24, the area of classic CNV, on average, decreased by approximately 0.4 DA in the two ranibizumab groups; in the sham injection group, it increased by approximately 1.4 DA ($P \leq 0.0002$ for treatment comparisons vs. sham injection group). The 24-month results in area of lesion, area of subretinal fluid, and significant growth of CNV also favored the ranibizumab groups. Ranibizumab, administered as 3 monthly ITV injections of 0.3 mg or 0.5 mg followed by injections every 3 months or more frequently over 24 months, was effective in maintaining visual acuity in subjects with minimally classic, occult, or predominantly classic subfoveal neovascular AMD. Ranibizumab, administered as three monthly ITV injections of 0.3 mg or 0.5 mg followed by injections every 3 months or more frequently over 24 months, was safe and well tolerated by subjects with minimally classic, occult, or predominantly classic subfoveal neovascular AMD (Table 17.1).

PrONTO Study

The Prospective OCT Imaging of Patients with Neovascular AMD Treated with intraocular Ranibizumab (PrONTO) Study assessed a variable dosing regimen mainly based on OCT findings. Patients received three consecutive monthly ITV injections of ranibizumab 0.5 mg and were then evaluated monthly for retreatment. Re-treatment with ranibizumab was performed at each monthly visit if any criterion was fulfilled such as a loss of five letters or more or an increase of at least 100 µm, during the first year, or if any qualitative increase in the amount of fluid was detected using OCT, during the 2nd year (38). The PrONTO Study demonstrated variable-dosing regimen to be as effective as a fixed-dosing regimen in improving visual acuity and OCT findings with a far lower number of injections over a period of 12 and even 24 months.

Table 17.1	RESULTS FOR THE 3 PHASE III STUDIES								
Study findings	Anchor study (N:423)			Marina study (N:716)			Pier study (N:184)		
	Classic CNV			Occult CNV			Quarterly dosing		
	0.3 mg	0.5 mg	PDT arm	0.3 mg	0.5 mg	Sham arm	0.3 mg	0.5 mg	Sham arm
Main change VA	(+)8.5	(+)11.3	(–)9.5	(+)5.4	(+)6.6	(–)14	(–)1.6	(–)0.2	(–)16.3
>15 Letters gain	36%	40%	6%	26%	33%	4%	12%	13%	10%
Lost <15 letters	94%	96%	64%	90%	92%	53%	83%	90%	49%
20/40 or better	31%	39%	3%	34%	42%	6%	30%	28%	11%

SAILOR Study (FVF3689g)

This phase III trial was designed to investigate the safety and tolerability of ranibizumab in naive and previously treated subjects with CNV secondary to AMD. This study enrolled a total of 4,313 subjects and was completed on July 16, 2007. Subjects in Cohort 1 (N = 2,378) were randomized (1:1) to receive ranibizumab at a dose level of 0.3 mg or 0.5 mg; subjects were masked to these dose levels. Treatment was administered monthly for three initial doses (Day 0, Month 1, and Month 2), with scheduled follow-up visits on Months 3, 6, 9, and 12. Retreatment after the first three injections was performed as needed, on the basis of predefined criteria with injections no more frequently than every 30 days. Retreatment in Cohort 1 was held in the event of either of the following; Central retinal thickness ≤225 μm, determined using OCT, with absence of intraretinal and subretinal fluid, BCVA of 20/20 or better in the study eye, determined using Early Treatment of Diabetic Retinopathy Study (ETDRS) chart Cohort 2 (N = 1,922) consisted of subjects enrolled after the majority of Cohort 1 subjects had been enrolled, with enrollment continuing until ranibizumab was approved or denied by the FDA for US marketing, and if approved, until commercially available or September 30, 2006, whichever was earlier. Subjects in Cohort 2 received open-label ranibizumab at the 0.5-mg dose level, with an initial injection on Day 0 followed by retreatment at the physician's discretion, no more frequently than every 30 days. Subjects were monitored for safety for a total of 12 months; safety information, including both serious and nonserious adverse events, was collected at every clinic visit, with two formal safety visits scheduled at Months 6 and 12. The study consisted of a 30-day screening period and a 1-year treatment period. Treatment duration was approximately 197 days for both dose groups in Cohort 1 and 144 days for subjects in Cohort 2. The mean follow-up time differed between Cohort 1 and Cohort 2, 337 days versus 254 days, respectively. Ranibizumab was well tolerated, and the incidence of ocular serious adverse events (SAEs) and adverse events (AEs) was low and unrelated to dose.

HARBOR Study (FVF4579g)

The HARBOR study is an ongoing 24-month, phase III, randomized, multicenter, double-masked, active treatment–controlled study evaluating the efficacy and safety of 2.0 mg and 0.5 mg ITV ranibizumab administered monthly and on an as-needed basis (PRN) in patients with subfoveal neovascular AMD. The first 12-month randomized treatment period was completed in August of 2011, and the primary analyses described here are based on these 12-month data. In total, 1098 patients were enrolled and randomized in a 1:1:1:1 ratio to one of four treatment arms: 0.5 mg monthly (n = 276), 0.5 mg PRN (n = 275), 2.0 mg monthly (n = 274), or 2.0 mg PRN (n = 273). Using the prespecified multiplicity adjustment approach (Hochberg-Bonferroni approach) and prespecified noninferior margin of four letters,

the 2.0-mg monthly dose was not superior to the 0.5-mg monthly dose, and the 0.5-mg PRN and 2.0-mg PRN doses were not noninferior to the 0.5-mg monthly dose. The mean change from baseline in BCVA at Month 12 for the 0.5-mg monthly, 0.5-mg PRN, 2.0-mg PRN, and 2.0-mg monthly arms were 10.1, 8.2, 8.6, and 9.2 letters, respectively. Although Study FVF4579g did not meet the prespecified statistical analyses for the primary end point, clinically meaningful visual and anatomic benefits of ITV ranibizumab (0.5 mg or 2 mg) administered monthly or PRN over 12 months were observed for all treatment groups (Fig. 17.6). The 0.5-mg PRN and 2.0-mg PRN groups achieved these results with a mean of 7.7 and 6.9 injections, respectively (out of 12 possible injections), compared with a mean of 11.3 and 11.2 injections in the 0.5-mg monthly and 2.0-mg monthly groups, respectively (Fig. 17.13).

There are two clinical trials developed by Novartis (June 2003—Novartis Ophthalmics and Genentech announced that they have entered into an agreement under which Novartis Ophthalmics will receive an exclusive license to develop and market Lucentis outside of North America) using Lucentis outside United States: EXCITE and SUSTAIN.

EXCITE Study (CRFB002A2302)

This study was a randomized, double-masked, active-controlled, stratified, multicenter study conducted by Novartis outside of the United States. The study was designed to compare the efficacy and safety of two alternative dosing regimens of ranibizumab with monthly dosing of ranibizumab. Patients were randomized in a 1:1:1 ratio to one of three different masked treatment arms. Treatment arm A: 0.3 mg ranibizumab was administered by ITV injections for 3 consecutive months, followed by quarterly injections (quarterly dosing). Treatment arm B: 0.5 mg of ranibizumab was administered by ITV injections for 3 consecutive months, followed by quarterly injections (quarterly dosing). Treatment arm C (the reference arm): 0.3 mg of ranibizumab was administered monthly by ITV injections for 12 consecutive months (monthly dosing). Patients randomized to treatment Arms A and B received a sham injection during the monthly visits when an ITV injection of ranibizumab was not scheduled for a total of six sham injections. The study was initiated December 22, 2005, enrolled 353 patients at 59 centers in Europe, South America, Australia, and the Middle East and was completed on January 9, 2008. The study population included male and female patients ≥50 years of age with predominantly classic, minimally classic, or occult lesions with no classic component and with primary or recurrent subfoveal CNV secondary to AMD. In addition to angiographically documented CNV, the lesion could contain additional components of subretinal hemorrhage, blocked fluorescence not from hemorrhage, and serous detachment of the RPE, but these additional components could not form ≥50% of the total lesion area. The primary efficacy end point was the mean change in BCVA

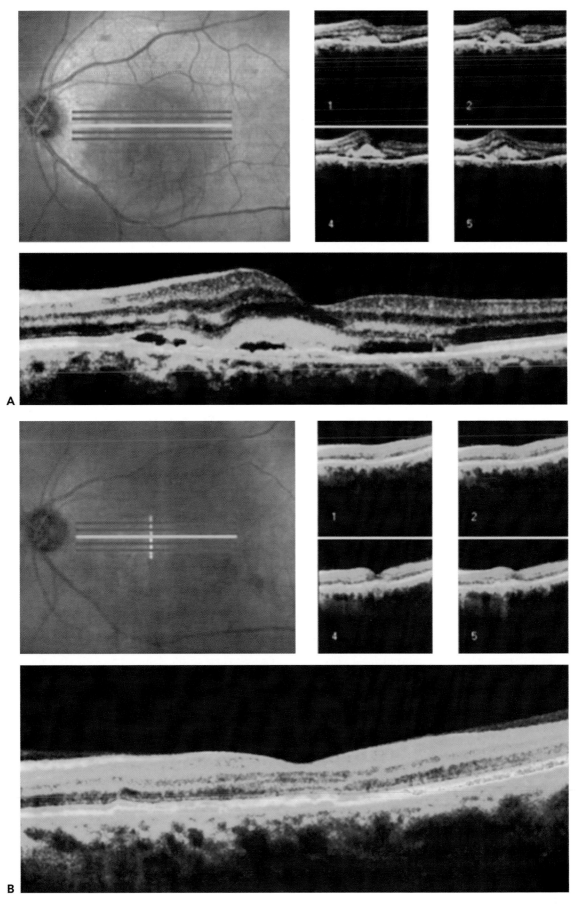

Figure 17.13 ■ **A.** HARBOR OCT pretreatment. **B.** HARBOR OCT posttreatment.

from baseline to Month 12. BCVA increased by a mean of 4.9 letters in the 0.3-mg quarterly group, 3.8 letters in the 0.5-mg quarterly group, and 8.3 letters in the 0.3-mg monthly groups. Compared with monthly dosing, the change in BCVA from baseline was 3.3 letters lower in the 0.3-mg quarterly group and 4.5 letters lower in the 0.5-mg quarterly group. During the maintenance phase (Month 3 to Month 12), BCVA decreased by 1.8 and 2.8 letters for the 0.3-mg and 0.5-mg quarterly groups, respectively, compared with an increase of 0.8 letters for the monthly group. The change in central retinal thickness from baseline to Month 12 was comparable between the three treatment groups, while the time points Month 5, 8, and 11 reflect the trough values of quarterly treatment, indicating superiority efficacy for the monthly treatment. After the loading phase in the quarterly treatment groups, a variation in change was seen from baseline over time in visual acuity and central retinal thickness. A decrease in visual acuity as well as increase in central retinal thickness was observed between quarterly ranibizumab injections. The protocol prespecified noninferiority margin of 6.8 letters is now considered to be too wide from a clinical and regulatory perspective. Given the current widely accepted margin of 5.0 letters, the 0.5-mg and 0.3-mg quarterly dosing could not be considered noninferior to monthly dosing. The data suggest the superiority of monthly treatment given the systematic pattern (in relation to the injections), the consistency in the VA time courses of the quarterly treatments, and statistically by CIs indicating such a treatment difference. Ranibizumab administered 0.3-mg monthly and 0.3-mg and 0.5-mg quarterly, after a 3-month loading phase, is safe and well tolerated in patients with CNV secondary to AMD.

SUSTAIN Study (CRFB002A2303)

This study was a phase IIIb, open-label, multicenter 12-month study conducted by Novartis outside of the United States to evaluate the safety, tolerability, and efficacy of ranibizumab (0.3 mg) in patients with subfoveal CNV secondary to AMD using a guided individualized PRN dosing regimen. The enrolled patients received three consecutive ITV injections of 0.3 mg ranibizumab monthly, and the eligibility for additional treatments was determined by the investigator based on the retreatment and/or dose-holding criteria (greater than 5-letter decrease in BCVA or greater than 100-μm increase in central retinal thickness on OCT). The study was initiated on April 7, 2006 at 60 centers in Europe and Australia and was completed on April 18, 2008. A total of 531 patients were enrolled and 519 patients were treated in this study. Participants included patients (except for those in the United States) who had completed the Core Treatment Phase of study protocol CRFB002A2301 (ANCHOR) and opted to continue in this study, newly diagnosed patients, and previously diagnosed patients who had had recent disease progression despite other prior therapy allowed by the exclusion criteria. Except for patients who

completed participation in study protocol CRFB002A2301, those previously treated with ranibizumab were not eligible to participate in this study. The study population consisted of male and female patients ≥50 years of age, with a diagnosis of active primary or recurrent CNV secondary to AMD, including those with predominantly classic, minimally classic, or occult lesions with no classic component. The total area of CNV (including both classic and occult components) encompassed by the lesion was to be ≥50% of the total lesion area, and the total lesion area was to be ≤12 disc areas. At baseline, mean visual acuity was 56.1 ± 12.19 letters, and mean central retinal thickness was 340.5 ± 113.19 μm. Mean (median) time since diagnosis of AMD was 1.3 (0.4) years. The study showed that BCVA increased from baseline to Month 3 by 5.8 letters and from baseline to Month 12 by 3.6 letters. The initial gain in BCVA observed after the loading phase at Month 3 was followed by a slight decrease of 2.3 letters during the maintenance phase. The mean change in central retinal thickness from baseline to Month 3 was 101.1 μm; from baseline to Month 12, the mean change in central retinal thickness was 91.5 μm. The change from baseline in BCVA reached its peak at Month 3; thereafter, VA on average appeared to stabilize with PRN treatment. A slight decrease in BCVA was observed from Month 3 to Month 9, and it stabilized during the last 3 months of the maintenance phase. Most of the reduction in central retinal thickness was observed 1 month after the first treatment and represented the level of stabilization reached during the second half of the study from Month 7 to 12. ANCHOR patients who participated in this study under maintenance phase conditions showed an increase in BCVA from baseline to Month 3 of 1.9 letters and from baseline to Month 12 of 1.6 letters. The mean changes in central retinal thickness from baseline to Month 3 and from baseline to Month 12 were +36.3 μm and +39.3 μm, respectively. For ANCHOR patients in this study, VA and central retinal thickness remained stable with PRN treatment. The efficacy results suggest that a flexible dosing regimen based on VA/OCT-guided re-treatment criteria and monthly monitoring can help to sustain and/or stabilize VA close to the values achieved after the three initial monthly (loading phase) injections. Favorable functional outcome (VA gain) over 12 months was achieved with a low average number of re-treatments in the maintenance phase.

CATT Study

In April 2011, the results of a National Eye Institute–funded trial were published online in The New England Journal of Medicine. The CATT trial (Comparison of AMD Treatments Trials) was a randomized study looking for the relative efficacy and safety of ranibizumab and bevacizumab and determining whether an as-needed regimen would compromise long-term visual acuity was compared with a monthly regimen. The study randomized patients to four groups: ranibizumab every 28 days (ranibizumab monthly), bevacizumab every 28 days (bevacizumab monthly), ranibizumab only when signs of active neovascularization were present (ranibizumab as needed), and bevacizumab only when signs of active neovascularization were present (bevacizumab as needed). The primary outcome was the mean change in visual acuity between baseline and 1 year. Secondary outcomes included the proportion of patients with a change in visual acuity of 15 letters or more, the number of injections, the change in fluid and foveal thickness on OCT (as measured by the OCT Reading Center), the change in lesion size on fluorescein angiography (as measured by the Fundus Photograph Reading Center), the incidence of ocular and systemic adverse events, and annual drug cost (per-dose cost, approximately $2,000 for ranibizumab and $50 for bevacizumab). In each of the head-to-head comparisons of ranibizumab with bevacizumab, the drugs had equivalent effects on visual acuity at all time points throughout the first year of follow-up. The mean number of letters gained, the proportion of patients in whom visual acuity was maintained (less than 15 letters lost), and the proportion of those who had a gain of at least 15 letters were nearly the same for each drug when the regimen was the same. Also, they found that excellent results for visual acuity could be achieved with less-than-monthly regimens for both drugs. Ranibizumab given as needed was equivalent to ranibizumab given monthly, with a mean difference of 1.7 letters. Bevacizumab given as needed was equivalent to bevacizumab given monthly at all time points through 36 weeks (with mean differences all within 1.6 letters); at 52 weeks, the difference of 2.1 letters yielded an inconclusive comparison. The mean gains of 5.9 letters with bevacizumab given as needed and of 6.8 letters with ranibizumab given as needed are the best outcomes observed with less-than-monthly regimens in any large, multicenter clinical trial of ranibizumab. Both bevacizumab and ranibizumab substantially and immediately reduced the amount of fluid in or under the retina. The proportion of patients who had complete resolution of fluid was greater with ranibizumab than with bevacizumab. This difference was evident after the first injection, with no fluid seen at 4 weeks in 27.5% of patients receiving ranibizumab and 17.3% of

those receiving bevacizumab, and the difference persisted throughout the first year. The absolute between-drug difference in the amount of residual fluid was small, and in the majority of patients, neither drug eliminated all fluid. The greater prevalence of fluid in the group given bevacizumab as needed led to an average of 0.8 more injections during the first year than in the group given ranibizumab as needed. Monthly injections of either drug resulted in no increase in the mean lesion area, whereas there was a small increase with injections given as needed. With a limited statistical power to detect important adverse events, the trial found no significant differences between the two drugs in rates of death, atherothrombotic events, or venous thrombotic events, findings that are consistent with the results of a study of Medicare claims involving more than 145,000 treated patients. However, in the study, the rate of serious systemic adverse events, primarily hospitalizations, was higher among bevacizumab-treated patients than among ranibizumab-treated patients (24.1% vs. 19.0%, $P = 0.04$).

RANIBIZUMAB SAFETY

The most common adverse reactions among patients treated with ranibizumab include conjunctival hemorrhage, eye pain, vitreous floaters, increased intraocular pressure, and intraocular inflammation. Serious adverse events related to the injection procedure occurred in less than 0.1% of ITV injections, including endophthalmitis, retinal detachments, and traumatic cataracts. Other serious ocular adverse events observed occurred in less than 2% of patients, included intraocular inflammation and increased intraocular pressure. The main ocular side effects of the ranibizumab are summarized in Table 17.2.

Arterial Thromboembolic Events

As part of the safety data review process, Genentech undertook a review of all Antiplatelet Trialist's Collaboration (APTC) arterial thromboembolic events (ATEs), which are

Table 17.2 MAIN ADVERSE EVENTS REPORT FOR THE 3 PHASE III STUDIES

Main adverse event	LUCENTIS arm	CONTROL arm
Conjunctival hemorrhage	77%–43%	66%–29%
Vitreous floaters	32%–3%	10%–3%
Retinal hemorrhage	26%–15%	56%–37%
Intraocular pressure increased	24%–8%	7%–3%
Intraocular inflammation	18%–5%	11%–3%
Eye irritation	19%–4%	20%–6%
Cataract	16%–5%	16%–6%
Foreign body sensation in eyes	19%–6%	14%–6%

defined as stroke, myocardial infarction (MI) or vascular death, and death of unknown origin. The clinical trial database was evaluated for APTC ATEs, and a meta-analysis, including the controlled phase II and III studies (FOCUS, ANCHOR, MARINA, PIER, and SAILOR), was performed. The objective of the meta-analysis was to clarify if there was an increased rate of stroke or other APTC ATEs with ranibizumab compared at 0.3-mg and 0.5-mg doses and with control subjects in the pooled data across trials. Initial safety analyses of individual Lucentis trials FVF2428g (FOCUS), FVF2587g (ANCHOR), FVF2598g (MARINA), FVF3192g (PIER), and FVF3689g (SAILOR) showed that a greater percentage of subjects experienced strokes in the 0.5-mg arms compared with control in MARINA and FOCUS, and that a greater percentage was seen in the 0.5-mg arm compared with the 0.3-mg arm in SAILOR Cohort 1. The numbers of events were small, and none of these differences approached statistical significance. No such differences were seen in ANCHOR or PIER. As reported in the Lucentis Company Core Datasheet (CDS), US package insert (USPI), and the Ranibizumab Investigator Brochure, there was a low annual percentage (less than 4%) of ATEs observed in the ranibizumab clinical trials; however, there is a potential risk of ATEs following ITV use of inhibitors of VEGF. In the oncology setting, for example, an increased rate of ATEs associated with systemic administration of AVASTIN (bevacizumab) has been observed.

Bevacizumab is a humanized monoclonal antibody targeted against VEGF that is administered intravenously, while ranibizumab, a fragment of this antibody with a lower molecular weight and a higher affinity for VEGF, is designed for intraocular use. A previous meta-analysis was performed to evaluate the rate of ATEs in subjects with cancer receiving intravenous bevacizumab plus chemotherapy versus chemotherapy alone. This meta-analysis found an approximately twofold higher relative risk of stroke in subjects who received bevacizumab compared with those receiving chemotherapy alone. The Lucentis APTC ATE meta-analysis included the results from the 2-year trials MARINA (sham vs. 0.3 mg vs. 0.5 mg), ANCHOR (PDT vs. 0.3 mg vs. 0.5 mg), FOCUS (PDT vs. 0.5 mg + PDT), PIER (sham vs. 0.3 mg vs. 0.5 mg), and the 1-year study SAILOR Cohort 1 (0.3 mg vs. 0.5 mg). It is important to note that PIER sham subjects crossed over to ranibizumab 0.5 mg early in the 2nd year of the study.

For all APTC ATEs and for all three comparisons, 0.3 mg versus 0.5 mg; 0.3 mg versus control; and 0.5 mg versus control, the pooled rates were similar among the treatment groups. The odds ratios for all comparisons were near 1.0, providing no evidence for a difference in ATE rates between groups. In the comparisons with control, the meta-analysis showed 2-year cumulative incidence rates that were similar in the 0.5-mg dose group (4.8% in MARINA, ANCHOR, and FOCUS pooled), the 0.3-mg dose group (4.5% in MARINA and ANCHOR pooled) and the control group (4.4% in

MARINA, ANCHOR, and FOCUS pooled; 4.0% in MARINA and ANCHOR pooled). For MIs, all three comparisons showed that the pooled rates were also similar among the treatment groups. The odds ratios for all comparisons were near 1.0, providing no evidence for a difference in MI rates between groups. In the comparisons with control, the 2-year cumulative MI rates were similar in the 0.5-mg dose group (1.7% in MARINA, ANCHOR, and FOCUS pooled); 0.3-mg dose group (2.4% in MARINA and ANCHOR pooled); and the control group (2.1% in MARINA, ANCHOR, and FOCUS pooled and 1.6% in MARINA and ANCHOR pooled). When comparing pooled stroke rates in the 0.5-mg dose group versus control, the stroke rate was higher in the pooled 0.5-mg group at 2.7% (13/484) compared with the control rate of 1.1% (5/435), with an odds ratio of 2.2 (95% CI 0.8–7.1), pooling the data from the MARINA, ANCHOR, and FOCUS studies. Comparing the 0.3-mg dose with control, the stroke rate in the pooled 0.3-mg group was 1.6% (6/375) compared with the control rate of 1.3% (5/379), with an odds ratio of 1.2 (95% CI 0.5–4.4), pooling the data from MARINA and ANCHOR because FOCUS did not include a 0.3-mg dose group. The numbers of events were small even in the pooled data, and the confidence intervals (CIs) for these odds ratios were wide and included 1.0. When comparing 0.3-mg versus 0.5-mg, the stroke rates were similar in both dose groups in the pooled 2-year data for MARINA, ANCHOR, and PIER. However, the rate of stroke was higher in the 0.5-mg dose group than in the 0.3-mg dose group in SAILOR Cohort 1. Pooling the data for all four studies in the stratified analysis, the estimated odds ratio was 1.5, with a 95% CI of 0.8 to 2.9, which included 1.0.

This meta-analysis had inherent limitations. The studies included had different designs, patient populations, and control groups, as well as varying durations of treatment. In addition, the treatment regimens included monthly dosing, quarterly dosing, protocol-defined re-treatment criteria, and ranibizumab combined with another active agent, verteporfin PDT. The heterogeneity across studies also placed limits on the interpretation of the pooled stratified analyses. Despite combining information across studies, the meta-analysis was still limited by the rare number of events overall, making it difficult to draw definitive conclusions.

CONCLUSION

The treatment of ocular neovascular diseases is being revolutionized by ITV therapies targeting vascular endothelial growth factor. Ranibizumab monotherapy remains the preferred therapy in the management of neovascular AMD at the present time. Ongoing clinical trials will help determine the efficacy of ranibizumab relative to bevacizumab, evaluate the long-term efficacy and safety of combination therapy modalities, and assess the role of new pharmacologic agents. The functional and anatomic outcomes achieved in the pivotal ranibizumab trials with monthly injections set the standard for comparison. Since then, various modified dosing regimens with the aim of lessening the treatment burden associated with monthly injections have been investigated. Combination therapy incorporating PDT and antivascular endothelial growth factor therapy may represent an alternative treatment approach, and randomized multicenter clinical trials are ongoing. In addition, new pharmacologic agents are being developed and investigated. The benefit of ITV ranibizumab applies to all angiographic subtypes of neovascular AMD and across all lesion sizes. The two original phase III studies (ANCHOR and MARINA) demonstrated sustained visual acuity gains over a 2-year monthly dosing schedule. Following these trials, several studies looked at ways to decrease the treatment burden while maintaining similar visual gains. These trials included PIER, PrONTO, EXCITE, SUSTAIN, HORIZON, and CATT. Visual acuity data show that monthly dosing of ranibizumab produces superior vision outcomes compared to a fixed-dosing schedule. ITV ranibizumab is well tolerated and shown to have a very low rate of adverse ocular or systemic side effects. Ranibizumab has been developed specifically for intraocular use, although this drug exhibits excellent safety profiles, ocular and systemic complications, particularly thromboembolic events, it still remains a concern in patients receiving therapy. Both the ophthalmologist and the medical physician to reassess the need for intraocular therapy and explore the feasibility of changing medications should carefully evaluate patients experiencing adverse events that may be related to VEGF suppression. Ranibizumab has positively altered the treatment of wet AMD and offers hope for millions of patients.

REFERENCES

1. Ferrara N, Davis-Smyth T. The biology of vascular endothelial growth factor. Endocr Rev. 1997;18:1–20.

2. Shibuya M, Yamaguchi S, Yamane A, et al. Nucleotide sequence and expression of a novel human receptor-type tyrosine kinase gene (flt) closely related to the fms family. Oncogene. 1990;5:519–524.

3. Matthews W, Jordan CT, Gavin M, et al. A receptor tyrosine kinase cDNA isolated from a population of enriched primitive hematopoietic cells and exhibiting close genetic linkage to c-kit. Proc Natl Acad Sci U S A. 1991;88:9026–9030.

4. Connolly DT, Heuvelman DM, Nelson R, et al. Tumor vascular permeability factor stimulates endothelial cell growth and angiogenesis. J Clin Invest. 1989;84:1470–1478.

5. Keck PJ, Hauser SD, Krivi G, et al. Vascular permeability factor, an endothelial cell mitogen related to PDGF. Science. 1989;246:1309–1312.

6. Plouet J, Schilling J, Gospodarowicz D. Isolation and characterization of a newly identified endothelial cell mitogen produced by AtT-20 cells. EMBO J. 1989;8:3801–3806.

7. Conn G, Bayne ML, Soderman DD, et al. Amino acid and c DNA sequences of a vascular endothelial cell mitogen that is homologous to platelet derived growth factor. Proc Natl Acad Sci U S A. 1990;87:2628–2632.

8. De Vries C, Escobedo JA, Ueno H, et al. The fms-like tyrosine kinase, a receptor for vascular endothelial growth factor. Science. 1992;255:989–991.

9. Terman BI, Crrion ME, Kovacs E, et al. Identification of a new endothelial cell growth factor receptor tyrosine kinase. Oncogene. 1991;6:1677–1683.

10. Millauer B, Wizigmann-Voos S, Schnurch H, et al. High affinity VEGF binding and development expression suggest Flk-1 as a major regulator of vasculogenesis and angiogenesis. Cell. 1993;72:835–846.

11. Quinn TP, Peters KG, de Vries C, et al. Fetal liver kinase 1 is a receptor for vascular endothelial growth factor and is selectively expressed in vascular endothelium. Proc Natl Acad Sci U S A. 1993;90:7533–7537.

12. Ferrera N, Henzel WJ. Pituitary follicular cells secrete a novel heparin-binding growth factor specific for vascular endothelial cells. Biochem Biophys Res Commun. 1989;161:851–858.

13. Leung DW, Cachianes G, Kuang WJ, et al. Vascular endothelial growth factor is a secreted angiogenic mitogen. Science. 1989;246:1306–1309.

14. Pepper MS, Wasi S, Ferrara N, et al. In vitro angiogenic and proteolytic properties of bovine lymphatic endothelial cells. Exp Cell Res. 1994;210:298–305.

15. Pepper MS, Ferrara N, Orci L, et al. Vascular endothelial growth factor (VEGF) induces plasminogen activators and plasminogen activator inhibitor-1 in microvascular endothelial cells. Biochem Biophys Res Commun. 1991;181:902–906.

16. Connolly DT, Olander JV, Heuvelman DM, et al. Human vascular permeability factor. Isolation from U937 cells. J Biol Chem. 1989;264:20017–20024.

17. Phillips GD, Stone AM, Jones BD, et al. Vascular endothelial growth factor (rhVEGF165) stimulates direct angiogenesis in the rabbit cornea. In Vivo. 1994;8:961–965.

18. Dvorak HF. Tumors: wounds that do not heal. Similarities between tumor stroma generation and wound healing. N Engl J Med. 1986;315:1650–1659.

19. Lopez PF, Sippy BD, Lambert HM, et al. Transdifferentiated retinal pigment epithelial cells are immunoreactive for vascular endothelial growth factor in surgically excised age-related macular degeneration-related choroidal neovascular membranes. Invest Ophthalmol Vis Sci. 1996;37:855–868.

20. Kvanta A, Algvere PV, Berglin L, et al. Subfoveal fibrovascular membranes in age-related macular degeneration express vascular endothelial growth factor. Invest Ophthalmol Vis Sci. 1996;37:1929–1934.

21. Dvorak HF, Harvey VS, Estrella P, et al. Fibron containing gels induce angiogenesis. Implications for tumor stroma generation and wound healing. Lab Invest. 1987;57:673–686.

22. Gerhardinger C, Brown LF, Mizutani M, et al. Expression of vascular endothelial growth factor in the human retina and in nonproliferative diabetic retinopathy. Am J Pathol. 1998;152:1453–1462.

23. Miller JW, Adamis AP, Aiello LP. Vascular endothelial growth factor in ocular neovascularization and proliferative diabetic retinopathy. Diabetes Metab Rev. 1997;13:37–50.

24. Kim I, Ryan AM, Rohan R, et al. Constitutive expression of VEGF, VEGFR-1 and VEGFR-2 in normal eyes. Invest Ophthalmol Vis Sci. 1999;40:2115–2121.

25. Kliffen M, Sharma HS, Mooy CM, et al. Increased expression of angiogenic growth factors in age-related maculopathy. Br J Ophthalmol. 2008;126:513–518.

26. Husain D, Miller JW, Kenney AG, et al. Photodynamic therapy and digital angiography of experimental iris neovascularization using liposomal benzoporphyrin derivative. Ophthalmology. 1997;104:242–250.

27. Okamoto N, Tobe T, Hackett SF, et al. Transgenic mice with increased expression of vascular endothelial growth factor in the retina: a new model of intraretinal and sub retinal neovascularization. Am J Pathol. 1997;151:281–291.

28. Schwesinger C, Yee C, Rohan RM, et al. Intrachoroidal neovascularization in transgenic mice overexpressing vascular endothelial growth factor in the retinal pigment epithelium. Am J Pathol. 2001;158:1161–1172.

29. Kim KJ, Li B, Houck K, et al. The vascular endothelial growth factor proteins: identification of biologically relevant regions by neutralizing monoclonal antibodies. Growth Factors. 1992;7:53–64.

30. Presta LG, Chen H, O'Connor SJ, et al. Humanization of an anti-vascular endothelial growth factor monoclonal antibody for the therapy of solid tumor and other disorders. Cancer Res. 1997;57:4593–4599.

31. Krzystolik MG, Afshari MA, Adamis AP, et al. Prevention of experimental choroidal neovascularization with intravitreal anti-vascular endothelial growth factor antibody fragment. Arch Ophthalmol. 2002;120:338–346.

32. Rosenfeld PJ, Schwartz SD, Blumenkranz MS, et al. Maximum tolerated dose of a humanized anti-vascular endothelial growth factor antibody fragment for treating neovascular age-related macular degeneration. Ophthalmology. 2005;112:1048–1053.

33. Heier JS, Antoszyk AN, Pavan PR, et al. Ranibizumab for treatment of neovascular age-related macular degeneration: a phase I/II multicenter, controlled, multidose study. Ophthalmology. 2006;113:642.

34. Rosenfeld PJ, Heier JS, Hantsbarger G, et al. Tolerability and efficacy of multiple escalating doses of ranibizumab (Ranibizumab) for neovascular age-related macular degeneration. Ophthalmology. 2006;113:632–642.

35. Heier JS, Boyer DS, Ciulla TA, et al.; for the FOCUS Study Group. Ranibizumab combined with verteporfin photodynamic therapy in neovascular age-related macular degeneration. Year 1 results of the FOCUS Study. Arch Ophthalmol. 2006;124:1532–1542.

36. Rosenfeld PJ, Brown DM, Heier JS, et al. Ranibizumab for neovascular age-related macular degeneration. N Engl J Med. 2006;355:1419–1431.

37. Brown DM, Kaiser PK, Michels M, et al. Comparison of ranibizumab and verteporfin photodynamic therapy for neovascular age-related macular degeneration. N Engl J Med. 2006;355:1432–1444.

38. Fung AE, Lalwani GA, Rosenfeld PJ, et al. An optical coherence tomography-guided, variable dosing regimen with intavitreal ranibizumab (Lucentis) for neovascular age-related macular degeneration. Am J Opthalmol. 2007;143(4):566–583.

18

BEVACIZUMAB FOR THE TREATMENT OF EXUDATIVE AGE-RELATED MACULAR DEGENERATION

LUCIENNE C. COLLET • BORJA F. CORCÓSTEGUI

INTRODUCTION

Age-related macular degeneration (AMD) is the main cause of irreversible blindness in developing countries (1–7). In the United States, AMD causes 46% of the cases of severe visual loss (visual acuity [VA] 20/200 or worse) in patients older than 40 years (7), affecting approximately 1.75 million people (6). In Europe, AMD is also the leading cause of blindness, and its prevalence in patients aged 65 to 75 years is reported to range between 9% and 25% (8). Visual impairment secondary to AMD varies among the European countries. Studies have shown a prevalence of 40% in France (9), 39% in Germany (10), 36% in the Netherlands (11), 16% in the European North of Russia (12), and 14% in Bulgaria (13). In China, the prevalence of early AMD is 9.2% and late AMD 1.9%. The prevalence of early AMD increased from 5% in the 65- to 69-year group to 24.4% in patients older than 80 years and for late AMD, from 1% to 9% (14). Age is the most significant factor associated with AMD.

AMD is classified into nonexudative and exudative forms. The nonexudative form is characterized by the presence of drusen, retinal pigment epithelium (RPE) abnormalities (hypo- or hyperpigmentation), and geographic atrophy. The exudative or neovascular form is characterized by choroidal neovascularization (CNV), serous or hemorrhagic detachment of the retina or RPE, hard exudates, subretinal and sub-RPE fibrovascular proliferation, and disciform scar.

VASCULAR ENDOTHELIAL GROWTH FACTOR

During the last two decades, different treatment modalities have been used for the treatment of AMD. In the beginning, thermal laser photocoagulation was used to destroy CNV, but it caused irreversible visual loss due to retinal burns and had a recurrence rate of 50% (15). Next, photodynamic therapy (PDT) with verteporfin was introduced, and the majority of the patients reduced the risk of visual loss but few gained vision (16,17).

In 1989, Ferrara and Henzel (18) isolated and purified an endothelial cell mitogen, and they named it vascular permeability factor or vascular endothelial growth factor (VEGF). In the last 20 years, intensive research on VEGF-mediated disease has increased our knowledge of neovascular ocular pathology. VEGF-A is a homodimeric glycoprotein that functions as a growth factor specific for endothelial cells (19). It induces vascular permeability and is a regulator of vasculogenesis and angiogenesis. Blood vessel formation involves both vasculogenesis and angiogenesis.

Vasculogenesis takes place in the embryo and is characterized by the differentiation of endothelial cell precursors, while angiogenesis describes the formation of new blood vessels from existing vessels. The process of angiogenesis is responsible for new blood vessel formation in adults. This may take place in biologic or pathologic situations, such as AMD, cancer, proliferative retinopathies, diabetic maculopathy, and retinal vein occlusion among others (20).

There are factors that promote angiogenesis and factors that inhibit it. The factors that activate angiogenesis are VEGF, transforming growth factor α, transforming growth factor β, fibroblast growth factor, angiopoietin-1, angiopoietin-2 (21–23), and cysteine-rich 61 (Cyr61) (24).

VEGF can activate angiogenesis, lymphangiogenesis, vascular permeability, and prevents apoptosis promoting survival of endothelial cells. Without VEGF, endothelial cells in immature vessels could not survive, grow, or proliferate (19,23,25,26). The VEGF gene family includes VEGF-A, VEGF-B, VEGF-C, and VEGF-D (23). There are four active VEGF-A isoforms: $VEGF_{121}$, $VEGF_{165}$, $VEGF_{189}$, and $VEGF_{206}$. The most frequently expressed isoform is $VEGF A_{165}$ (27).

VEGF receptors are located on the surface of endothelial cells. Three receptor tyrosine kinases have been identified for VEGF: VEGFR-1, VEGFR-2, and VEGFR-3. VEGFR-1 (fms-like tyrosine kinase-1) has both positive and negative angiogenic effects; VEGFR-2 (fetal liver kinase-1 and kinase insert domain–containing receptor) is the main mediator of angiogenic, mitogenic, and vascular permeability effects of VEGF A; VEGFR-3 promotes angiogenic effects on lymphatic vessels (19,28).

VEGF-A binds to receptors: VEGFR-1 and VEGFR-2. Studies on humans and primates have shown that VEGF-A is important in the pathogenesis of AMD and other eye diseases (29–31).

In fact, increased concentrations of VEGF-A have been found in exudative AMD. VEGF-A has been found to be expressed in RPE cells, suggesting their involvement in new vessel formation (30). Additionally, high levels of VEGF-A, along with increased $VEGF_{121}$ and $VEGF_{165}$ expression, have been detected in CNV from AMD patients (31,32) as well as increased levels of VEGF in the vitreous humor of patients with CNV (33). VEGF-A is a target for the treatment of eye diseases in which angiogenesis is important, such as AMD. Treatment strategies are aimed at inhibition of VEGF.

■ THERAPIES TO INHIBIT VEGF

Therapies to inhibit VEGF include an aptamer (pegaptanib sodium), specific antibodies (bevacizumab and ranibizumab), the immunoglobulin G—VEGF receptor fusion protein (VEGF trap), and fragment antibodies of small interfering RNA (siRNA, bevasiranib) (34).

Bevacizumab

Bevacizumab is a full-length recombinant humanized monoclonal immunoglobulin-G that binds to all isoforms of VEGF and prevents VEGF from binding to its receptors (35). In 1997, bevacizumab (Avastin: Genentech, South San Francisco, CA) was first introduced and was the first antiangiogenic agent approved by the US Food and Drug Administration (FDA) to inhibit tumor growth (Fig. 18.1). In 2004, bevacizumab was approved for treatment of metastatic colorectal cancer.

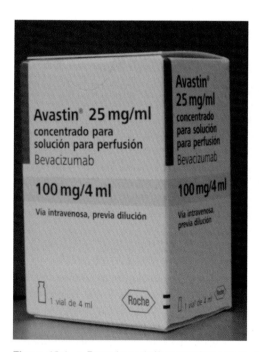 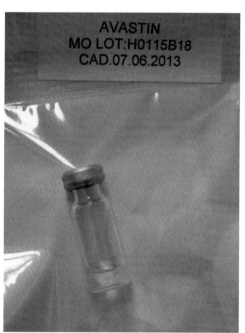

Figure 18.1 ■ Bevacizumab (Avastin: Genentech, South San Francisco, CA) was first introduced and was the first antiangiogenic agent approved by the U.S. Food and Drug Administration (FDA) to inhibit tumor growth.

The off-label use of intravenous bevacizumab for neovascular AMD showed promising results (36). Preclinical studies on pharmacokinetics of *intravenous* bevacizumab show a serum half-life of 1 to 2 weeks (37), and clinical studies in patients show a half-life of 21 days (38).

Pharmacokinetics studies of *intravitreal* bevacizumab in rabbit models have shown that after an injection of 1.25 mg bevacizumab, a peak concentration of free bevacizumab (400 µg/mL) is achieved in the vitreous humor. Vitreous concentrations decline with a half-life of 4.32 days, but concentrations ≥10 µg/mL were maintained in the vitreous for 30 days. A peak concentration in the aqueous humor reached at day 3 after drug administration. Low concentrations were detected in the serum after intravitreal injection and in the aqueous humor of the fellow eye (39). In another study done in macaques, the aqueous humor and serum bevacizumab concentration were measured after intravitreal bevacizumab injection. At day 1, a peak in the aqueous humor was observed while the peak concentration in the serum was at 1 week. VEGF levels returned to preinjection concentrations after 42 days (40). In humans treated with intravitreal bevacizumab, a study showed decrease in VEGF concentration within 7 days of treatment (41).

SANA (Systemic Avastin for Neovascular AMD) was the first prospective study in patients with exudative AMD treated with intravenous bevacizumab. Eighteen patients with subfoveal CNV were enrolled in an open-label study in which bevacizumab 5 mg/kg was injected *intravenously* every 2 weeks for two or three infusions. VA improved from 54 letters (Snellen VA 20/80) at baseline to 68 letters (Snellen VA 20/40) at 24 weeks, an increase of 14 letters (P ≤ 0.001). Additionally, retinal thickness decreased from 392 to 280 µm at week 24. Adverse events occurred in 18.5% of the patients. At week 3, increased blood pressure was observed and controlled with antihypertensive drugs (36,42). Additionally, bevacizumab was also associated with increased risk of venous thromboembolism in cancer patients (43). Intravenous bevacizumab improved VA and decreased retinal thickness as early as 1 week after therapy; however, its potential systemic side effects outweighed its benefits.

The first anti-VEGF drug designed for intraocular use in the treatment of AMD was pegaptanib sodium (Macugen). Pegaptanib is a 28-base RNA oligonucleotide ligand or aptamer that binds to human $VEGF_{165}$ with high specificity and affinity. Pegaptanib showed efficacy for the treatment of AMD; however, the VISION study concluded that intravitreal pegaptanib injection at 6-week intervals stabilized vision in 70% of cases and improved it in only 6% (44,45).

In 2006, phase III clinical trials, MARINA and ANCHOR, demonstrated that the use of anti-VEGF ranibizumab (Lucentis, Genentech, Inc. South San Francisco, CA) promoted VA improvement in patients with neovascular AMD, stabilizing vision in 95% of patients and improving VA between 7.2 and 11.3 letters in 30% to 40% of patients (46,47). While these trials were still in progress,

Rosenfeld et al. (48) showed that bevacizumab could also lead to VA improvement at a considerably lower cost and became the first to report the use of intravitreal bevacizumab for the treatment of exudative AMD to minimize the risk of systemic treatment (48). Consequently, bevacizumab was and is used worldwide by clinicians for the treatment of neovascular AMD. Exudative AMD is the most common indication for intravitreal bevacizumab. However, the use of bevacizumab developed in the absence of formal protocols. Many papers, including retrospective and prospective studies, uncontrolled case series, and uncontrolled randomized trials, have shown improvement in VA as well as decrease in macular thickness after treatment.

Subsequently, intravitreal injection of bevacizumab achieved worldwide success because of its safety profile, availability, short-term effects, and low cost compared to other anti-VEGF drugs. Since ranibizumab and bevacizumab are derived from the same monoclonal antibody and have a similar mechanism of action, it was suggested that they have similar efficacy and safety in treating AMD. Despite the lack of large-scale clinical trials, bevacizumab is the most commonly used treatment in the United States for exudative AMD (49). In an analysis of 222,886 Medicare beneficiaries from 2008, 146,276 (64.4%) received bevacizumab and 80,929 (35.6%) received ranibizumab (49).

In the beginning, there were many issues to resolve, such as retinal penetration, toxicity, and schedule for retreatment. A question of particular interest was whether intravitreal bevacizumab could penetrate the retina given its large size, but some reports concluded full retina penetration after injection (50). In fact, an animal study using confocal immunohistochemistry demonstrated full retinal thickness penetration 24 hours after intravitreal injection (51). With regard to toxicity, several experimental animal studies confirmed no retinal toxicity even at doses of 5 mg of intravitreal bevacizumab (52,53). Electrophysiologic and histologic studies have not demonstrated toxicity as well (52–56). Studies in patients with AMD have shown improvement in mf-ERG responses and its correlation with improvement in VA. Specifically, improvement in P1 amplitude was observed and correlated with decreased leakage on fluorescein angiography. These results may explain an increase in neural activity in the retina.

By 2006, level 1 evidence has supported the safety and efficacy of Lucentis. Level 1 evidence is evidence obtained from properly conducted well-designed, randomized, controlled trials (46,47). In the case of bevacizumab, no level 1 evidence existed until 2011. During this time, data were limited to case series and randomized controlled trials with small numbers of patients or short follow-up periods. El-Mollayes et al. (57) reviewed 571 articles involving bevacizumab use and AMD between 1997 and 2010 (57). Of these articles, only eight included at least 30 patients with AMD treated with bevacizumab for at least 12 months of follow-up (58–65). These studies were characterized by small number of patients (from 37–147 subjects), different concentrations of intravitreal bevacizumab (1.25, 2.5, and 1 mg), and different treatment protocols (three monthly injections followed by as-needed treatment or as-needed injections 4 or 8 weeks after the first injection). The studies reported an average number of 4.3 injections over 12 months, and best-corrected visual acuity (BCVA) improvement of 8 letters (from 39.9 letters at baseline to 47.95 letters by 12 months), additionally central retinal thickness improved from 375.2 to 249.9 μm by the end of 12 months (57).

It is important to understand that phase III trials enroll large number of patients to ensure enough strength of evidence with meaningful differences from active or control cases and to characterize safety profile of the treatment. The PDT trials, TAP and VIP, enrolled 948 patients. The VISION trial of pegaptanib enrolled 1,186 patients. MARINA enrolled 716 patients, and ANCHOR enrolled 423 patients. In the case of bevacizumab, phase III clinical trials had not been conducted, and the best evidence was a level 2 evidence obtained from well-designed controlled trials without randomization, series with or without intervention, and multicenter case–control studies, until 2010 and 2011 with ABC and CATT studies.

THE ABC AND CATT STUDIES

Presently, there are results and ongoing phase III, randomized clinical trials on bevacizumab in AMD. The ABC trial was conducted in Saudi Arabia. The CATT study (Comparison of AMD Treatments Trials), which compares intravitreal bevacizumab to ranibizumab, was conducted in the United States, and similar studies are being conducted in Germany (VIBERA), United Kingdom (IVAN), Austria (MANTA), Norway (LUCAS), and France (GEFAL).

The ABC trial reported the first level 1 evidence for the efficacy of bevacizumab in the treatment of neovascular AMD. The treatment schedule was based on an as-required strategy. In this prospective, randomized, multicenter, double-masked trial, more than 45% of patients treated with bevacizumab improved 10 or more letters while 32% of the patients treated with bevacizumab gained 15 or more letters from baseline VA. Mean VA increased 7.0 letters in the treatment group with a median of seven injections during a 54-week period. These results are comparable to those in the MARINA and ANCHOR studies, and the retreatment approach used was not a fixed monthly but an as-required one (66).

Limitations of the ABC trial are that it does not compare bevacizumab with ranibizumab and the number of patients enrolled is small. Bevacizumab remains not approved by the FDA for intraocular use, and this may have medicolegal implications

In 2011, CATT study (Comparison of Age-Related Macular Degeneration Treatment Trials) was published (67). It is a multicenter, single-blind, noninferiority trial that enrolled 1,208 patients with exudative AMD at 44 clinical centers. The patients were treated with 0.50 mg ranibizumab or 1.25 mg bevacizumab on either a monthly schedule or as needed with monthly evaluation. There were four study groups: ranibizumab every 28 days (ranibizumab monthly), bevacizumab every 28 days (bevacizumab monthly), ranibizumab only with active CNV (ranibizumab as needed), and bevacizumab only with active CNV (bevacizumab as needed). Every 28 days, an optical coherence tomography (OCT) was performed, and signs of active CNV were defined as decreased VA compared to previous examination, new or persistent hemorrhage, fluid seen on OCT, or dye leakage on fluorescein angiography.

Among the 1,161 patients who were alive 1 year after enrollment, VA was available for 1,105 (95.2%) patients. All four study groups showed VA improvement from baseline to 1 year, with most improvement during the first 6 months. At 1 year, bevacizumab was comparable to ranibizumab (99.2% confidence interval for the difference in the mean change in VA within –5 to +5 letters) when both were given monthly and when they were administered as needed. Additionally, ranibizumab given as needed was comparable to ranibizumab given monthly. When comparing bevacizumab administered as needed and bevacizumab administered monthly, the data were inconclusive. No inferiority or noninferiority was established in the two study groups. Ranibizumab administered as needed was comparable with bevacizumab given monthly. However, the comparison between ranibizumab administered monthly and bevacizumab given as needed was also inconclusive.

At 1 year, patients treated with ranibizumab monthly gained 8.5 letters, whereas ranibizumab administered as needed led to a gain of 6.8 letters. Additionally, patients treated with bevacizumab monthly gained 8.0 letters, whereas bevacizumab administered as needed led to a gain of 5.9 letters. The proportion of patients who did not show a decrease in VA of 15 letters or more from baseline was 94.4% in the group treated with ranibizumab monthly, 94% in the group treated with bevacizumab monthly, 95.4% in the group treated with ranibizumab as needed, and 91.5% in the group treated with bevacizumab as needed. The patients who gained at least 15 letters increased during the first 36 weeks in all four groups but did not differ at 1 year among the groups. Fixed monthly retreatment improved VA, and the differences were not significant in the ranibizumab group and inconclusive for the bevacizumab groups. In relation to the cost of treatment, the average cost per patient for the first year in the ranibizumab-monthly group was $23.500; in the ranibizumab as-needed group, the cost was $13.800; $595 in the bevacizumab-monthly group and $385 in the bevacizumab as-needed group (67).

The results from the ABC and CATT studies are based on 1-year follow-up and are encouraging; however, longer follow-ups are needed. Longer follow-ups may show surprising results. In the HORIZON study, patients who were treated on a monthly schedule during year 1 and afterward with an as-needed schedule show a decrease in median VA by five letters after 1 year and by an additional three letters after 2 years (68).

PROTOCOLS OF TREATMENT: RETREATMENT ALGORITHMS AND MAINTENANCE THERAPY

Fixed Monthly Injections

Initially, there was no clear consensus on retreatment strategies. In the MARINA and ANCHOR studies of ranibizumab, patients received monthly intravitreal injections during 2 years, so each patient received a total of 24 injections. Today, the fixed monthly ranibizumab retreatment schedule has not been widely accepted (46,47). Later, large clinical trials such as PIER, SAILOR, and EXCITE have evaluated less frequent retreatment strategies. Patients were at first treated with three monthly injections of ranibizumab, termed the *"loading phase,"* followed by a quarterly injection regimen. The results observed were positive but did not equal the MARINA and ANCHOR results. In fact, patients showed less mean gain in VA, and fewer patients experienced 15 or more letters of visual gain. Additionally, if after the loading phase there was a gain in VA, it was not maintained during the study (69–71). EXCITE, PIER, and SAILOR studies evaluated monthly maintenance therapy compared to reduced frequency schedule of injections and found that reduced schedule is insufficient for optimal monitoring of disease progression (70,71).

As-Required Injections

PrONTO study introduced a dosing regimen characterized by three consecutive monthly intravitreal injections followed by as-needed retreatment based upon signs of recurrence, ophthalmoscopy, OCT, or fluorescein angiography, called the as-needed or PRN protocol (72). It seems that the PRN dosing regimen is the most widely used today. Ranibizumab was used in PrONTO study, and the dosing regimen was OCT guided and variable. Patients received three monthly intravitreal injections, and retreatment was based upon loss of five letters of VA, new-onset hemorrhage or CNV, increase of central retinal thickness of more than 100 μm documented with OCT, or intraretinal fluid. The 2nd year of study added as retreatment criteria evidence of recurrent intraretinal, subretinal, or sub-RPE fluid (72,73). In the first year of PrONTO study, patients received an average of 5.6 injections of ranibizumab. The results of PrONTO study suggest that 70% of the patients treated with intravitreal ranibizumab showed resolution of edema within 1 month after the first injection, and 90% of the patients showed resolution of fluid after the loading phase (72).

The ABC trial used a loading phase and then an as-required retreatment schedule, based on criteria for retreatment: subretinal fluid on OCT, new hemorrhage, CNV, decreased vision by five or more letters with new intraretinal fluid on OCT, and injections performed at six weekly intervals. By using this retreatment schedule, the results of ABC trial showed that after 54 weeks, 32% of participants receiving bevacizumab gained 15 or more letters of VA, the results are comparable to those in the MARINA and ANCHOR studies (66).

The CATT study compared ranibizumab and bevacizumab using monthly and as-required retreatment schedules (67). In this study, bevacizumab administered monthly led to a gain of 8.0 letters at 12 months, and bevacizumab administered as-required led to a gain of 5.9 letters. Similarly, ranibizumab administered monthly led to a gain of 8.5 letters at 12 months, and ranibizumab in as-required schedule led to a gain of 6.8 letters. It is clear that a monthly retreatment schedule showed greater gain in VA, but the differences were "inconclusive" for the bevacizumab groups and were not significant for the ranibizumab groups. These studies follow up patients for 12 months, but other studies with longer follow-ups, such as HORIZON and SUSTAIN, have shown that significant visual gain is achieved with monthly injections and the as-required schedule is not as effective as the monthly fixed schedule.

Treat and Extend

Other retreatment schedules are used, in order to minimize the number of injections and visits to the hospital. In the treat-and-extend schedule, the patients are treated with monthly injections until macula is dry and without fluid seen with OCT. The follow-up between injections is lengthened by 1 to 2 weeks until recurrence of fluid is observed. If recurrent fluid is detected on a follow-up visit, the treatment interval is reduced to the previous interval. Treatment schedule is variable and subject to change at every visit, but the time between visits in individualized based on each patient's response to treatment (74–76).

Combination Therapy

The findings of PrONTO study revealed that 70% of patients show resolution of macular edema within 1 month of intravitreal ranibizumab, and after the loading phase, 90% of patients show resolution of all fluid (72). However, in some patients, bevacizumab or ranibizumab may be insufficient to resolve neovascularization associated with AMD. Patients either may be refractory to these treatment modalities or may develop resistance to therapy. One study reported that resistance to bevacizumab is observed in 6 out of 59 eyes with 14 months of follow-up and after median number of 8 injections (77). Several factors may be involved in the resistance of treatment with bevacizumab. For instance, the development of neutralizing antibodies against bevacizumab molecule was confirmed in serum of patients treated with intravitreal injections (78). Additionally, inflammation and hypoxia may play a role in this resistance probably due to an independent pathway that may stimulate CNV formation through release of pro-angiogenic factors (79). An increased number of macrophages have been observed in excised human CNV treated with intravitreal bevacizumab (80). There is evidence that the basement membrane of endothelial cells persist after their death, acting as a scaffold for regrowth of CNV (81). Consequently, it has been suggested that combining treatments with different mechanisms of action may result beneficial (82). One of the combination therapies suggested is verteporfin PDT in combination with anti-VEGF (84). This treatment strategy may reduce the number of treatments required. Some studies have shown that combining PDT with bevacizumab stabilized VA, decreased the number of injections per year, and decreased pigment epithelium detachment (84–87). Also anti-VEGF therapy may be combined with macular radiation therapy, and it can be delivered through an external device on the sclera or through an internal device after pars plana vitrectomy (88). Also, severe submacular hemorrhage cases may be treated with vitrectomy and coapplication of subretinal injection of rtPA and bevacizumab followed by intravitreal fluid–gas exchange and after the procedure repeated postoperative intravitreal injections of anti-VEGF (89). However, large-scale, multicenter, double-blind studies are necessary to confirm combination therapy's efficacy and safety.

Treatment Every 2 Weeks

The majority of patients benefit from a monthly treatment schedule, but some eyes will show no improvement and signs of CNV getting worse (90). In a recent study, authors create a mathematical model that predicts, by increasing the number of bevacizumab injections from monthly to every 14 days, the resulting trough levels of VEGF-binding activity of bevacizumab and other anti-VEGF molecules. They found that bevacizumab administered every 14 days showed a binding activity to be 6.5-fold higher, and they conclude that the theoretical increase in trough binding levels when anti-VEGF drugs are dosed every 2 weeks may benefit patients who show response to treatment within 2 weeks but rebound with increased macular thickness after a month (91).

▌ SECONDARY EFFECTS

In chemotherapy treatments, systemic bevacizumab has been associated with an increased risk of thromboembolic events (43,92). In the case of AMD, intravitreal bevacizumab is administered at a dose of 1 to 2.5 mg that is 150 times less than the systemic chemotherapy dosage (93). Consequently, in relation to AMD, studies have shown no correlation between the number of bevacizumab injections and the incidence of adverse effects such as thromboembolic disease, new-onset hypertension, myocardial infarction, cerebrovascular accident, hemorrhage, and death (94). An international Internet survey of 70 centers in 12 countries reported on 7,113 injections given to 5,228 patients. The ocular adverse events observed included endophthalmitis in 0.01%, one case of traumatic lens injury

(0.01%), and three cases of retinal detachment (0.04%). Potential drug-related ocular adverse events included intraocular inflammation (0.14%), acute vision loss (0.07%), nontraumatic cataract progression (0.01%), and central retinal artery occlusion (0.01%). Potential drug-related systemic adverse events included acute blood pressure rise (0.21%), stroke (0.07%), deep venous thrombosis (0.01%), transient ischemic attack (0.01%), and death (0.03%) (95). An analysis of eight studies reported the adverse events following intravitreal bevacizumab injection to be uveitis (0.11%), preretinal bleeding (0.11%), macular hole (0.11%), cataract (0.11%), RPE rip (0.014), endophthalmitis (0.6%), transient rise in intraocular pressure (0.86%), myocardial infarction (0.08%), and death (0.31%) (57).

Retrobulbar hemodynamics of 43 patients with AMD was examined with color Doppler ultrasonography after injection of 1.25 mg bevacizumab. Intravitreal bevacizumab induced a significant decrease in the peak systolic velocity and end-diastolic velocity and a significant rise in the resistive index of the central retinal artery and short posterior ciliary artery of the injected eye. Consequently, it seems that bevacizumab intravitreal injection significantly affects ocular hemodynamic parameters of both the injected and uninjected eyes (96). More studies are needed to understand the consequences of this observation.

▌ SAFETY OF REPEATED INTRAVITREAL INJECTIONS

Fortunately, repeated intravitreal injections for an extended period of time show low incidence of ocular adverse events. It has been recommended that the injection technique used should avoid vitreal reflux, either by changing the needle gauge or injection technique (97). Also, the preparation of bevacizumab syringes should be done carefully, following aseptic guidelines.

▌ PREPARATION

Bevacizumab for intravitreal administration has to be prepared from the intravenous chemotherapy formulation. The guidelines recommend preparation of individual syringes using aseptic technique and adequate sterilization procedures (98,99). Usually the syringes are prepared containing 0.12 mL (3 mg). Immediately prior to intravitreal injection, the plunger is advanced to 0.05 mL (Fig. 18.2). A study reported that syringes under 4°C show 10% degradation of the drug concentration at 3 months and 12% degradation when frozen in a syringe at –10°C (100). Other reports have described storage and reuse of a single vial for multiple doses under refrigeration with no ocular adverse events (101,102).

Patients must be informed about the risks and benefits of bevacizumab intravitreal injection, highlighting potential ophthalmic and systemic adverse events (103).

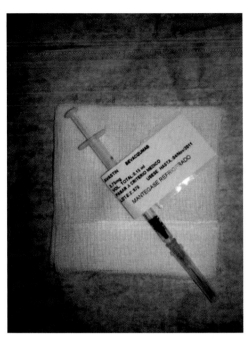

Figure 18.2 ■ The preparation of individual syringes requires a strict aseptic technique with adequate sterilization procedures.

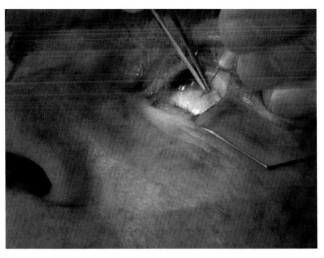

Figure 18.3 ■ The use of an oblique injection technique may help minimize reflux of bevacizumab preventing reflux and subconjunctival bleb formation.

Additionally, the American Academy of Ophthalmic Executives (AAOE) recommends consideration of FDA-approved drugs before off-label bevacizumab. Patients must sign an informed consent and should be aware of the off-label indication of intravitreal bevacizumab. Also patients should be instructed for symptoms that should be reported immediately (104).

■ NEEDLE GAUGE AND TECHNIQUE

Other complications described are temporary increase in intraocular pressure and reflux of bevacizumab with the formation of a subconjunctival bleb (105–107). Some ophthalmologists have adopted different intravitreal injection techniques in order to decrease the incidence of reflux taking into consideration intraocular pressure (108,109). Some patients may experience elevation of intraocular pressure 30 minutes after the injection.

Reflux of the drug may occur following an injection (107,110,111). To minimize the amount of reflux, authors have recommended an anterior chamber paracentesis immediately after an injection. The use of a "mercury bag" placed over the eye 20 minutes before injection may prevent bleb formation, ensuring that bevacizumab or any other intravitreal anti-VEGF remains in the vitreous. Small needle diameter, such as a 32-gauge needle, and an oblique injection technique may further minimize reflux after intravitreal injection (Figs. 18.3 and 18.4) (97,112).

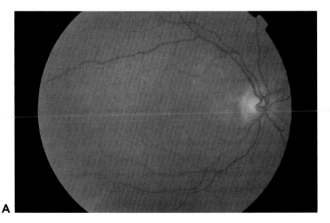

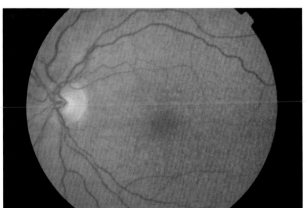

A   B

Figure 18.4 ■ Seventy-eight-year-old patient, VA OD: 20/100, OS: 20/25. **A,B.** Pretreatment color fundus photography.

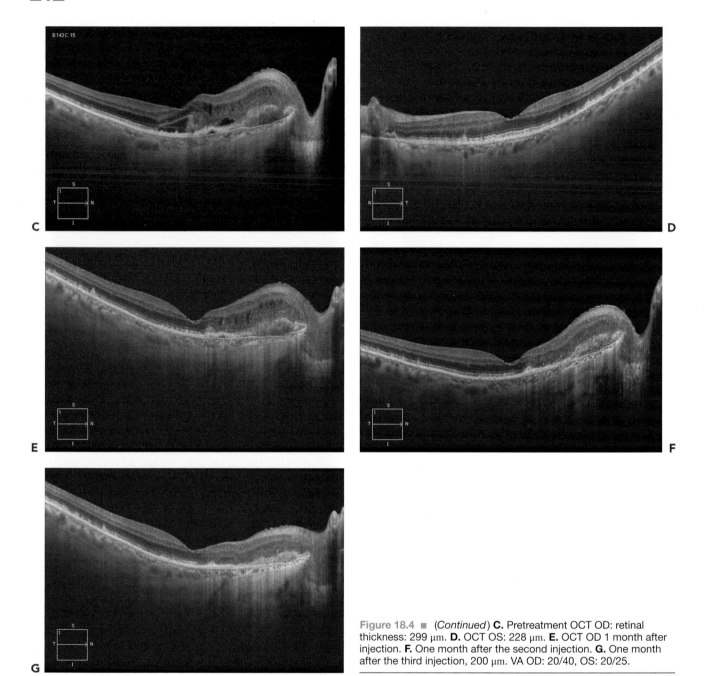

Figure 18.4 ■ (Continued) **C.** Pretreatment OCT OD: retinal thickness: 299 μm. **D.** OCT OS: 228 μm. **E.** OCT OD 1 month after injection. **F.** One month after the second injection. **G.** One month after the third injection, 200 μm. VA OD: 20/40, OS: 20/25.

CONCLUSION

Numerous clinical trials have studied the efficacy and safety of bevacizumab. At the time of this chapter being written, two intravitreal anti-VEGF drugs were used in clinical practice: ranibizumab and bevacizumab. Both can be used for exudative AMD, and both have level 1 evidence that are effective and safe. Studies have not detected clinical superiority of one drug over the other; however, larger clinical trials with extended follow-ups are necessary. The most important factor that determines drug selection is cost. The cost of ranibizumab is 40 times the cost of bevacizumab. Bevacizumab is safe, cost-effective, and efficacious in the treatment of exudative AMD. However, it is administered in an off-label manner. In the future, new anti-VEGF drugs will appear as well as combination therapies.

REFERENCES

1. National Advisory Eye Council (US). Vision research: a national plan 1994-1998. NIH publication no. 93-3186. Bethesda, MD: US Department of Health and Human Services; 1993.

2. National Institute for Neurological Diseases and Blindness, Section on Blindness Statistics. Statistics on blindness in the model reporting area, 1969-1970. DHEW publication no. (NIH) 73-427: US Department of Health, Education and Welfare. Washington, DC: US Government Printing Office; 1973.

3. Klein R, Klein BE, Linton KL. Prevalence of age-related maculopathy. The Beaver Dam Eye Study. Ophthalmology. 1992;99:933–943.

4. Kahn HA, Leibowitz HM, Ganley JP, et al. The Framingham Eye Study. I. Outline and major prevalence findings. Am J Epidemiol. 1977;106:17–32.

5. Sommer A, Tielsch JM, Katz J, et al. Racial differences in the cause-specific prevalence of blindness in east Baltimore. N Engl J Med. 1991;325:1412–1417.

6. Friedman DS, O'Colmain BJ, Munoz B, et al. Prevalence of age-related macular degeneration in the United States. Arch Ophthalmol. 2004;122:564–572.

7. Congdon N, O'Colmain B, Klaver CC, et al. Causes and prevalence of visual impairment among adults in the United States. Arch Ophthalmol. 2004;122:477–485.

8. van Leeuwen R, Klaver CC, Vingerling JR, et al. The risk and natural course of age-related maculopathy: follow-up at 6 1/2 years in the Rotterdam study. Arch Ophthalmol. 2003;121:519–526.

9. Cohen D, Sartral M, Nounou P, et al: Evaluation of moderate and severe visual impairments in patients attending an ophthalmology clinic. A prospective study of 1,172 patients (in French). J Fr Ophtalmol. 2000;23:437–443.

10. Gruener F. Prävalenz, Inzidenz und Ursache von Blindheit und wesentlicher Sehbehinderung in. Hessen, Marburg; Diss, Marburg: 2001.

11. Despriet DD, Klaver CC, Witteman JC, et al. Complement factor H polymorphism, complement activators, and risk of age-related macular degeneration. JAMA. 2006;296:301–309.

12. Bannikova RV, Sannikov AL, Konovalov AV: Characteristics of ophthalmic pathology under the conditions of the European North of Russia (in Russian). Probl Sotsialnoi Gig Zdravookhranenniiai Istor Med. 2002;(3):35–36.

13. Kocur I, Resnikoff S. Visual impairment and blindness in Europe and their prevention. Br J Ophthalmol. 2002;86:716–722.

14. Chen S, Cheng C, Peng K, et al. Prevalence and associated risk factors of age-related macular degeneration in an elderly Chinese population in Taiwan: the Shihpai Eye Study. Invest Ophthalmol Vis Sci. 2008;49(7):3126–3133.

15. Macular Photocoagulation Study Group. Argon laser photocoagulation for neovascular maculopathy Five year results from randomized clinical trials Macular Photocoagulation Study Group. Arch Ophthalmol. 1991;109(8):1109–1114.

16. Treatment of Age-Related Macular Degeneration with Photodynamic Therapy (TAP) Study Group. Photodynamic therapy of subfoveal choroidal neovascularization in age-related macular degeneration with verteporfin: one-year results of 2 randomized clinical trials—TAP report. Arch Ophthalmol. 1999;117:1329–1345.

17. Verteporfin in Photodynamic Therapy Study Group. Verteporfin therapy of subfoveal choroidal neovascularization in age related macular degeneration: two-year results of a randomized clinical trial including lesions with occult with no classic choroidal neovascularization—verteporfin in photodynamic therapy report 2. Am J Ophthalmol. 2001;131:541–560.

18. Ferrara N, Henzel WJ. Pituitary follicular cells secrete a novel heparin-binding growth factor specific for vascular endothelial cells. Biochem Biophys Res Commun. 1989;161:851–858.

19. Ferrara N, Gerber HP, LeCouter J. The biology of VEGF and its receptors. Nat Med. 2003;9(6):669–676.

20. Ferrara N. Role of vascular endothelial growth factor in physiologic and pathologic angiogenesis: therapeutic implications. Semin Oncol. 2002;29:1014.

21. Ferrara N, Chen H, Davis-Smyth T, et al. Vascular endothelial growth factor is essential for corpus luteum angiogenesis. Nat Med. 1998;4:336–340.

22. Veikkola T, Alitalo K. VEGFs, receptors and angiogenesis. Semin Cancer Biol. 1999;9(3):211–220.

23. Leung DW, Cachianes G, Kuang WJ, et al. Vascular endothelial growth factor is a secreted angiogenic mitogen. Science. 1989;246:1306–1309.

24. You J, Yang CM, Yang CH. Elevation of angiogenic factor cysteine-rich 61 levels in vitreous of patients with proliferative diabetic retinopathy. Retina. 2012;32(1):103–111.

25. Nagy JA, Vasile E, Feng D, et al. Vascular permeability factor/vascular endothelial growth factor induces lymphangiogenesis as well as angiogenesis. J Exp Med. 2002;196:1497–1506.

26. Ferrara N. Vascular endothelial growth factor: basic science and clinical progress. Endocr Rev. 2004;25:581–611.

27. Houck KA, Ferrara N, Winer J, et al. The vascular endothelial growth factor family: identification of a fourth molecular species and characterization of alternative splicing of RNA. Mol Endocrinol. 1991;5:1806–1814.

28. Karkkainen MJ, Makinen T, Alitalo K. Lymphatic endothelium: a new frontier of metastasis research. Nat Cell Biol. 2002;4(1):E2–E5.

29. Tolentino MJ, Miller JW, Gragoudas ES, et al. Vascular endothelial growth factor is sufficient to produce iris neovascularization and neovascular glaucoma in a nonhuman primate. Arch Ophthalmol 1996;114:964–970.

30. Kliffen M, Sharma HS, Mooy CM, et al. Increased expression of angiogenic growth factors in age-related maculopathy. Br J Ophthalmol. 1997;81:154–162.

31. Kvanta A, Algvere PV, Berglin L, et al. Subfoveal fibrovascular membranes in age-related macular degeneration express vascular endothelial growth factor. Invest Ophthalmol Vis Sci. 1996;37:1929–1934.

32. Rakic JM, Lambert V, Devy L, et al. Placental growth factor, a member of the VEGF family, contributes to the development of choroidal neovascularization. Invest Ophthalmol Vis Sci. 2003;44:3186–3193.

33. Wells JA, Murthy R, Chibber R, et al. Levels of vascular endothelial growth factor are elevated in the vitreous of patients with subretinal neovascularisation. Br J Ophthalmol. 1996;80:363–366.

34. Bhisitkul RB. Vascular endothelial growth factor biology: clinical implications for ocular treatments. Br J Ophthalmol. 2006;90(12):1542–1547.

35. van Wijngaarden P, Coster DJ, Williams KA. Inhibitors of ocular neovascularization: promises and potential problems. JAMA. 2005;293:1509–1513.

36. Michels S, Rosenfeld PJ, Puliafito CA, et al. Systemic bevacizumab (avastin) therapy for neovascular age-related macular degeneration: twelve-week results of an uncontrolled open-label clinical study. Ophthalmology. 2005;112:1035–1047.

37. Presta LG, Chen H, O'Connor SJ, et al. Humanization of an anti-vascular endothelial growth factor monoclonal antibody for the therapy of solid tumors and other disorders. Cancer Res. 1997;57:4593–4599.

38. Gordon MS, Margolin K, Talpaz M, et al. Phase I safety and pharmacokinetic study of recombinant human anti-vascular endothelial growth factor in patients with advanced cancer. J Clin Oncol. 2001;19:843–850.

39. Bakri S, Snyder M, Reid J, et al. Pharmacokinetics of intravitreal Bevacizumab (Avastin). Ophthalmology. 2007;114:855–859.

40. Miyake T, Sawada O, Kakinoki M, et al. Pharmacokinetics of bevacizumab and its effect on vascular endothelial growth factor after intravitreal injection of bevacizumab in macaque eyes. Invest Ophthalmol Vis Sci. 2010;51(3):1606–1608.

41. Matsuyama K, Ogata N, Jo N, et al. Levels of vascular endothelial growth factor and pigment epithelium-derived factor in eyes before and after intravitreal injection of bevacizumab. Jpn J Ophthalmol. 2009;53(3):243–248.

42. Moshfegui AA, Rosenfeld PJ, Puliafito CA, et al. Systemic bevacizumab therapy for neovascular age-related macular degeneration twenty-four-week results of an uncontrolled open-label clinical study. Ophthalmology. 2006;113:e1–e12.

43. Rani S, Chu D, Keresztes R, et al. Risk of venous thromboembolism with the angiogenesis inhibitor bevacizumab in cancer patients. JAMA. 2008;300(19):2277–2285.

44. Gragoudas ES, Adamis AP, Cunningham ET Jr, et al. Pegaptanib for neovascular age-related macular degeneration. N Engl J Med. 2004;351:2805–2816.

45. Chakravarthy U, Adamis AP, Cunningham ET Jr, et al. VEGF Inhibition Study in Ocular Neovascularization (V.I.S.I.O.N.) Clinical Trial Group. Year 2 efficacy results of 2 randomized controlled clinical trials of pegaptanib for neovascular age-related macular degeneration. Ophthalmology. 2006;113(9):1508.e1–1508.e25.

46. Brown DM, Kaiser PK, Michels M, et al. Ranibizumab versus verteporfin for neovascular age-related macular degeneration. N Engl J Med. 2006;355(14):1432–1444.

47. Rosenfeld PJ, Brown DM, Heier JS, et al. Ranibizumab for neovascular age-related macular degeneration. N Engl J Med. 2006;355(14):1419–1431.

48. Rosenfeld PJ, Moshfegui AA, Puliafito CA. Optical coherence tomography findings after an intravitreal injection of bevacizumab (avastin) for neovascular age-related macular degeneration. Ophthalmic Surg Lasers Imaging. 2005;36:331–335.

49. Brechner RJ, Rosenfeld PJ, Babish JD, et al. Pharmacotherapy for neovascular age-related macular degeneration: an analysis of the 100% 2008 Medicare fee for-service Part B claims file. Am J Ophthalmol. 2011;151:887–895.

50. Scharaermeyer UA, Henke-Fahle S, Grisanti S, et al. Evidence for transport of bevacizumab through the retina by muller cells in rabbits. ARVO. 2006;Abstract 4169.

51. Shahar J, Avery RL, Hellwell G, et al. Electrophysiologic and retinal penetration studies following intravitreal injection of bevacizumab (avastin). Retina. 2006;26:262–269.

52. Manzano RP, Peyman GA, Khan P, et al. Testing intravitreal toxicity of bevacizumab (Avastin). Retina. 2006;26:257–261.

53. Feiner L, Barr EE, Shui YB, et al. Safety of intravitreal injection of bevacizumab in rabbit eyes. Retina. 2006;26:882–888.

54. Maturi RK, Bleau LA, Wilson DL. Electrophysiologic findings after intravitreal bevacizumab (Avastin) treatment. Retina. 2006;26:270–274.

55. Pedersen K, Moller F, Sjølie A, et al. Electrophysiological assessment of retinal function during 6 months of bevacizumab treatment in neovascular age-related macular degeneration. Retina. 2010;30(7):1025-1033.

56. Karanjia R, Eng K, Gale J, et al. Electrophysiological effects of intravitreal Avastin (bevacizumab) in the treatment of exudative age related macular degeneration Br J Ophthalmol. 2008;92:1248–1252.

57. El-Mollayess G. Bevacizumab and neovascular age related macular degeneration: pathogenesis and treatment. Semin Ophthalmol. 2011;26(3):69–76.

58. Wu L, Arevalo JF, Maia M, et al. for the Pan-American Collaborative Retina Study Group (PACORES). Comparing outcomes in patients with subfoveal choroidal neovascularization secondary to age-related macular degeneration treated with two different doses of primary intravitreal bevacizumab: Results of the Pan-American Collaborative Retina Study Group (PACORES) at the 12-month follow-up. Jpn J Ophthalmol. 2009;53:125–130.

59. Carneiro AM, Falcão MS, Brandão EM, et al. Intravitreal bevacizumab for neovascular age-related macular degeneration with or without prior treatment with photodynamic therapy: one-year results. Retina. 2010;30(1):85–92.

60. Mekjavic PJ, Kraut A, Urbancic M, et al. Efficacy of 12-month treatment of neovascular age-related macular degeneration with intravitreal bevacizumab based on individually determined injection strategies after three consecutive monthly injections. Acta Ophthalmol. 2009; DOI 10.1111/j.1755-3768.2009.01740.x.

61. Costagliola C, Romano M, Corte MD, et al. Intravitreal bevacizumab for treatment-naive patients with subfoveal occult choroidal neovascularization secondary to age-related macular degeneration: a 12-month follow-up study. Retina. 2009;29(9):1227–1234.

62. Leydolt C, Michels S, Prager F, et al. Effect of intravitreal bevacizumab (Avastin(R)) in neovascular age-related macular degeneration using a treatment regimen based on optical coherence tomography: 6- and 12-month results. Acta Ophthalmol. 2010;88(5):594–600.

63. Fong KC, Kirkpatrick N, Mohamed Q, et al. Intravitreal bevacizumab (Avastin) for neovascular age related macular degeneration using a variable frequency regimen in eyes with no previous treatment. Clin Exp Ophthalmol. 2008;36(8):748–755.

64. Bashshur ZF, Haddad ZA, Schakal A, et al. Intravitreal bevacizumab for treatment of neovascular age-related macular degeneration: a one-year prospective study. Am J Ophthalmol. 2008;145(2):249–256.

65. Arevalo JF, Fromow-Guerra J, Sanchez JG, et al. Pan-American Collaborative Retina Study Group. Primary intravitreal bevacizumab for subfoveal choroidal neovascularization in age-related macular degeneration: Results of the Pan-American Collaborative Retina Study Group at 12 months follow-up. Retina. 2008;28(10):1387–1394.

66. Tufail A, Patel PJ, Egan C, et al. Bevacizumab for neovascular age related macular degeneration (ABC Trial): multicentre randomised double masked study. Br Med J. 2010;340(7761): article c2459.

67. Martin DF, Maguire MG, Ying GS, et al. The CATT Research Group. Ranibizumab and Bevacizumab for Neovascular Age-Related Macular Degeneration. N Engl J Med. 2011;364:1897–1908.

68. Bressler NM. Antiangiogenic approaches to age-related macular degeneration today. Ophthalmology. 2009;116(10):S15–S23.

69. Abraham P, Yue H, Wilson L. Randomized, double-masked, sham-controlled trial of ranibizumab for neovascular age-related macular degeneration: PIER study year 2. Am J Ophthalmol. 2010;150(3):315–324.

70. Regillo CD, Brown DM, Abraham P, et al. Randomized, double-masked, sham-controlled trial of ranibizumab for neovascular age-related macular degeneration: PIER Study Year 1. Am J Ophthalmol. 2008;145(2):239–248.

71. Schmidt-Erfurth U, Eldem B, Guymer R, et al. Efficacy and safety of monthly versus quarterly ranibizumab treatment in neovascular age-related macular degeneration. The EXCITE Study. Ophthalmology. 2011;118:831–839.

72. Fung AE, Lalwani GA, Rosenfeld PJ, et al. An optical coherence tomography-guided, variable dosing regimen with intravitreal ranibizumab (Lucentis) for neovascular age-related macular degeneration. Am J Ophthalmol. 2007;143:566–583.

73. Lalwani GA, Rosenfeld PJ, Fung AE, et al. A variable dosing regimen with intravitreal ranibizumab for neovascular age-related macular degeneration: year 2 of the PrONTO Study. Am J Ophthalmol. 2009;148(1):43–58.

74. Gupta OP, Shienbaum G, Patel AH, et al. A treat and extend regimen using ranibizumab for neovascular age-related macular degeneration clinical and economic impact. Ophthalmology. 2010;117:2134–2140.

75. Engelbert M, Zweifel SA, Freund KB. Treat and extend dosing of intravitreal antivascular endothelial growth factor therapy for type 3 neovascularization/ retinal angiomatous proliferation. Retina. 2009;29(10):1424–1431.

76. Oubraham H, Cohen SY, Samimi S, et al. Inject and extend dosing versus dosing as needed: a comparative retrospective study of ranibizumab in exudative age-related macular degeneration. Retina. 2011;31:26–30.

77. Forooghian F, Cukras C, Meyerle CB, et al. Tachyphylaxis after intravitreal bevacizumab for exudative age-related macular degeneration. Retina. 2009;29(6):723–731.

78. Forooghian F, Chew EY, Meyerle CB, et al. Investigation of the role of neutralizing antibodies against bevacizumab as mediators of tachyphylaxis. Acta Ophthalmol. 2009;89(2):e206–e207.

79. Sheridan CM, Pate S, Hiscott P, et al. Expression of hypoxia-inducible factor-1-alpha and -2alpha in human choroidal neovascular membranes. Graefes Arch Clin Exp Ophthalmol. 2009;247(10):1361–1367.

80. Tatar O, Yoeruek E, Szurman P, et al. Effect of bevacizumab on inflammation and proliferation in human choroidal neovascularization. Arch Ophthalmol. 2008;126:782–790.

81. Stahl A, Paschek L, Martin G, et al. Combinatory inhibition of VEGF and FGF2 is superior to solitary VEGF inhibition in an in vitro model of RPE-induced angiogenesis. Graefes Arch Clin Exp Ophthalmol. 2009;247(6):767–773.

82. Spaide RF. Perspectives: rationale for combination therapies for choroidal neovascularization. Am J Ophthalmol. 2006;141(1):149–156.

83. Kaiser PK. Combination therapy with verteporfin and anti- VEGF agents in neovascular age-related macular degeneration: where do we stand? Br J Ophthalmol. 2010;94(2):143–145.

84. Schaal S, Kaplan HJ, Tezel TH. Is there tachyphylaxis to intravitreal antivascular endothelial growth factor pharmacotherapy in age-related macular degeneration? Ophthalmology. 2008;115(12):2199–2205.

85. Shima C, Gomi F, Sawa M, et al. One-year results of combined photodynamic therapy and intravitreal bevacizumab injection for retinal pigment epithelial detachment secondary to age-related macular degeneration. Graefes Arch Clin Exp Ophthalmol. 2009;247(7):899–906.

86. Augustin AJ, Puls S, Offermann I. Triple therapy for choroidal neovascularization due to age-related macular degeneration: verteporfin PDT, bevacizumab, and dexamethasone. Retina. 2007;27(2):133–140.

87. Bakri SJ, Couch SM, McCannel CA, et al. Same-day triple therapy with photodynamic therapy, intravitreal dexamethasone, and bevacizumab in wet age-related macular degeneration. Retina. 2009;29(5):573–578.

88. A´vila MP, Farah ME, Santos A, et al. Twelve-month short-term safety and visual-acuity results from a multicentre prospective study of epiretinal strontium-90 brachytherapy with bevacizumab for the treatment of subfoveal choroidal neovascularization secondary to age-related macular degeneration. Br J Ophthalmol. 2009;93(3):305–309.

89. Treumer F, Roider J, Hillenkamp J. Long-term outcome of subretinal coapplication of rtPA and bevacizumab followed by repeated intravitreal anti-VEGF injections for neovascular AMD with submacular haemorrhage. Br J Ophthalmol. 2012;96(5):708–703.

90. Rosenfeld PJ, Shapiro H, Tuomi L, et al. Characteristics of patients losing vision after 2 years of monthly dosing in the phase III ranibizumab clinical trials. Ophthalmology. 2011;118:523–530.

91. Stewart M, Rosenfeld P, Penha F, et al. Pharmacokinetic rationale for dosing every 2 weeks versus 4 weeks with intravitreal ranibizumab, bevacizumab, and aflibercept (Vascular Endothelial Growth Factor Trap-Eye). Retina. 2012;32(3):434–457.

92. US Food and Drug Administration (FDA) MedWatch. Safety: Avastin (bevacizumab). January 2005. http://www.fda.gov/Safety/MedWatch/Safety Information/SafetyAlertsforHumanMedicalProducts/ucm150721.htm. Accessed August 19, 2009.

93. Michels S. Is intravitreal bevacizumab (Avastin) safe? Br J Ophthalmol. 2006;90(11):1333–1334.

94. Sheybani A, Kymes S, Schlief S, et al. Vascular events in patients with age-related macular degeneration treated with intraocular bevacizumab. Retina. 2009;29(10):1404–1408.

95. Fung AE, Rosenfeld PJ, Reichel E. The International Intravitreal Bevacizumab Safety Survey: using the internet to assess drug safety worldwide. Br J Ophthalmol. 2006;90(11):1344–1349.

96. Hosseini H, Lotfi M, Heidari M, et al. Effect of intravitreal Bevacizumab on retrobulbar Blood flow in injected and uninjected fellow eyes of patients with neovascular age-related macular degeneration. Retina. 2012;32(5):967–971.

97. Cortez RT, Ramirez G, Collet L, et al. Intravitreal bevacizumab injection: an experimental study in White New Zealand Rabbits. Arch Ophthalmol. 2010;128(7):884–887.

98. ASHP technical assistance bulletin on pharmacy-prepared ophthalmic products. Am J Hosp Pharm. 1993;50:1462–1463.

99. Trissel L. An update on USP chapter 797: the new national standard for sterile preparation. www.ashpadvantage.com/website_images/pdf/hospira797.pdf. Accessed March 6, 2006.

100. Bakri SJ, Snyder MR, Pulido JS, et al. Six-month stability of bevacizumab (Avastin) binding to vascular endothelial growth factor after withdrawal into a syringe and refrigeration or freezing. Retina. 2006;26:519–522.

101. Guerrero-Naranjo J, Bueno-Garcia R, Quiroz-Mercado H, et al. Security and side effects of intravitreal Avastin using two methods of storage (poster B447). Program 4501. Presented at: Association for Research in Vision and Ophthalmology 2006 Annual Meeting, Fort Lauderdale, FL, 2006.

102. Wu L, Martinez-Castellanos M, Quiroz-Mercado H, et al. Safety of an intravitreal injection of bevacizumab (Avastin): results of a multicenter trial. Program PA018. Presented at: 2006 American Academy of Ophthalmology/Asia Pacific Academy of Ophthalmology Joint Meeting, Las Vegas, NV, 2006.

103. Statement on Avastin. Position statement released by AMD Alliance International. www.amdalliance.org/information/treatments/treatments.php. Accessed September 20, 2006.

104. Risk management recommendations for off-label, intravitreal use of Avastin. American Academy of Ophthalmic Executives. www.omic.com/resources/risk_man/forms.cfm. Accessed September 20, 2006.

105. Benz MS, Albini TA, Holz ER, et al. Short-term course of intraocular pressure after intravitreal injection of triamcinolone acetonide. Ophthalmology. 2006;113:1174–1178.

106. Morlet N, Young SH. Prevention of intraocular pressure rise following intravitreal injection. Br J Ophthalmol. 1993;77:572–573.

107. Boon CJ, Crama N, Klevering BJ, et al. Reflux after intravitreal injection of bevacizumab. Ophthalmology. 2008;115:1270.

108. Rodriguez EB, Meyer CH, Grummann A Jr, et al. Tunneled scleral incision to prevent vitreal reflux after intravitreal injection. Am J Ophthalmol. 2007;143:1035–1037.

109. Aiello LP, Brucker AJ, Chang S, et al. Evolving guidelines for intravitreal injections. Retina. 2004;24(5 Suppl):S3–S19.

110. Hollands H, Wong J, Bruen R, et al. Short-term 410 intraocular pressure changes after intravitreal injection of bevacizumab. Can J Ophthalmol. 2007;42:807–811.

111. Bakri SJ, Pulido JS, McCannel CA, et al. Immediate intraocular pressure changes following intravitreal injections of triamcinolone, pegaptanib, and bevacizumab. Eye. 2009;23:181–185.

112. Rodriguez G, Meyer CH, Grummann A Jr, et al. Tunneled scleral incision to prevent vitreal reflux after intravitreal injection. Am J Ophthalmol. 2007;143:1035–1037.

19

VEGF TRAP-EYE FOR NEOVASCULAR AGE-RELATED MACULAR DEGENERATION

CLAUDIA M. KRISPEL • QUAN DONG NGUYEN • DIANA V. DO

INTRODUCTION

The advent of anti–vascular endothelial growth factor (anti-VEGF) therapies has revolutionized the treatment of neovascular age-related macular degeneration (AMD) as well as other retinopathies driven by VEGF. In recent years, a multitude of studies has provided evidence that therapy with intravitreal monoclonal antibodies directed against VEGF improves visual outcome in patients with exudative macular degeneration (1–3).

VASCULAR ENDOTHELIAL GROWTH FACTOR

The family of VEGF proteins includes multiple subtypes including VEGF-A, VEGF-B, VEGF-C, VEGF-D, and PIGF (placental growth factor). The VEGF family members predominantly involved in ocular neovascularization are VEGF-A and PIGF. VEGF-A and PIGF increase permeability of choroidal neovascular tissues through the action of the VEGF receptors, which are tyrosine kinase receptors with an extracellular binding domain and an intracellular tyrosine kinase domain. Upon ligand (VEGF) binding to the receptor, the receptors dimerize, and the tyrosine kinase domain initiates phosphorylation at the C-terminus of the molecule. This initiates an intracellular signaling cascade that ultimately leads to changes in gene transcription. Many forms of ocular neovascularization

are currently treated with intravitreal monoclonal antibodies (ranibizumab and bevacizumab), which target all isoforms of VEGF-A but do not target PIGF. The VEGF Trap-Eye (aflibercept) offers an alternate to the standard anti-VEGF therapies used in ocular neovascular disease and may have several advantages over the monoclonal antibodies.

VEGF TRAP-EYE (AFLIBERCEPT)

The VEGF Trap-Eye (aflibercept) is a 110 kDa fusion protein that was engineered to have several potential advantageous properties over monoclonal antibodies, including increased intravitreal half-life compared to ranibizumab, high binding affinity for VEGF-A, and broader activity including binding of PIGF (4). VEGF Trap-Eye consists of the extracellular portions of the normally membrane-bound VEGF receptors 1 and 2, fused to the Fc portion of human immunoglobulin G. The rationale is that this drug has a low likelihood of inciting an immune response against itself and will be more effective at decreasing the pathologic activity of choroidal neovascular membranes.

Stewart et al. (5,6) have used mathematical modeling to predict the biologic activity of VEGF Trap-Eye. This model shows that due to the increased binding affinity of VEGF Trap-Eye (140× that of ranibizumab) and the increased intravitreal half-life compared to ranibizumab (estimated at 4–5 days for aflibercept), the biologic activity of VEGF

216

Trap-Eye 10 weeks after injection is roughly equivalent to the biologic activity of ranibizumab 30 days after injection (5).

Stewart et al. (6) more recently applied their mathematical model to determine the theoretical peak and trough binding activities of ranibizumab, bevacizumab, and aflibercept if injected every 14 days or every 28 days. This model shows that increased frequency of ranibizumab and bevacizumab injections results in increased trough anti-VEGF binding. The authors suggest that patients who do not respond well to monthly anti-VEGF injections with bevacizumab or ranibizumab fail because the trough binding activity falls so low that the VEGF overwhelms the antibody. When the authors modeled the binding activity for VEGF Trap-Eye, they found that both the peak and trough binding activities are vastly higher than either ranibizumab or bevacizumab given monthly or even every 14 days. These modeling studies suggest that VEGF Trap-Eye may be equally or more efficacious than the monoclonal antibodies and may require less frequent dosing.

CLINICAL EXPERIENCE WITH VEGF TRAP-EYE

Clinical use of VEGF Trap-Eye has shown promising results both for the treatment of neovascular macular degeneration and diabetic macular edema. The CLEAR-IT 2 trial (Clinical Evaluation of Antiangiogenesis in the Retina Intravitreal Trial) (7) investigated VEGF Trap-Eye in the treatment of subfoveal choroidal neovascularization secondary to neovascular AMD. In this multicenter, randomized, phase 2, double-masked trial, 159 patients with subfoveal choroidal neovascularization secondary to exudative AMD were randomized into five treatment groups. These groups included 0.5 or 2 mg VEGF Trap-Eye every 4 weeks during

a fixed-dosing period, which extended from weeks 1 through 12, after which treatments were given on an as-needed basis. The remaining three groups received 0.5, 2, or 4 mg VEGF Trap-Eye initially and every 12 weeks during the 12-week fixed-dosing period, after which treatments were given on an as-needed basis. The average number of injections given during the "prn" phase of the treatment was two. The investigators in the study found a substantial decrease in lesion thickness and improvements in best-corrected visual acuity (BCVA) in all groups that were sustained throughout the as-needed phase of the trial. This study showed promising results that control of choroidal neovascular activity can be achieved with fewer injections compared to the standard monthly injections of ranibizumab.

Following the CLEAR-IT 2 trial, phase 3 clinical trials comparing the safety and efficacy of VEGF Trap-Eye to that of ranibizumab in the United States (VIEW 1) and in Europe, Asia, and Latin America (VIEW 2) were completed. Although the final manuscripts have not been published, the results of these studies have been released and presented at various meetings (8–10). VIEW 1 and VIEW 2 each enrolled over 1,200 patients with previously untreated subfoveal neovascular AMD, with an average baseline BCVA letter score of approximately 54. The patients were randomized to one of four treatment groups, which are as follows: VEGF Trap-Eye 2 mg every 4 weeks, VEGF Trap-Eye 2 mg every 8 weeks, VEGF Trap-Eye 0.5 mg every 4 weeks, and ranibizumab 0.5 mg every 4 weeks. Each arm (including the VEGF Trap-Eye 2 mg every 8 weeks) initially received a loading dose of a monthly injection for the first 3 months.

At the 52-week evaluation, the percentage of patients who avoided severe vision loss (greater than 15 ETDRS letters) was equivalent among the four groups (94%–96% of patients; Fig. 19.1). The percentage of patients who gained

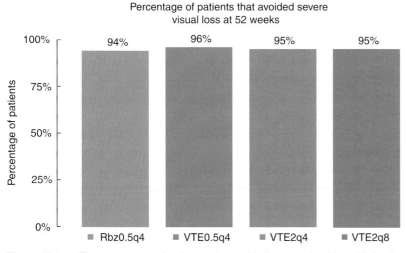

Figure 19.1 ■ The percentage of patients who avoided severe visual loss (defined as loss of ≥15 ETDRS letters) was not different among the four treatment arms (ranibizumab 0.5 mg every 4 weeks [Rbz0.5q4]; VEGF Trap-Eye 0.5 mg every 4 weeks [VTE0.5q4]; VEGF Trap-Eye 2 mg every 4 weeks [VTE2q4]; VEGF Trap-Eye 2 mg every 8 weeks [VTE2q8]).

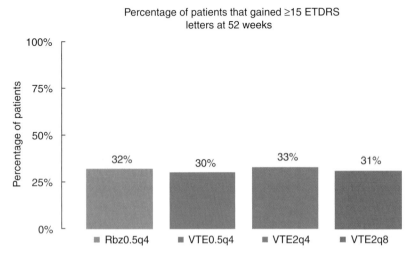

Figure 19.2 ■ The percentage of patients who gained ≥15 ETDRS at 52 weeks was not different among the four treatment arms (abbreviations as in Fig. 19.1).

ETDRS letters at 52 weeks was also equivalent among the four treatment arms (Fig. 19.2). At 52 weeks, 47% to 51% of eyes randomized to VEGF Trap-Eye gained 10 or more letters compared to 50% of eyes randomized to ranibizumab. Structural changes in the retina were also assessed in the VIEW 1 and VIEW 2 trials. Time-domain optical coherence tomography (OCT) showed that the central retinal thickness decreased 123 to 139 μm in the VEGF Trap-Eye groups and decreased by 128 μm in the ranibizumab group at week 52. In addition, the proportion of eyes without evidence of fluid on OCT was 73% in the VEGF Trap-Eye 2 mg every 4 weeks, 68% in the VEGF Trap-Eye 2 mg every 8 weeks, 60% in VEGF Trap-Eye 0.5 mg every 4 weeks, and 62% in the ranibizumab every 4 weeks.

Rates of adverse effects including endophthalmitis were not different among the treatment groups. There were three cases of injection-related endophthalmitis among the eyes treated with ranibizumab and three cases of endophthalmitis among the eyes randomized to VEGF Trap-Eye. Rates of systemic complications including vascular death, stroke, and myocardial infarction were low (approximately 1%–2% rate of arteriothrombotic events) and were not different among the four treatment arms. There did not appear to be any unexpected ocular or systemic safety concerns with VEGF Trap-Eye.

The VIEW 1 and 2 studies demonstrated that all doses and dosing regimens of VEGF Trap-Eye were equivalent to every 4-week dosing of ranibizumab, with comparable ocular and systemic safety profiles. These results are promising and may change the standard of care for neovascular AMD.

Although diabetes is not covered in the scope of this text, it should be mentioned that VEGF Trap-Eye has also undergone rigorous investigation for the treatment of diabetic macular edema. The DA VINCI (DME and VEGF Trap Eye: Investigation of Clinical Impact) (11) is a multicenter, randomized, double-masked phase 2 trial investigating VEGF Trap-Eye compared to standard focal

laser for diabetic macular edema. This study enrolled 221 patients with diabetic macular edema who were randomized to one of five treatment arms. The treatment arms included four arms receiving VEGF Trap-Eye, either 0.5 or 2 mg every 4 weeks, 2 mg monthly for three doses then every 8 weeks, or 2 mg monthly for three doses and then "prn." The fifth treatment arm received macular laser treatment. The VEGF Trap-Eye arms received sham laser, while the laser group received sham injections. At the 24-week end point, mean visual acuity gains in the VEGF Trap-Eye groups ranged from 8.5 to 11.4 ETDRS letters, compared to 2.5 ETDRS letters in the macular laser arm. Additionally, 4.5% of patients in the VEGF Trap-Eye 0.5-mg arms lost greater than 15 ETDRS letters compared to 9.1% in the laser group. None of the patients in the 2 mg VEGF Trap-Eye suffered this degree of loss. This phase 2 study suggests that VEGF Trap-Eye is superior to standard focal laser for the treatment of diabetic macular edema. A phase 3 clinical trial is now underway to further investigate VEGF Trap-Eye in diabetic macular edema.

In November 2011, VEGF Trap-Eye was approved by the United States Food and Drug Administration (FDA) for the treatment of neovascular AMD, and many retina specialists have begun to incorporate this medicine into their clinical practices.

CONCLUSIONS

VEGF Trap-Eye will likely have a significant role in treating neovascular AMD, given its efficacy, durability, and safety. Decreased dosing frequency may significantly improve the quality of life of patients requiring treatment and reduce burden of cost and time on health care systems and providers. Long-term outcomes and the role of VEGF Trap-Eye in other VEGF-driven ocular disease will undoubtedly be the focus of many future studies.

REFERENCES

1. Martin DF, et al. Ranibizumab and bevacizumab for neovascular age-related macular degeneration. N Engl J Med. 2011;364(20):1897–1908.

2. Brown DM, et al. Ranibizumab versus verteporfin for neovascular age-related macular degeneration. N Engl J Med. 2006;355(14):1432–1444.

3. Rosenfeld PJ, et al. Ranibizumab for neovascular age-related macular degeneration. N Engl J Med. 2006;355(14):1419–1431.

4. Holash J, et al. VEGF-Trap: a VEGF blocker with potent antitumor effects. Proc Natl Acad Sci U S A. 2002;99(17):11393–11398.

5. Stewart MW, Rosenfeld PJ. Predicted biological activity of intravitreal VEGF Trap. Br J Ophthalmol. 2008;92(5):667–668.

6. Stewart MW, et al. Pharmacokinetic rationale for dosing every 2 weeks versus 4 weeks with intravitreal ranibizumab, bevacizumab, and aflibercept (vascular endothelial growth factor trap-eye). Retina. 2012;32(3):434–487.

7. Heier JS, et al. The 1-year results of CLEAR-IT 2, a phase 2 study of vascular endothelial growth factor trap-eye dosed as-needed after 12-week fixed dosing. Ophthalmology. 2011;118(6):1098–1106.

8. Schmidt-Erfurth U. VEGF Trap-eye phase III trial results. VIEW 2 results. Paper presented at Angiogenesis, Exudation, and Degeneration 2011; 2011; Miami, FL.

9. Heier JS. VEGF Trap-eye phase III trial results. VIEW 1 results. Paper Presented at Angiogenesis, Exudation, and Degeneration 2011; Miami, FL, 2011.

10. Nguyen QD. Neovascular age related macular degeneration: Aflibercept Update. Paper presented at Macula 2012; New York, NY, 2012.

11. Do DV, et al. The DA VINCI Study: phase 2 primary results of VEGF trap-eye in patients with diabetic macular edema. Ophthalmology. 2011;118(9):1819–1826.

20

RADIATION FOR THE TREATMENT OF WET AGE-RELATED MACULAR DEGENERATION

ROBERT PETRARCA • TIMOTHY L. JACKSON

■ INTRODUCTION

At present, most patients with wet age-related macular degeneration (AMD) are treated with regular, intravitreal injections of drugs directed against vascular endothelial growth factor (VEGF), namely ranibizumab, bevacizumab, and aflibercept (1–5). While these drugs offer visual outcomes far better than the natural history, all require an expensive and burdensome course of treatment. The large phase III studies of ranibizumab used monthly dosing. For pragmatic and cost reasons, most clinicians use an as-required (PRN) (6) or "treat and extend" dosing regimen (7) that entails regular hospital visits and usually several injections per year. Further, not all patients respond fully, and many of those who do respond initially, subsequently lose vision (8). There is therefore a need for a more durable treatment modality that can reduce the cost and burden of treatment, while maintaining or improving vision. This chapter explores the early attempts to use radiation as a treatment for wet AMD, and more recent attempts to revisit this treatment modality.

■ BACKGROUND TO RADIATION THERAPIES

Radiation is energy emitted from a source and can be classified into nonionizing radiation (visible light, infrared, and radio waves), and ionizing radiation (alpha, beta, gamma, and x-rays). Radiation is ionizing if it creates an ion (a charged particle) when it interacts with an atom. This will only occur if the particle or photon of radiation has sufficient energy to detach electrons from another atom or molecule (9).

Ionizing radiation creates free radicals, which are highly reactive charged molecules or atoms. In the context of radiation therapy, these free radicals are usually generated from the interaction of radiation and water molecules. If this occurs within a living organism, then the free radicals can damage DNA. In addition, radiation can ionize DNA itself, breaking its molecular bonds. Alpha and beta particles are directly ionizing, in that they carry a charge and directly interact (via coulombic forces) with atomic electrons, causing excitation. Gamma and x-rays are indirectly ionizing, because they are electrically neutral and do not directly interact with atomic electrons but instead transfer energy to charged particles (via electromagnetic or nuclear interaction) (9).

The Gray (Gy) is the basic unit of measurement for the "absorbed dose," which refers to the total energy absorbed per unit mass (kg), and has replaced the previous unit of measurement, the rad (1 Gy = 100 rad) (9,10).

Radiation used for medical therapies can be divided into two main categories, depending on its method of delivery to the tissue. Brachytherapy from the Greek word *brachy*, meaning "short distance," places the source of radiation close to the target lesion. The source is usually an isotope that produces ionizing radiation as it decays and emits energy. Teletherapy (external beam therapy) from the Greek word *tele*, meaning "from afar," uses radiation formed into a beam that can be projected at an internal body tissue from an external source. The source can also be an isotope, but more recently, electronically produced ionizing radiation has been used (11).

RADIATION AND NEOVASCULAR AMD

There are biologic principles suggesting radiation may have potential as a treatment for wet AMD. Neovascular AMD is similar to a proliferative wound healing process, and proliferating cells are known to be sensitive to the effects of ionizing radiation. Localized radiotherapy causes irreparable damage to DNA and protein synthesis, preventing further replication, while still maintaining cellular integrity (12–14). All cells in the treatment zone are affected; however, radiation has a selective effect. This is because nondividing cells are able to repair the damage to their DNA, while the rapidly proliferating cells discontinue the cell division cycle and undergo apoptosis (15).

The retina and optic nerve are relatively resistant to the effects of radiation, as they consist of highly stable cells with minimal mitotic activity (16,17). By contrast, choroidal neovascularization (CNV) is propagated by mitotic activity, with rapidly replicating endothelial cells that are more sensitive to radiation than are the nonproliferating capillary endothelial cells seen in mature retinal vessels (18,19). There is a potential therapeutic range where the radiation can be safely administered and yet inhibit the CNV vascular endothelium proliferation, causing regression or selective cell death. Fibroblast proliferation is also inhibited (20). Therefore, radiation has the potential to prevent both the vascular leakage and scarring associated with neovascular AMD and vision loss (21).

In addition to its selective action, radiation may also have synergy with anti-VEGF therapy. Anti-VEGF agents have a rapid onset of action, but only limited durability in many patients. In general, disease activity tends to recur as they are eliminated from the eye. By contrast, radiotherapy produces a delayed response but has a much longer duration of action. Therefore, there is rationale for a synergistic response when a combination approach is utilized as both therapies target the disease in different ways (22). The anti-VEGF therapy inhibits growth factors in the local area, while the radiotherapy disables the local inflammatory cell population and induces an apoptotic effect on the vascular endothelium. The overall result from these two approaches has the potential to bring a faster and more complete recovery of functional vision. This hypothesis is supported by clinical evidence from oncology, in which bevacizumab and radiotherapy were combined to treat colon cancer (23,24).

EARLY CLINICAL TRIALS

Radiotherapy as a treatment for neovascular AMD was first proposed in 1993, after initial animal studies and a phase 1 study that demonstrated significant regression of subfoveal CNV lesions (20,25). Initial ophthalmology case series investigated fractionated external beam radiotherapy, dividing the dose into smaller treatments (typically 2–3 Gy) over several days, to reduce damage to off-target tissue, with a total dose of 10 to 50 Gy (26–32). The results of these early, small, nonrandomized studies were somewhat inconclusive, especially given the variable natural course of AMD. Therefore, multiple randomized controlled trials were undertaken, using various fractionated radiotherapy doses from 7.5 to 24 Gy (33–41). Overall, a small but statistically significant reduction in the risk of vision loss was found (42). Although most studies reported that radiotherapy had a favorable effect, the difference was not always significant, and there was considerable inconsistency between the trials. Dose fractionation was not proven to offer an advantage over single-dose treatment (43).

Although the efficacy data were sometimes inconclusive, the majority of studies observed a reduction in scarring compared with the natural history of neovascular AMD. One study comparing bilateral disease showed an improvement in vision compared to the untreated fellow eyes for as long as 40 months after treatment (44).

The other technique investigated during these early studies was brachytherapy plaque irradiation. Various doses were used, with beta radiation sources such as strontium-90, in a single fraction dose of 12.6, 29, or 32.4 Gy (45,46) (doses differ from those published, based on recent recalibration measurements) (47). A radioactive source was introduced using an applicator positioned on the episcleral surface under the macula and held in place for up to 54 minutes. Favorable efficacy results were reported with the 29 Gy and 32.4 Gy doses, but not with 12.6 Gy.

Palladium-103 was another brachytherapy isotope investigated, with doses in the range of 12.5 to 24 Gy, delivered over 18 to 65 hours. The authors reported that 62% of patients had regression or stabilization of their exudative disease after 7 years (48–50).

A Cochrane review of radiation for the treatment of wet AMD was conducted in 2010. It did not include the recent epimacular brachytherapy and stereotactic radiotherapy studies but instead analyzed 14 early external beam radiotherapy trials and one plaque brachytherapy trial. It identified that the incidence of adverse events was low and that there was some evidence for an effect of radiotherapy in cases of severe visual acuity loss (6+ lines lost) over 12 months; however, this was not seen in the moderate visual loss groups (3+ lines lost) and was not maintained at 24 months' follow-up. With only a small number of trials included in the meta-analysis, with different investigational dosages and clinical and statistical inconsistency between trials, the analyses were limited and firm conclusions could not be made. It recommended that further trials be conducted with sufficient sample sizes to detect any moderate effects and that the results of all the visual acuity outcomes were reported to allow further meta-analysis review (42).

While some radiotherapy studies showed results better than the natural history, the results do not compare favorably to those in the anti-VEGF era (42,46,51). This may be because of collateral damage to ocular tissue and difficulty targeting macular lesions using technology that was designed for cancerous lesions that are usually several orders of magnitude larger than AMD lesions. Another factor may have been the time delay before radiation has an effect. This meant the disease progressed before the benefit of radiation occurred.

Another disadvantage of early external beam therapy relates to the linear accelerators and nuclear laboratory facilities required to generate the radiation. These required large power supplies and cooling measures and produced extremely high levels of energy, which are tightly regulated and require special precautions to prevent the escape of radiation, including lead-lined concrete walls (52).

OCULAR ADVERSE EVENTS OF RADIATION THERAPY

Despite attempts to minimize collateral damage, radiation therapy can cause damage to normal, healthy cells within, or neighboring, the treatment area. The susceptibility to the effect of ionizing radiation varies widely depending on the sensitivity of a particular tissue, in relation to the total dose delivered (Table 20.1).

Tear Film Disruption

Studies have described epiphora or transient conjunctival irritation and dry eye syndrome following radiotherapy (35,49). The symptoms may result from radiation damage to the lacrimal and meibomian glands, the conjunctiva itself, or its goblet cells (53,54). Deficiencies in any of the tear-film components (lipid layer, aqueous layer, mucinous layer) can result in unstable tear film, leading to dry eye symptoms, with secondary changes of the corneal and conjunctival surface. These effects are usually transient, typically lasting for a few months (55).

Cataract

The crystalline lens is the ocular structure with the highest susceptibility to radiation (48), with a reported threshold of 2 Gy (46). Lens opacities may develop within months or years, depending on the dose administered (56).

Radiation Optic Neuropathy

The threshold for clinically observable radiation damage to the optic nerve is reported to be greater than 55 Gy (19,57), with patients typically presenting after 8 to 16 months and very occasionally after 3 years (58). It is believed to be caused by damage to the vascular endothelial cells at the level of the choriocapillaris. This leads to vascular occlusions and vascular insufficiency of the optic nerve, which is then unable to meet the metabolic demands of the damaged tissue (59). Patients present with an anterior optic neuropathy that may manifest as papillitis and optic atrophy, characterized by initial disk swelling, hemorrhage, and cotton-wool spots (60). The prognosis is poor, often with a final visual acuity of less than 20/200, and many eyes become completely blind (61).

Table 20.1	CLINICALLY OBSERVABLE RADIATION DAMAGE THRESHOLDS FOR OCULAR STRUCTURES AND THE CALCULATED DOSES FOR EPIMACULAR BRACHYTHERAPY AND STEREOTACTIC RADIOSURGERY (48,57,65,66,79,80)			
Tissue	Effect	Reported thresholds for clinically observable radiation damage (gray)	Dose delivered during epimacular brachytherapy (gray)	Dose delivered during stereotactic radiosurgery (gray)
Lens	Cataract	2	0.00056	0.12–0.13
Retina	Radiation retinopathy	35–55	24	16–24
Optic nerve	Optic neuropathy	>55	2.4	0.2–0.37

Adapted from Finger PT, Berson A, Ng T, Szechter A. Ophthalmic plaque radiotherapy for age-related macular degeneration associated with subretinal neovascularization. Am J Ophthalmol. 1999;127(2):170–177.

Radiation Retinopathy

Radiation retinopathy is an occlusive microangiopathy, secondary to endothelial cell loss and capillary closure. It leads to the formation of small, dilated collateral channels that bypass the area of ischemia and assume a telangiectatic-like form (62). It was first described in 1933 following the use of radon seeds to treat retinal tumors (63). Patients developed retinal inflammation and degeneration, with exudates, hemorrhages, retinal pigment epithelium changes, and optic disk edema. The retinopathy was slowly progressive with a delayed onset, typically 6 months to 3 years after radiation treatment, with the severity dependent on the total dose of radiation administered (64). It is believed that the retina can usually tolerate doses up to 35 to 50 Gy, beyond which radiation retinopathy may occur (57,65,66).

Clinically, radiation retinopathy has an appearance similar to that of diabetic retinopathy, with the development of microaneurysms, followed by retinal hemorrhages, telangiectatic vessels, capillary nonperfusion, infarcts of the nerve fiber layer, and vascular obliterations at the level of the choriocapillaris (67–69). The earliest clinical features are discrete foci of occluded capillaries and irregular dilatation of the neighboring microvasculature. Fundus fluorescein angiography can confirm the extent of capillary dropout and the general capillary competence at this early stage (70). Indocyanine green angiography at an early stage shows atrophy of the retinal pigment epithelium and choriocapillaris, and eventually, the larger choroidal vessels became nonperfused (71). Vision loss is caused by macular edema, exudation, and retinal ischemia. In the late stages, secondary ischemic complications may lead to proliferative retinopathy, neovascularization, and subsequent vitreous hemorrhages, rubeosis iridis, and tractional retinal detachments (72–74). Patients who develop proliferative radiation retinopathy have a poor prognosis, with most achieving only 20/200 vision or worse after 6 years (75).

Studies using newer treatment modalities have described a non–vision-threatening form of radiation retinopathy (76–78). This is characterized by a nonprogressive, nonproliferative retinopathy and often favorable visual outcomes; indeed, it has been reported that the visual outcomes were better than those in participants who did not develop radiation retinopathy, at least over the 2- to 3-year time frames of the studies that have reported to date (77,78). This suggests that some patients may be more sensitive to the effects or radiation—both its beneficial and deleterious effects (77). Key clinical findings were macular intraretinal hemorrhages and telangiectatic dilatations of the perifoveolar capillaries and small areas of capillary nonperfusion that are best detected using fluorescein angiography (Fig. 20.1) (78).

CURRENT RADIOTHERAPY TREATMENTS

There has been renewed interest in the use of radiation to treat wet AMD, with three methods of delivery undergoing clinical trials: epimacular brachytherapy, stereotactic radiotherapy, and proton beam irradiation (Table 20.2).

Epimacular Brachytherapy

Unlike previous attempts using external beam radiation, epimacular brachytherapy was specifically developed to deliver intraocular radiation. The device (VIDION; NeoVista Inc., Fremont, CA) uses beta radiation from a strontium-90/yttrium-90 source. Beta radiation has a rapid decline in dose with increasing distance from the source (Fig. 20.2). This limits radiation exposure to a defined region, minimizing the risk of damage to adjacent normal tissue. The central macular lesion receives 24 Gy, the optic nerve receives 2.4 Gy, and the lens receives 0.00056 Gy (Fig. 20.3) (Table 20.2) (48,57,65,66,79–81).

The beta radiation used in epimacular brachytherapy is delivered via a pars plana vitrectomy (Fig. 20.4). Once the vitreous has been removed, the surgeon positions the probe over the CNV lesion (Fig. 20.5). A preoperative fundus fluorescein angiogram is used to ensure that the area of maximum dosage is directed over the area of greatest disease activity. The probe is held in position for approximately 4 minutes and then removed. Surgery is usually undertaken using local anesthetic in a day case setting.

In the initial published trials of epimacular brachytherapy, patients received an anti-VEGF injection at or near to the time of surgery and again 1 month later to treat any preexisting disease activity at the time of surgery. Thereafter, they had anti-VEGF therapy as needed, based on disease activity (79,82).

The combination of vitrectomy and radiation may be uniquely suited to the treatment of AMD. It has been proposed that removal of the vitreous increases the level of oxygen available to the inner layers of the retina via diffusion from the aqueous humor (83–85). A reduced oxygen tension may play a role in the initial CNV formation, and elevated oxygenation is likely to reduce VEGF levels (86). Increasing oxygenation in the treatment area at the time of brachytherapy may increase the formation of free radicals and therefore the double-stranded DNA breaks required to treat CNV lesions (87,88). The disadvantage of vitrectomy is that it may reduce the half-life of ranibizumab, as animal studies using other drugs indicate that vitrectomy may increase the rate of drug elimination from the vitreous (89–92).

CLINICAL TRIALS OF EPIMACULAR BRACHYTHERAPY

Two key studies provided the early data on the safety and efficacy of epimacular brachytherapy.

NVI-068

The first, NVI-068, was a nonrandomized multicentre feasibility study that recruited 34 treatment-naive participants in Mexico and Brazil. Subjects received either 15 Gy (eight participants) or 24 Gy (26 participants) of beta

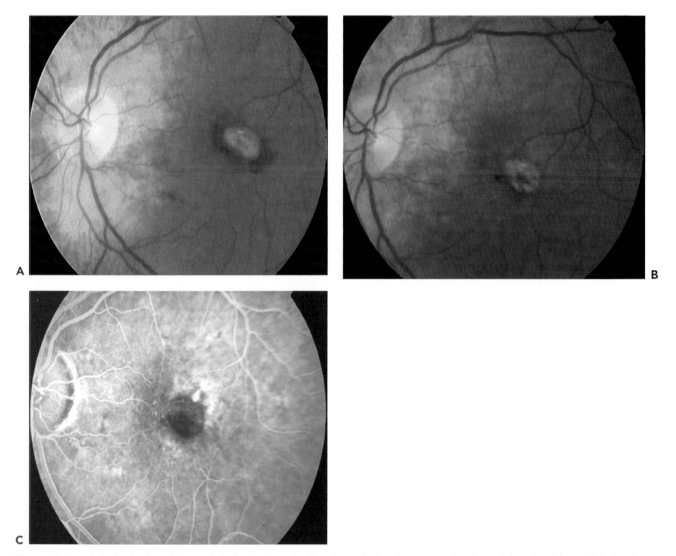

Figure 20.1 ■ **A.** Color fundus photograph before treatment with epimacular brachytherapy, showing subfoveal CNV associated with subretinal hemorrhage. **B.** Color fundus photograph 19 months after the initial treatment. The image shows fibrotic CNV surrounded by small superficial hemorrhages. **C.** Fluorescein angiography showing telangiectatic dilatation of the perifoveal capillaries, consistent with mild, nonproliferative radiation retinopathy. The CNV appears inactive, with no signs of leakage. (Reprinted with permission from Navarro R, Bures-Jelstrup A; Vasquez LM, et al. Radiation maculopathy after epimacular brachytherapy for the treatment of subfoveal choroidal neovascularization secondary to age-related macular degeneration. Retin Cases Brief Rep. 2011;5(4):352–354.)

radiation. Twelve months after treatment, there were no radiation-related adverse events recorded. There was however a significant difference in ETDRS visual acuity between the two groups. In the 24-Gy group, the mean visual acuity improved by 10.3 letters (approximately two Snellen lines), while the 15-Gy group lost 1.0 letters (82).

NVI-111

The second trial, NVI-111, was a prospective, nonrandomized, multicentre study that enrolled 34 treatment-naive participants in Mexico and Brazil. Participants were treated with a single dose of 24 Gy epimacular brachytherapy and two injections of anti-VEGF therapy. The first injection was given either at approximately 10 days before surgery or at the conclusion of epimacular brachytherapy. The second injection

was given 1 month later. Thereafter, anti-VEGF therapy was administered monthly PRN. Twelve months after treatment, there were no reported cases of radiation retinopathy. ETDRS visual acuity showed a mean improvement of 8.9 letters (approximately two Snellen lines), with 91% maintaining vision (defined as a loss of fewer than 15 ETDRS letters) and 68% having stable or improved visual acuity (improved by ≥0 letters) (79). Approximately three-quarters of participants required no further anti-VEGF therapy over the first year. By comparison, the Comparison of AMD Treatment Trials (CATT) study found that participants required an average of 7.7 anti-VEGF injections over this interval (4).

Subsequent review of the NVI-111 participants at 24 months revealed a mean visual acuity of –4.9 ETDRS letters (approximately one Snellen line), but the authors attributed this loss of vision to the development of cataract

Table 20.2	SUMMARY OF THE EPIMACULAR BRACHYTHERAPY AND STEREOTACTIC RADIOTHERAPY CLINICAL TRIALS				
Study name	Radiotherapy	Dose (gray)	Prior anti-VEGF therapy	Study phase	Number of participants
NVI-068	Epimacular brachytherapy	15 or 24	Treatment naive	Noncontrolled	34
NVI-111	Epimacular brachytherapy	24	Treatment naive	Noncontrolled	34
CABERNET	Epimacular brachytherapy	24	Treatment naive	Randomized controlled	457
MERITAGE	Epimacular brachytherapy	24	Previously treated	Noncontrolled	53
MERLOT	Epimacular brachytherapy	24	Previously treated	Randomized controlled	363
CLH001	Stereotactic radiotherapy	16 or 24	Treatment naive and previously treated	Noncontrolled	62
INTREPID	Stereotactic radiotherapy	16 or 24 or Sham	Previously treated	Randomized controlled	226
Proton beam pilot	Proton beam radiotherapy	2 × 12	Treatment naive and previously treated	Noncontrolled	6
PBAMD2	Proton beam radiotherapy	2 × 8, 2 × 12 or sham	Previously treated	Randomized controlled	45

in the phakic participants. This appeared to be supported by the 36-month data that revealed a final mean visual acuity of +3.9 ETDRS letters, and a mean of only three retreatment injections during this time (76). There was one case of nonproliferative retinopathy identified in the 36-month report, with relatively subtle microvascular changes (telangiectatic vessels, vessel beading, and microaneurysms). The changes were detected in the parafoveal region of a patient who had no adverse effect on visual acuity (improved one line from baseline) and who remained

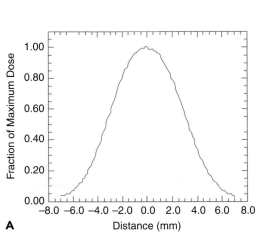 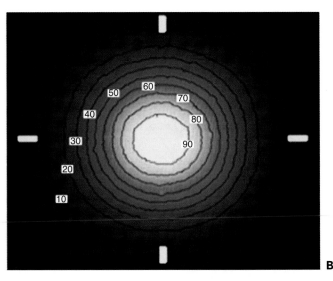

Figure 20.2 ■ Dose attenuation with distance. **A.** Graph showing the attenuation in the dose of radiation delivered, in relation to distance from the source. In general, it can be seen that the dose is inversely related to the square of the distance from the probe.
B. —Radiochromic Film Contour Plot for the strontium-90 radiation source. White boxes represent the percent of maximum dose. The yellow hash marks on the image correspond to the horizontal and vertical (top-down) dose rate profiles as displayed in the left image. The inside edge of each hash mark is equidistant to the radiation center of the source. (Courtesy of NeoVista.)

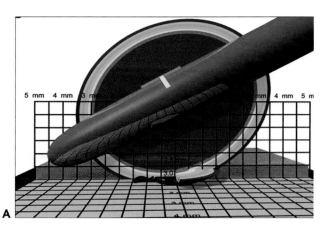
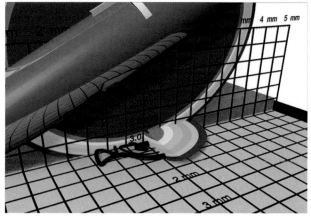

Figure 20.3 ■ **A,B.** Computer-generated images showing the dose attenuation with distance from the probe to the retinal surface (red = 24 Gy) and in 0.1-mm increments (orange = 20 Gy; yellow = 17 Gy; light green = 14 Gy; dark green = 11 Gy; light blue = 10 Gy; and dark blue = 9 Gy). (Courtesy of NeoVista.)

stable at 43 months of follow-up with only one additional anti-VEGF injection administered at the first month after brachytherapy (76).

The promising results of these pilot studies led to the larger studies of epimacular brachytherapy.

MERITAGE

The Macular EpiRetinal brachytherapy in Treated AGE-related macular degeneration (MERITAGE) study (ClinicalTrials.gov Identifier: NCT00809419) was a multicentre, noncontrolled Phase II study evaluating the safety and efficacy of epimacular brachytherapy in participants who required persistent anti-VEGF injections. MERITAGE enrolled 53 participants from five sites in the United States, Israel, and the United Kingdom. The objective was to investigate if visual acuity could be maintained while reducing the demand of retreatment with anti-VEGF therapy. Unlike the preceding studies, MERITAGE enrolled participants who

were already receiving treatment with ranibizumab or bevacizumab. In addition, participants were required to meet minimum prior injection criteria to be eligible, namely three rescue injections in the 6 months preceding enrollment or five rescue injections in the 12 months preceding enrollment.

Prior to enrollment, the participants had a mean duration of disease of 28 months and had received an average of 12.5 anti-VEGF treatments, with one participant receiving a maximum of 38 prior injections. As a result, this study selectively recruited participants with the most active disease, who might otherwise be predicted to have a poor outcome. This differs from previous studies on radiotherapy that recruited treatment-naive disease, where the case mix may have been more typical. Because participants have already commenced treatment, the MERITAGE study did not expect to show visual gains, unlike studies that recruit untreated disease.

The MERITAGE study reported that after 12 months of follow-up, the mean change in visual acuity was –4.0 ETDRS letters (approximately one Snellen line) with a mean of 3.2

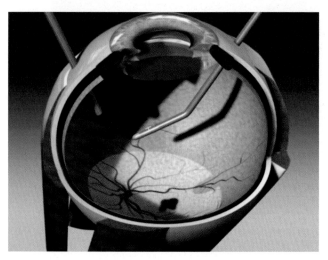

Figure 20.4 ■ Intraocular probe in the midvitreous cavity, prior to placement on the retinal surface. (Courtesy of NeoVista.)

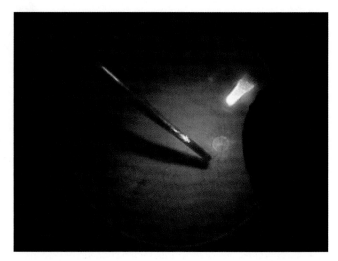

Figure 20.5 ■ Epimacular brachytherapy probe positioned on the retinal surface, during surgery.

anti-VEGF injections. The proportion of participants maintaining vision (losing fewer than 15 ETDRS letters) was 81%, and the rate of administration of anti-VEGF injections had reduced from 0.45 injections per participant per month prior to enrollment to 0.27 injections per participant per month over 12 months (47).

Microperimetry and indocyanine green angiography were performed on all participants at one of the MERITAGE recruiting sites, to determine if the radiotherapy causes reduced retinal sensitivity or choroidal ischemia. The site reported similar results to previous investigations using strontium-90 (93), with no loss of retinal sensitivity or evidence of choroidal damage after 12 months. There appeared to be a positive dose response, with a statistically significant correlation between proximity to the radioactive source and improvement in retinal sensitivity (Fig. 20.6). This response was most significant within the neovascular lesion area. This suggests that the benefit of epimacular brachytherapy is due, at least in part, to the effect of radiation, and not

some other confounding variable, such as the vitrectomy procedure, as the areas that received the higher doses demonstrated the greatest functional improvement. The authors speculated that it might be possible to offer a more customized dose delivery, rather than offering a standard dose of 24 Gy, regardless of the lesion type, size, or topography (94).

A subsequent report analyzed the optical coherence tomography (OCT) and fundus fluorescein angiograms of the MERITAGE participants at 12 months. OCT center thickness increased by 50 μm over this time frame, but the median increase was only 1.8 μm, reflecting the fact that the mean increase was driven by a minority of eyes with relatively large increases (95). The angiographic lesion size was substantially larger than most other trials, and this would be expected to result in worse visual outcome (96).

Both the OCT and visual outcomes suggested that classic lesions responded better than occult lesions. Over half of the participants had occult lesions (with no classic) with a mean center thickness increase of 62 μm and loss

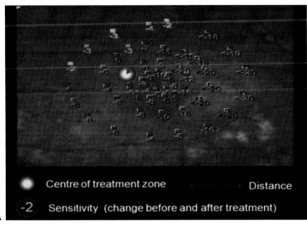

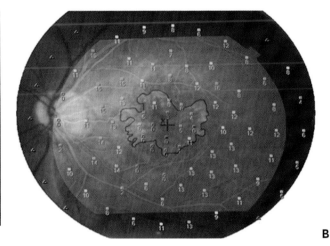

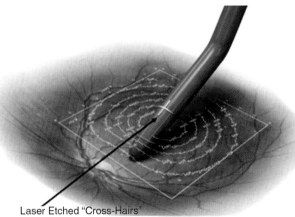

Figure 20.6 ■ Determining the relationship between radiation dose and retinal sensitivity. **A.** The change in sensitivity was calculated for areas within and outside the AMD lesion area. This boundary was defined using the fundus fluorescein angiogram images and included all components of the AMD lesion, including any hemorrhage, fibrosis, or leakage. This was then superimposed onto the microperimetry fundus photograph so that data points could be mapped. **B.** Positioning of the probe was planned prior to surgery, to ensure delivery of the maximum dose to the most active part of the AMD lesion. Probe position was recorded at the end of the operation by marking the FFA. Once the FFA was overlaid on the microperimetry field, it was possible to calculate the distance from the probe for each sensitivity data point. It was thus possible to correlate the change in retinal sensitivity to the dose of radiation received. **C.** The epimacular brachytherapy probe is etched with a cross that corresponds to the position of the radioactive pellet within the probe. The retina beneath this cross receives the maximum 24-Gray dose.

of 5 ETDRS letters (one Snellen line). Minimally classic lesions had an increase of 51 μm and lost 6 ETDRS letters. Predominately classic lesions decreased by 43 μm and gained 2 ETDRS letters (95).

The adverse events reported in the first 12 months of the MERITAGE study were mainly related to the development of postvitrectomy cataract, with no radiation retinopathy identified. The study will however monitor participants for 3 years, as radiation retinopathy may occur at a later stage (47).

In summary, the MERITAGE study recruited patients with active disease, who were losing vision despite frequent anti-VEGF therapy. It demonstrated stabilization of vision in a majority of participants and a reduced frequency of reinjection. Subgroup analysis suggested classic lesions were the most responsive.

CABERNET

The CNV Secondary to AMD Treated with BEta RadiatioN Epiretinal Therapy (CABERNET) study (ClinicalTrials.gov Identifier: NCT00454389) was the first multinational, pivotal, randomized controlled trial evaluating the safety and efficacy of epimacular brachytherapy in treatment-naive participants. CABERNET enrolled 457 participants across 45 sites in the United States, Europe, Israel, and South America. The 302 participants in the epimacular brachytherapy (24 Gy) treatment arm had two mandatory ranibizumab injections. The 155 participants in the control arm received ranibizumab injections following a modified PIER protocol, which included three initial monthly injections followed by injections every 3 months. Participants in both arms were seen on a monthly basis, and rescue therapy was permitted according to protocol-specific retreatment criteria.

At the 24-month end point, the CABERNET study failed to meet its primary outcomes using a predefined 10% noninferiority margin and 97% confidence interval, indicating that in treatment-naive participants, the use of epimacular brachytherapy was not shown to be noninferior to anti-VEGF monotherapy, in terms of vision maintenance (77). The epimacular brachytherapy group received a mean of 6.2 injections of ranibizumab treatments and had a mean change in visual acuity of –2.5 ETDRS letters, while the control group received a mean of 10.4 injections and had a mean change in visual acuity of +4.4 ETDRS letters (approximately one Snellen line) (77).

In the epimacular brachytherapy arm, 42% of participants received no injections after 12 months and only one injection up to 24 months, with a mean gain of 3.3 ETDRS letters; 27% of participants received no rescue injections throughout the 24-month course of the study and achieved a gain of 5.7 ETDRS letters. These results suggested there were some lesions that were particularly sensitive to the treatment (77).

Post hoc analysis, at a 20% noninferiority margin and a 95% confidence interval, found that epimacular brachytherapy was noninferior for lesions smaller than 3.5 disk areas and for classic or minimally classic lesions, as judged by the investigator. It was observed that the large occult lesions drove the mean visual acuity results down. The authors speculated that the edge of these larger lesions may have received a subtherapeutic dose due to the rapid tapering of the treatment dose from the center, which, although advantageous in terms of safety, may lead to parts of larger lesions being undertreated. Furthermore, positioning of the probe over the area of greatest disease activity may have been difficult with occult lesions, due to their indistinct boundaries and their variable shape, which makes it difficult to define a geometric centre (77).

CABERNET demonstrated that epimacular brachytherapy had an acceptable safety profile over a 2-year interval. The most frequent adverse event reported was cataract, occurring in 40% of the participants who were phakic at enrollment, and which was most likely related to the vitrectomy rather than the radiotherapy. There were ten cases (3%) of suspected nonprogressive, nonproliferative, radiation retinopathy, but interestingly, these participants tended to have a positive clinical outcome, with a mean gain in vision of 4.4 ETDRS letters (approximately one Snellen line) and a mean of only two rescue injections over 2 years. Further follow-up is planned, as radiation retinopathy can occur beyond a 24-month window.

RETINAL ANGIOMATOUS PROLIFERATION

Although there is little clinical evidence to date, theoretically, epimacular brachytherapy may be well suited to the treatment of retinal angiomatous proliferation (RAP). These lesions often have rapid and aggressive growth (97,98), and assuming then that they are highly mitotic, they should be more susceptible to the effects of the ionizing radiation. Further, their small size and easily defined centre means it is possible to accurately administer the maximum dose (24 Gy) to almost the entire lesion.

A single case of RAP treated with epimacular brachytherapy has been reported, with a positive clinical outcome. Preoperatively, the patient had received eight ranibizumab injections over a 10-month period and had active leakage during angiography. At 12 months after epimacular brachytherapy, she had gained 16 ETDRS letters (approximately three Snellen lines), with resolution angiographic leakage (Fig. 20.7) with only one further anti-VEGF injection over 21 months (99).

IDIOPATHIC POLYPOIDAL CHOROIDAL VASCULOPATHY

The efficacy of epimacular brachytherapy in cases of idiopathic polypoidal choroidal vasculopathy (IPCV) (100,101) is unknown, but it is possible that IPCV may be amenable

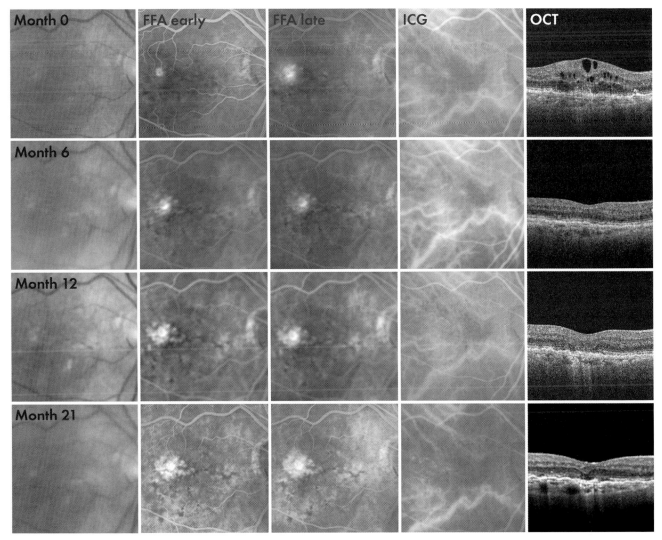

Month 0	FFA early	FFA late	ICG	OCT
Month 6				
Month 12				
Month 21				

Figure 20.7 ■ Treatment of a RAP lesion: The top row shows fundus photographs, early fundus fluorescein angiography (FFA), late fundus fluorescein angiography, indocyanine green angiography (ICG), and optical coherence tomography (OCT) results at baseline (preoperative). The second row shows results at 6 months after epimacular brachytherapy. The third row shows results at 12 months. The bottom row shows the results at further follow-up of 21 months. The FFAs show persisting late staining of fibrous tissue but a loss of active leakage seen at baseline, following treatment with epimacular brachytherapy. ICG fails to show any deleterious effects of radiation on the choroidal circulation. OCT shows a marked reduction in intraretinal fluid that persists over 21 months. (Reprinted with permission from Petrarca R, Nau J, Dugel P, et al. Epimacular brachytherapy for the treatment of retinal angiomatous proliferation. Retin Cases Brief Rep. 2012;6(4):353–357.)

to radiation, and furthermore, these lesions often show a suboptimal response to anti-VEGF injections. Conversely, radiation has been associated with the development of IPCV (102).

There have been two identified cases of IPCV treated by epimacular brachytherapy, both within the MERITAGE study. In both cases, the lesions were seen using indocyanine green angiography, with one lesion located at the macular and the other in a peripapillary location (94). Prior to enrollment in the study, the participants had received a mean of 21 injections over a mean of 29 months. At 12 months following treatment with epimacular brachytherapy, the mean change in vision was +3.0 ETDRS letters, with a mean of only three anti-VEGF treatments.

MERLOT

The Macular EpiRetinal Brachytherapy versus Lucentis Only Treatment (MERLOT) study (ClinicalTrials.gov Identifier: NCT01006538) is a pivotal, multicenter, randomized controlled trial in the United Kingdom, recruiting participants who have already commenced anti-VEGF therapy. It has completed recruitment with a total of 363 participants who were randomized in a 2:1 ratio, to either epimacular brachytherapy (24 Gy) with as-required ranibizumab or as-required ranibizumab monotherapy. The MERLOT study, like MERITAGE, targets participants requiring regular anti-VEGF injections. The rationale is that there are limited surgical resources, and these resources are best directed to those who have not fully responded to ranibizumab therapy or whose response is short-lived. These participants have the most to gain from a therapy that may reduce their frequency of anti-VEGF retreatment (103). The 12-month results are expected in early 2013.

Stereotactic Radiotherapy

More recently, investigators have revisited external beam therapy, using a technique called Stereotactic Radiosurgery or Stereotactic Radiotherapy. The IRay system (Oraya Therapeutics, Newark, CA, USA) uses a low-voltage x-ray source that does not require the same degree of radiation shielding as the early linear accelerators. The system is designed to fit in a standard clinical environment and runs off a 220 to 240 V wall socket, without the need for room shielding or expensive safety precautions (Fig. 20.8) (80).

The system is designed to overcome the traditional disadvantages of external beam therapy by dividing the dose into separate beams that pass into the eye via different locations and overlap on the CNV lesion (104). The beams pass through the inferior pars plana region of the sclera, at the 5-, 6-, and 7-o'clock positions (Fig. 20.9). These overlap on the predicted foveal center, dispersing the scleral entry dose and minimizing exposure of the lens and optic nerve (80,104,105). The patient is secured in position with a head restraint that also contains a lead backing to prevent radiation traveling beyond the patient. Exposure to the lower lid is limited by a lid retractor. The operator is separated from the patient during treatment via a lead-lined glass shield, which allows the operator to monitor the patient (Fig 20.5) (80,106). The patient's eye is then secured in position with a vacuum-coupled contact lens interface with suction; the system can detect any eye motion and stabilizes the eye during treatment (Fig. 20.10). The eye is then continually tracked during treatment, and an inbuilt safety feature

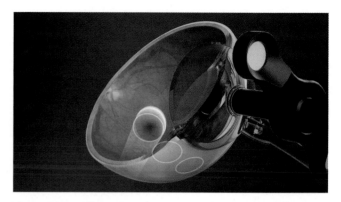

Figure 20.9 ■ Illustration of the trajectory of the stereotactic radiotherapy beams that pass through the pars plana, overlapping on the macula, and avoiding the lens and optic nerve. (Courtesy of Oraya.)

interrupts the radiation treatment if the eye moves out of position. The system can treat most AMD lesions centered on the fovea, with an average accuracy of 0.6 mm and a precision of 0.4 mm (107,108).

CLINICAL TRIALS OF STEREOTACTIC RADIOTHERAPY

CLH001 Study

The CLH001 study (Safety and tolerability of the IRay system in subjects with exudative CNV secondary to AMD; ClinicalTrials.gov Identifier: NCT01217762) was a single-center, noncontrolled pilot study in Mexico that included 62 participants with neovascular AMD. The study recruited participants who had already commenced anti-VEGF therapy and also those who were treatment naive. It investigated two radiation doses, 16 and 24 Gy. Induction involved anti-VEGF therapy at baseline and month 1, with the radiotherapy administered during the first 2 weeks after baseline. Both regimens then administered anti-VEGF as required, based on protocol-specific retreatment criteria.

In the 16-Gy group, 28 participants were originally recruited (one was later excluded due to wrong diagnosis). Of these, 11 had been previously treated with anti-VEGF therapy, and in this group, the mean change in visual acuity was +8.2 ETDRS letters at 12 months. Sixteen participants were treatment-naive, with a mean change of +8.6 ETDRS letters. With both groups combined, participants received a mean of only 1.0 additional anti-VEGF treatment, with 52% (14) of the participants not requiring any further retreatment (109).

In the 24-Gy group, 19 participants were recruited; 11 had been previously treated with anti-VEGF therapy, while eight were treatment-naive participants and the mean change of visual acuity at 12 months was +7.5 ETDRS letters and +8.3 ETDRS letters, respectively. The group as a whole received a mean of 1.0 retreatment injection over the 12 months, with 58% (11) of the participants requiring no further treatment.

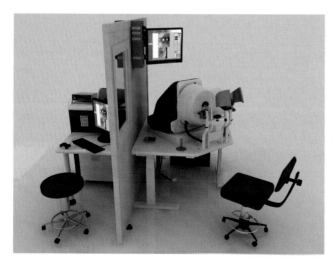

Figure 20.8 ■ The photograph shows the IRay system used to deliver stereotactic radiotherapy. The patient and operator site on opposite sides of a lead-lined glass screen. (Courtesy of Oraya.)

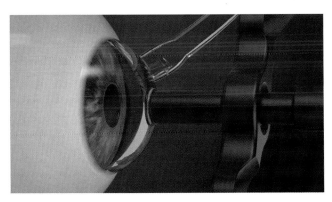

Figure 20.10 ■ During stereotactic radiotherapy, the participant's eye position is controlled using a contact lens system, with markers that can be tracked by the robotically positioned device that generates the radioactive beams. This ensures that the radiation is delivered to the appropriate target area and enables the system to halt the delivery of radiation if the eye moves out of position. (Courtesy of Oraya.)

Overall, 100% of the participants maintained vision (losing fewer than 15 ETDRS letters) and 79% achieved a gain in vision, with a mean change in OCT central retinal thickness of –87 µm (110).

After the preliminary 12-month follow-up, there were no significant ocular or nonocular adverse events attributed to the stereotactic radiotherapy device, except for one case of transient asymptomatic superficial punctate keratopathy due to the contact lens eye stabilizer. In particular, there were no radiation-related adverse events, including retinopathy, optic neuropathy, and cataract advancement (109,110). In summary then, CLH001 suggested that 16 and 24 Gy doses achieve a similar outcome in terms of visual acuity and demand for anti-VEGF retreatment.

INTREPID STUDY

The IRay plus anti-VEGF treatment for patients with wet AMD (INTREPID) study (ClinicalTrials.gov Identifier: NCT01016873) is a double-masked, sham-controlled, randomized controlled trial, evaluating the safety and effectiveness of stereotactic radiotherapy in participants who have commenced anti-VEGF therapy. It has completed recruitment of 226 participants across 21 European sites. Participants were randomized to 16, 24 Gy, or sham therapy, with as-required ranibizumab in all groups. Results are expected toward the middle of 2012. The primary efficacy outcome measure is the posttreatment demand for anti-VEGF retreatment.

Proton Beam Radiotherapy

Fractionated proton beam radiotherapy continues to be evaluated, in facilities with a cyclotron nuclear laboratory (38). Initial reports used proton beam radiotherapy as a monotherapy, but more recently, it has been combined with anti-VEGF therapy. Compared to epimacular

brachytherapy, proton beam radiotherapy has the potential to target large lesions, and in comparison to stereotactic radiotherapy, it is not limited to treating lesions within a central 4-mm treatment zone. In addition, a comparably sized single proton beam should limit the lateral spread of radiation to surrounding tissues, such as the lens and optic nerve (111).

CLINICAL TRIALS OF PROTON BEAM RADIOTHERAPY

Pilot Proton Beam with Anti-VEGF Study

A pilot study of ranibizumab combined with proton beam irradiation (ClinicalTrials.gov Identifier: NCT01213082) recruited six participants—four were treatment naive and two had previously been treated with anti-VEGF therapy. Participants were treated with four consecutive monthly ranibizumab injections and 24 Gy proton beam irradiation in two 12 Gy fractions, given 24 hours apart, within 6 weeks of the first injection. After 12 months, the mean change in visual acuity was +9.2 ETDRS letters (approximately two Snellen lines) with a mean of six anti-VEGF treatments. After 24 months, the mean change in visual acuity had dropped to –0.4 ETDRS letters with a mean of 10.6 anti-VEGF treatments. There were no cases of radiation retinopathy, over a mean follow-up of 28 months.

PBAMD2 Study

The prospective randomized trial of Proton Beam combined with anti-VEGF therapy for exudative Age-related Macular Degeneration (PBAMD2) study (ClinicalTrials. gov Identifier: NCT01213082) aims to recruit 45 previously treated participants in the United States. Participants will be randomized to receive either 16 Gy or 24 Gy proton beam therapy given in two fractions, 24 hours apart, with anti-VEGF therapy, compared with sham irradiation and anti-VEGF therapy. The trial is currently recruiting, and results are expected in late 2013.

CONCLUSION

The ongoing management of patients with neovascular AMD presents a considerable challenge to health care providers. The ideal treatment for this sight-threatening condition would maintain or improve a patient's vision, while eliminating, or at least limiting, the number of anti-VEGF injections and follow-ups. Theoretically, radiation therapy has the potential to meet both these requirements, but large clinical studies have yet to prove this is the case.

The initial studies of epimacular brachytherapy were very encouraging, but the results of the CABERNET study of treatment-naive disease failed to replicate the early data, and further analysis is needed to determine which subsets of patients may benefit. The MERLOT study should overcome some of the design issues of CABERNET, in that both arms receive the same anti-VEGF retreatment, and this study will also target the largest patient group, namely those who have already commenced anti-VEGF therapy.

Preliminary studies of stereotactic radiotherapy were also very positive, but pivotal trials have yet to be completed. The INTREPID study was designed to determine whether or not stereotactic radiotherapy reduces the demand for anti-VEGF therapy, and it remains to be determined if it will have sufficient statistical power to conclude on the treatment's visual efficacy.

Studies investigating the proton beam radiotherapy with anti-VEGF are at an early stage, with a pilot study showing similar results to the preliminary studies of epimacular brachytherapy and stereotactic radiotherapy. Larger studies are required.

Given that radiation retinopathy may occur beyond the usual 1- or 2-year reporting window of many clinical trials, extended follow-up will be needed to determine its true incidence and its visual prognosis.

In summary, it is too early to conclude on the safety and efficacy of modern radiation therapy for wet AMD. Further, the three candidate technologies have important differences, such that the findings from one cannot be applied to the others. Taken together, the MERLOT and CABERNET studies should ultimately enable clinicians to conclude on the risks and benefits of epimacular brachytherapy. The INTREPID study may possibly do likewise for stereotactic radiotherapy, and if not it will at least indicate whether larger studies of stereotactic radiotherapy are justified. Modern proton beam therapy is certainly of interest, but at a relatively early stage of development.

REFERENCES

1. Rosenfeld PJ, Brown DM, Heier JS, et al. Ranibizumab for neovascular age-related macular degeneration. N Engl J Med. 2006;355(14):1419–1431.

2. Brown DM, Kaiser PK, Michels M, et al. Ranibizumab versus verteporfin for neovascular age-related macular degeneration. N Engl J Med. 2006; 355(14):1432–1444.

3. Tufail A, Patel P, Egan C, et al. ABC Trial Investigators. Bevacizumab for neovascular age related macular degeneration (ABC Trial): multicentre randomised double masked study. BMJ. 2010;340:c2459. Available at: http://www.bmj.com/content/340/bmj.c2459?view=long&pmid=20538634. Accessed December 31, 2011.

4. Martin DF, Maguire MG, et al.; CATT Research Group. Ranibizumab and bevacizumab for neovascular age-related macular degeneration. N Engl J Med. 2011;364(20):1897–1908.

5. Heier JS, Boyer D, Nguyen QD, et al. The 1-year Results of CLEAR-IT 2, a phase 2 study of vascular endothelial growth factor trap-eye dosed as-needed after 12-week fixed dosing. Ophthalmology. 2011;118(6):1098–1106.

6. Lalwani G, Rosenfeld P, Fung A, et al. A variable-dosing regimen with intravitreal ranibizumab for neovascular age related macular degeneration: year 2 of the PrONTO Study. Am J Ophthalmol. 2009;148:43–58.

7. Engelbert M, Zweifel S, Freund K. Long-term follow-up for type 1 (subretinal pigment epithelium) neovascularization using a modified "treat and extend" dosing regimen of intravitreal antivascular endothelial growth factor therapy. Retina. 2010;30:1368–1375.

8. Holz F, Amoaku W, Donate J, et al.; SUSTAIN Study Group. Safety and efficacy of a flexible dosing regimen of ranibizumab in neovascular age-related macular degeneration: the SUSTAIN Study. Ophthalmology. 2011;118:663–671.

9. Attix F. Introduction to radiological physics and radiation dosimetry. New York: John Wiley & Sons; 1986.

10. Gazda M, Coia L. Principles of radiation therapy. In: Pazdyr R, Coia L, Hoskins W, et al., eds. Cancer management: a multidisciplinary approach. New York: PRR, Melville; 2001:9–20.

11. Barnhard HJ. Supervoltage therapy comes of age. N Engl J Med. 1958; 258(6):275–277.

12. Krishnan L, Krishnan EC, Jewell WR. Immediate effect of irradiation on microvasculature. Int J Radiat Oncol Biol Phys. 1988;15(1):147–150.

13. Mooteri SN, Podolski JL, Drab EA, et al. WR-1065 and radioprotection of vascular endothelial cells. II. Morphology. Radiat Res. 1996;145(2):217–224.

14. Rosander K, Zackrisson B. DNA damage in human endothelial cells after irradiation in anoxia. Acta Oncol. 1995;34(1):111–116.

15. Kirwan JF, Constable PH, Murdoch IE, et al. Beta irradiation: new uses for an old treatment: a review. Eye (Lond). 2003;17(2):207–215.

16. Engerman RL, Pfaffenbach D, Davis MD. Cell turnover of capillaries. Lab Invest. 1967;17(6):738–743.

17. Sharma NK, Gardiner TA, Archer DB. A morphologic and autoradiographic study of cell death and regeneration in the retinal microvasculature of normal and diabetic rats. Am J Ophthalmol. 1985;100(1):51–60.

18. Archer DB, Amoaku WM, Gardiner TA. Radiation retinopathy—clinical, histopathological, ultrastructural and experimental correlations. Eye (Lond). 1991;5(Pt 2):239–251.

19. Parsons JT, Fitzgerald CR, Hood CI, et al. The effects of irradiation on the eye and optic nerve. Int J Radiat Oncol Biol Phys. 1983;9(5):609–622.

20. Chakravarthy U, Gardiner TA, Archer DB, et al. A light microscopic and autoradiographic study of non-irradiated and irradiated ocular wounds. Curr Eye Res. 1989;8(4):337–348.

21. Gelisken O, Yazici B. Radiation therapy in exudative age-related macular degeneration. Semin Ophthalmol. 1999;14(1):27–34.

22. Woodward BW. Comparison of efficacy of proton beam and 90Sr/90Y beta radiation in treatment of exudative age-related macular degeneration. Fremont, CA: NeoVista Inc.; 2008.

23. Willett CG, Boucher Y, di Tomaso E, et al. Direct evidence that the VEGF-specific antibody bevacizumab has antivascular effects in human rectal cancer. Nat Med. 2004;10(2):145–147.

24. Senan S, Smit EF. Design of clinical trials of radiation combined with antiangiogenic therapy. Oncologist. 2007;12(4):465–477.

25. Chakravarthy U, Houston RF, Archer DB. Treatment of age-related subfoveal neovascular membranes by teletherapy: a pilot study. Br J Ophthalmol. 1993;77(5):265–273.

26. Bergink GJ, Deutman AF, van den Broek JE, et al. Radiation therapy for age-related subfoveal choroidal neovascular membranes. A pilot study. Doc Ophthalmol. 1995;90(1):67–74.

27. Holz FG, Bellmann C, Engenhart R, et al. External stereotaxic focal irradiation therapy for subfoveal choroidal neovascularization. Invest Ophthalmol Vis Sci. 1996;37:550–550.

28. Matsuhashi H, Noda Y, Takahashi D, et al. Radiation therapy for small choroidal neovascularization in age-related macular degeneration. Jpn J Ophthalmol. 2000;44(6):653–660.

29. Haas A, Papaefthymiou G, Langmann G, et al. Gamma knife treatment of subfoveal, classic neovascularization in age-related macular degeneration: a pilot study. J Neurosurg. 2000;93:172–176.

30. Schittkowski M, Schneider H, Gruschow K, et al. 3 years experience with low dosage fractionated percutaneous teletherapy in subfoveal neovascularization. Clinical results. Strahlenther Onkol. 2001;177(7):345–353.

31. Eter N, Schuller H, Spitznas M. Radiotherapy for age-related macular degeneration: is there a benefit for classic CNV? Int Ophthalmol. 2001;24(1):13–19.

32. Gripp S, Stammen J, Petersen C, et al. Radiotherapy in age-related macula degeneration. Int J Radiat Oncol Biol Phys. 2002;52(2):489–495.

33. Bergink GJ, Hoyng CB, van der Maazen RW, et al. A randomized controlled clinical trial on the efficacy of radiation therapy in the control of subfoveal choroidal neovascularization in age-related macular degeneration: radiation versus observation. Graefes Arch Clin Exp Ophthalmol. 1998;236(5):321–325.

34. Char DH, Irvine AI, Posner MD, et al. Randomized trial of radiation for age-related macular degeneration. Am J Ophthalmol. 1999;127(5):574–578.

35. The radiation Therapy for age-related Macular Degeneration (RAD) Study Group. A prospective, randomized, double-masked trial on radiation therapy for neovascular age-related macular degeneration (RAD Study). Radiation therapy for age-related macular degeneration. Ophthalmology. 1999;106(12):2239–2247.

36. Kobayashi H, Kobayashi K. Age-related macular degeneration: long-term results of radiotherapy for subfoveal neovascular membranes. Am J Ophthalmol. 2000;130(5):617–635.

37. Valmaggia C, Ries G, Ballinari P. Radiotherapy for subfoveal choroidal neovascularization in age-related macular degeneration: a randomized clinical trial. Am J Ophthalmol. 2002;133(4):521–529.

38. Ciulla TA, Danis RP, Klein SB, et al. Proton therapy for exudative age-related macular degeneration: a randomized, sham-controlled clinical trial. Am J Ophthalmol. 2002;134(6):905–906.

39. Hart PM, Chakravarthy U, Mackenzie G, et al. Visual outcomes in the sub-foveal radiotherapy study: a randomized controlled trial of teletherapy for age-related macular degeneration. Arch Ophthalmol. 2002;120(8):1029–1038.

40. Marcus DM, Peskin E, Maguire M, et al. The age-related macular degeneration radiotherapy trial (AMDRT): one year results from a pilot study. Am J Ophthalmol. 2004;138(5):818–828.

41. Prettenhofer U, Haas A, Mayer R, et al. Long-term results after external radiotherapy in age-related macular degeneration. A prospective study. Strahlenther Onkol. 2004;180(2):91–95.

42. Evans JR, Sivagnanavel V, Chong V. Radiotherapy for neovascular age-related macular degeneration. Cochrane Database Syst Rev. 2010;(5):CD004004.

43. Archambeau JO, Mao XW, Yonemoto LT, et al. What is the role of radiation in the treatment of subfoveal membranes: review of radiobiologic, pathologic, and other considerations to initiate a multimodality discussion. Int J Radiat Oncol Biol Phys. 1998;40(5):1125–1136.

44. Hart PM, Archer DB, Chakravarthy U. Asymmetry of disciform scarring in bilateral disease when one eye is treated with radiotherapy. Br J Ophthalmol. 1995;79(6):562–568.

45. Jaakkola A, Heikkonen J, Tommila P, et al. Strontium plaque irradiation of subfoveal neovascular membranes in age-related macular degeneration. Graefes Arch Clin Exp Ophthalmol. 1998;236(1):24–30.

46. Jaakkola A, Heikkonen J, Tommila P, et al. Strontium plaque brachytherapy for exudative age-related macular degeneration: three-year results of a randomized study. Ophthalmology. 2005;112(4):567–573.

47. Dugel P, Petrarca R, Bennett M, et al. Twelve month safety and feasibility study of epimacular brachytherapy for the treatment of neovascular age-related macular degeneration in subjects treated with chronic anti-VEGF therapy: The MERITAGE Study. Ophthalmology. 2012;119(7):1425–1431.

48. Finger PT, Berson A, Ng T, et al. Ophthalmic plaque radiotherapy for age-related macular degeneration associated with subretinal neovascularization. Am J Ophthalmol. 1999;127(2):170–177.

49. Finger PT, Berson A, Sherr D, et al. Radiation therapy for subretinal neovascularization. Ophthalmology. 1996;103(6):878–889.

50. Finger PT, Gelman YP, Berson AM, et al. Palladium-103 plaque radiation therapy for macular degeneration: results of a 7 year study. Br J Ophthalmol. 2003;87(12):1497–1503.

51. Chakravarthy U, MacKenzie G. External beam radiotherapy in exudative age-related macular degeneration: a pooled analysis of phase I data. Br J Radiol. 2000;73(867):305–313.

52. Rokni SH, Fassò A, Liu JC. Operational radiation protection in high-energy physics accelerators. Radiat Prot Dosimetry. 2009;137(1–2):3–17.

53. Karp LA, Streeten BW, Cogan DG. Radiation-induced atrophy of the meibomian glands. Arch Ophthalmol. 1979;97(2):303–305.

54. Stephens LC, Schultheiss TE, Peters LJ, et al. Acute radiation injury of ocular adnexa. Arch Ophthalmol. 1988;106(3):389–391.

55. Eter N, Schüller H. External beam radiotherapy for age-related macular degeneration causes transient objective changes in tear-film function. Graefes Arch Clin Exp Ophthalmol. 2001;239(12):923–926.

56. Macfaul PA, Bedford MA. Ocular complications after therapeutic irradiation. Br J Ophthalmol. 1970;54(4):237–247.

57. Parsons JT, Bova FJ, Fitzgerald CR, et al. Radiation retinopathy after external-beam irradiation: analysis of time-dose factors. Int J Radiat Oncol Biol Phys. 1994;30(4):765–773.

58. Jiang GL, Tucker SL, Guttenberger R, et al. Radiation-induced injury to the visual pathway. Radiother Oncol. 1994;30(1):17–25.

59. Levy RL, Miller NR. Hyperbaric oxygen therapy for radiation-induced optic neuropathy. Ann Acad Med Singapore. 2006;35(3):151–157.

60. Kline LB, Kim JY, Ceballos R. Radiation optic neuropathy. Ophthalmology. 1985;92(8):1118–1126.

61. Miller NR. Radiation-induced optic neuropathy: still no treatment. Clin Exp Ophthalmol. 2004;32(3):233–235.

62. Archer DB. Responses of retinal and choroidal vessels to ionising radiation. Eye (Lond). 1993;7(1):1–13.

63. Stallard HB. Radiant energy as (a) a pathogenic and (b) a therapeutic agent in ophthalmic disorders. Br J Ophthalmol. 1933;6:1.

64. Zamber RW, Kinyoun JL. Radiation retinopathy. West J Med. 1992;157(5):530–533.

65. Boozalis GT, Schachat AP, Green WR. Subretinal neovascularization from the retina in radiation retinopathy. Retina. 1987;7(3):156–161.

66. Gordon KB, Char DH, Sagerman RH. Late effects of radiation on the eye and ocular adnexa. Int J Radiat Oncol Biol Phys. 1995;31(5):1123–1139.

67. Brown GC, Shields JA, Sanborn G, et al. Radiation retinopathy. Ophthalmology. 1982;89(12):1494–1501.

68. Irvine AR, Wood IS. Radiation retinopathy as an experimental model for ischemic proliferative retinopathy and rubeosis iridis. Am J Ophthalmol. 1987;103(6):790–797.

69. Chee PH. Radiation retinopathy. Am J Ophthalmol. 1968;66(5):860–865.

70. Amoaku WMK, Archer DB. Fluorescein angiographic features: natural course and treatment of radiation retinopathy. Eye (Lond). 1990;4:657–667.

71. Amoaku WMK, Lafaut B, Sallet G, et al. Radiation choroidal vasculopathy: an indocyanine green angiography study. Eye (Lond). 1995;9(6):738–744.

72. Hayreh SS. Post-radiation retinopathy. A fluorescence fundus angiographic study. Br J Ophthalmol. 1970;54(11):705–714.

73. Kinyoun JL, Kalina RE, Brower SA, et al. Radiation retinopathy after orbital irradiation for graves' ophthalmopathy. Arch Ophthalmol. 1984;102(10):1473–1476.

74. Chaudhuri PR, Austin DJ, Rosenthal AR. Treatment of radiation retinopathy. Br J Ophthalmol. 1981;65(9):623–625.

75. Kinyoun JL, Lawrence BS, Barlow WE. Proliferative radiation retinopathy. Arch Ophthalmol. 1996;114(9):1097–1100.

76. Avila MP, Farah ME, Santos A, et al. Three-year safety and visual acuity results of epimacular 90 strontium/90 yttrium brachytherapy with bevacizumab for the treatment of subfoveal choroidal neovascularization secondary to age-related macular degeneration. Retina. 2012;32(1):10–18.

77. Dugel P, Bebchuk J, Nau J, et al. Epimacular brachytherapy for neovascular age-related macular degeneration: a randomized, controlled trial (CABERNET). Ophthalmology. 2013;120(2):317–327.

78. Navarro R, Burés-Jelstrup A, Vásquez LM, et al. Radiation maculopathy after epimacular brachytherapy for the treatment of subfoveal choroidal neovascularization secondary to age-related macular degeneration. Retin Cases Brief Rep. 2011;5(4):352–354.

79. Ávila MP, Farah ME, Santos A, et al. Twelve-month short-term safety and visual-acuity results from a multicentre prospective study of epiretinal strontium-90 brachytherapy with bevacizumab for the treatment of subfoveal choroidal neovascularisation secondary to age-related macular degeneration. Br J Ophthalmol. 2009;93(3):305–309.

80. Hanlon J, Lee C, Chell E, et al. Kilovoltage stereotactic radiosurgery for age-related macular degeneration: assessment of optic nerve dose and patient effective dose. Med Phys. 2009;36(8):3671–3681.

81. Timke C, Zieher H, Roth A, et al. Combination of vascular endothelial growth factor receptor/platelet-derived growth factor receptor inhibition markedly improves radiation tumor therapy. Clin Cancer Res. 2008;14(7):2210–2219.

82. Avila MP, Farah ME, Santos A, et al. Twelve-month safety and visual acuity results from a feasibility study of intraocular, epiretinal radiation therapy for the treatment of subfoveal CNV secondary to AMD. Retina. 2009;29(2):157–169.

83. Stefansson E, Landers MB III, Wolbarsht ML. Increased retinal oxygen supply following pan retinal photocoagulation and vitrectomy and lensectomy. Trans Am Ophthalmol Soc. 1981;79:307–334.

84. Jampol LM. Oxygen therapy and intraocular oxygenation. Trans Am Ophthalmol Soc. 1987;85:407–437.

85. Hashimoto E, Hirakata A, Hotta K, et al. Unusual macular retinal detachment associated with vitreomacular traction syndrome. Br J Ophthalmol. 1998;82(3):326.

86. Stefansson E. The therapeutic effects of retinal laser treatment and vitrectomy. A theory based on oxygen and vascular physiology. Acta Ophthalmol Scand. 2001;79(5):435–440.

87. Nordsmark M, Overgaard M, Overgaard J. Pretreatment oxygenation predicts radiation response in advanced squamous cell carcinoma of the head and neck. Radiother Oncol. 1996;41(1):31–39.

88. Brizel DM, Scully SP, Harrelson JM, et al. Tumor oxygenation predicts for the likelihood of distant metastases in human soft tissue sarcoma. Cancer Res. 1996;56(5):941–943.

89. Ficker L, Meredith T, Gardner S, et al. Cefazolin levels after intravitreal injection. Invest Ophthalmol Vis Sci. 1990;31(3):502–505.

90. Lee SS, Ghosn C, Yu Z, et al. Vitreous VEGF clearance is increased after vitrectomy. Invest Ophthalmol Vis Sci. 2010;51(4):2135–2138.

91. Beer PM, Bakri SJ, Singh RJ, et al. Intraocular concentration and pharmacokinetics of triamcinolone acetonide after a single intravitreal injection. Ophthalmology. 2003;110(4):681–686.

92. Chin H, Park T, Moon Y, et al. Difference in clearance of intravitreal triamcinolone acetonide between vitrectomized and nonvitrectomized eyes. Retina. 2005;25(5):556–560.

93. Jaakkola A, Vesti E, Immonen I. Correlation between octopus perimetry and fluorescein angiography after strontium-90 plaque brachytherapy for subfoveal exudative age related macular degeneration. Br J Ophthalmol. 1998;82(7):763–768.

94. Petrarca R, Richardson M, Nau J, et al. Safety testing of epimacular brachytherapy with microperimetry and indocyanine green angiography: 12 month results. Retina. 2013;33:1232–1240.

95. Petrarca R, Dugel P, Nau J, et al. Macular EpiRetinal brachytherapy in Treated AGE-related macular degeneration (MERITAGE): 12 month optical coherence tomography and fluorescein angiography analysis. Ophthalmology. 2013;120(2):328–333.

96. Blinder KJ, Bradley S, Bressler NM, et al. Effect of lesion size, visual acuity, and lesion composition on visual acuity change with and without verteporfin therapy for choroidal neovascularization secondary to age-related macular degeneration: TAP and VIP report no. 1. Am J Ophthalmol. 2003;136(3):407–418.

97. Yannuzzi L, Negrao S, Lida T, et al. Retinal angiomatous proliferation in age-related macular degeneration. Retina. 2001;21:416–434.

98. Yannuzzi L, Freund K, Takahashi B. Review of retinal angiomatous proliferation or type 3 neovascularization. Retina. 2008;28:375–384.

99. Petrarca R, Nau J, Dugel PU, et al. Epimacular brachytherapy for the treatment of retinal angiomatous proliferation. Retin Cases Brief Rep. 2012;6(4):353–357.

100. Yannuzzi L, Wong D, Sforzolini B, et al. Polypoidal choroidal vasculopathy and neovascularized age-related macular degeneration. Arch Ophthalmol. 1999;117(11):1503–1510.

101. Ciardella A, Donsoff I, Huang S, et al. Polypoidal choroidal vasculopathy. Surv Ophthalmol. 2004;49(1):25–37.

102. Spaide R, Leys A, Herrman-Delemazure B, et al. Radiation associated choroidal neovasculopathy. Ophthalmology. 1999;106:2254–2260.

103. Petrarca R, Jackson T. Radiation therapy for neovascular age-related macular degeneration. Clin Ophthalmol. 2011;5:57–63.

104. Lee C, Chell E, Gertner M, et al. Dosimetry characterization of a multi-beam radiotherapy treatment for age-related macular degeneration. Med Phys. 2008;35(11):5151–5160.

105. Hanlon J, Firpo M, Chell E, et al. Stereotactic radiosurgery for AMD: a monte carlo-based assessment of patient-specific tissue doses. Invest Ophthalmol Vis Sci. 2011;52(5):2334–2342.

106. Moshfeghi DM, Kaiser PK, Gertner M. Stereotactic low-voltage x-ray irradiation for age-related macular degeneration. Br J Ophthalmol. 2011;95(2):185–188.

107. Gertner M, Chell E, Pan KH, et al. Stereotactic targeting and dose verification for age-related macular degeneration. Med Phys. 2010;37(2):600–606.

108. Taddei PJ, Chell E, Hansen S, et al. Assessment of targeting accuracy of a low-energy stereotactic radiosurgery treatment for age-related macular degeneration. Phys Med Biol. 2010;55(23):7037.

109. Morales-Canton V, Quiroz-Mercado H, Velez-Montoya R, et al. 16 and 24 Gy, low-voltage, x-ray irradiation with ranibizumab therapy for neovascular age-related macular degeneration: 12 month outcomes. Am J Ophthalmol. 2013;155(6):1000–1008.

110. Morales-Canton V, Quiroz-Mercado H, Velez-Montoya R, et al. 24 Gy low-voltage x-ray irradiation with ranibizumab therapy for age-related macular degeneration: 12 month outcomes. Am J Ophthalmol. 2013;155(6):1000–1008.

111. Park S, Daftari I, Phillips T, et al. Three-year follow-up of a pilot study of ranibizumab combined with proton beam irradiation as treatment for exudative age-related macular degeneration. Retina. 2012;32(5):956–966.

21

COMBINATION THERAPY FOR NEOVASCULAR AGE-RELATED MACULAR DEGENERATION

FRANCIS CHAR DECROOS • ANDRE J. WITKIN • CARL D. REGILLO

■ INTRODUCTION

Age-related macular degeneration (AMD) is the most frequent cause of blindness among individuals aged 55 years or older in developed countries, and thus AMD is a major health problem worldwide (1). This impact of AMD is expected to grow in magnitude in the upcoming decade owing to progressive increases in both life expectancy and the proportion of elderly persons. In the United States alone, it is estimated that the number of persons having late AMD will increase to 2.95 million by 2020 (1). The choroidal neovascular (CNV) lesions of AMD lead to the vast majority of severe visual loss from this ocular disease (2). In a meta-analysis of 53 studies of eyes with untreated neovascular AMD, the mean vision loss was three lines after 1 year and four lines after 2 years of follow-up. In this same work, after 3 years after CNV onset, 75.7% of patients demonstrated 20/200 or worse vision and 41.9% of patients lost more than six lines of vision from baseline (3).

The exact pathophysiology of CNV is complex and not completely understood. In eyes with AMD, oxidative stress and inflammation at the level of the retinal pigment epithelium (RPE) and Bruch's membrane may imbalance the homeostatic equilibrium and lead to up-regulation of angiogenic and inflammatory factors (4). These factors in turn may lead to promotion of a CNV membrane composed of inflammatory, vascular, and nonvascular components

such as glial cell, fibroblasts, and a remodeled extracellular matrix (5).

Targeted modulation of the proangiogenic cascade in neovascular AMD through inhibition of vascular endothelial growth factor (VEGF) has been one of the triumphs of modern medicine. Off-label monthly intravitreal injection of bevacizumab (Avastin, Roche, Basel, Switzerland), a full-length humanized monoclonal antibody targeted against VEGF-A, demonstrated the ability to improve visual acuity in eyes with neovascular AMD (6–9). The landmark MARINA (Minimally Classic/Occult Trial of the Anti-VEGF Antibody Ranibizumab in the Treatment of Neovascular AMD) and ANCHOR (Anti-VEGF Antibody for the Treatment of Predominantly Classic Choroidal Neovascularization in AMD) studies demonstrated the ability of monthly injections of ranibizumab (Lucentis, Roche, Basel, Switzerland), a monoclonal antibody fragment, to improve visual acuity in eyes with neovascular AMD after 2 years of serial treatment (10,11). One-year results from the Comparison of AMD Treatments Trial (CATT) showed that monthly treatment with bevacizumab was not inferior to ranibizumab monthly treatment at 1 year and that *pro re nata* (PRN) injection of ranibizumab and bevacizumab using strict retreatment criteria was not inferior to monthly treatment (9). More recently, in November 2011, intravitreal aflibercept (Eylea, Regeneron Pharmaceuticals, Tarrytown, NY) was FDA approved for the treatment of neovascular AMD based on results from the phase III studies VIEW-1 and VIEW-2 (VEGF Trap: Investigation of Efficacy and Safety in Wet AMD). These trials showed aflibercept to be equivalent to monthly ranibizumab injections in treatment of neovascular AMD with aflibercept dosed either monthly or every 2 months (after three monthly loading doses) (12,13). The results of the VIEW-1 and VIEW-2 studies are not yet published.

Ranibizumab and bevacizumab have been revolutionary advances in the treatment of neovascular AMD; however, the burden of repeated monthly clinic visits and injections remains significant. Investigators attempted to decrease the number of injections by using various individualized protocols. Using optical coherence tomography (OCT) and strict retreatment criteria, monthly follow-up in conjunction with PRN dosing of intravitreal ranibizumab has demonstrated visual acuity results comparable to monthly ranibizumab dosing (9,14,15). However, monthly follow-up with PRN dosing schedules does not address the burden of frequent clinic visits on patients and caregivers (16,17).

The newly FDA-approved aflibercept may also theoretically decrease the need for monthly injections, as data from phase III trials suggest that injections of aflibercept every 8 weeks after three monthly loaded doses resulted in comparable visual acuity and anatomic results to monthly injections with ranibizumab. However, clinical experience with this newly approved medication is thus far limited, and patients receiving aflibercept will still continue to require close follow-up and frequent treatments.

In addition to the burden of frequent clinic visits and serial intravitreal injections, VEGF blockade does not directly address the inflammatory and mesenchymal remodeling components of CNV development (18). Though inhibition of VEGF may also have some effect on these alternate mechanisms of CNV formation, concomitant treatment of neovascular AMD with a variety of therapeutic modalities theoretically offers the potential to decrease treatment burden and improve outcomes (5). Combination therapy with one or more treatment modalities such as photodynamic therapy (PDT), intraocular corticosteroid, radiation therapy, or anti–platelet-derived growth factor (PDGF) therapy, in conjunction with VEGF inhibition, is an example of an approach that may more broadly target both vascular and extravascular pathways of CNV formation. This type of multifaceted approach has been successfully utilized by oncologists when treating cancer and thus may also be a reasonable conceptual approach when treating neovascular AMD (5).

Prior to development of anti-VEGF medications, PDT was the standard of care for treatment of some forms of neovascular AMD. In 2000, the FDA approved the use of PDT for treatment of predominantly classic CNV secondary to AMD. PDT reduced the rate of vision loss but did not offer vision gain for the vast majority of treated patients with neovascular AMD. The standard PDT protocol utilizes intravenous infusion of verteporfin (Visudyne, QLT, Menlo Park, CA) activated by subsequent administration of nonthermal low-energy red laser light over 83 seconds. Photoactivation of verteporfin with laser results in free radical formation within the CNV lesion, resulting in damage to the vascular endothelium and subsequent vessel occlusion (19,20). Compared to thermal laser, PDT is less destructive; however, PDT can still induce choroidal hypoperfusion (21). Free radical release may be the causative mechanism that leads to some damage to the choroid (21). Additionally, PDT has also been shown to up-regulate intraocular VEGF production from the choroidal endothelial cells (22). One method to limit the toxicity of PDT is to reduce the fluence by either decreasing the power of laser light (less than 50 J/cm^2) or reducing overall treatment time (less than 83 seconds). Studies have demonstrated that reduced-fluence PDT has similar therapeutic efficacy for CNV but potentially reduces the amount of choroidal toxicity seen with standard-fluence PDT (20,23).

Intravitreal corticosteroids may be a way to minimize unwanted inflammation produced during PDT treatment for neovascular AMD. Combining corticosteroid and PDT has been shown to reduce the need for retreatment with PDT in several studies (24–27). In addition to their potent anti-inflammatory effects, corticosteroids have been shown to demonstrate antiproliferative, antiangiogenic, and antifibrotic effects (28,29). In particular, intraocular steroids can decrease intraocular VEGF levels while also reducing levels of several other inflammatory cytokines (18). Triamcinolone acetonide and dexamethasone are examples of two commonly used steroids for intraocular therapy. The half-life of intraocular triamcinolone is approximately 3 weeks with a clinical effect lasting months. In contrast, dexamethasone is more potent but has a shorter half-life of approximately 3 days (30). Compared to triamcinolone, dexamethasone is less lipophilic, which leads to decreased trabecular meshwork adhesion and potentially a more favorable side effect profile (31).

Radiation therapy may be another approach to address the multifactorial etiology of CNV. Radiation therapy can partly inhibit angiogenic, inflammatory, and fibrotic pathways (32–34). The antiangiogenic effect of radiation therapy on endothelial cells in particular has been well established (35,36). Aside from their atypical location, blood vessels within CNV membranes demonstrate uncontrolled growth, atypical orientation, and increased permeability, which may make them more susceptible to radiation. Radiation therapy has been shown to promote a return to more normal vascular morphology in vascular membranes (37). The anti-inflammatory properties of radiation may also limit the continuous inflammatory cycle of CNV initiation, growth, involution, and reactivation (38). In addition, the antifibrotic effects of radiation (39) may decrease the potential for metaplastic transformation from CNV to macular scar (38).

Prevention of CNV maturation through inhibition of PDGF may result in CNV regression and lead to improved visual and anatomical outcomes in patients with neovascular AMD. Immature CNV is comprised mainly of endothelial cells that mature in part through PDGF-mediated recruitment of pericytes (40). The pericytes support survival and development (41) of endothelial cells through a variety of physical and chemical mechanisms including production of VEGF (42). Pericyte stabilization of CNV endothelial cells may result in some innate resistance to VEGF blockade (43), and thus, preventing this pericyte recruitment through PDGF inhibition might result in CNV instability and regression (40). For example, PDGF inhibition in one animal model resulted in complete prevention of pericyte recruitment (44). Another animal study demonstrated that inhibition of both PDGF and VEGF was more effective in causing CNV regression than was anti-VEGF monotherapy (44).

PDT + ANTI-VEGF

PDT promotes neovascular regression via a vaso-occlusive mechanism of action, and the combination of VEGF blockage with PDT has potential for additive or synergistic effects. In particular, combined therapy may allow for longer treatment-free intervals and decreased number of intravitreal injections over time (45). Several prospective studies have examined the utility of standard-fluence PDT + bevacizumab (46–48). These studies all have shown stability or modest improvement in visual acuity and reduced number of treatments for the PDT + bevacizumab groups. More recently, investigators retrospectively compared 139 eyes with bevacizumab-treated neovascular AMD to 236 eyes treated with PDT + bevacizumab. At 12 months, the monotherapy group demonstrated a +5.1-letter gain compared to +4.8 letters in the combination treatment group. No significant difference in number of injections between groups was noted (49).

For AMD patients with predominantly classic CNV, the RhuFab V2 Ocular Treatment Combining the Use of Visudyne to Evaluate Safety (FOCUS) study examined the efficacy of standard-fluence PDT with and without the addition of monthly intravitreal ranibizumab injections. In the FOCUS study, all patients underwent standard-fluence PDT but were randomized to receive ranibizumab or sham injection 7 days after. Intravitreal ranibizumab was administered monthly, and PDT was repeated only if persistent leakage was observed on fluorescein angiography performed on a quarterly basis. At 12 months, patients in the PDT + ranibizumab treatment group demonstrated a mean +4.9 letter gain compared to a –8.2 letter loss in the PDT + sham injection group (50). Similar results of mean +4.6 letter gain versus –7.8 letter loss were observed for the PDT + ranibizumab treatment group and the PDT + sham injection group after 24 months of follow-up, respectively (51). However, the FOCUS trial was not designed to ascertain the differential efficacy between PDT + ranibizumab and ranibizumab monotherapy.

The SUMMIT clinical trial program was conducted to better define the role of PDT in conjunction with anti-VEGF agents, as well as to better understand the role of reduced-fluence PDT in the treatment of neovascular AMD. This clinical trial program included a North American study (DENALI), European study (MONT BLANC), and an Asian study (EVEREST). Both the DENALI and MONT BLANC trials were designed to show the noninferiority of PDT + ranibizumab to intravitreal ranibizumab monotherapy. Of note, ranibizumab was dosed monthly for 3 successive months then administered on a PRN basis. In addition, DENALI was designed to quantify the percentage of trial participants with treatment-free interval greater than 3 months, and MONT BLANC was designed to investigate superiority of standard-fluence PDT + ranibizumab to ranibizumab monotherapy (52).

The 12-month results of the DENALI trial showed that the standard-fluence PDT + ranibizumab group gained on average +5.3 letters from baseline, and patients in the reduced-fluence PDT + ranibizumab combination group gained on average +4.4 letters. However, patients in the monthly ranibizumab monotherapy group gained on average +8.1 letters at month 12, and thus, DENALI did not demonstrate noninferiority between the groups. Most patients in the PDT + ranibizumab combination groups (93% for standard fluence and 84% for reduced fluence) demonstrated a ranibizumab treatment-free interval of at least 3 months during the study. The 12-month results of MONT BLANC trial showed a mean change in baseline visual acuity at 12 months of +4.4 letters for the ranibizumab monotherapy group and +2.5 letters for the standard-fluence PDT + ranibizumab group, suggesting that combination therapy was not superior to monotherapy. A similar proportion of treatment-free intervals were observed for both the combination group (96%) and the monotherapy group (92%) (30). The EVEREST trial differs in that it is designed to compare standard-fluence PDT combined + ranibizumab and ranibizumab monotherapy in the treatment of polypoidal choroidal vasculopathy. Final published reports of these trials in the peer-reviewed literature are pending.

STEROID + ANTI-VEGF

Combination therapies that target both the inflammatory and angiogenic components of the CNV cascade have been investigated as another approach to treat neovascular AMD. Two small series report short-term functional and anatomical benefit of bevacizumab and triamcinolone combination therapy (53,54). Tao and Jonas (55) performed a prospective noncomparative interventional case series of high-dose (20–25 mg) intravitreal triamcinolone and bevacizumab in 31 patients with neovascular AMD and persistent macular fluid despite at least three prior monthly bevacizumab treatments. Interestingly, vision significantly improved at the 2-month follow-up, though this visual gain was not maintained at the final 7-month follow-up visit. el Matri et al. (56) treated seven eyes with CNV associated with a large pigment epithelial detachment with 4 mg intravitreal triamcinolone. This treatment was followed by bevacizumab 1 week later with subsequent combination or bevacizumab treatments as needed. The mean duration of follow-up was 11 months in this prospective study. Visual acuity improved from 20/125 at baseline to 20/80 at final follow-up, and four pigment epithelial detachments flattened completely. Further studies are required before investigators can support a clear role for combination steroid + anti-VEGF therapy in the treatment of neovascular AMD.

PDT + STEROID

PDT can induce a localized tissue inflammatory response, and combination therapy with PDT and an intravitreal corticosteroid might be a way to mitigate this undesirable inflammation after PDT. In several clinical studies, PDT + intravitreal steroid therapy decreased the need for retreatment but lacked consistent ability to improve visual acuity from pretreatment levels (57–60). As several randomized, prospective trials have since demonstrated the ability of VEGF inhibitors to significantly improve visual acuity in eyes with neovascular AMD (9–13), anti-VEGF therapy has become the mainstay of therapy for neovascular AMD, and the role of combination PDT + steroid therapy is mostly historical at the present time.

TRIPLE THERAPY

Despite the lack of evidence to support the superior efficacy of combination PDT + steroid or PDT + VEGF inhibition compared to anti-VEGF monotherapy, a plausible biologic basis exists for triple therapy combining an intravitreal corticosteroid, anti-VEGF, and PDT. CNV secondary to AMD is complex multifactorial process combining angiogenesis, inflammation, and mesenchymal cell infiltration (5), and triple therapy may favorably alter this cascade at multiple critical points. PDT promotes the undesired effects of choroidal hypoperfusion, inflammation, and VEGF up-regulation (21,22), which may be mitigated through concurrent steroid and anti-VEGF use. Triple therapy may also prove a useful therapeutic approach in eyes with AMD and persistent exudation despite multiple serial anti-VEGF treatment or for patients unable to comply with the frequent clinic evaluations and injections required for optimal anti-VEGF dosing.

Studies investigating triple therapy can be divided into those using intravitreal dexamethasone (61–64), intravitreal triamcinolone (65,66), and one study utilizing sub-Tenon's triamcinolone (67). Several challenges exist when critically examining these reports, including varying levels of PDT fluence, differing anti-VEGF agents, and the fact that none of these published studies are randomized or controlled. Additionally, some groups included

only treatment-naive patients, while others included both treatment-naive patients and patients who had previously undergone treatment. Fortunately, the Reduced Fluence Visudyne Anti-VEGF-Dexamethasone in Combination for AMD Lesions (RADICAL) trial was a prospective, multicenter, randomized trial of combination therapy for the treatment of wet AMD that may help better delineate the role of triple therapy with reduced-fluence PDT, dexamethasone, and ranibizumab after final results are released. Each of the previously mentioned studies allowed all types of CNV lesions to be included. Results from these studies are summarized in Table 21.1.

Dexamethasone, Bevacizumab, and PDT

Augustin and Schmidt-Erfurth (25) performed a prospective noncomparative interventional case series of triple therapy in 104 treatment-naive patients with neovascular AMD. This study employed reduced-fluence PDT (70 vs. 83 seconds), with same-day single-port 25-gauge limited vitrectomy (removal of 0.5 mL) and injection of 0.8 mg dexamethasone and 1.5 mg of bevacizumab. Patients were followed at 6-week intervals, with a mean follow-up of 40 weeks. Eighteen eyes (17%) received a single additional intravitreal injection of bevacizumab for persistent macular fluid on OCT without detectable angiographic leakage, and in an additional five cases (5%), a second cycle of triple therapy was used to treat recurrent angiographic CNV activity. Mean visual acuity improved significantly from 20/126 to 20/85 ($P < 0.01$), and 39.4% of the patients gained three or more lines of vision, while mean retinal thickness decreased from 464 to 281 μm ($P < 0.01$). No patients demonstrated significant intraocular pressure (IOP) elevation.

Forte et al. (63) performed retrospective case series comparing triple therapy in 61 eyes of 56 treatment-naive patients to anti-VEGF monotherapy in 40 eyes of 40 treatment-naive patients (63). The investigators utilized standard-fluence PDT followed by same-day intravitreal injections of 0.4 mg dexamethasone and either 1.25 mg bevacizumab (26 eyes) or 0.5 mg ranibizumab (35 eyes). Patients were followed at 1- to 2-month intervals with a mean follow-up of 14.1 months in the triple therapy group. A mean of 0.92 retreatments with triple therapy were given over 12 months at the managing physician's discretion. At 12 months, the triple therapy group demonstrated improvement in mean visual acuity from baseline of 20/174 to 20/120 ($P = 0.02$), and likewise, mean retinal thickness improved from 323 to 212 μm ($P < 0.01$). Compared to the anti-VEGF monotherapy group, the triple therapy group required significantly fewer total number of treatments during follow-up (1.92 vs. 3.12), significantly fewer monthly treatments (0.13 vs. 0.19), and demonstrated a longer interval prior to first retreatment (5.4 vs. 3.6 months).

Ehmann and Garcia (64) reported a retrospective interventional case series in 32 eyes of 30 treatment-naive patients. The authors studied reduced-fluence PDT

Table 21.1 TRIPLE THERAPY FOR NEOVASCULAR AMD

Manuscript and year	Design	Triple therapy medications	Eyes (patients)	Follow-up	Previous treatments	Visual acuity (baseline to final)	OCT (μm) (baseline to final)	Increased IOP	Retreatments
Ahmadieh et al. (2007)	Prospective	SF-PDT 2 mg TA 1.25 mg IVB	17 (17)	50.4 wk (results given at 24 wk)	No	20/110–20/51 ($P < 0.01$)	395–221 ($P = 0.05$)	1 eye	10 (58%) IVB
Augustin et al. (2007)	Prospective case series	RF-PDT 0.8 mg DM 1.5 mg IVB	104 (104)	40 wk	No	20/126–20/85 ($P < 0.01$)	464–281 ($P < 0.01$)	0	18 (17%) IVB 5 (5%) triple
Bakri et al. (2009)	Retrospective	RF-PDT 0.2 mg DM 1.25 mg IVB	31 (31)	13.7 mo	Anti-VEGF 18 (58%)	20/81–20/76 ($P = 0.7$)	293–245 ($P = 0.05$)	0	Mean/patient: 3.3 IVB 1.3 triple
Ehmann et al. (2010)	Retrospective	RF-PDT 0.8 mg DM 1.25 mg IVB (×2)	32 (30)	12 mo	No	20/110–20/68 ($P < 0.01$)	328–216 ($P < 0.01$)	0	Mean/patient: 1.4 triple
Forte et al. (2011)	Retrospective	SF-PDT 0.4 mg DM 1.25 mg IVB or 0.5 mg IVR	61 (56)	14.1 mo	No	20/174–20/120 ($P = 0.02$)	Not reported	0	Mean/patient: 1.92 triple
Kovacs et al. (2011)	Retrospective	RF-PDT 40 mg (ST) TA 1.25 mg IVB	26 (26)	56.7 wk	No	20/243–20/218 ($P = 0.21$)	–102 decrease from baseline at 12 mo (n = 10)	1 eye	13 (50%) IVB
RADICAL trial Hudson et al Unpublished	Prospective Randomized Controlled (compared to IVR)	RF-PDT 0.5 mg DM 0.5 mg IVR	162 (162)	24 mo	No	+6.8 letter gain from baseline after 12 mo	Not reported	Not reported	4.2 retreatment visits at 24 mo
Yip et al. (2009)	Prospective case series	SF-PDT 4 mg TA 1.25 mg IVB	36 (36)	14.7 mo	SF-PDT 15 (42%)	20/332–20/303 ($P = 0.60$)	Not reported	3 eyes	8 (22%) IVB

RF-PDT, reduced-fluence photodynamic therapy; SF-PDT, standard-fluence photodynamic therapy; DM, dexamethasone; TA, triamcinolone acetonide; IVB, bevacizumab; IVR, ranibizumab; ST, sub-Tenon; OCT, central foveal thickness optical coherence tomography from baseline to the final follow-up unless otherwise specified; IOP, intraocular pressure; VEGF, vascular endothelial growth factor; Reduced Fluence Visudyne Anti-VEGF-Dexamethasone in Combination for AMD Lesions trial, RADICAL trial.

(25 J/cm^2) followed by an intravitreal injection of 0.8 mg dexamethasone the same day, with subsequent intravitreal injections of 1.25 mg bevacizumab at 1 and 7 weeks after PDT. All patients were followed for 12 months. At 13 weeks after initial PDT and dexamethasone, repeat OCT and fluorescein angiography were performed to assess CNV activity. The mean number of treatment cycles was 1.4, with 22 (69%) eyes requiring only one cycle of treatment. Mean visual acuity improved from 20/110 at baseline to 20/68 at 12 months ($P < 0.01$), with associated foveal thickness decreased from 328 to 216 µm ($P < 0.01$). No patients demonstrated a significant IOP elevation.

Bakri et al. (62) compiled a retrospective case series of 31 patients treated with triple therapy for AMD, of which 18 patients (58%) had received anti-VEGF therapy prior to enrollment (mean 3.6 injections). This study examined reduced-fluence PDT (25 J/cm^2) followed by same-day intravitreal injections of 0.2 mg dexamethasone and 1.25 mg bevacizumab. Patients were followed at 1- to 2-month intervals with a mean follow-up of 13.7 months. Retreatment was given in all patients based on physician-dependent retreatment criteria. A mean of 1.7 bevacizumab injections and 0.2 repeat triple therapy treatments per patient were given in the first 6 months, and a mean of 2.3 bevacizumab injections and 0.3 repeat triple therapy treatments were given throughout follow-up. In all patients, change in mean visual acuity from baseline (20/80) to final follow-up (20/60) was not statistically significant ($P = 0.69$). Subgroup analysis of treatment-naive eyes and previously treated eyes likewise revealed no significant improvement in visual acuity. For all patients, there was a borderline improvement in mean retinal thickness (293 µm at baseline to 245 µm at final follow-up, $P = 0.053$). No patients demonstrated significant IOP elevation.

Triamcinolone, Bevacizumab, and PDT

Ahmadieh et al. (65) performed a prospective interventional case series in 17 treatment-naive eyes. They studied standard-fluence PDT followed by intravitreal injections of 2 mg triamcinolone and 1.25 mg bevacizumab 48 hours after PDT. Patients were followed at 6-week intervals for a mean follow-up of 50.4 weeks. CNV activity on angiography required retreatment with intravitreal bevacizumab. Seven eyes (41%) did not require retreatment, while 10 eyes (59%) were retreated, and most eyes required two additional bevacizumab injections. Mean visual acuity in the triple therapy group improved from 20/110 at baseline to 20/51 (P < 0.01) after 24 weeks, and similarly, mean retinal thickness improved from 395 at baseline to 221 µm ($P = 0.05$) at the same time points. IOP elevation was noted in one patient, but the IOP was controlled with topical medications.

Yip et al. (66) performed a prospective interventional case series in 36 eyes, 15 (42%) of which had undergone prior PDT. The investigators utilized standard-fluence PDT followed by same-day intravitreal injections of 4 mg triamcinolone and 1.25 mg bevacizumab. Follow-up was 1 week, 6 weeks, 3 months, and then every 3 months after treatment for a mean follow-up of 14.7 months. Retreatment with bevacizumab was required if fluorescein angiography demonstrated CNV activity at 3 months, and eight eyes (22%) required repeat injections. Mean visual acuity demonstrated no significant improvement from 20/332 at baseline to 20/303 ($P = 0.60$) at 6 months. Foveal thickness on OCT was not followed. Multiple complications were reported including one RPE rip, significant cataract requiring surgery in three eyes, and IOP elevations in three eyes that were controlled with eyedrops.

Kovacs et al. (67) collected a retrospective case series of triple therapy in 26 treatment-naive patients. This group studied reduced-fluence PDT (25 J/cm^2) followed by an intravitreal injection of 1.25 mg bevacizumab and a sub-Tenon's injection of 40 mg triamcinolone at the same visit. Patients were followed at variable intervals for a mean of 56.7 weeks, and retreatment with intravitreal bevacizumab was at the physician's discretion. By the end of the study, 13 of 26 eyes (50%) needed retreatment; 11/18 eyes (61.1%) required retreatment by 12 months. Mean visual acuity demonstrated no significant improvement from 20/243 at baseline to 20/218 ($P = 0.21$) at 6 months. In one patient, an increase in IOP after treatment was controlled with topical medications.

Dexamethasone, Ranibizumab, and PDT

The RADICAL study was a single-masked, randomized, multicenter phase II trial that compared the efficacy of reduced-fluence PDT and ranibizumab combination therapy, with or without dexamethasone, with ranibizumab monotherapy in 131 treatment-naive patients with neovascular AMD. The trial comprised four study groups, comparing half-fluence PDT with ranibizumab, half-fluence PDT with ranibizumab and dexamethasone, and quarter-fluence PDT with ranibizumab and dexamethasone to ranibizumab monotherapy. Doses of 0.5 mg ranibizumab and 0.5 mg dexamethasone are used for all treatment groups. Patients were followed monthly for the first year and quarterly or more frequently at the physician's discretion for the 2nd year. At 12 months, triple therapy with half-fluence PDT, ranibizumab, and dexamethasone demonstrated a visual improvement of +6.8 letters compared with +6.5 letters in the ranibizumab monotherapy group. After 24 months, triple therapy required a mean of 4.2 retreatments compared to 8.9 retreatments in the ranibizumab monotherapy group. The outcomes of the RADICAL trial were presented at the 2010 American Society of Retinal Specialist's meeting, but a final published report in the peer-reviewed literature is pending (68).

▌ RADIATION + ANTI-VEGF

Brachytherapy and external beam therapy are the two radiation delivery methods that have been utilized for treatment of neovascular AMD. Brachytherapy requires a radiation source placed close to the macula. During epimacular brachytherapy, a probe is inserted through the pars plana and held over the macula for a short period of time for radiation delivery. Alternatively, plaque brachytherapy utilizes a radioactive plaque sewn onto the sclera adjacent to the macula for radiation delivery. External beam radiotherapy utilizes radiation from a source outside the body directed at the lesion of concern. Delivery systems for external beam radiotherapy vary from hospital-based to office-based systems.

The Cochrane collaboration reviewed 13 randomized controlled trials that investigated external beam radiation monotherapy in 1,154 eyes with neovascular AMD. The radiation dose in the studies varied from 7.5 to 25 grays (Gy). The primary outcome of this review was loss of visual acuity defined as the dichotomous variable "more than six lines of vision loss," and secondary outcomes included change in visual acuity from baseline as a continuous variable. This review noted a 40% relative risk reduction of more than six lines of vision loss at 12 months; however, this finding was not maintained at 24 months. Importantly, this review also noted no significant adverse events with 2 Gy radiation fractions up to a total dose of 20 Gy, though some ocular complications were noted at a dose of 25 Gy. The authors concluded that meta-analysis did not support the use of external beam radiation monotherapy for neovascular AMD (34). Similarly, results were reported from a randomized, controlled, 36-month trial of Strontium plaque brachytherapy for 88 eyes with neovascular AMD. This study investigated two different dosages of radiation, with a maximum dosage of 15 Gy. The primary trial outcome was change in visual acuity, and no significant difference between observation and plaque radiation was reported after 12 months of follow-up (69).

Though current evidence does not support external beam or plaque radiation as monotherapy for neovascular AMD, combination therapy with VEGF blockade and two innovative methods of radiation delivery is currently being investigated. Epimacular brachytherapy (Epi-Rad, Neovista, Fremont, CA) is one such method of radiation delivery that uses a probe surgically placed through the pars plana and held over the area of neovascularization. Another is an office-based external beam device (IRay, Oraya Therapeutics, Inc., Newark, CA).

Epimacular brachytherapy requires a pars plana vitrectomy, placement of a proprietary epimacular radiation applicator adjacent to the CNV, and delivery of 24 Gy of beta radiation over approximately 4 minutes. The radiation applicator houses the Strontium-90 isotope in a shielded container, and the isotope can be deployed to the minimally shielded applicator tip intraoperatively (70). Avila et al. (71) investigated the effects of radiation applicator treatment in combination with two bevacizumab treatments in 34 eyes. Intravitreal bevacizumab was dosed either 10 days prior to radiation treatment or immediately after the radiation treatment. Outcomes were reported at 12 months, and 36-month

follow-up is planned. After 12 months, the mean change from baseline was a gain of +8.9 Early Treatment Diabetic Retinopathy Study (ETDRS) letters, with 38% of patients demonstrating a ≥15 letter gain in vision. Likewise, the mean baseline thickness at the foveal center was 322 μm and improved to 250 μm at 12 months. Maximal vision gain and reduction in foveal center thickness from baseline were noted at 3 and 6 months, respectively. No cases of radiation retinopathy or radiation optic neuropathy were reported.

The noteworthy findings reported by Avila et al. are undergoing current investigation in other larger trials combining vitrectomy, epimacular brachytherapy, and intravitreal ranibizumab in comparison to ranibizumab monotherapy for treatment-naive patients with neovascular AMD. These studies include the CABERNET and MERITAGE trials based in the United States and the United Kingdom, respectively. The MERLOT study is also investigating the efficacy of Epi-Rad for patients requiring persistent anti-VEGF treatments.

The CABERNET trial 24-month results were presented at the Angiogenesis 2012 meeting (72). In the vitrectomy + epimacular brachytherapy + ranibizumab combination therapy group, ranibizumab was administered at baseline, 1 month, and then as needed during monthly follow-up visits. In the monotherapy group, ranibizumab was administered during each of the first three monthly visits and then as needed during remaining monthly visits. The epimacular brachytherapy combination therapy group demonstrated a mean loss of −2.5 letters at 24 months compared to a +4.4 letter gain for the ranibizumab monotherapy group. Patients in the combination therapy group received an average of 6 injections over 24 months, while the ranibizumab monotherapy group received 11 injections over the same duration. The epimacular brachytherapy combination therapy group failed to meet the 10% noninferiority margin compared to ranibizumab monotherapy. Of the 310 patients undergoing epimacular brachytherapy combination therapy, there were 10 patients with signs of possible early radiation retinopathy by 24 months and no patients with definitive proliferative radiation retinopathy. The preliminary results of the CABERNET trial do not currently support a role for epimacular brachytherapy combination therapy as a first-line treatment of neovascular AMD.

The IRay is an office-based, stereotactic, robotic, radiotherapy platform designed to deliver low-energy x-ray radiation through the pars plana to the macula. The device features eye tracking to accurately direct radiation and cease radiation delivery in the event of excess eye movement. After standard A-scan ultrasound, radiation is delivered at three separate locations through the inferior pars plana to overlap on the macula. Exposure to adjacent structures is minimized by a lid speculum, and appropriate radiation angulation prevents radiation to the lens (73). In a preliminary prospective study of 19 patients undergoing ranibizumab injections and 24-Gy macular radiation via the office-based external beam system, a mean change in visual acuity of +6.4 letters from baseline at 6 months was noted. After the initial two required injections, a mean of 0.4 ranibizumab injections were administered to each patient over 6 months (74). In another small prospective study of 26 patients undergoing ranibizumab injections and 16-Gy macular radiation via the office-based external beam system, a mean change in visual acuity of +9.5 letters from baseline after 6 months was noted. After the initial two required injections, a mean of 0.5 ranibizumab injections were administered to each patient over 6 months (75). No radiation-related adverse events were reported in either preliminary study. Combination therapy using the office-based external beam system in conjunction with ranibizumab is currently undergoing phase II study as part of the Investigation of Nontransplant-Eligible Patients Who Are Inotrope Dependent (INTREPID) trial in Europe as well as another trial in Mexico.

ANTI-PDGF + ANTI-VEGF

Combining PDGF and VEGF inhibition has replicated animal model CNV regression (44) in human subjects. E10030 (Ophthotech, Princeton, NJ) is an PDGF blocking aptamer that has completed phase I testing in 22 patients with results presented at ARVO 2009 (76). Treatment-naive patients were given separate sequential injections of 0.5 mg ranibizumab and E10030 as one of four different doses on a monthly basis. At the 12-week primary endpoint, the mean change in visual acuity was +15.7 letters, and 60% of patients gained 15 letters from baseline overall. Over the same time frame, the mean center point retinal thickness decreased from 395 µm at baseline to 229 µm, and 85% of lesions demonstrated CNV regression on fluorescein angiography. No adverse events were reported in this initial series. Of note, 12-week follow-up was reported for only 15 patients at the ARVO 2009 meeting. Combination therapy with E10030 and ranibizumab is currently undergoing phase II study.

CONCLUSION

Monthly intravitreal injections with ranibizumab remain the gold standard for treatment of neovascular AMD, although 1-year results from the CATT trial suggest that PRN treatment with monthly follow-up, and OCT-guided dosing can produce comparable visual outcomes with a mean of approximately seven and eight injections of ranibizumab and bevacizumab, respectively (9). Results from the VIEW-1 and VIEW-2 trials demonstrate equivalence between monthly ranibizumab and injection of aflibercept every 2 months after three initial monthly injections; however, it remains to be seen how aflibercept will be used clinically and how often patients will require follow-up. Frequent injections and even frequent clinic visits without injections

are burdensome to patients, so the need remains for other therapeutic innovation. Additionally, some patients with neovascular AMD have persistent decreased visual acuity or persistent signs of active exudation despite prolonged serial anti-VEGF therapy. These patients may benefit from a combination therapy approach to either improve efficacy or decrease treatment burden. Neovascular AMD is a multifactorial process involving angiogenic stimulus, inflammation, and mesenchymal cell alteration. Selective inhibition at multiple points of this cascade offers potential theoretical benefits over VEGF blockade alone.

Several studies reviewed above, including unpublished results from the RADICAL trial, suggest a potential role for triple therapy to reduce treatment burden for selected cases of neovascular AMD. However, decreasing treatment frequency may sacrifice some of the visual acuity benefit seen with monthly anti-VEGF therapy. Further investigations will be needed to delineate optimal PDT fluence, choice and dose of steroid, and anti-VEGF dosing and follow-up interval. The preliminary results of the DENALI and CABERNET trials do not support a role for combination PDT + anti-VEGF or epimacular radiation brachytherapy + anti-VEGF in patients with new-onset neovascular AMD. Combination therapy with one or more therapeutic modalities such as PDT, steroid, radiation, and PDGF inhibition in conjunction with VEGF inhibition remains an incompletely evaluated, but potentially useful, alternative approach to anti-VEGF monotherapy in selected patients with neovascular AMD. Anti-VEGF therapy combined with anti-PDGF treatment offers the potential for CNV regression and the possibility of enhanced visual improvement over anti-VEGF treatment alone. Larger, phase II studies are currently underway to evaluate this combination therapy approach.

REFERENCES

1. Friedman DS, O'Colmain BJ, Munoz B, et al. Prevalence of age-related macular degeneration in the United States. Arch Ophthalmol. 2004;122:564–572.

2. Ferris FL III, Fine SL, Hyman L. Age-related macular degeneration and blindness due to neovascular maculopathy. Arch Ophthalmol. 1984;102:1640–1642.

3. Wong TY, Chakravarthy U, Klein R, et al. The natural history and prognosis of neovascular age-related macular degeneration: a systematic review of the literature and meta-analysis. Ophthalmology. 2008;115:116–126.

4. Ohno-Matsui K, Morita I, Tombran-Tink J, et al. Novel mechanism for age-related macular degeneration: an equilibrium shift between the angiogenesis factors VEGF and PEDF. J Cell Physiol. 2001;189:323–333.

5. Spaide RF. Rationale for combination therapy in age-related macular degeneration. Retina. 2009;29:S5–S7.

6. Avery RL, Pieramici DJ, Rabena MD, et al. Intravitreal bevacizumab (Avastin) for neovascular age-related macular degeneration. Ophthalmology. 2006;113:363–372 e5.

7. Aisenbrey S, Ziemssen F, Volker M, et al. Intravitreal bevacizumab (Avastin) for occult choroidal neovascularization in age-related macular degeneration. Graefes Arch Clin Exp Ophthalmol. 2007;245:941–948.

8. Fong KC, Kirkpatrick N, Mohamed Q, et al. Intravitreal bevacizumab (Avastin) for neovascular age-related macular degeneration using a variable frequency regimen in eyes with no previous treatment. Clin Exp Ophthalmol. 2008;36:748–755.

9. Martin DF, Maguire MG, Ying GS, et al. Ranibizumab and bevacizumab for neovascular age-related macular degeneration. N Engl J Med. 2011;364:1897–1908.

10. Rosenfeld PJ, Brown DM, Heier JS, et al. Ranibizumab for neovascular age-related macular degeneration. N Engl J Med. 2006;355:1419–1431.

11. Brown DM, Kaiser PK, Michels M, et al. Ranibizumab versus verteporfin for neovascular age-related macular degeneration. N Engl J Med. 2006;355:1432–1444.

12. VIEW_1. Double-Masked Study of Efficacy and Safety of IVT VEGF Trap-Eye in Subjects with Wet AMD (VIEW 1) ClinicalTrials. gov identifier: NCT00509795 ClinicalTrials.gov. Available from: http//clinicaltrials.gov/ct2/show/NCT00509795.

13. VIEW_2. VEGF Trap-Eye: Investigation of Efficacy and Safety in Wet AMD (VIEW 2). ClinicalTrials.gov identifier: NCT00637377 ClinicalTrials.gov. Available from: http//clinicaltrials.gov/ct2/show/NCT00637377.

14. Fung AE, Lalwani GA, Rosenfeld PJ, et al. An optical coherence tomography-guided, variable dosing regimen with intravitreal ranibizumab (Lucentis) for neovascular age-related macular degeneration. Am J Ophthalmol. 2007;143:566–583.

15. Lalwani GA, Rosenfeld PJ, Fung AE, et al. A variable-dosing regimen with intravitreal ranibizumab for neovascular age-related macular degeneration: year 2 of the PrONTO Study. Am J Ophthalmol. 2009;148:43–58.

16. Gupta OP, Shienbaum G, Patel AH, et al. A treat and extend regimen using ranibizumab for neovascular age-related macular degeneration clinical and economic impact. Ophthalmology. 2011;117:2134–2140.

17. Shienbaum G, Gupta OP, Fecarotta C, et al. Bevacizumab for neovascular age-related macular degeneration using a treat-and-extend regimen: clinical and economic impact. Am J Ophthalmol. 2012;153:468–473 e1.

18. Sohn HJ, Han DH, Kim IT, et al. Changes in aqueous concentrations of various cytokines after intravitreal triamcinolone versus bevacizumab for diabetic macular edema. Am J Ophthalmol. 2011;152:686–694.

19. Treatment_of_age-related_macular_degeneration_with_photodynamic_therapy_Study_Group. Photodynamic therapy of subfoveal choroidal neovascularization in age-related macular degeneration with verteporfin: one-year results of 2 randomized clinical trials–TAP report. Treatment of age-related macular degeneration with photodynamic therapy (TAP) Study Group. Arch Ophthalmol. 1999;117:1329–1345.

20. Azab M, Boyer DS, Bressler NM, et al. Verteporfin therapy of subfoveal minimally classic choroidal neovascularization in age-related macular degeneration: 2-year results of a randomized clinical trial. Arch Ophthalmol. 2005;123:448–457.

21. Schmidt-Erfurth U, Michels S, Barbazetto I, et al. Photodynamic effects on choroidal neovascularization and physiological choroid. Invest Ophthalmol Vis Sci. 2002;43:830–841.

22. Schmidt-Erfurth U, Schlotzer-Schrehard U, Cursiefen C, et al. Influence of photodynamic therapy on expression of vascular endothelial growth factor (VEGF), VEGF receptor 3, and pigment epithelium-derived factor. Invest Ophthalmol Vis Sci. 2003;44:4473–4480.

23. Michels S, Hansmann F, Geitzenauer W, Schmidt-Erfurth U. Influence of treatment parameters on selectivity of verteporfin therapy. Invest Ophthalmol Vis Sci. 2006;47:371–376.

24. Spaide RF, Sorenson J, Maranan L. Photodynamic therapy with verteporfin combined with intravitreal injection of triamcinolone acetonide for choroidal neovascularization. Ophthalmology. 2005;112:301–304.

25. Augustin AJ, Schmidt-Erfurth U. Verteporfin therapy combined with intravitreal triamcinolone in all types of choroidal neovascularization due to age-related macular degeneration. Ophthalmology. 2006;113:14–22.

26. Chan WM, Lai TY, Wong AL, et al. Combined photodynamic therapy and intravitreal triamcinolone injection for the treatment of subfoveal choroidal neovascularisation in age related macular degeneration: a comparative study. Br J Ophthalmol. 2006;90:337–341.

27. Sacu S, Varga A, Michels S, et al. Reduced fluence versus standard photodynamic therapy in combination with intravitreal triamcinolone: short-term results of a randomised study. Br J Ophthalmol. 2008;92:1347–1351.

28. Tano Y, Chandler D, Machemer R. Treatment of intraocular proliferation with intravitreal injection of triamcinolone acetonide. Am J Ophthalmol. 1980;90:810–816.

29. Antoszyk AN, Gottlieb JL, Machemer R, et al. The effects of intravitreal triamcinolone acetonide on experimental pre-retinal neovascularization. Graefes Arch Clin Exp Ophthalmol. 1993;231:34–40.

30. Couch SM, Bakri SJ. Review of combination therapies for neovascular age-related macular degeneration. Semin Ophthalmol. 2011;26:114–120.

31. Thakur A, Kadam R, Kompella UB. Trabecular meshwork and lens partitioning of corticosteroids: implications for elevated intraocular pressure and cataracts. Arch Ophthalmol. 2011;129:914–920.

32. Finger PT, Berson A, Sherr D, et al. Radiation therapy for subretinal neovascularization. Ophthalmology. 1996;103:878–889.

33. Finger PT, Berson A, Ng T, et al. Ophthalmic plaque radiotherapy for age-related macular degeneration associated with subretinal neovascularization. Am J Ophthalmol. 1999;127:170–177.

34. Evans JR, Sivagnanavel V, Chong V. Radiotherapy for neovascular age-related macular degeneration. Cochrane Database Syst Rev. 2010:CD004004.

35. Garcia-Barros M, Paris F, Cordon-Cardo C, et al. Tumor response to radiotherapy regulated by endothelial cell apoptosis. Science. 2003;300:1155–1159.

36. Imaizumi N, Monnier Y, Hegi M, et al. Radiotherapy suppresses angiogenesis in mice through TGF-betaRI/ALK5-dependent inhibition of endothelial cell sprouting. PLoS One. 2010;5:e11084.

37. Hori K, Saito S, Tamai M. Effect of irradiation on neovascularization in rat skinfold chambers: implications for clinical trials of low-dose radiotherapy for wet-type age-related macular degeneration. Int J Radiat Oncol Biol Phys. 2004;60:1564–1571.

38. Silva RA, Moshfeghi AA, Kaiser PK, et al. Radiation treatment for age-related macular degeneration. Semin Ophthalmol. 2011;26:121–130.

39. Ivanov VN, Zhou H, Ghandhi SA, et al. Radiation-induced bystander signaling pathways in human fibroblasts: a role for interleukin-33 in the signal transmission. Cell Signal. 2010;22:1076–1087.

40. Jo N, Mailhos C, Ju M, et al. Inhibition of platelet-derived growth factor B signaling enhances the efficacy of anti-vascular endothelial growth factor therapy in multiple models of ocular neovascularization. Am J Pathol. 2006;168:2036–2053.

41. Benjamin LE, Hemo I, Keshet E. A plasticity window for blood vessel remodelling is defined by pericyte coverage of the preformed endothelial network and is regulated by PDGF-B and VEGF. Development. 1998;125:1591–1598.

42. Reinmuth N, Liu W, Jung YD, et al. Induction of VEGF in perivascular cells defines a potential paracrine mechanism for endothelial cell survival. FASEB J. 2001;15:1239–1241.

43. Mitchell TS, Bradley J, Robinson GS, et al. RGS5 expression is a quantitative measure of pericyte coverage of blood vessels. Angiogenesis. 2008;11:141–151.

44. Uemura A, Ogawa M, Hirashima M, et al. Recombinant angiopoietin-1 restores higher-order architecture of growing blood vessels in mice in the absence of mural cells. J Clin Invest. 2002;110:1619–1628.

45. Cruess AF, Zlateva G, Pleil AM, et al. Photodynamic therapy with verteporfin in age-related macular degeneration: a systematic review of efficacy, safety, treatment modifications and pharmacoeconomic properties. Acta Ophthalmol. 2009;87:118–132.

46. Lazic R, Gabric N. Verteporfin therapy and intravitreal bevacizumab combined and alone in choroidal neovascularization due to age-related macular degeneration. Ophthalmology. 2007;114:1179–1185.

47. Navea A, Mataix J, Desco MC, et al. One-year follow-up of combined customized therapy. Photodynamic therapy and bevacizumab for exudative age-related macular degeneration. Retina. 2009;29:13–19.

48. Ladewig MS, Karl SE, Hamelmann V, et al. Combined intravitreal bevacizumab and photodynamic therapy for neovascular age-related macular degeneration. Graefes Arch Clin Exp Ophthalmol. 2008;246:17–25.

49. Rudnisky CJ, Liu C, Ng M, et al. Intravitreal bevacizumab alone versus combined verteporfin photodynamic therapy and intravitreal bevacizumab for choroidal neovascularization in age-related macular degeneration: visual acuity after 1 year of follow-up. Retina. 2010;30:548–554.

50. Heier JS, Boyer DS, Ciulla TA, et al. Ranibizumab combined with verteporfin photodynamic therapy in neovascular age-related macular degeneration: year 1 results of the FOCUS Study. Arch Ophthalmol. 2006;124:1532–1542.

51. Antoszyk AN, Tuomi L, Chung CY, et al. Ranibizumab combined with verteporfin photodynamic therapy in neovascular age-related macular degeneration (FOCUS): year 2 results. Am J Ophthalmol. 2008;145:862–874.

52. Kaiser PK. Combination therapy with verteporfin and anti-VEGF agents in neovascular age-related macular degeneration: where do we stand? Br J Ophthalmol. 2010;94:143–145.

53. Jonas JB, Libondi T, Golubkina L, et al. Combined intravitreal bevacizumab and triamcinolone in exudative age-related macular degeneration. Acta Ophthalmol. 2010;88:630–634.

54. Colucciello M. Intravitreal bevacizumab and triamcinolone acetonide combination therapy for exudative neovascular age-related macular

degeneration: short-term optical coherence tomography results. J Ocul Pharmacol Ther. 2008;24:15–24.

55. Tao Y, Jonas JB. Intravitreal bevacizumab combined with intravitreal triamcinolone for therapy-resistant exudative age-related macular degeneration. J Ocul Pharmacol Ther. 2010;26:207–212.

56. el Matri L, Chebil A, Kort F, et al. Intravitreal injection of triamcinolone combined with bevacizumab for choroidal neovascularization associated with large retinal pigment epithelial detachment in age-related macular degeneration. Graefes Arch Clin Exp Ophthalmol. 2010;248:779–784.

57. Iwama D, Otani A, Sasahara M, et al. Photodynamic therapy combined with low-dose intravitreal triamcinolone acetonide for age-related macular degeneration refractory to photodynamic therapy alone. Br J Ophthalmol. 2008;92:1352–1356.

58. Ruiz-Moreno JM, Montero JA, Zarbin MA. Photodynamic therapy and high-dose intravitreal triamcinolone to treat exudative age-related macular degeneration: 2-year outcome. Retina. 2007;27:458–461.

59. Gilson MM, Bressler NM, Jabs DA, et al. Periocular triamcinolone and photodynamic therapy for subfoveal choroidal neovascularization in age-related macular degeneration. Ophthalmology. 2007;114:1713–1721.

60. Chaudhary V, Mao A, Hooper PL, et al. Triamcinolone acetonide as adjunctive treatment to verteporfin in neovascular age-related macular degeneration: a prospective randomized trial. Ophthalmology. 2007;114:2183–2189.

61. Augustin AJ, Puls S, Offermann I. Triple therapy for choroidal neovascularization due to age-related macular degeneration: verteporfin PDT, bevacizumab, and dexamethasone. Retina. 2007;27:133–140.

62. Bakri SJ, Couch SM, McCannel CA, et al. Same-day triple therapy with photodynamic therapy, intravitreal dexamethasone, and bevacizumab in wet age-related macular degeneration. Retina. 2009;29:573–578.

63. Forte R, Bonavolonta P, Benayoun Y, et al. Intravitreal ranibizumab and bevacizumab in combination with full-fluence verteporfin therapy and dexamethasone for exudative age-related macular degeneration. Ophthalmic Res. 2011;45:129–34.

64. Ehmann D, Garcia R. Triple therapy for neovascular age-related macular degeneration (verteporfin photodynamic therapy, intravitreal dexamethasone, and intravitreal bevacizumab). Can J Ophthalmol. 2010;45:36–40.

65. Ahmadieh H, Taei R, Soheilian M, et al. Single-session photodynamic therapy combined with intravitreal bevacizumab and triamcinolone for neovascular age-related macular degeneration. BMC Ophthalmol. 2007;7:10.

66. Yip PP, Woo CF, Tang HH, et al. Triple therapy for neovascular age-related macular degeneration using single-session photodynamic therapy combined with intravitreal bevacizumab and triamcinolone. Br J Ophthalmol. 2009;93:754–758.

67. Kovacs KD, Quirk MT, Kinoshita T, et al. A retrospective analysis of triple combination therapy with intravitreal bevacizumab, posterior sub-tenon's triamcinolone acetonide, and low-fluence verteporfin photodynamic therapy in patients with neovascular age-related macular degeneration. Retina. 2011;31:446–452.

68. Hudson H. RADICAL: 24-Month Results of a Phase II Exploratory Randomized Clinical Trial of Reduced Fluence vPDT–Anti-VEGF–Dexamethasone in AMD. 2010 Annual ASRS Meeting, Vancouver, CA.

69. Jaakkola A, Heikkonen J, Tommila P, et al. Strontium plaque brachytherapy for exudative age-related macular degeneration: three-year results of a randomized study. Ophthalmology. 2005;112:567–573.

70. Avila MP, Farah ME, Santos A, et al. Twelve-month safety and visual acuity results from a feasibility study of intraocular, epiretinal radiation therapy for the treatment of subfoveal CNV secondary to AMD. Retina. 2009;29:157–169.

71. Avila MP, Farah ME, Santos A, et al. Twelve-month short-term safety and visual-acuity results from a multicentre prospective study of epiretinal strontium-90 brachytherapy with bevacizumab for the treatment of subfoveal choroidal neovascularisation secondary to age-related macular degeneration. Br J Ophthalmol. 2009;93:305–309.

72. Dugel P. CABERNET: For Treatment of Naive Neovascular Macular Degeneration. 2012 Angiogenesis, Exudation and Degeneration Meeting, Miami, FL. February 2–4, 2012.

73. Moshfeghi DM, Kaiser PK, Gertner M. Stereotactic low-voltage x-ray irradiation for age-related macular degeneration. Br J Ophthalmol. 2011;95: 185–188.

74. Canton VM, Quiroz-Mercado H, Velez-Montoya R, et al. 24-Gy low-voltage x-ray irradiation with ranibizumab therapy for neovascular AMD: 6-month safety and functional outcomes. Ophthalmic Surg Lasers Imaging 2011;43:20–24.

75. Canton VM, Quiroz-Mercado H, Velez-Montoya R, et al. 16-Gy low-voltage x-ray irradiation with ranibizumab therapy for AMD: 6-month safety and functional outcomes. Ophthalmic Surg Lasers Imaging. 2011;42:468–473.

76. Boyer D. Ophthotech_Anti-PDGF_in_AMD_Study_Group. Combined inhibition of platelet derived (PDGF) and vascular endothelial (VEGF) growth factors for the treatment of neovascular age-related macular degeneration (NV-AMD)—results of a phase 1 study. ARVO 2009. Invest Ophthalmol Vis Sci. 50: E-Abstract 12602009.

22

FOVISTA, A PEGYLATED ANTI-PDGF APTAMER IN WET AMD

MARY ALEXANDER DEAS-HAMRICK • SAMIR PATEL
ISOBEL V.L. GOLDSMITH • D. VIRGIL ALFARO III

Anti-VEGF therapy remains the standard of care in the management of wet age-related macular degeneration (AMD). Currently, the market is dominated by three drugs that are injected intravitreally: Lucentis, Eylea, and Avastin. The causes of visual loss in wet AMD remain multifactorial and include intraretinal cysts, subretinal fluid, subretinal blood, subretinal scarring, retinal pigment epithelium (RPE) loss, and tears and rips of the RPE. Combination therapy in the treatment of wet AMD has attempted to address this multifactorial element by combining anti-VEGF agents with intravitreal steroids and/or photodynamic therapy (PDT). Nevertheless, the results published in small clinical studies have failed to support the use of combined therapy for wet AMD.

Fovista, a pegylated aptamer with anti-PDGF function, appears to be a distinct and fundamentally different approach to combination therapy, by targeting pericytes, those cells important for the long-term stability and function of new vessels seen in wet AMD. Indeed, a uniquely large phase 2 multicentered, randomized, and double-masked clinical trial showed superiority of Fovista combined with Lucentis over Lucentis alone in patients with classic subfoveal choroidal neovascular membranes (CNVMs). In this chapter, the authors have three main objectives: (i) presenting the basic science of aptamers; (ii) discussing the pericytes in new vessel formation seen in tumors and in ocular angiogenesis; and (iii) presenting and discussing the data from the phase 2 Fovista study.

APTAMERS

An aptamer (from the Latin *aptus*, to fit, and the Greek *meros,* meaning part or region) is a single-stranded oligonucleotide that folds into a unique three-dimensional structure and, as a result of this spatial structure, is able to bind with high affinity and specificity to a target molecule such as a protein. Aptamers are larger than small molecule drugs but smaller than antibodies. They are obtained via in vitro selection from combinatorial oligonucleotide libraries, a process that allows for the selection of aptamers with specificity for almost any protein target. Since 1990, aptamers have been generated against hundreds of molecular targets, from small molecules and peptides to many proteins of therapeutic interest and even to cells and tissues (1,2).

Aptamers are typically 15 to 40 nucleotides in length and can be made of DNA, RNA, or nucleotides with a chemically modified sugar backbone. The secondary structure of aptamers is defined by complementary base pairing, which generates stable tertiary structure. The large amount of possible tertiary structures enables aptamers to bind with high affinity via van der Waals, hydrogen bonding, and electrostatic interactions to most small-molecule, peptide, or protein targets (3).

Aptamers have the potential for superior binding capabilities compared to naturally occurring RNA or DNA molecules because they are selected solely on the basis of their binding affinity. Furthermore, high-resolution, three-dimensional structural analyses have shown that adaptive recognition (involving conformational alteration of either the protein or the aptamer) is possible (4,5). This adaptive recognition produces an even tighter fit between the aptamer and protein, further increasing binding affinity. Aptamers display dissociation constants in the picomolar to low nanomolar range (6,9).

In addition to high binding affinity, aptamers are able to recognize their targets with great specificity. They are able to distinguish between protein isoforms as well as between different functional or conformational forms of the same protein (7). Many aptamers that are selected to bind to a specific protein also inhibit the protein's function. Most, but not all, therapeutically useful aptamers are inhibitors, binding and inhibiting enzyme activities or protein–protein interactions, and thereby function as antagonists (8,13).

Aptamers are randomly synthesized by an iterative process known as SELEX (systematic evolution of ligands by exponential enrichment), which was concurrently developed by the Gold and Szostak laboratories in 1990 (2). The SELEX method begins with a population of randomly synthesized RNA or DNA oligonucleotides, usually 20 to 40 nucleotides in length. In vitro selection allows the specificity and affinity of the aptamer to be tightly controlled. The randomized oligomer region is flanked by specific sequences needed for enzymatic manipulation (8). These regions contain binding sequences for reverse transcriptase (RT) and polymerase chain reaction (PCR) primers, a promoter sequence for T7 RNA polymerase, and possibly restriction endonuclease sites for cloning (9).

In practice, a standard randomized 40-nucleotide library generates as many as 10^{15} distinct aptamers (9). During the selection process, the library is enriched in sequences possessing increased affinity to the target. The sequences in the library that do not bind to the target ligand are removed, typically by affinity chromatography (10). Aptamers that bind to a target are selected, amplified by RT-PCR and then reselected. This process can be repeated if necessary to achieve the desired affinity and specificity. Depending on the dissociation constant values of the aptamer–target complex, five to fifteen rounds of selection (in which the stringency of the elution conditions is increased to identify the tightest-binding sequences) are typically performed to obtain aptamers (11). After cloning and sequencing, selected aptamer sequences can be synthesized chemically using solid-phase phosphoramidite chemistry (9).

Most of the targets for therapeutic aptamers are in solution in the blood plasma or on the surface of cells that are accessible from the blood plasma. These aptamers are subject to nuclease degradation, renal filtration, and uptake by the liver, as well as other tissues such as the spleen (8,12). As aptamers are chemically synthesized and lack many of the functional groups commonly present in proteins, a single functional group can be site-specifically introduced and used as a unique site for conjugation of other molecules to the aptamer without disrupting structure or function. Thus, aptamers can be modified in ways that enhance pharmacokinetic properties, avoiding the losses of activity that are often seen for stochastically modified therapeutic protein conjugates.

Unmodified RNA and DNA molecules are too susceptible to nuclease-mediated degradation to be useful for most therapeutic applications and therefore require some manner of chemical modification, before, after, or during selection. For example, the phosphodiester backbone of RNA-based aptamers is vulnerable to serum ribonucleases at pyrimidine residues, and the 5' and 3'-termini are vulnerable to exonucleases. To avoid degradation, chemically synthesized aptamers can be capped with modified or inverted nucleotides (13). Modified nucleotides can be introduced into libraries before initiation of SELEX by polymerases that can accept modified nucleotide triphosphates. By incorporating these modified nucleotides into aptamers, they become more resistant to nucleases, thereby improving their biological efficacy. To date, the highest affinity aptamers that have been reported contain modified nucleotides that bind in the single-digit picomolar range (8).

Even with extensive modification to block nuclease degradation, stabilized molecules must exhibit molecular weights of greater than 40 kDa (30–50 kDa is the molecular mass cutoff for the renal glomerulus) in order to remain in circulation for extended durations (3,8,14). This optimal molecular weight is most commonly realized by pegylation. To prolong renal clearance, high molecular weight polyethylene glycols (PEGs) can be covalently attached to aptamers, which typically have a molecular mass of 5 to 15 kDa (8), without significantly altering their ability to tightly bind to targets. Such modifications have a significant effect on the half-life of an aptamer, extending it from minutes to several hours (3).

This amenability to chemical modification is one property that distinguishes aptamers from monoclonal antibodies, which are only receptive to very limited chemical modification. For example, protein–PEG conjugation often results in a mixture of products and a loss of activity (8). Although aptamers are frequently referred to as "chemical antibodies," and although both aptamers and antibodies are able to bind with high specificity and high affinity ($K_d \approx 10^{-10}$–10^{-7} M) (1) to target molecules, there are certain aptamer properties that make them preferable to antibodies in both diagnostic and therapeutic applications.

Aptamers have exhibited little or no toxicity or immunogenicity, even when administered in excess of therapeutic doses (15). In fact, producing antibodies to aptamers is extremely hard (most likely because aptamers cannot be presented by T cells via the major histocompatibility complex and the immune response is not normally programmed to recognize nucleic acid fragments). In contrast, the efficacy of many peptides and monoclonal antibodies can be severely limited by immune responses. In fact, even antibodies whose nonhuman component has been replaced with human sequence (i.e., "humanization") can elicit immune responses (9).

Therapeutic antibodies are also more difficult to administer than aptamers. Because of their comparatively low solubility, comparatively large volumes are necessary when administrating most therapeutic monoclonal antibodies. Thus, most therapeutic antibodies require administration by intravenous infusion (generally over 2–4 hours). Conversely, aptamers have both good solubility and low molecular weight and therefore have the advantage of being able to be administered by either intravenous or subcutaneous injection (3).

Therapeutic aptamers are chemically robust. They are able to quickly regain activity following exposure to heat and denaturants. In addition, they can be stored in ambient temperatures as lyophilized powders for extended periods (more than 1 year) (3). Antibodies, however, are not as chemically stable. They are susceptible to irreversible denaturation and have a limited shelf life. The manufacturing of antibodies, which requires the use of cell-based expression systems, is far more complicated and less cost-effective than the commercial synthesis of aptamers (9). Furthermore, viral or bacterial contamination of the manufacturing process can affect the quality of the antibodies produced. The chemical production process of aptamers is not disposed to viral or bacterial contamination (8).

The first RNA aptamer to be successfully developed as a therapeutic agent in humans was pegaptanib sodium (Macugen), approved by the US Food and Drug Administration in December 2004 for the treatment of neovascular AMD (9). Pegaptanib, a 28-nucleotide RNA aptamer that is covalently linked to two PEG moieties, is an anti-vascular endothelial growth factor (anti-VEGF) RNA aptamer that is administered via intravitreal injection (4). It binds to all isoforms of human extracellular VEGF except for the smallest (VEGF121) (8). In particular, it binds with high affinity and selectivity to the VEGF165 isoform. VEGF is an endogenous proangiogenic protein involved in macular degeneration and in some cancers. Furthermore, VEGF has been associated with the leakage of blood vessels (3). Once pegaptanib is bound to VEGF, it inhibits the interaction of VEGF with its receptors, VEGFR1 and VEGFR2. Pegaptanib is used to improve the loss of visual acuity (VA) caused by the abnormal angiogenesis that is characteristic of AMD, the leading cause of blindness in people over 50 years of age in developed nations (4).

Fovista is a pegylated aptamer containing 32 monomeric units (32-mer) arranged as a linear sequence of three oligonucleotide segments connected by nonnucleotide hexaethylene glycol spacers. The aptamer terminates in a hexylamino linker to which two 20-kDa monomethoxy PEG units are covalently attached via the two amino groups on a lysine residue (16).

PERICYTES

Pericytes are branched cells that envelop the surface of the vascular tube. They possess a cell body with a prominent, round nucleus and a small amount of cytoplasm with several long finger-like extensions embracing the endothelium wall. They are thought to be the cells that stabilize the vessel wall, controlling endothelial cell proliferation and thus the growth of new capillaries. Research suggests that they communicate with endothelial cells by direct physical contact and paracrine signaling pathways (17). In addition, they can produce vasoconstriction and vasodilation within capillary beds to regulate vascular diameter and capillary blood flow. When vessels lose pericytes, they become hemorrhagic and hyperdilated, which leads to conditions such as edema, diabetic retinopathy, and even embryonic lethality (18).

Pericytes have been shown to perform specific functions in several organs including the brain, liver and kidneys and have therefore been given additional names in these organs (18). Furthermore, pericyte density differs in respect to the function of vessels and organs in which they are found. They are abundant on small venules and arterioles but are relatively sparse on capillaries. Pericyte density is dependent on blood pressure levels. In humans, for example, pericytes are more abundant further down the torso and legs, where increased pressure is necessary to pump the blood upward (19).

In addition to their involvement in hemodynamic processes, pericytes also have an active role in angiogenesis, the physiological process of new blood vessel formation from preexisting vessels. Angiogenesis not only depends on endothelial cell invasion and proliferation but also requires pericyte coverage of vascular sprouts for vessel stabilization (20). These processes are coordinated by vascular endothelial growth factor (VEGF) and platelet derived growth factor (PDGF) via their cognate receptors on endothelial cells and vascular smooth muscle cells (VSMCs), respectively. PDGF induces neovascularization by preparing VSMCs/pericytes to release proangiogenic mediators (20).

In vessel sprouting, VEGF-stimulated endothelial cells secrete proteases to degrade the vessel basement membrane. This enables the endothelial cells to invade the surrounding endothelial cell membrane and form a migration column consisting of proliferating and migrating endothelial cells. As seen in the retina, this column is guided by a migrating endothelial cell at the tip, which progresses toward a VEGF gradient. Newly formed sprouts cease proliferation behind this migration zone, adhere to each other, and form a new, lumen-containing vessel. Endothelial cells then secrete growth factors, partly to attract pericytes that envelop the vessel wall and promote vessel maturation (21,22). These views of pericyte and endothelial cell interactions are largely based on the concept that pericyte recruitment lags behind endothelial sprouting. The resulting "window of pericyte absence" allows for vascular plasticity, which results in growth, survival, remodeling, or regression of the endothelium, depending on the presence or absence of angiogenic growth factors such as VEGF (23).

Angiogenesis also occurs under pathological conditions like diabetic retinopathy and tumor growth. The difference between physiological and pathological angiogenesis lies in the tightly regulated balance of proangiogenic and antiangiogenic factors. During physiological neovascularization, newly formed vessels mature quickly, stabilize, and cease proliferation. Under pathological conditions, blood vessel growth loses the normal regulatory balance. Vessels formed during pathological angiogenesis do not stop growing and are under constant reconstruction, leading to an irregular vascular system (18).

Angiogenesis in tumors leads to disorganized vasculature with irregularly shaped and leaky vessels that are often unable to support efficient blood flow. And just as tumor endothelial cells differ from the normal endothelium, tumor pericytes also differ from normal pericytes. In general, pericytes in tumors appear to be more loosely attached to the vasculature, and their cytoplasmic processes can extend into the tumor tissue and can change their pericyte expression profile (24).

The exact reasons for abnormal pericyte behavior are still unknown but may result from imbalanced endothelial cell/pericyte signaling circuits. Recent data suggest that tumors employ the same signal mechanisms that are used in developmental angiogenesis (18). This also implies that tumor pericytes, though less abundant and more loosely attached than normal pericytes, still regulate vessel integrity, maintenance, and function. The fact that tumor vessels without pericytes appear more vulnerable suggests that they may be more responsive to antiendothelial drugs. Indeed, combinations of receptor tyrosine kinase inhibitors that target endothelial cells and pericytes by blocking VEGF and PDGF signaling, respectively, more efficiently diminished tumor blood vessels and tumors than any of the inhibitors individually (25). The same effect was achieved when PDGF inhibitors were combined with an antiangiogenic chemotherapy regimen that targeted endothelial cells. Targeting PDGFR signaling disrupted pericyte support, while the antiangiogenic chemotherapy targeted the sensitized endothelial cells, collectively destabilizing the preexisting tumor vasculature (17).

The vessels of the neural tissues, such as the brain and the retinas, contain high pericyte density. In fact, the retina has the highest density of pericytes in the body (18). Diabetic patients often develop diabetic retinopathy, of which an early characteristic is the loss of retinal pericytes (26). As a result, the vascular walls weaken and generate microaneurysms. Structural analyses of microaneurysms in the retina reveal a significant absence of pericytes. This suggests that the loss of vessel integrity due to the absence of pericytes leaves vessels vulnerable to aneurysms. When progressive vascular occlusions in diabetic eyes lead to blindness, the retina responds with either a progressive increase of vascular permeability, which leads to macular edema, or the formation of new, proliferating vessels. Also, diabetic retinas have an increased expression of VEGF-A and its receptors (18).

Normal vessels, surprisingly, seem to be able to withstand a substantial reduction in the density of pericytes, at least in mice (20). Although a reduction in pericyte density produces functionally and structurally abnormal vessels, only pericyte reductions of greater than 90% are lethal (18). This observation suggests that even small numbers of pericytes and pericytes with structural abnormalities, as observed in tumors, can still be functional and important for vessel stability and endothelial cell survival. These findings have led to a new concept of antiangiogenic therapy: combined targeting of endothelial cells and pericytes to more efficiently diminish blood vessels and halt subsequent tumor growth (20).

FOVISTA

Intravitreal anti-VEGF therapy has become the international standard of care in the management of subfoveal CNVMs secondary to AMD. Large multicentered clinical trials have shown ranibizumab to be superior to PDT in the management of classic lesions, and other publications have demonstrated that occult and less defined lesions respond to intravitreal anti-VEGF therapy (27). The CATT trial demonstrated that the safety and efficacy of ranibizumab versus bevacizumab are almost identical. A head-to-head trial has not been done comparing Eylea to Lucentis (28).

Since the initial use of anti-VEGF therapy in wet AMD, clinicians, and investigators have attempted to improve the efficacy of treatment through combination therapy. The ANCHOR study treated patients with intravitreal Lucentis and PDT but did not show an improvement of VA compared to monotherapy with bevacizumab alone (29). Other investigators have combined ranibizumab or bevacizumab with intravitreal triamcinolone acetate with or with PDT, attempting a multifactorial approach to CNVM treatment. The rationale for this approach has been based upon the documented presence of inflammatory components of wet AMD as well as known long-lasting effects of PDT on the activity of subfoveal CNVMs. None of these combined therapeutic approaches have been shown to be superior to monotherapy in terms of patients of VA of 20/40 or better.

The results of a phase 2, randomized, double-masked, controlled clinical trial were recently reported that showed superiority of combined Lucentis and Fovista over Lucentis alone in the treatment of subfoveal CNVMs. The results of this study show compelling evidence that intravitreal injection of an anti-PDGF aptamer that binds and strips pericytes that are associated with CNVMs in combination with Lucentis is superior to Lucentis alone.

Study design of the phase 2 study: Patients with active, classic subfoveal choroidal neovascularization (CNV) were randomized to one of three treatment groups: Fovista 1.5 mg + Lucentis 0.5 mg ($N = 152$); Fovista 0.3 mg + Lucentis 0.5 mg ($N = 149$); and Sham + Lucentis 0.5 mg ($N = 148$). Patients were given monthly injections over a 24-week period (Fig. 22.1). Demographically,

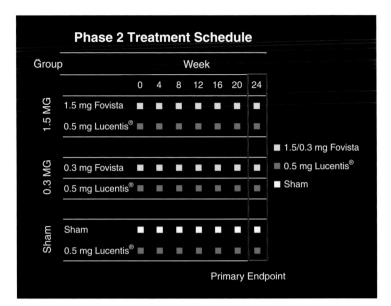

Figure 22.1 ■ Study design of the phase 2 study describes the three patient groups randomized for treatment and the monthly dosing scheme.

the patients were distributed evenly in terms of gender, race, age, lesion size, baseline vision, and smoking status (Table 22.1).

The investigators studied and documented safety issues to include ocular and systemic adverse events (AE) and serious adverse events (SAE). Ocular AE were reported as conjunctival hemorrhage, punctate keratitis, eye pain, conjunctiva hyperemia, subretinal fibrosis, and increased intraocular pressure. These were reported in less than 5% of patients and were evenly distributed among the three groups. SAE involving the eye, including corneal erosion, uveitis, and reduced VA, were seen in less than 1% of patients. In regards to systemic safety issues, cardiac disorders, nonfatal myocardial infarctions (MI), nonfatal strokes, and vascular deaths were equally distributed among the three groups of patients (Tables 22.2, to 22.4).

The efficacy of combination therapy of intravitreal Fovista and Lucentis and its superiority over Lucentis monotherapy were demonstrated in this study, when the investigators evaluated change in VA from baseline, improvement in vision over time, significant visual gain, optical coherence tomography (OCT) studies, and fluorescein angiography.

At the 24-week end point, Fovista combined with Lucentis met its prespecified primary end point with both Fovista/Lucentis groups achieving a mean change in vision from baseline greater than that of monotherapy (Fig. 22.2). In evaluating dose–response curves of the three groups, those patients receiving Fovista and Lucentis had demonstrable mean change in vision for all time points during the study (Fig. 22.3). Most compelling was the significant visual gain, defined as gaining more than three, four, or five lines of vision, as patients on combination therapy showed a 190% relative benefit in those patients gaining greater than five lines. OCT studies of the three groups showed similar findings when evaluating subretinal fluid, intraretinal cystic fluid, and sub-RPE fluid (Fig. 22.4). An interesting finding was the diminished percentage of patients who developed subretinal hyperreflective material (SHRM), in those eyes receiving combination therapy (Fig. 22.5). On angiography, there was a greater reduction in the CNV size seen in patients receiving combination therapy (Fig. 22.6).

Table 22.1	BASELINE DEMOGRAPHICS		
	Monotherapy Lucentis *N* = 148	0.3 mg Fovista (anti-PDGF) + Lucentis *N* = 149	1.5 mg Fovista (anti-PDGF) + Lucentis *N* = 152
Female	93 (62.8%)	90 (60.4%)	92 (60.5%)
Caucasian	144 (97.3%)	145 (97.3%)	149 (98.0%)
Mean age (years)	78	77.6	77.8
Lesion size (DA)	1.8	1.9	1.5
Baseline VA (letters)	50.6	50.6	49.3
Active smoker	13 (8.8%)	21 (14.1%)	17 (11.3%)

Table 22.2   OCULAR ADVERSE EVENTS REPORTED IN ≥5% OF PATIENTS

	Monotherapy Lucentis N = 148	0.3 mg Fovista + Lucentis N = 149	1.5 mg Fovista + Lucentis N = 152
Patients with ≥1 AE	**75 (50.7%)**	**79 (53.0%)**	**79 (52.0%)**
Conjunctival hemorrhage	37 (25.0%)	34 (22.8%)	51 (33.6%)
Punctate keratitis	10 (6.8%)	19 (12.8%)	15 (9.9%)
Eye pain	8 (5.4%)	10 (6.7%)	13 (8.6%)
Conjunctival hyperemia	13 (8.8%)	9 (6.0%)	13 (8.6%)
Subretinal fibrosis	8 (5.4%)	6 (4.0%)	5 (3.3%)
Intraocular pressure (IOP) increased	4 (2.7%)	8 (5.4%)	9 (5.9%)

Table 22.3   OCULAR SERIOUS ADVERSE EVENTS

	Monotherapy Lucentis N = 148 N (%)	0.3 mg Fovista + Lucentis N = 149 N (%)	1.5 mg Fovista + Lucentis N = 152 N (%)
Eye disorders	**1 (0.7%)**	**1 (0.7%)**	**1 (0.7%)**
Corneal erosion	0 (0.0%)	0 (0.0%)	1 (0.7%)
Uveitis	0 (0.0%)	1 (0.7%)	0 (0.0%)
Visual acuity reduced	1 (0.7%)	0 (0.0%)	0 (0.0%)

Table 22.4   SYSTEMIC SERIOUS ADVERSE EVENTS

	Monotherapy Lucentis N = 148 N (%)	0.3 mg Fovista + Lucentis N = 149 N (%)	1.5 mg Fovista + Lucentis N = 152 N (%)
Patients with ≥1 systemic SAE	**11 (7.4%)**	**13 (8.7%)**	**9 (5.9%)**
MedDRA system organ class[a]			
Cardiac disorders	2 (1.4%)	2 (1.3%)	2 (1.3%)
Gastrointestinal disorders	1 (0.7%)	2 (1.3%)	3 (2.0%)
Infections	1 (0.7%)	2 (1.3%)	0 (0.0%)
Musculoskeletal disorders	1 (0.7%)	0 (0.0%)	2 (1.3%)
Neoplasms	3 (2.0%)	3 (2.0%)	1 (0.7%)
Nervous system disorders	3 (2.0%)	1 (0.7%)	0 (0.0%)
Respiratory disorders	0 (0.0%)	3 (2.0%)	2 (1.3%)
Any APTC event[b]	**3 (2.0%)**	**1 (0.7%)**	**0 (0.0%)**
Nonfatal MI	0 (0.0%)	0 (0.0%)	0 (0.0%)
Nonfatal stroke	2 (1.4%)	1 (0.7%)	0 (0.0%)
Vascular death	1 (0.7%)	0 (0.0%)	0 (0.0%)

[a]Data are listed for organ classes with three or more events.
[b]Antiplatelet Trialists' Collaboration.

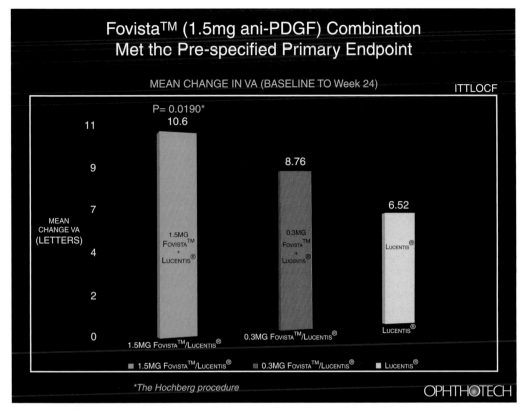

Figure 22.2 ■ Combination therapy with Fovista and Lucentis was superior to Lucentis alone when evaluating letters gained from baseline.

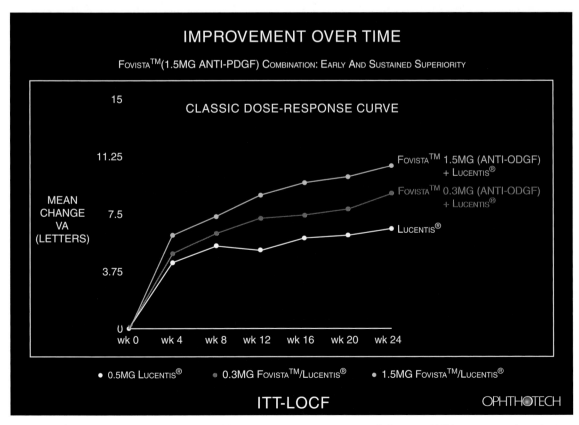

Figure 22.3 ■ The dose–response curves of the three treatment groups reveals increased VA improvement in patients treated with Fovista in combination with Lucentis.

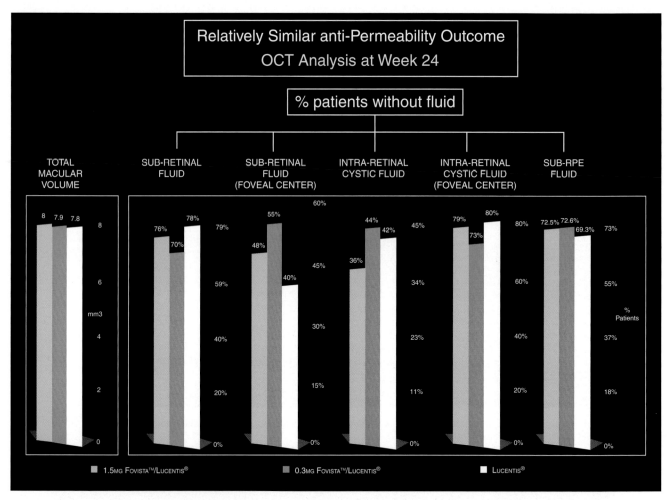

Figure 22.4 ■ OCT of all three treatment groups showed comparable results in the analysis of subretinal fluid and intraretinal cysts.

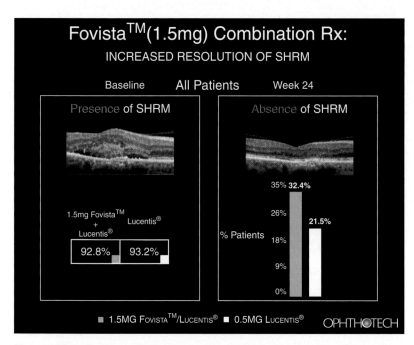

Figure 22.5 ■ An interesting finding was the diminished percentage of patients who developed sub-retinal hyper-reflective material (SHRM), in those eyes receiving combination therapy.

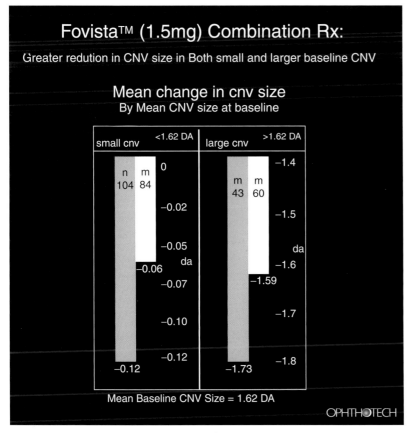

Figure 22.6 ■ On angiography, there was a greater reduction in the CNV size seen in patients receiving combination therapy.

REFERENCES

1. Davydova AS, Vorobjeva MA, Venyaminova AG. Escort aptamers: new tools for the targeted delivery of therapeutics into cells. Acta Naturae. 2011;3(4):12–29.

2. Dausse E, Gomes SDR, Toulmé JJ. Aptamers: a new class of oligonucleotides in the drug discovery pipeline? Curr Opin Pharmacol. 2009;9:602–607.

3. Pendergrast PS, Marsh HN, Grate D, et al. Nucleic acid aptamers for target validation and therapeutic applications. J Biomol Tech. 2005;16(3):224–234.

4. Alfaro DV, Liggett PE, Mieler WF, et al. Age related macular degeneration: a comprehensive textbook. Philadelphia, PA: Lippincott; 2006:272.

5. Herman T, Patel DJ. Adaptive recognition by nucleic acid aptamers. Science. 2000;287:820–825.

6. Valentino TL, Kaplan HJ, Del Priore LV, et al. Retinal pigment epithelial repopulation in monkeys after submacular surgery. Arch Ophthalmol. 1995;113:932–938.

7. Sekiya S, Nishikawa F, Noda K, et al. In vitro selection of RNA aptamers against cellular and abnormal isoform of mouse prion protein. Nucleic Acids Symp Ser. 2005;49:361–362.

8. Keefe AD, Pai S, Ellington A. Aptamers as therapeutics. Nat Rev Drug Discov. 2010;9:537–550.

9. Ng EWM, Shima DT, Calias P, et al. Pegaptanib, a targeted anti-VEGF aptamer for ocular vascular disease. Nat Rev Drug Discov. 2006;5:123–132.

10. Jarosch F, Buchner K, Klussmann S. In vitro selection using a dual RNA library that allows primerless selection. Nucleic Acids Res. 2006;34(12):e86.

11. Zimbres FM, Támok A, Ulrich H. Aptamers: novel molecules as diagnostic markers in bacterial and viral infections? BioMed Res Int. 2013;2013:731516.

12. Watson SR, Chang YF, O'Connell D, et al. Anti-L-selection aptamers: binding characteristics, pharmacokinetic parameters, and activity against an intravascular target in vivo. Antisense Nucleic Acid Drug Dev. 2000;10:63–75.

13. Ni X, Castanares M, Mukherjee A, et al. Nucleic acid aptamers: clinical applications and promising new horizons. Curr Med Chem. 2011;18(27):4206–4214.

14. Healy JM, Lewis SD, Kurz M, et al. Pharmacokinetics and biodistribution of novel aptamer compositions. Pharm Res. 2004;21:2234–2246.

15. White RR, Sullenger BA, Rusconi CP. Developing aptamers into therapeutics. J Clin Invest. 2000;106:929–934.

16. Mandarino L, Sundarraj N, Finlayson J, et al. Regulation of fibronectin and laminin synthesis by retinal capillary endothelial cells and pericytes in vitro. Exp Eye Res. 1993;57:609–621.

17. Bergers G, Song S. The role of pericytes in blood-vessel formation and maintenance. Neuro Oncol. 2005;7:452–464.

18. Sims DE. Diversity within pericytes. Clin Exp Pharmacol Physiol. 2000;27:842–846.

19. Greenberg J, Shields D, Barillas S, et al. A role for VEGF as a negative regulator of pericyte function and vessel maturation. Nature. 2008;456:809–813.

20. Mones J. Inhibiting VEGF and PDGF to treat AMD: drugs that combine regression of CNV with resolution permeability in wet AMD may enhance visual outcomes. Rev Ophthalmol. 2011;9:56–59.

21. Gerhardt H, Golding M, Fruttiger M, et al. VEGF guides angiogenic sprouting utilizing endothelial tip cell filopodia. J Cell Biol. 2003;161:1163–1177.

22. Bondjers C, Kalen M, Hellstrom M, et al. Transcription profiling of platelet-derived growth factor-B-deficient mouse embryos identifies RGS5 as a novel marker for pericytes and vascular smooth muscle cells. Am J Pathol. 2003;162:721–729.

23. Bergers G, Benjamin L. Tumorigenesis and the angiogenic switch. Nat Rev Cancer. 2003;3:401–410.

24. Ribatti D, Nico B, Crivellato E. The role of pericytes in angiogenesis. Int J Dev Biol. 2011;55:261–268.

25. Abramsson A, Lindblom P, Betsholtz C. Endothelial and nonendothelial sources of PDGF-B regulate pericytes recruitment and influence vascular pattern formation in tumors. J Clin Invest. 2003;112:1142–1151.

26. Cai J, Boulton M. The pathogenesis of diabetic retinopathy: old concepts and new questions. Eye (Lond). 2002;16:242–260.

27. Martin DF, Maguire MG, Fine SL, et al. Ranibizumab and bevacizumab for treatment of neovascular age-related macular degeneration: two-year results. Ophthalmology. 2012;119(7):1388–1398.

28. Heier JS, Boyer DS, Ciulla TA, et al. Ranibizumab combined with verteporfin photodynamic therapy in neovascular age-related macular degeneration: year 1 results of the FOCUS study. Arch Ophthalmol. 2006;124(11): 1532–1542.

29. Brown DM, Michels M, Kaiser PK, et al. Ranibizumab versus verteporfin photodynamic therapy for neovascular age-related macular degeneration: two-year results of the ANCHOR study. Ophthalmology. 2009;116(1): 57–65.

23

COMPLICATIONS OF INTRAVITREAL INJECTIONS

MARIA LOZANO-VAZQUEZ • JOSE M. GARCIA-GONZALEZ •
VEERAL SHETH • HARIT K. BHATT • SUNDEEP GRANDHE •
MADHU AMARA • RAMA D. JAGER

Intravitreal (IVT) injections have been used in the treatment of ocular diseases for over a century since being initially reported in 1911 by Ohm (1) as a means to introduce air for retinal tamponade and repair of detachment. In the 1940s, the IVT administration of pharmaceutical agents was pioneered with the use of penicillin to treat endophthalmitis (2). During the 1950s and 1960s, the use of IVT injections still was limited to the administration of air or silicone oil, in the treatment of retinal detachment (3,4). However, by the 1970s, the advent of newer antimicrobial agents led to renewed interest in IVT therapy for endophthalmitis. The gradual increase in confidence in the safety of IVT injection led to the evaluation of IVT administration of a number of agents throughout the 1990s such as dexamethasone (5) in diabetic retinopathy, triamcinolone acetonide (6) as a treatment of exudative age-related macular degeneration (AMD), methotrexate (7,43) for treatment of ocular lymphoma, tPA (8) for the management of submacular hemorrhage, and fomivirsen sodium (9) to treat CMV retinitis. In 1998, the U.S. Food and Drug Administration (FDA) approved the use of the first agent for IVT injections, fomivirsen sodium for the treatment of CMV retinitis. During the 2000s, new applications for IVT injection continued to accelerate with vascular endothelial growth factor (VEGF) inhibitors for exudative AMD (10–12) and ovine hyaluronidase (13).

Over the last decade, the use of IVT injection has exploded in the therapeutic management of AMD and many other intraocular diseases. An examination of the risks associated with IVT therapy is paramount, given its exponentially increasing usage.

Although efforts have been made to distinguish the risks associated with the specific agents being administered from risks related to the IVT injection procedure, per se, in some instances, making such distinctions has proven difficult. It is important to note that some compounds administered by IVT injection have not been approved for intraocular use and may contain harmful excipients, have improper pH balance, or include unacceptably high levels of contaminants, such as endotoxin.

Drug concentrations in the vitreous are determined not only by the amount of drug given but also by the distribution and clearance of such compounds (14,15). As with other routes of drug administration, pharmacokinetic characteristics are dependent on the anatomical and physiologic features of the site of administration (14,15) and physiochemical properties of agents administered (16). Although several investigators have explored the pharmacokinetic properties of the IVT injection of selected compounds in animal models (14–17) and to a limited extent in humans (18,19), this topic remains complex and incompletely understood.

Descriptions of some variables related to IVT injection that may influence the results do not always get mentioned. These variables may include preoperative prophylactic antibiotics, pre- or postoperative procedures to control elevations in intraocular pressure (IOP) (digital massage, paracentesis), preparation of the injection site (anesthetic,

255

antibiotics, mydriatics, antiseptics), immobilization of the eye (the use of forceps, digits, or lid specula), and postoperative therapy (topical antibiotics).

Risk assessment of IVT injection is undoubtedly complex. Several potential complications of IVT injection, such as endophthalmitis, retinal detachment, and intraocular hemorrhage, can be vision threatening. The following section provides an estimation of the prevalence of each complication within the context of overall risk of IVT injection. Whenever possible, complications caused by the IVT injection procedure were distinguished from those attributable to the condition being treated or those related to the administration of specific therapeutic compounds (Tables 23.1 to 23.3). We have included the results of the extensive review of risks of IVT injection performed by Jager et al. 2004 (23).

ENDOPHTHALMITIS

The overall prevalence of endophthalmitis after IVT injection is low. Retrospective reports indicate a per-injection endophthalmitis risk between 0% and 0.87% (29–32). Jager et al. (23) 2004 reported an overall prevalence of endophthalmitis, excluding cases reported as noninfectious endophthalmitis or pseudoendophthalmitis, of 0.5% per eye and 0.2% per injection. Endophthalmitis was reported very rarely after IVT injection of gas or other compounds other than antiviral agents and triamcinolone acetonide, with a combined prevalence of 0.1% per eye and 0.1% per injection for all other compounds (10,23,33,34). The trials for ranibizumab, ranibizumab versus verteporfin for neovascular AMD (ANCHOR) (35) and ranibizumab for neovascular AMD (MARINA) (36), also demonstrated a low rate of endophthalmitis. At 1 year, ANCHOR reported a 0.07% per-injection endophthalmitis rate, and by 2 year, there were only three cases of endophthalmitis out of 5,921 injections (0.05%) (35).

Singerman et al. (VISION Trial: VEGF Inhibition Study in Ocular Neovascularization) (37) reported a low rate of serious ocular events during 3 years of pegaptanib sodium for treatment of neovascular AMD with a rate of endophthalmitis from 0.16% per injection (12 of 7,545 injections) in the first year to 0.10% per injection (4/4091) in the 2nd year and to 0.06% per injection (2/3227) in the 3rd year ($P < 0.0001$). This decrease in the rate of endophthalmitis may result at least partially from a protocol emphasizing the importance of adherence to aseptic technique when performing IVT injections. Other reasons for lower rates of endophthalmitis may also be the widespread adoption of and increasing familiarity with IVT injections by retina specialists over the 3 years of this study.

The Pan American Collaborative Retina Study Group (PACORES, 2008) mentioned seven cases of bacterial endophthalmitis of a total of 4,303 IVT injections of bevacizumab during 12 months of safety monitoring (28). The cultures yielded five cases of coagulase-negative staphylococci and one case each of *Staphylococcus aureus* and *Streptococcus*.

Noninfectious (sterile) endophthalmitis and pseudoendophthalmitis may also occur after IVT triamcinolone injections. Some studies (Table 23.2) have reported incidents of 0.5% to 0.9% per IVT triamcinolone injections (32,37,38).

RETINAL DETACHMENT

Retinal detachment is uncommon (23,27,28,32,36,37) after IVT injection. The VISION trial (27) described an incidence of rhegmatogenous retinal detachment of 0.03% per injection (1/3227) (27). ANCHOR and MARINA studies demonstrated a 0.01% per-injection detachment rate (35,36).

Jager et al. (23) mentioned an overall prevalence of retinal detachment of 3.9% per eye and 0.9% per injection. The majority of cases identified in this review appeared to be related to patients underlying condition, principally CMV retinitis and vitreous hemorrhage in the setting of diabetic retinopathy (23).

IRITIS/UVEITIS

Secondary uveitis is an uncommon complication of IVT injection. Ocular inflammation has been observed in 26.9% of eyes with CMV retinitis treated with IVT cidofovir (22,39), in 38.2% of eyes treated with IVT fomivirsen (9), and in 48.4% of eyes treated with IVT ovine hyaluronidase (13) for the treatment of vitreous hemorrhage. Taskintuna et al. (22) reported a high prevalence of intraocular inflammatory reactions in the fellow (untreated) eyes of some patient, many of whom previously had been treated with systemic antiviral agents. Moreover, acute intraocular inflammation has been reported to occur after intravenous administration of cidofovir. These findings suggest that the occurrence of noninfectious intraocular inflammation in patients receiving IVT cidofovir is a consequence of the therapeutic agent itself and not the IVT injection. Another confounding factor in identifying the cause of intraocular inflammation in patients receiving cidofovir is the condition known as immune recovery uveitis in which patients with CMV retinitis develop inflammation when their CD4 count increases after beginning treatment with HAART (39,40).

OCULAR HYPERTENSION

Increases in IOP after IVT injection may be transient or sustained. Although transient IOP responses to IVT injection were described inconsistently in many reports, sustained ocular hypertension was associated primarily with the administration of triamcinolone acetonide (23,29,30,41). Prevalence of ocular hypertension after IVT injection of triamcinolone varies between studies (38%–52%) (23–25,29,30).

Table 23.1 SERIOUS ADVERSE EVENTS (SAES) REPORTED FROM STUDIES INVOLVING ADMINISTRATION OF ANTIVIRAL COMPOUNDS

Study	Study type	Indication	Compound	No. of eyes	No. of injections	EO	RD	I/U	HE	OH	CY	HP	Other SAEs
Cochereau-Massin et al. 1991 (20)	POS	CMV retinitis	Ganciclovir	64	710	–	5	–	2	–	–	–	5 optic disk atrophy
Rahhal et al. 1996 (21)	CS	CMV retinitis	Cidofovir	53	168	–	1	29	–	–	–	4	2 transient and 2 irreversible HP
Taskintuna et al. 1997 (22)	CS	CMV retinitis	Cidofovir	27	46	–	–	1	–	–	–	–	—
Vitravene, 2002 (9)	RCT	CMV retinitis	Fomivirsen	330	1,791	2	33	126	21	54	33	6	4 CME; 3 RAO; 5 retinal tears; 1 RVO; 4 macular degeneration; 1 optic atrophy; 1 orbital cellulitis
Jager et al. 2004 (23)	RS	CMV retinitis	Ganciclovir	909	10,839	12	54	179	24	54	44	28	6 optic disk atrophy 13 Transient and 3 irreversible HP
			Cidofovir			1.3[a]	5.9[a]	19.7[a]	2.6[a]	5.9[a]	4.8[a]	3.1[a]	
			Fomivirsen			0.1[b]	0.5[b]	1.7[b]	0.2[b]	0.5[b]	0.4[b]	0.3[b]	4 CME; 3 RAO; 5 retinal tears; 1 RVO; 4 macular degeneration; 1 orbital cellulitis

Blank spaces indicate no reported events.
[a]Prevalence per eye (%).
[b]Prevalence per injection (%).
IVT, intravitreal; EO, endophthalmitis; RD, retinal detachment; I/U, iritis/uveitis/vitritis/anterior chamber inflammation; HE, hemorrhage; OH, ocular hypertension; CT, cataract; HP, hypotony; CS, case series; RCT, randomized controlled trial; POS, prospective open study; RS, retrospective study; CMV, cytomegalovirus; CME, cystoids macular edema; RAO, retinal artery occlusion; RVO, retinal vein occlusion.

Table 23.2 SERIOUS ADVERSE EVENTS (SAES) REPORTED FROM STUDIES INVOLVING ADMINISTRATION OF TRIAMCINOLONE ACETONIDE (TCA)

Study	Study type	Indication	Compound	No. of eyes	No. of injections	EO	RD	I/U	HE	OH	CT	HP	Other SAEs
Jager et al. 2004 (23)	RS	AMD DME CME CNV	TCA	1,703	1,739	24 0.6[a] 0.6[b]	—	—	—	38.3[a] 36.6[b]	100 9.9[a] 9.9[b]	13	14 P-EO 1 HRVO
DRCR, 2008 (24)	RCT	CSDME	TCA	510	1,583	0	6	—	—	126	148	—	3 RVO 1 Anterior ischemic optic neuropathy 0 P-EO
SCORE, 2009 (25)	RCT	BRVO	TCA	274	—	1	1	—	3	68	65	—	0 P-EO
SCORE, 2009 (26)	RCT	CRVO	TCA	183	—	0	0	—	4	42	55	—	0 P-EO

Blank spaces indicate no reported events.
[a]Prevalence per eye (%).
[b]Prevalence per injection (%).
IVT, intravitreal; EO, endophthalmitis; P-EO, pseudoendophthalmitis; RD, retinal detachment; I/U, iritis/uveitis/vitritis/anterior chamber inflammation; HE, hemorrhage; OH, ocular hypertension; CT, cataract; HP, hypotony; TCA, triamcinolone acetonide; RS, retrospective study; RCT, randomized controlled trial; DME, diabetic macular edema; POS, prospective open study; AMD, age-related macular degeneration; CME, cystoid macular edema; CRVO, central retinal vein occlusion; BRVO, branch retinal vein occlusion; HRVO, hemiretinal vein occlusion; CSDME, clinically significant macular edema; CNV, choroidal neovascularization.

Table 23.3 SERIOUS ADVERSE EVENTS (SAES) REPORTED FROM STUDIES INVOLVING ADMINISTRATION OF ANTI-VEGF

Study	Study type	Indication	Compound	No. of eyes	No. of injections	EO	RD	I/U	HE	OH	CT	HP	Other SAEs
Eyetech Study Group, 2003 (11)	POS	AMD	Pegaptanib sodium	21	61	—	—	7	—	1	—	—	—
VISION, 2008 (27)	RCT	AMD	Pegaptanib sodium	422	3,227	2	1	14	1	32	23	—	41 punctate keratitis 15 conjunctival hemorrhage 17 cardiac disorders 23 gastrointestinal disorders 15 vascular disorders 2 MI
PACORES, 2008 (28)	RS	RVO AMD DME PDR	Bevacizumab	1,310	4,303	7	7	4	1	7	—	1	7 acute HTN 6 CVA 5 MI

Blank spaces indicate no reported events.
EO, endophthalmitis; P-EO, pseudoendophthalmitis; RD, retinal detachment; I/U, iritis/uveitis/vitritis/anterior chamber inflammation; HE, hemorrhage; OH, ocular hypertension; CT, cataract; HP, hypotony; RS, retrospective study; RCT, randomized controlled trial; CS, case series; POS, prospective open study; DME, diabetic macular edema; AMD, age-related macular degeneration; CME, cystoid macular edema; CRVO, central retinal vein occlusion; CMV, cytomegalovirus; HRVO, hemiretinal vein occlusion; RVO, retinal vein obstruction; anti-VEGF, vascular endothelial growth factor inhibitor; HTN, systemic hypertension; MI, myocardial infarction; CVA, cerebrovascular accident; PDR, proliferative diabetic retinopathy.

Excluding IVT injection of triamcinolone acetonide, Jager et al. (23) described a prevalence of ocular hypertension of 2.4% per eye and 0.4% per injection, with most these events having been reported in association with fomivirsen (9,23).

Transiently elevated IOP, in contrast, is common and may occur after IVT administration of any agent. Although most studies make no mention of transient ocular hypertension, some studies have reported a transient increase in IOP when injecting simultaneous expansile gas and recombinant tPA (tissue plasminogen activator) (4.7% of eyes) (33) and pegaptanib sodium (4.8% of eyes) (11). This transient increase in IOP was likely related to the amount of volume injected in the eye, which was 0.09 mL of pegaptanib in the VISION study rather than the standard 0.5 mL, and the use of 0.05 mL of 100% sulfur hexafluoride expansile gas plus 0.05 mL of tPA in the former study.

Gillies et al. (41) reported that 21 of 75 eyes (28%) treated with 4 mg triamcinolone required glaucoma drops at some point during a 3-year period. Over a mean period of 8 months, 71% of eyes discontinued treatment as the IOP normalized, but six eyes (8%) required continued IOP-lowering therapy. In the Diabetic Retinopathy Clinical Research Network (DRCR.net) study comparing IVT triamcinolone acetonide and focal–grid photocoagulation for diabetic macular edema, 102 of 254 eyes (40%) in the 4-mg triamcinolone group, 51 of 256 eyes (20%) in the 1-mg triamcinolone group, and 34 of 330 eyes (10%) in the laser group developed some adverse IOP-related event (defined as an IOP elevation greater than 10 mmHg from baseline, IOP greater than 30 mmHg, initiation of IOP-lowering medications, or a diagnosis of glaucoma) in a 2-year follow-up (24). The Standard of Care versus Corticosteroid for Retinal Vein Occlusion (SCORE) study compared IVT triamcinolone with standard of care for both branch retinal vein occlusion (BRVO) and central retinal vein occlusion (CRVO). In the first year of the BRVO study, IOP-lowering medications were initiated in 57 of 138 (41%) eyes in the 4-mg triamcinolone group, 11 of 136 (8%) eyes in the 1-mg group, and 3 of 137 (2%) eyes in the standard care group (26). In the CRVO study, IOP-lowering therapy started in 32 of 91 (35%) eyes in the 4-mg triamcinolone group, 18 of 92 (20%) eyes in the 1-mg group, and 7 of 88 (8%) eyes in the observation group (25).

INTRAOCULAR HEMORRHAGE

Intraocular hemorrhage (i.e., retinal hemorrhage, vitreous hemorrhage, or hyphema) was reported occasionally after IVT injection, and although the etiology was unclear, in most instances, it was probably attributable to the underlying pathologic condition for which the injection was administered and not the IVT injection procedure per se. Jager et al. reported an overall prevalence of intraocular hemorrhage after IVT injections of 6% (176/2,940) per eye and 1.3% (176/13,400) per injection in an extensive review of the literature from 1966 to 2004.

More recent studies are consistent with a low prevalence of intraocular hemorrhage after IVT injection (25,26). Mason et al. (42) reported no hemorrhagic complications (choroidal hemorrhage, vitreous hemorrhage, or increased submacular hemorrhage) in a single-center retrospective case series review of 520 patients (675 eyes) receiving anti-VEGF injections in patient on systemic anticoagulants.

CATARACT

Cataract development and/or progression has been reported rarely after IVT injection, with exception of eyes treated with triamcinolone acetonide, fomivirsen, cidofovir, and methotrexate (9,23,43). The studies that reported the greatest number of cataract development were those evaluating the off-label use of triamcinolone acetonide. Early reports demonstrated cataract formation, most notably posterior subcapsular cataract, in 7% to 50% of patients (24,31,44). These early reports are limited by short follow-up periods that underestimated long-term cataract progression (44,45). By year 2 of the DRCR.net Study comparing IVT triamcinolone acetonide and focal–grid photocoagulation, 74% of eyes in the steroid injection arm, 23% (47 of 256 eyes) receiving 1 mg and 51% (101 of 254 eyes) receiving 4 mg, underwent cataract surgery (24). By year 3, the cumulative probability of cataract surgery was 31% in the laser group, 46% in the 1-mg triamcinolone group, and 83% in the 4-mg triamcinolone group (P < 0.001) (46). In the SCORE BRVO study, 60% of patients injected with triamcinolone, 25% (27 of 136 eyes) receiving 1 mg and 35% (38 of 138 eyes) receiving 4 mg, versus 13% (15 of 137 eyes) of laser-treated patients had onset or progression of lens opacity. Similar progression of lens opacity was seen in the SCORE CRVO study, where 59% of patients injected with triamcinolone, 26% (20 of 92 eyes) receiving 1 mg and 33% (25 of 91 eyes) receiving 4 mg, versus 18% (12 of 88 eyes) of observation patients had onset or progression of lens opacity (25,26).

Cataract formation was also common in eyes treated with antiviral agents, with a prevalence of 4.8% (44/909) per eye and 0.4% (44/10,839) per injection. Most of these cases were reported after administration of IVT fomivirsen (9).

IVT methotrexate administration was associated with an increased prevalence of cataract. A case series by Smith et al. (43), involving 494 IVT injections of methotrexate in 26 eyes, described cataract progression in 19 eyes (73%) when followed for 180 to 1,050 days. It was not described whether these were newly formed or existing cataracts; however, 12 of these eyes had undergone vitrectomy before initial IVT methotrexate therapy, and four additional eyes underwent vitrectomy before an additional course of IVT injection was administered.

HYPOTONY

Hypotony occurred rarely after IVT injection. Some studies described hypotony in 3.1% of eyes treated with IVT antiviral therapy, including 22 cases reporting low IOP after administration of cidofovir (21,22) and 6 cases after injecting fomivirsen (9). Cidofovir is known to have a direct toxic effect on the ciliary body, which may explain the occurrence of hypotony in patients receiving this compound. Low IOP was also described after IVT injection of ovine hyaluronidase (13).

OTHER UNCOMMONLY REPORTED SERIOUS COMPLICATIONS

Retinal vein occlusion was observed in 1 of 75 eyes after using IVT triamcinolone acetonide (24), in 1 of 330 eyes after using fomivirsen (9), and in 1 of 1,344 eyes after ovine hyaluronidase (13). Three of 1,791 eyes were reported to have retinal artery occlusions after IVT injection of fomivirsen (9). Optic disk atrophy was described in five eyes treated with ganciclovir (20). Corneal epitheliopathy (15/26 eyes) has been described after using intraocular methotrexate (43). Maculopathy, in the form of various pigment epithelial disturbances, has been described after using methotrexate (11/26 eyes) (43) and macular edema in 46 of 966 eyes that received ovine hyaluronidase (13).

Systemic

Certain agents, such as anti-VEGF agents and corticosteroids, have significant and potentially life-threatening complications when given systemically. The potential systemic side effects of anti-VEGF agents include thromboembolic events such as stroke, myocardial infarction, angina, gastrointestinal perforation, hemorrhage, hypertensive crisis, and congestive heart failure.

The primary benefit of IVT injection is that the therapeutic agent can work directly in the eye while minimizing systemic absorption. Recent studies have included systemic adverse effects as part of the IVT injection analysis. Campbell et al. (47) did not appreciate any changes in the rate of hospitalization for stroke in patients receiving bevacizumab and ranibizumab for AMD between 2002 and 2010 in older patient (median age 77 years) in Ontario (Canada). This study was limited to strokes requiring hospitalization, and it did not include milder vascular events not requiring hospitalization. Martin et al. (48) described thromboembolic events (nonfatal stroke, nonfatal myocardial infarction, vascular death) in 28 of 599 patients (4.7%) with ranibizumab and in 29 of 586 patients (5.0%) with bevacizumab after 2-year follow-up. Gastrointestinal disorder (nauseas, vomiting, hemorrhage, hernia) was described by Martin et al. (48) in 11 of 599 (1.8%) patients treated with ranibizumab and in 28 of 586 (62%) patients treated with bevacizumab.

A potential complication of IVT injection is the occurrence of an anaphylactic reaction to compounds; at least one report exists in the literature in which anaphylaxis occurred after IVT administration of cefazolin (49).

INTRAVITREAL INJECTION TECHNIQUE

To date, there has been no universal technique for IVT injections. Different techniques may include the use of preoperative prophylactic antibiotic therapy, the implementation of preoperative or postoperative procedures to control elevations in IOP (digital massage, paracentesis), preparation of the injection site (anesthetics, antibiotics, mydriatics, or antiseptics), location of the injection site (quadrant or distance from limbus), immobilization of the eye (use of forceps, lid specula, digits), and postoperative therapy (antibiotics or ocular antihypertensive). Some authors have suggested a variety of approaches that may reduce the prevalence of serious adverse events after IVT injection (50). These include the use of povidone–iodine, face masks, and topical antibiotics before IVT; lowering concentration of triamcinolone to reduce the rate of ocular hypertension; decreasing the injection volume from 0.1 to 0.05 mL to reduce the amount of transient elevations in IOP after IVT; and using smaller gauge needles to minimize risk of vitreous or medication reflux (24,32,51–54).

CONCLUSION

IVT injections have increasingly been incorporated into routine patient management. To date, clinical experience suggests that the procedure itself is associated with a low incidence of serious adverse events while the majority of ocular and systemic side effects are primarily due to the injected agent.

REFERENCES

1. Ohm J. Uber die behandlung der netzhautablosung durch operative entleerung der subretinalen flussigkeit und einspritzung von luft in den glaskorper. Albrecht von Graefes Arch Ophthalmol. 1911;79:442–450.

2. Schneider J, Frankel SS. Treatment of late postoperative intraocular infections with intraocular injection of penicillin. Arch Ophthalmol. 1947;37:304–307.

3. Rosengren B. 300 cases operated upon for retinal detachment; method and results. Acta Ophthalmol (Copenh). 1952;30:117–122.

4. Cibis PA, Becker B, Okun E, et al. The use of liquid silicone in retinal detachment surgery. Arch Ophthalmol. 1962;68:590–599.

5. Blankenship GW. Evaluation of a single intravitreal injection of dexamethasone phosphate in vitrectomy surgery for diabetic retinopathy complications. Graefes Arch Clin Exp Ophthalmol. 1991;229:62–65.

6. Penfold PL, Gyory JF, Hunyor AB, et al. Exudative macular degeneration and intravitreal triamcinolone. A pilot study. Aust N Z J Ophthalmol. 1995;23:293–298.

7. Fishburne BC, Wilson DJ, Rosenbaum JT, et al. Intravitreal methotrexate as an adjunctive treatment of intraocular lymphoma. Arch Ophthalmol. 1997;115:1152–1156.

8. Hassan AS, Johnson MW, Schneiderman TE, et al. Management of submacular hemorrhage with intravitreal tissue plasminogen activator injection and pneumatic displacement. Ophthalmology. 1999;106:1900–1907.

9. Vitravene Injection (fomivirsen sodium intravitreal injection). Approval letter, pages 1–4. Vol. 2004. U.S. Food and Drug Administration web site. Available at: http://www.fda.gov/cder/foi/nda/98/20961_Vitravene_Approve.pdf

10. The Eyetech Study Group. Preclinical and phase 1A clinical evaluation of an anti-VEGF pegylated aptamer (EYE001) for the treatment of exudative age-related macular degeneration. Retina. 2002;22:143–152.

11. The Eyetech Study Group. Anti-vascular endothelial growth factor therapy for subfoveal choroidal neovascularization secondary to age-related macular degeneration: phase II study results. Ophthalmology. 2003;110:979–986.

12. Gragoudas ES. Pegaptanib for neovascular age related macular degeneration, for the VEGF Inhibition Study in Ocular Neovascularization Clinical Trial Group. N Engl J Med. 2004;351:2805–2816.

13. Kuppermann B, Thomas E, Smet M, et al. the Vitrase for Vitreous Hemorrhage Study Groups. Safety results of the two phase III trials of an Intravitreous Injection of highly purified Ovine Hyaluronidase (Vitrase) for the Management of Vitreous Hemorrhage. Am J Ophthalmol. 2005;140(4):585–597.

14. Coco RM, Lopez MI, Pastor JC, et al. Pharmacokinetics of intravitreal vancomycin in normal and infected rabbit eyes. J Ocul Pharmacol Ther. 1998;14:555–563.

15. Wingard LB Jr, Zuravleff JJ, Doft BH, et al. Intraocular distribution of intravitreally administered amphotericin B in normal and vitrectomized eyes. Invest Ophthalmol Vis Sci. 1989;30:2184–2189.

16. Stay MS, Xu J, Randolph TW, et al. Computer simulation and diffusive transport of controlled-release drugs in the vitreous humor. Pharm Res. 2003;20:96–102.

17. Scholes GN, O'Brien WJ, Abrams GW, et al. Clearance of triamcinolone from vitreous. Arch Ophthalmol. 1985;103:1567–1569.

18. Jonas JB. Concentration of intravitreally injected triamcinolone acetonide in aqueous humour. Br J Ophthalmol. 2002;86:1066.

19. Beer PM, Bakri SJ, Singh RJ, et al. Intraocular concentration and pharmacokinetics of triamcinolone acetonide after a single intravitreal injection. Ophthalmology. 2003;110:681–686.

20. Cochereau-Massin I, Lehoang P, Lautier-Frau M, et al. Efficacy and tolerance of intravitreal ganciclovir in cytomegalovirus retinitis in acquired immune deficiency syndrome. Ophthalmology. 1991;98:1348–1355.

21. Rahhal FM, Arevalo JF, Munguia D, et al. Intravitreal cidofovir for the maintenance treatment of cytomegalovirus retinitis. Ophthalmology. 1996;103:1078–1083.

22. Taskintuna I, Rahhal FM, Arevalo JF, et al. Low-dose intravitreal cidofovir (HPMPC) therapy of cytomegalovirus retinitis in patients with acquired immune deficiency syndrome. Ophthalmology. 1997;104:1049–1057.

23. Jager RD, Aiello LP, Patel SC, et al. Risks of intravitreous injection: a comprehensive review. Retina. 2004;5:676–698.

24. Diabetic Retinopathy Clinical Research Network. A randomized trial comparing intravitreal triamcinolone acetonide and focal-grid photocoagulation for diabetic macular edema. Ophthalmology. 2008;115:1447–1449.

25. Ip MS, Scott IU, VanVeldhuisen PC, et al. A randomized trial comparing the efficacy and safety of intravitreal triamcinolone with observation to treat vision loss associated with macular edema secondary to central retinal vein occlusion: the Standard Care vs Corticosteroid for Retinal Vein Occlusion (SCORE) study report 5. Arch Ophthalmol. 2009;127:1101–1114.

26. Scott IU, Ip MS, VanVeldhuisen PC, et al. A randomized trial comparing the efficacy and safety of intravitreal triamcinolone with standard care to treat vision loss associated with macular edema secondary to branch retinal vein occlusion: the Standard Care vs Corticosteroid for Retinal Vein Occlusion (SCORE) study report 6. Arch Ophthalmol. 2009;127:1115–1128.

27. Singerman LJ, Masonson H, Patel M, et al. Pegaptanib sodium for neovascular age-related macular degeneration: third-year safety results of the VEGF inhibition Study in Ocular Neovascularization (VISION) trial. Br J Ophthalmol. 2008;92:1606–1611.

28. Wu L, Martinez-Castellanos MA, Quiroz-Mercado H, et al. Twelve-month safety of intravitreal injections of bevacizumab (Avastin): results of the Pan-American Collaborative Retina Study Group (PACORES). Graefes Arch Clin Exp Ophthalmol. 2008;246:81–87.

29. Konstantopoulos A, Williams CP, Newson RS, et al. Ocular morbidity associated with intravitreal triamcinolone acetonide. Eye (Lond). 2007;21:317–320.

30. Khairallah M, Zeghidi H, Ladjimi A, et al. Primary intravitreal triamcinolone acetonide for diabetic massive macular hard exudates. Retina. 2005;25:835–839.

31. Ozkiris A, Erkilic K. Complications of intravitreal injection of triamcinolone acetonide. Can J Ophthalmol. 2005;40:63–68.

32. Nelson ML, Tennant MT, Sivalingam A, et al. Infectious and presumed non infectious endophthalmitis after intravitreal triamcinolone acetonide injection. Retina. 2003;23:686–691.

33. Hattenbach LO, Klais C, Koch FH, et al. Intravitreous injection of tissue plasminogen activator and gas in the treatment of submacular hemorrhage under various conditions. Ophthalmology. 2001;108:1485–1492.

34. Brown DM, Kaiser PK, Michels M, et al. Ranibizumab versus verteporfin for neovascular age-related macular degeneration. N Engl J Med. 2006;355:1432–1444.

35. Brown DM, Kaiser PK, Michels M, et al. Ranibizumab versus verteporfin photodynamic therapy for neovascular age-related macular degeneration. Two-year results of the ANCHOR study. Ophthalmology. 2009;116:57–65.e5.

36. Rosenfeld PJ, Brown DM, Heier JS, et al. MARINA Study Group. Ranibizumab for neovascular age-related macular degeneration. N Engl J Med. 2006;355:1419–1431.

37. Roth DB, Chieh J, Spirn MJ, et al. Non infectious endophthalmitis after intravitreal triamcinolone injection. Arch Ophthalmol. 2003;121:1279–1282.

38. Jonish J, Lai JC, Deramo VA, et al. Increased incidence of sterile endophthalmitis following intravitreal preserved triamcinolone acetonide. Br J Ophthalmol. 2008;92:1501–1054.

39. Robinson MR, Reed G, Csaky KG, et al. Immune-recovery uveitis in patients with cytomegalovirus retinitis taking highly active antiretroviral therapy. Am J Ophthalmol. 2000;130:49–56.

40. Cunnigham ET Jr. Uveitis in HIV positive patients (editorial). Br J Ophthalmol. 2000;84:233–235.

41. Gillies MC, Simpson JM, Bilson FA, et al. Safety of an intravitreal injection of triamcinolone: results from a randomized clinical trial. Arch Ophthalmol. 2004;122:336–340.

42. Mason J, Frederick P, Neimkin M, et al. Incidence of hemorrhagic complications after intravitreal bevacizumab (avastin) or ranibizumab (lucentis) injections on systemically anticoagulated patients. Retina. 2010;30:1386–1389.

43. Smith JR, Rosenbaum JT, Wilson DJ, et al. Role of intravitreal methotrexate in the management of primary central nervous system lymphoma with ocular involvement. Ophthalmology. 2002;109:1709–1716.

44. Avitabile T, Longo A, Reibaldi A. Intravitreal triamcinolone compared with macular laser grid photocoagulation for the treatment of cystoids macular edema. Am J Ophthalmol. 2005;140:695–702.

45. Gillies MC, Kuzniarz M, Craig J, et al. Intravitreal triamcinolone-induced elevated intraocular pressure is associated with the development of posterior subcapsular cataract. Ophthalmology. 2005;112:139–143.

46. Diabetic Retinopathy Clinical Research Network. Three-Year Follow-up of a randomized trial comparing Focal/Grid Photocoagulation and intravitreal triamcinolone for diabetic macular edema. Arch Ophthalmol. 2009;127(3):245–251.

47. Campbell RJ, Bell CM, Paterson MP, et al. Stroke rates after introduction of vascular endothelial growth factor inhibitors for macular degeneration: a time series analysis. Ophthalmology. 2012;119:1604–1608.

48. Martin DF, Maguire MG, Fine SL, et al. Ranibizumab and Bevacizumab for treatment of neovascular age-related macular degeneration, two years results. Ophthalmology. 2012;119:1388–1398.

49. Kraushar MF, Nussbaum P, Kisch AL. Anaphylactic reaction to intravitreal cefazolin. Retina. 1994;14:187–188.

50. Aiello LP, Brucker AJ, Chang S, et al. Evolving guidelines for intravitreous injections. Retina. 2004;24:S3–S19.

51. Schimel AM, Scott IU, Flynn HW. Endophthalmitis after intravitreal injections: Should the use of face masks be the standard of care? Arch Ophthalmol. 2011;129(12):1607–1609. doi:10.1001/archophthalmol.2011.370.

52. Sebag J, Tang M. Pneumatic retinopexy using only air. Retina. 1993;13:8–12.

53. Kramar M, Vu L, Whitson JT, et al. The effect of intravitreal triamcinolone on intraocular pressure. Curr Med Res Opin. 2007;23:1253–1258.

54. Androudi S, Leiko E, Meniconi M, et al. Safety and efficacy of intravitreal triamcinolone acetonide for uveitic macular edema. Ocul Immunol Inflamm. 2005;13:205–212.

24

INTRODUCTION TO GENE THERAPY AND RELATED TECHNIQUES FOR RETINAL DISORDERS AND AGE-RELATED MACULAR DEGENERATION

HENRY ALEXANDER LEDER • KEISUKE MORI • PETER L. GEHLBACH

◼ INTRODUCTION

Gene therapy is the introduction of exogenous nucleic acids into a host's cells with subsequent expression for the treatment of disease. Gene therapy can be thought of as a pharmacologic method by which nucleic acids and ultimately bioactive proteins become the therapeutic agents delivered to the target tissues. Among the therapeutic benefits arising from gene transfer are gene repair, gene activation or inactivation, and the expression of proteins that are therapeutic to the disease state. Gene expression cassettes are designed for the production of therapeutic proteins, noncoding RNAs, or the constituents of other novel treatment strategies. Many of these strategies are currently in the basic or preclinical stages of development. Gene expression cassettes can be transferred into target cells by a variety of methods, one of the most frequent being viral transfection. Once the expression cassette is introduced into the target tissue, the foreign DNA is expressed by the host cell. Bioactive products that result may be therapeutic to the host cell or in the case of secreted proteins may be therapeutic to adjacent cells or distant diseased tissues.

Gene therapy had received much of its early theoretical support by the early 1970s (before the recombinant DNA era) from knowledge of the mechanisms of cell transformation by tumor viruses. Classes of DNA and RNA tumor viruses have evolved that carry out precisely those functions crucial to gene therapy, that is, the heritable and stable introduction of functional new genetic information into mammalian cells. Thus, it was proposed that such viruses or other like agents, deprived of their own deleterious functions, could be used as vehicles to introduce normal and functional genes into human cells to correct cellular defects and cure genetic diseases (1).

The first human gene therapy trial was begun in September 1990 and involved transfer of the adenosine deaminase (ADA) gene into lymphocytes of a patient having an otherwise lethal defect in this enzyme; the disease produces immune deficiency. The results of this initial trial were encouraging and have helped to stimulate further clinical trials (2).

It is essential to know the precise structure, function, and regulation of a target gene for successful gene therapy. General steps for gene therapy include the following: First, identifying the defective gene and isolating a normal counterpart. Second, the normal gene must be inserted into a cell where it must function properly. This may require integration into the host cell chromosome or deletion of the defective gene. An isolated, cloned gene can either be directly injected into a cell or be packaged into a vector by recombinant DNA techniques and then introduced. Once in the cell, it may become integrated into the nuclear DNA or remain free in the cytoplasm as a self-replicating, extrachromosomal element (3). Finally, the transferred DNA must be expressed by the host cells, resulting in a bioactive product. Some gene therapy techniques require cell mitosis for efficient incorporation of the therapeutic gene into the host chromosome. Retroviral vectors (e.g., lentivirus, a modified HIV vector) have a demonstrated ability to transfect postmitotic adult retinal neurons.

A number of ocular diseases are amenable to gene therapy approaches, and the eye has characteristics that are potentially advantageous to these strategies. In brief, the eye is a small compartment and is relatively isolated by virtue of its ocular coats and a blood–ocular barrier. Therefore, intraocular injection of a small amount of vector results in transduction of a relatively large proportion of susceptible ocular cells and relatively little entry into cells outside of the eye. This makes it possible to minimize systemic side effects.

An important application of gene transfer techniques is in the replacement of mutated genes that code for proteins needed for the normal functioning of ocular cells. In the case of defective photoreceptors or retinal pigment epithelial cells, gene transfer provides a way to replace the defective gene product and potentially treat various retinal degenerations (4–6). This type of gene therapy holds great promise for the treatment of inherited disorders causing blindness such as retinitis pigmentosa and Leber congenital amaurosis (LCA) and may someday play a role in treating the genetic aspects of age-related macular degeneration (AMD) (7).

An alternative gene transfer strategy is to transduce cells within the eye in order produce therapeutic proteins that do not replace specific defective proteins. Rather, the overexpressed protein may serve as a survival factor that rescues or protects, for example, photoreceptor cells from a variety of neurodegenerative processes that might result in retinal degeneration. Alternatively, the expression of an antiangiogenic factor might be expected to broadly inhibit a number of diseases via inhibition of angiogenesis as a final common pathway for a number of ocular diseases. Pigment epithelium–derived factor (PEDF) is an example of a molecule that has been shown to be of protective value

in preclinical evaluation using a number of animal models of angiogenesis and neurodegeneration, following ocular transduction with viral vectors (8–12). Both adenovirus-vectored PEDF and a lentivirus-vectored somatostatin have been in phase I clinical evaluation.

THE RETINA AS A GENE TRANSFER TARGET

Retinogenesis is a developmental process that is tightly regulated both temporally and spatially and is therefore an excellent model for studying the molecular and cellular mechanisms of neurogenesis in the central nervous system (13).

The retina has unique properties that make it particularly amenable for gene transfer. It is a thin laminar structure that is accessible by multiple routes; consequently, different areas of the eye and various cell types are accessible to therapeutic intervention. Fortuitously, the fact that the eye is small and enclosed limits the dose of vector necessary to achieve a local therapeutic effect. There are physical barriers to the retina, such as the blood–retinal barrier, that further protect from widespread dissemination of the vector into the systemic circulation. The subretinal space is separated from its choroidal blood supply by the retinal pigment epithelium (RPE) and its intercellular junctions and is protected from the interior of the eye by the internal limiting membrane and the retina itself. These barriers provide a beneficial effect in protecting the retina from the immune response by sequestering antigens from the systemic circulation but also can make access to subretinal space more challenging. The eye as a treatment target possesses experimental advantages for viral vector delivery; for example, due to the size of the globe, one can reasonably extrapolate a treatment dose from an animal experiment to a human study. This extrapolation is more reliable than for other organ systems. In addition, there are a number of sophisticated means to evaluate retinal therapeutic efficacy over time. Retinal function can be monitored with noninvasive and quantitative tests that include but are not limited to ophthalmoscopy, electroretinography, optical coherence tomography, the measurement of afferent pupillary responses, and visual evoked potentials. Finally, a number of genes responsible for retinal disease have been identified, and a number of animal models of retinal disease exist and continue to improve and new models based on increasing understanding of disease continue to evolve (14).

RETINAL DEGENERATION

Retinal diseases amenable to gene therapy are often characterized by neuronal degeneration such as retinitis pigmentosa or Stargardt's disease or by complications of disease such as ocular neovascularization in AMD and other retinal diseases. A significant advance has been the discovery of the ABCR (retina-specific, ATP-binding cassette transporter) gene and its mutation in autosomal recessive Stargardt's macular dystrophy and fundus flavimaculatus (15). The ABCR gene is expressed in rods; its gene product, rim protein, is thought to function in the recycling of rod outer segment components between the RPE and the retina (1). Carriers of heterozygous gene defects may be at increased risk for AMD; several ABCR gene mutations have been identified in some populations of patients with AMD. In addition, mutations in TIMP3 lead to Sorsby's fundus dystrophy, a retinal disease that exhibits characteristics of AMD, including thickened Bruch's membrane, high risk for neovascularization, and photoreceptor degeneration (16).

DOMINANT AND RECESSIVE RETINAL DEGENERATIONS

Retinal diseases may have multifactorial causes. Inherited retinal degenerations may be sporadic, dominant, recessive, X-linked, or maternal (mitochondrial). In addition, they differ in onset, function of the gene product, pattern and level of gene expression, region of the retina affected, primary and secondary cells involved, and clinical manifestations. Ideally, it would be beneficial to develop a therapy that would permanently correct the defect at the genomic level. To date, researchers have largely focused on a gene replacement approach for recessive mutations and a gene inactivation approach for dominant mutations (14).

Recessively inherited retinal degenerations represent a group of retinal abnormalities whose phenotype is due to the lack of function of a gene; in other words, they are characterized by the inability to produce a functional gene product. The absence of the normal gene product, such as a structural protein of the outer segment or an enzyme in the phototransduction cascade, results in expression of the mutant phenotype. The principle of gene therapy in recessive degeneration is to "cure" the disease by replacing the missing gene with a wild-type copy in each photoreceptor. The goal of photoreceptor rescue requires efficient transduction of most of the photoreceptor cells because, in theory, any cell expressing a wild-type gene will survive. Ali et al. (17) reported the first successful rescue in rds null mice. These animals fail to form outer segments, develop an early loss of retinal function, and their degeneration is characterized by progressive photoreceptor cell death. Following adeno-associated vector delivery of peripherin/RDS, functional and morphologic studies revealed that there was outer segment restoration and proper disc formation. Somatic therapies aimed at enhancing survival using growth factors, and antiapoptosis genes have also been shown to improve photoreceptor cell survival in recessive degenerations but are not curative.

On the other hand, autosomal dominant retinal degenerations are characterized by the production of abnormal protein in photoreceptor cells. The abnormal, mutant form of the protein is, in some way, toxic to the retina and causes progressive retinal degeneration, with the final common pathway being apoptotic cell death. For this reason, gene therapy for dominant disease is focused on inhibiting the translation of the mutant protein, for example, by direct cleavage of the mutant messenger RNA (mRNA) transcript.

Several animal models of dominant retinal diseases have been generated. These transgenic animals carry one copy of a mutated gene that encodes a misfolded or mislocalized protein. The expression of these proteins in photoreceptors results in toxicity, which leads to cell death through an apoptotic mechanism. Therefore, it is strategic to eliminate or correct the mutated gene in order to restore function. The former has been successfully achieved with ribozymes in the P23H transgenic rat. Ribozymes are RNA-cleaving RNA molecules that specifically remove defective mRNAs or replace them with the correct sequence. The ribozymes were designed to target the mutant P23H transcript and be placed into an adeno-associated vector, under the regulation of a rhodopsin promoter. The treatment resulted in morphologic and functional rescue (14).

In general, retinal degenerations are variable entities varying from early to late onset and with rapid to slowly progressive courses. Slowly progressive variants may have a much wider therapeutic window than those with an earlier onset, such as Leber's congenital amaurosis. In the former case, it is critical to use a delivery vehicle that allows for expression over extended periods of time, understanding that an eventual readministration could be necessary. It remains to be understood how best to optimize these treatments once begun. Consequently, it will be necessary to fully determine the mechanisms by which these molecules exert their protective function as well as the best routes of administration (e.g., subretinal or intravitreal) and the therapeutic/toxic dose ratio and therefore a great deal of work is ongoing.

TYPES OF POTENTIAL HUMAN GENETIC INTERVENTION

For the sake of discussion of human genetic intervention, four general categories of procedures have been outlined in accordance with their goal and target cells (18).

Somatic gene therapy: As applied to the treatment or prevention of disease, this type of intervention involves the correction of genetic defects in any of the body's cells, with the exception of the germ or reproductive cells. Given the recent developments in the field of somatic gene therapy, it is appropriate to broaden the definition to include genes that can be introduced into cells to provide a new function. One example of such an approach involves the insertion of a cytokine gene, such as interleukin-2 or tumor necrosis factor, into a patient's malignant cells to produce an immune response against the tumor. Depending on the location and orientation of the recombination targets, the recombination result could be the integration, excision, inversion, or translocation of the nuclear DNA (13).

Germinal gene therapy: This genetic intervention involves the correction or prevention of genetic deficiencies through the transfer of properly functioning genes into reproductive cells. To achieve the desired results from this approach, it may be necessary to replace or suppress the faulty gene rather than simply add a new gene. In germ-line alteration, gene addition would be unsatisfactory because it is not yet possible to predict the effects of a mixture of the normal gene and the mutated gene with respect to regulatory signals necessary for normal growth and development. Germ-line genetic modification could be effected either before fertilization or in the early postfertilization stages of embryogenic development.

Somatic cell or germ-line gene modifications may also be considered in order to affect selected physical and mental characteristics, with the aim of influencing such features as physical appearance or physical abilities. A principal difference in these uses of genetic modification is that they could be directed toward healthy people who have no evidence of genetic deficiency disease. Further, germ-line genetic intervention, if successful, could allow the enhancement to be passed on to succeeding generations.

STRATEGIES IN GENE THERAPY

Three general approaches are currently utilized:

1. Ex vivo: A procedure in which the new gene is transferred to cells in the laboratory and the modified cells are then administered to the recipient. This technique overcomes the problem of intraocular cell targeting. This cell therapy approach has several potential advantages. First, it improves the efficiency of transduction, selection, and cloning of transduced cells, which are more easily accomplished in vitro. Second, this approach permits assessment of safety profiles of modified cells prior to medical application. The main disadvantages of ex vivo transduction is that certain cells, such as photoreceptors, cannot yet be removed and surgically reintroduced into the retina.
2. In vivo: This gene transfer generally relies on a vector to introduce a therapeutic gene into the target cell. The vector is generally delivered remote from the target cell; for instance, the vector is delivered intravitreously, and the target cells may be the photoreceptors in the retina.
3. In situ: The gene or the vectors are delivered in the vicinity of the target cells.

In these strategies, the transfer process is usually aided by a vector that helps deliver the gene to the intracellular site where it can function appropriately (19).

The choice of an ex vivo, in vivo, or in situ strategy and of the vector used to carry the gene is dictated by the clinical target.

Gene Replacement, Correction, or Augmentation

One form of gene therapy would involve specific removal of the mutant gene sequence and its replacement with normal, functional genomic material. An ideal approach, gene correction, would entail specific correction of a mutant gene sequence without any additional changes in the target genome (1). An alternative strategy is gene augmentation, which is modifying the content or expression of mutant genes in defective cells by introducing a foreign normal genetic sequence. During the past decade, a number of efficient methods have been developed to introduce functional new genes into mammalian cells. In many cases, it is possible to restore a genetic function by the addition of nontargeted but functional genetic information into nonspecific sites of the genome without the removal or correction of a resident, nonfunctional mutant gene. During the creation of animal models for human genetic disease, inactivation of the target gene, so-called *gene knockout*, has been shown to be a successful methodology.

GENE THERAPY TECHNIQUES

There are a number of advantages to utilizing a gene transfer approach to therapy. One advantage is that the protein of interest may be continuously expressed over an extended duration, following a single injection of vector. The duration of protein expression varies depending on a number of factors including the type of vector used. In general, however, the duration of increased protein expression greatly exceeds the period of elevated protein levels that are achieved by a single injection of purified protein.

Currently, a number of viral vector platforms are in development and are being evaluated for potential use in ocular gene therapy. Of these, adenovirus, adeno-associated virus (AAV), retrovirus, and lentivirus are being intensively investigated by a number of laboratories around the world. Each vector is characterized by a unique biology as well as a unique set of advantages and disadvantages that relate to their potential utility as gene therapy vectors. A full discussion of each vector is beyond the scope of this chapter, but it is evident that with greater understanding and continued technologic innovation, each continues to evolve as a potential therapeutic strategy in the eye.

■ VIRAL VECTORS

Adenovirus Vectors

Adenoviruses are nonenveloped, double-stranded DNA viruses that infect a broad range of human and nonhuman cell types by binding to specific cell surface receptors. By a process of endocytosis, the virus gains access inside the target cell, then the virus binds to the nuclear envelope, and enters the nuclear space. The virus is not incorporated into the host genome but remains as a transcriptionally active episome within the nucleus. Concerns about the infectious nature of adenoviral vectors have led to the development of replication-deficient (helper-dependent) adenoviruses for gene transfer. Deletion of the replication-specific genes and nonessential DNA sequences from these viral vectors prevents viral replication. Adenoviral vectors can infect both dividing and nondividing cells, which makes them particularly useful to transfer genes to postmitotic cells. Adenoviruses have been effective in transducing retinal photoreceptors, ganglion cells, Müller cells, and RPE cells but do have some inherent limitations with respect to potential clinical application in the eye. For instance, peak transgene expression is typically limited to a few weeks as there is no integration into the host DNA. The broad range of target cells is a potential disadvantage if only one cell layer or cell type is targeted. Adenoviral transduction can also induce inflammatory responses and a significant immune response to viral proteins in the host. This may in turn limit the duration of gene expression and also expose transduced cells to immunologic responses. Modified adenoviral vectors may improve the duration of gene expression by reducing the number of viral proteins presented to the host immune system (20).

Several advantageous properties of adenovirus vectors have increased their potential utility as gene therapy vectors in recent years. Pioneering "proof of principle" work in retinal gene transfer has been conducted with adenoviral vectors (4,5). Among the advantages of this vector platform are the relative ease of production and purification, resulting in purification of high titers in large quantities; their ability to accept a large cloning capacity; an ability to transduce a variety of noncycling cells; the potential for high expression levels and comparatively rapid transgene expression. The use of adenoviral vector is, however, potentially complicated by significant inflammation as well as a shorter duration of expression than other available vectors (21–25). Inflammation and immune responses induced by adenovirus vectors may result in destruction of transduced cells. Vector modifications to reduce the immunogenicity of this vector, such as deletion of the E1A, E1B, E3, E4 virus genes, or the use of helper-dependent adenoviral vectors that are deleted in all viral protein–coding sequences (26–30) results in less cytotoxicity and potentially longer duration of transgene expression.

Despite some limitations, the adenoviral DNA vectors have been shown to be effective. They are easy to apply experimentally in vitro and in vivo, and they may be particularly useful for gene therapy in which transgene expression of limited duration is sufficient to achieve the desired clinical effect (31). In addition, clinical grade second-generation Ad vectors have been shown to be well tolerated in human eyes (32).

Adeno-Associated Virus Vectors

The potential for gene delivery to the eye using AAV vectors has received much attention. AAV is a member of the Parvovirinae subfamily of Parvoviridae. It is nonenveloped, with icosahedral symmetry and a diameter of 18 to 26 nm. It was originally isolated as a contaminant of adenoviral cultures and thus given the name AAV. This human nonpathogenic virus is replication defective in the absence of a *helper virus*. AAV is packaged as a 4.7 kb single-stranded DNA molecule. In the absence of a helper virus or helper function, the AAV genome integrates in the host cell genome entering the latent phase of its cycle (14).

Different AAV serotypes have different virion shell proteins and, as a consequence, vary in their ability to bind to and transfect different host cell types. To date, eight different AAV serotypes have been isolated, and possibly many more may be harbored in the genome of different mammalian tissues. The most divergent AAV sequence belongs to serotype 5, which was isolated from a condylomatous lesion. AAV 7 and 8 sequences were isolated from rhesus monkey tissues. All others to date have been isolated as contaminants of adenoviral cultures (14).

AAVs have a number of important advantages over other vectors that make them suitable for ocular studies; in particular, a relative lack of pathogenicity and their ability to induce long-term transgene expression in the eye. AAV vectors can be used to transfect a variety of ocular cell types including photoreceptors, RPE cells, Müller cells, retinal ganglion cells, trabecular meshwork cells, and corneal endothelial cells.

AAV vectors and lentivirus vectors each induce little immune response and mediate long-term expression (33,34). AAV vectors are promising because they are not considered pathogenic in humans and because transduction of a wide variety of postmitotic cells, including muscle cells and certain neuronal cells, is possible. The duration of AAV-mediated expression of proteins in the human eye is not yet fully defined and varies depending on a variety of factors some of which are known and some of which are still not well understood. In rodents, there is evidence that in some settings, expression can occur for the entire life of the animal. Although such extended periods of expression are theoretically advantageous in the setting of chronic disease, the effects of excessive and prolonged expression of various transgenes in retinal cells remains largely unknown. By way of example, it is known that increased expression of wild-type rhodopsin or peripherin/rds can result in degeneration of photoreceptors (35,36). A brief profile of the advantages of AAV as a vector platform for ocular gene therapy reveals significant advantages including highly efficient transduction of some retinal cells, stable transduction of a variety of cell types, including neurons, and the potential for prolonged duration of expression. Some of the potential benefits and risks of each of the highlighted vector platforms are shown in Table 24.1.

At present, there are two general approaches by which therapeutic AAV-mediated gene transfer might be useful in the context of ocular disease. First, AAV-mediated gene therapy has the potential to correct the specific gene defect in conditions where the defect is well understood. Correction of an ocular genetic defect requires gene delivery to the defective cells and has been successfully used to slow photoreceptor loss in several rodent models of primary photoreceptor diseases. Nevertheless, there are many ocular conditions where no specific genetic defect has been characterized. It is likely that many of these diseases will turn out to involve pathology more complex than a well-characterized mutation in a single gene. In such circumstances, a second strategy for gene therapy may be useful. This involves using gene transfer to reduce loss of function by ameliorating the effect of the primary defect. For instance, AAV-mediated transfection of retinal cells with the gene for basic fibroblast growth factor-2 (FGF-2), glial cell line–derived neurotrophic factor, and ciliary neurotrophic factor have been demonstrated to slow photoreceptor loss in rat models of retinitis pigmentosa (37).

Transduction of RPE cells and photoreceptors is most efficiently achieved by subretinal injection of AAV. The subretinal space has a relatively high degree of immune privilege, and typically, very little evidence of inflammation is seen in the vicinity of the injection site. Subretinal injection induces a bleb of concentrated virus in intimate contact with photoreceptors and RPE cells. On the other hand, intravitreal injection can be used to transfect Müller cells and retina ganglions cells (38). The barrier and binding qualities of the internal limiting barrier, however, appear to limit easy access to the subretinal space, from the vitreous, for rAAV. In theory, the potential for a host immune response to AAV is greater following intravitreal injection, and the possibility exists of an AAV-specific systematic antibody response.

Several developmental processes, including mitosis, migration, differentiation, cell death, and synaptic formation, may affect the cellular uptake of the virus vector, the distribution of the particles, and the persistence of transgene expression. On the other hand, the time of virus administration profoundly affects the tropism, efficiency, and distribution of the transgene (14).

One of the major limitations of AAV as a useful therapeutic vector is the relatively small amount of passenger DNA that can be incorporated. Although genes up to 6.0 kb have been packaged into AAV, these overstuffed viruses were not active. The usual packaging limit for AAV appears to be 5.1 to 5.3 kb. Nevertheless, by exploiting the intermolecular rearrangement, it is possible to overcome this problem. By way of example, genes larger than 4.7 kb can be split between two different AAV vectors.

Beltran et al. (39) reported the use of AAV-2/5–vectored human RPGR with human IRBP or GRK1 promoters in a canine model of X-linked retinitis pigmentosa cased by a GTPase regulator (RPGR) gene, which encodes a photoreceptor ciliary protein. They were able to show with in vivo imaging, preserved photoreceptor nuclei, and inner/outer segments that were limited to treated areas. Both rod and cone photoreceptor function were greater in treated (three of four) than in control eyes. Histopathology indicated normal photoreceptor structure and reversal of opsin mislocalization in treated areas expressing human RPGR protein in rods and cones. Postreceptoral remodeling was also

Table 24.1	VIRAL VECTORS			
	Retrovirus	**Adenovirus**	**Adeno-associated virus**	**Lentivirus**
Nucleic acid	RNA	DNA	DNA	RNA
Pathogenicity	+	+	−	+
Cytotoxicity	−	+	−	−
Transduction in nondividing cells	−	+	+	+
Integration into the host chromosome	+	−	+(±)	+
Transduction efficiency	Low	Extremely high	Moderate	High
Expression level	Low	Strong	Moderate	Moderate
Duration of expression	Long (months to years)	Short (weeks to months)	Long (months to years)	Long (months to years)

corrected: there was reversal of bipolar cell dendrite retraction evident with bipolar cell markers and preservation of outer plexiform layer thickness. At this time, no clinical trials have begun.

Herpes Simplex Virus Vectors

The herpes simplex virus (HSV) is a DNA virus that has natural tropism for neurons. Thus, it may be useful in applying gene therapy to diseases of the nervous system, including the retina. HSV can infect nonneuronal tissue as well and does not require cell division to integrate into the host genome. Gene transfer using HSV utilizes either replication-defective mutants or multiple deletion mutants that have a limited capacity for replication, but they may be able to deliver genes locally within tissue with a limited infection. The ability of HSV to exist in a latent state likely makes this vector efficacious in producing stable transgene expression within host neurons. Moreover, the HSV viral genome is large and has the capacity to carry more than 30 kb of foreign DNA, significantly more than other vectors.

The HSV thymidine kinase gene (HSV-tk) has been used extensively in suicide gene therapy studies. The viral thymidine kinase has a markedly higher affinity for the prodrug ganciclovir than does the cellular thymidine kinase. Ganciclovir is converted to a cytotoxic metabolite with significantly higher efficiency by HSV-tk–transduced cells, and thus preferentially kills the transduced cell (31).

RNA Virus Vectors

Retroviruses are a family of RNA viruses that can infect cells and integrate into the genome of the host cell. RNA viruses are surrounded by a lipid envelope. Upon entry into the target cell, the RNA is released and reverse transcribed into double-stranded DNA that is stably integrated into the host DNA. Transgenes delivered by retroviruses demonstrate long-term stable gene expression and may be vertically transferred to daughter cells. Most retroviral vectors cannot enter the nucleus directly; they require cell division to infect the host cell following breakdown of the nuclear envelope.

To date, retroviral vectors are the most frequently employed platform in human clinical trials. The retrovirus vector transduces primarily proliferating cells of rodent and human origin that express the cellular receptor Ram-1 (40,41). They have been used as effective gene delivery tools in cells from the liver, retina, skeletal muscle, and the central nervous system. Retrovirus does not, however, transduce nondividing cells with an efficiency that translates into clinical utility at this time. Therefore, most retroviral vectors have limited application for targeting neural retinal cells or other ocular cells, which are largely postmitotic, in the postnatal period.

Lentiviruses are a subclass of retroviruses that includes the HIV family. Like all retroviruses, lentiviruses integrate a DNA copy into the host genome, but they encode proteins that allow them to form a complex with the nuclear envelope and to transit the pores of an intact nuclear membrane. Thus, lentiviruses can infect dividing and nondividing cells.

The ability of lentiviruses to integrate into nondividing cells relies on nuclear localization signals present in the preintegration complex that allow its entry into the nucleus without the need for nuclear membrane fragmentation. Transgenes integrate into the host genome, but viral genes do not; thus, there is less risk of generating recombinant retrovirus. Despite modifications to render the virus replication incompetent, there is appropriate concern about the clinical use of such vectors because of the theoretical possibility of generating a wild-type HIV virus during production or from viral recombination in the host (31). Bovine immunodeficiency virus (BIV) is a lentivirus that is not known to cause human disease. Subretinal injection of a BIV.*GFP* vector has been shown to produce a quick and prolonged transduction of RPE cells without an evident inflammatory response (42).

Table 24.1 summarizes the characteristics of gene transfer with viral vectors.

VIRAL VECTOR DELIVERY

Intravenous Vector Delivery

At the time of this writing, intravenous delivery of gene therapy vectors remains synonymous with systemic gene therapy. It is conceivable that advances in vector targeting, development of tissue-specific promoters, and further narrowing of vector tropism will lead to intravenous delivery of vectors that are highly specific for distant cell types, in the future. At this time, however, intravenous delivery is generally attended by systemic distribution of vector, transgene, and the products of transgene expression. The potential for both local and distant therapeutic effect as well as toxicity must be considered. Intravenous injection of adenoviral vectors expressing a transgene sequence coding for endostatin has been reported to inhibit systemic angiogenesis and tumor growth (43) as well as choroidal neovascularization (CNV) in a mouse model (8). Intravenous delivery of viral vector in the mouse has been previously described (8,43). Intravenous delivery of vector exposes the vascular endothelial cells of the retinal and choroidal vessels directly to the vector.

Intravitreous Vector Delivery

Intravitreous delivery of viral vectors exposes the cells that line the interior of the eye to vector. In mice, intravitreous injection is carried out on anesthetized animals under a dissecting microscope. The procedure has been described in detail elsewhere (5) (Fig. 24.1).

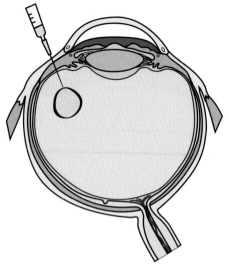

Figure 24.1 ■ Intravitreous injection in the mouse eye.

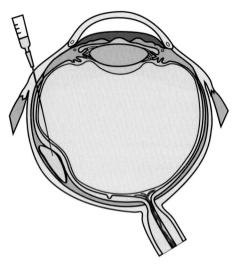

Figure 24.2 ■ Subretinal injection in the mouse eye. Following subretinal delivery, viral vectors have direct access to the subretinal space including photoreceptor outer segments and the RPE.

Following intravitreous delivery, viral vectors have direct access to the vitreous cavity and the cells that line the posterior and anterior ocular cavity.

In rats and larger animals, intravitreous delivery can be carried out in a manner analogous to intravitreous delivery in humans. Intravitreal injection is much more convenient in humans than it is in small animals. It is done routinely in the clinic, with only rare complications, chiefly, endophthalmitis and retinal detachment.

Subretinal Vector Delivery

Subretinal injection exposes both the photoreceptors and RPE directly to the vector. Various approaches to carrying out subretinal injection in mice have been described (4,8,44,45). Success has been achieved with a transscleral and transchoroidal approach (4,44,45), and with a transscleral and transvitreal approach as described by Mori et al. (8). The transscleral and transvitreal approach requires direct visualization of the retina and has been described elsewhere and is shown in Figure 24.2.

Periocular Injection of Vectors

Periocular gene transfer provides an alternative to intraocular vector delivery when the vectored transgene results in a secreted protein and the protein has properties that allow it to diffuse into the eye. In prior work, Gehlbach et al. (9) have shown that periocular vector delivery results in levels of pigment epithelium–derived growth factor or the secreted extracellular domain of vascular endothelial growth factor (VEGF) receptor 1 that are significantly elevated in the choroid and sufficient to inhibit choroidal neovascular membrane formation in mice. Periocular injection in mice has been described elsewhere and is depicted in Figure 24.3.

Ribozyme Therapy

Ribozymes are RNA-based enzymes that can cleave specific mRNA sequences. Mutation-specific cleavage of the transcript functionally silences the mutant allele by preventing synthesis of the abnormal protein from the transcript. The strategy used is to construct ribozymes that identify unique mutations or that permit binding to targeted, accessible sites in the mRNA transcript. Ribozyme therapy is effective in delaying retinal degeneration in animal models of dominant retinal degeneration, even after the degenerative process has begun.

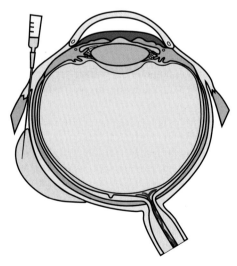

Figure 24.3 ■ Periocular injection in the mouse eye. Following periocular delivery, viral vectors have direct access to the subconjunctival space including episclera and conjunctiva. Access to orbital tissues including muscle, connective tissue, and lacrimal gland is also present.

Growth Factor Gene Therapy

Gene therapy using trophic growth factors is another approach to enhancing the survival of retinal photoreceptors in dominant retinal generation. For instance, the intravitreal injection of basic fibroblast growth factor (bFGF) delays retinal degeneration in some animal models (46).

Successful treatment with growth factors may also be achieved by genetically modifying cells ex vivo and then implanting them within the eye to act as a reservoir of trophic factors that bathe the retina by slow release into the vitreous.

Apoptosis has been implicated in retinal development and degeneration, but the specific apoptotic pathways are incompletely understood. Apoptosis is a process of programmed cell death without an ensuing inflammatory response. This neat packaging of cellular components allows for the precise removal of tissue during developmental remodeling, particularly in the retina. The retina develops from a single layer of undifferentiated ventricular neuroectoderm to a mature retina containing three cell layers of postmitotic, fully differentiated cells: the ganglion cell layer, the inner nuclear layer, and the outer nuclear layer. Extraneous cells unable to make functional neural connections are eliminated by apoptosis. Beyond this involvement in ocular development, apoptosis rarely occurs in a normal, healthy retina but has been implicated in both inherited and acquired retinal degenerations. The molecular pathogenesis of these retinal degenerations is still unclear, but apoptosis is the final common pathway in many retinal diseases, ranging from glaucoma to AMD, retinitis pigmentosa, and retinal detachment (47). Several proapoptotic and antiapoptotic genes have been identified. The use of growth factor gene therapy could help in rescue and/or prevent the apoptotic phenomenon in the target cells.

Antisense Gene Therapy

Antisense gene therapy is based on the use of synthetic, short DNA sequences that are designed to be complementary to a targeted mRNA molecule. This short DNA sequence is capable of forming a stable DNA–mRNA heteroduplex that prevents the translation of the associated protein from the transcript.

GENE THERAPY IN CLINICAL USE

Several retinal diseases have been proposed as targets for gene therapy. Retinal degenerations are particularly appealing since many have little or no conventional therapy, poor visual prognosis, and well-established genetic causes. In 2012, Jacobson et al. (48) reported on the 3-year results of a phase I/II clinical trial of the rAAV2-RPE65 vector injected subretinally for the treatment of LCA caused by RPE65 mutations. The study included 15 eyes from 15 patients 11 to 30 years old. The patients were broken into five cohorts that represented four dose levels and two different injection strategies. No systemic toxicity was reported, and ocular toxicity was related to surgical implantation. Visual improvement was seen in all patients but was modest. Improvement was also seen in the contralateral, control eyes, but this was statistically less than that of the experimental eyes. The study concluded that extrafoveal implantation is safer for these patients than foveal treatment. Additional studies are in progress to quantify the treatment benefit and long-term side effects.

GENE THERAPY AND AGE-RELATED MACULAR DEGENERATION

In wet AMD, a destabilization of the retinal and choroidal microenvironments leads to the formation of new blood vessels, which ultimately results in a decrease of visual acuity. Degenerative changes of the RPE and Bruch's membrane are the primary factors responsible for the disease. The pathophysiology of the disease is still incompletely understood. The putative role of specific genes in the degenerative process in AMD is less clear. Although certain genes may predispose some patients to develop AMD, the genetic linkage remains controversial and, to date, the genetics of AMD are emerging. Genetic susceptibility to AMD is probably multifactorial and thus will probably not be amenable to single gene therapy directed at the germinal line. In the absence of a well-defined genetic defect that gives rise to AMD, gene therapy will likely focus on somatic therapy using growth factors and antiapoptosis therapy to prolong the survival of the RPE and retinal photoreceptors, and these studies supported by the research community and commercial interests are under way.

Growth Factor Gene Therapy for AMD

There is experimental evidence that growth factors play an important role in maintaining the health of RPE cells and in enabling them to respond to injury. RPE cells express growth factors, and their receptors demonstrate the autocrine and paracrine functions of these substance. Theoretically, it may be possible to enhance RPE cell survival by somatic modulation of growth factor gene expression in patients with AMD. For instance, age-related phagocytic dysfunction and incomplete digestion of photoreceptor membranes by the RPE result in loss of RPE cells and in geographic atrophy, perhaps due in part, to the cytotoxicity of these deposits on the surrounding cells. Enhancing phagocytic activity in aging RPE cells using gene therapy is one potential approach to the treatment of AMD. bFGF has been shown to stimulate phagocytic activity and prolong retinal survival in animal models (31). An important number of other growth factors and secondary messengers of the intracellular signaling pathways have demonstrated protective effects on the retinal neurons in animal models of retinal degeneration. Gene transfer and expression of these growth factor proteins may similarly inhibit retinal degeneration by a neuroprotective effect in AMD (49).

The RPE synthesizes proteins that are antiangiogenic, such as tissue inhibitors of metalloproteinases and PEDF. Thus, potential gene therapy applications to CNV include antiangiogenic growth factor gene therapy, antisense or ribozyme therapy directed at angiogenic factors, and suicide gene therapy directed at neovascular tissue. Moreover, it was demonstrated that expression of angiostatin in experimental CNV significantly reduces the size of CNV lesions (50).

Transplantation of Genetically Modified Iris Pigment Epithelial Cells

Submacular transplantation of autologous iris pigment epithelial (IPE) cells has been proposed to replace the damaged RPE following surgical removal of the CNV (51). The IPE is anatomically contiguous with the RPE and has the same embryonic origin. In vitro, IPE cells share functional properties with the RPE cells, such as phagocytosis, degradation of rod outer segments, and synthesis of trophic factors. However, autologous transplantation of IPE cells alone has not yet resulted in a prolonged improvement of vision in patients with AMD, potentially because the lack of expression of one or several factors that are an important part of RPE function. Semkova et al. (51) have suggested a treatment for AMD based on transplantation of genetically modified autologous IPE cells. The most significant findings are summarized as follows: First, IPE cells were readily transduced with a high-capacity adenovirus (HC-ad) vector. Second, IPE cells secreted functionally active PEDF after HC-ad–mediated gene transfer. Third, subretinal transplantation of PEDF-expressing IPE cells inhibited neovascularization in models of retinal neoangiogenesis and prevented photoreceptor degeneration.

Antiangiogenic Gene Therapy for AMD

Ocular neovascularization is a central feature of AMD and diabetic retinopathy. CNV occurring in AMD commonly causes severe vision loss in elderly patients, and retinal neovascularization resulting from progression of diabetic retinopathy is still the most common cause of new blindness in the working-aged population (52,53). Anti-VEGF therapy has been a breakthrough therapy for ocular neovascular disease, including AMD. As discussed elsewhere, monthly intraocular injections of ranibizumab or bevacizumab have been shown to be highly effective in preserving and improving vision in neovascular AMD (54–56). Limitations of ranibizumab and bevacizumab therapy include frequent injections, risk of ocular complications (primarily endophthalmitis and retinal detachment), and a possible increased systemic risk of vaso-occlusive events. As such, a longer acting therapy, with fewer injections, may be desirable. In addition, not all patients respond fully to current anti-VEGF drugs and/or monthly peaks and troughs of therapy.

Characterization of the molecular and cellular events involved in angiogenesis has led to the identification of a number of angiostatic molecules with potential therapeutic value. Preclinical and clinical evaluation of each of these is required in order to determine potential therapeutic utility. Interferon-α2a causes dramatic involution of hemangiomas and inhibits iris neovascularization in a model of ischemic retinopathy (57,58). However, multicenter, randomized, placebo-controlled trial demonstrated that patients with CNV who received interferon-α2a do not have any involution of CNV and end up with worse vision than those treated with placebo.

VEGF is an endothelial cell mitogen that plays a central role in ocular angiogenesis (59–61). Inhibition of VEGF using anti-VEGF antibodies or soluble receptors can prevent the development of experimental iris or retinal neovascularization (62,63). VEGF kinase inhibitors, that block VEGF signaling, prevent the development of retinal and CNV (64). These are among the many indicators suggesting that anti-VEGF strategies play a role in treatment of CNV.

A novel method of posttranscriptional silencing of gene expression, called RNA interference (RNAi), was discovered (65). RNAi is a conserved cellular mechanism that silences the expression of a protein in a specific and potent fashion by utilizing double-strand RNA (dsRNA) molecules that target a particular mRNA. One dsRNA can destroy and inhibit transcriptional process of hundreds of targeted mRNA by activating the RNAi mechanism. This can result in the targeted silencing of thousands of protein molecules (66). Intravitreal injection of VEGF RNAi has been shown to inhibit the growth and vascular permeability of laser-induced CNV in a nonhuman primate, but the approach has not translated successfully into human application (67).

In addition to anti-VEGF strategies, other endogenous inhibitors of angiogenesis have been also described including angiostatin (67), endostatin (68,69), antithrombin III (70), and PEDF (71). Several lines of evidence indicate that these endogenous inhibitors are likely to be well tolerated in the eye and that they may have potential therapeutic value in the setting of pathologic ocular neovascularization. However, achieving therapeutic levels of drugs or proteins in the retina is complicated by the presence of a blood–retinal barrier. The systemic delivery of proteins to the retina is particularly problematic and at this time may alternatively require repeated intraocular injections. The patient risk and acceptance of this approach must be considered in this decision. Concern regarding toxicity associated with systemic delivery increases the appeal of local delivery approaches. Gene transfer offers novel means for local delivery of therapeutic proteins to intraocular tissues.

At this time, a variety of viral vectors are under intensive investigation and hold promise for clinical ocular gene therapy. Among those currently attracting attention are adenovirus, AAV, and lentivirus vectors. The choice of a vector depends on many factors that includes but is not limited to tropism of target cells, efficiency of transduction, size of the transgene, and needs regarding latency and duration of expression. Many endogenous, as well as synthetic, factors have been shown to possess potent antiangiogenic activity, including endostatin, angiostatin, and soluble VEGF receptor inhibitors. Currently, there are two phase I clinical trials, one using an AAV vector to express a VEGF-binding protein and another using a lentiviral vector to express endostatin and angiostatin (32). Results from these proof of concept studies are not yet published.

Adenoviral Vector–Mediated Antiangiogenic Gene Therapy

Preclinical proof using either recombinant adenovectors to carry the genes encoding PEDF and endostatin or recombinant AAVs carrying the transgene encoding for angiostatin have been published and demonstrate significant inhibition of CNV in various animal models. The intravenous administration of an adenoviral construct carrying the murine endostatin gene was tested in a murine model of CNV and found almost complete inhibition of neovascular activity. Similarly, subcutaneous injection of an AAV carrying a truncated angiostatin gene resulted in significant inhibition of retinal neovascularization. These encouraging results with endostatin and angiostatin suggest a potential role of antiangiogenesis in ocular disease.

PEDF has received major attention. PEDF was first described in 1989 by Tombran-Tink (72) in conditioned medium from cultured, fetal RPE cells; it was found to be a potent neurotrophic factor. Subsequently, PEDF has been purified and cloned both from humans and mice (73). The gene is expressed as early as 17 weeks in human fetal RPE cells, suggesting that PEDF is intimately involved in early neuronal development. PEDF attracted even more attention when Dawson et al. (71) demonstrated that PEDF is one of the most potent natural inhibitors of angiogenesis. In addition, PEDF is an inhibitor of endothelial cell migration. The amount of inhibitory PEDF produced by retinal cells was positively correlated with oxygen concentrations, suggesting that retinal cell loss plays a permissive role in ischemia-driven retinal neovascularization. Moreover, a correlation between changes in VEGF/PEDF ratio and the degree of retinal neovascularization in a rat model was demonstrated.

The AdVPEDF.11 is a replication-deficient adenovirus vector designed to deliver the human PEDF gene. Intravitreous injection of AdPEDF resulted in increased expression of PEDF mRNA in the eye, compared with AdNull (the same vector without the transgene) or with uninjected controls. PDEF trail was present not only in the retina but also in other parts of the eye, including the iris, lens, and corneal epithelium. After subretinal injection of AdPEDF, it was strongly detected in the RPE cells compared with other ocular structures (73).

SAFETY AND OBSTACLES IN GENE TRANSFER

The theoretical safety concerns regarding human gene transfer are not trivial. For the individual recipient, there is the possibility of vector-induced inflammation and immune responses. There are also theoretical issues that are important to society, including concerns about modifying the human germ line and about protecting the environment from new infectious agents generated from gene transfer vectors carrying expression genes with powerful biologic functions.

There have been serious adverse events in human gene transfer trials, including inflammation induced by the administration of adenovirus vectors and by administration to the central nervous system of a xenogenic producer cell line releasing a retrovirus vector (19). However, compared with the total numbers of individuals undergoing gene transfer, adverse events have been rare and have been related mostly to the dose and the manner in which the vectors were administered.

Two potential problems with retroviral vectors warrant discussion: insertional mutagenesis and helper virus production. Problems with insertional mutagenesis, such as activation of cellular oncogenes, are shared with any gene transfer technique that results in integration of new sequences into the cellular genome, with the possible exception of AAV. Although there are many examples of retroviral activation of cellular oncogenes in mice, these events occur in the context of a spreading infection by replication-competent virus. On the other hand, the potential for production of replication-competent (helper) virus during the production of retroviral vectors remains a concern.

No novel infectious agents generated from recombination of the transferred genome and the host genome or other genetic information have yet been detected, nor has any replication-competent virus related to the vector. Cells modified ex vivo with retrovirus vectors have been infused repetitively without adverse effects. While human gene transfer has not been implicated in initiating malignancy, the number of recipients and time of observation have not been great enough to allow definitive conclusions regarding this issue. Finally, with gene therapy used to induce production of drugs in vivo, the risk for local and systemic side effects from uncontrolled drug delivery is significant.

With the successes of the human gene transfer trials have come the sobering realities of the drug development process. Some of the following problems are generic for the field, and some are specific to the vector (19):

1. Inconsistent results: The majority of the human gene transfer studies have inconsistent results, and in some cases, the basis for them is unclear. One of the more important problems is obtaining homogeneous results in the different studies.

2. Results extrapolation: There have been several surprise examples in which predictions from gene transfer studies in experimental animals have not been borne out in human safety and efficacy trials.

3. Production problems: There are some hurdles in vector production that must be overcome before large clinical trials can be initiated. Generation of replication-competent virus is observed in production of clinical-grade retrovirus and adenovirus vectors. Lack of reproducibility, aggregation, and contamination with endotoxin also complicate production of clinical-grade plasmid liposome complexes.

4. The perfect vector: The ideal gene transfer vector would be capable of efficiently delivering one or more genes of the size needed for the clinical application. The vector would be specific for its target, not recognized by the immune system, stable and easy to reproducibly produce, and could be purified in large quantities at high concentrations. It would not induce inflammation and would be safe for the recipient and the environment. Finally, it would express the gene or genes it carries for as long as required in an appropriately regulated fashion. Clinical experience to date suggests that retrovirus, adenovirus, and plasmid–liposome vectors all need refinement. There is considerable interest in developing new vectors, but there is controversy as to which vector class is most likely to succeed, particularly for use in vivo applications.

There are two philosophical camps in vector design: viral and nonviral. The viral proponents believe that the most efficient means to deliver an expression gene in vivo is to package it in a replication-deficient recombinant virus. The logic supporting this approach is the knowledge that viruses are masterful at reproducing themselves and thus have evolved strategies to efficiently express their genetic information in the cells they infect. The nonviral proponents concede this argument, but believe that the redundant immune and inflammatory host defenses against viruses may be a risk to recipients, will limit the duration of expression as the infected cells are recognized by the immune system, and may hinder repeat administration of the vectors.

Intraocular Gene Delivery of Pigment Epithelium-Derived Factor: Human Clinical Trial in Exudative Age-Related Macular Degeneration

Previously, the investigational agent, $Ad_{GV}PEDF.11D$, an E1-, E3-, E4-deleted replication-deficient, second-generation adenovirus serotype 5, gene delivery vector, was tested for safety in a phase I clinical trial. The transgene in this vector is the cDNA for human PEDF. Intravitreous administration of $Ad_{GV}PEDF.11D$ provides a means of sustained delivery of PEDF within the eye (73). PEDF has been shown in animal models to both inhibit growth of CNV membranes and to induce regression of established CNV (8,74).

The primary objectives of the investigation were (a) to assess the safety, tolerability, and feasibility of intravitreous injection of $Ad_{GV}PEDF.11D$ in patients with severe, neovascular AMD; (b) to identify the maximum tolerated dose (MTD) of $Ad_{GV}PEDF.11D$; and (c) to get some indication of potential activity of $Ad_{GV}PEDF.11D$ in this clinical setting (73). The trial was an open-label, dose-escalation study. Eight dose levels were evaluated. The lowest injected dose was 1×10 (6) particle units (pu) with doses increasing to $1 \times 10^{9.5}$ in half log unit increments. Each patient enrolled was followed for 2 weeks for signs of dose-limiting toxicity prior to enrollment of the next patient. Following successful enrollment of three patients, the next one-half log unit higher dose was administered. In this stepwise fashion, all eight doses were evaluated with no evidence of dose-limiting toxicity (73). Early data suggested PEDF biologic activity in these patients with very advanced or severe "wet" AMD.

CONCLUSIONS AND FUTURE DIRECTIONS

Progress in gene therapy has offered patients the hope for treatment for retinal degeneration. Research has identified candidate genes and suitable delivery vehicles. Over the last decade, viral vector technology has grown and the use of AAV as a delivery vehicle for gene therapy has been accepted for broad applications, and lentivirus platforms are in further development. The development of novel technologies for gene delivery allows scientists to overcome a number of the limitations that were previously posed by the vector, such as packaging capacity and the ability to regulate gene expression, thus expanding the vector's applications. In the retina, it will be important to track and optimize the different steps of vector transduction, at both the cellular and molecular levels, to gain an understanding of the transduction entry pathways, intracellular trafficking, and mechanism of episomal expression and integration. Viral delivery of secreted therapeutic proteins has also been used to provide a potential treatment for ocular neovascularization associated with the exudative stages of macular degeneration. Several clinical trials for the treatment of AMD are currently under way that utilize vectors encoding antiangiogenic factors while vectors containing neuroprotective factors and regenerative factors are in development.

REFERENCES

1. Freidman T. Progress toward human gene therapy. Science. 1989;244:1275–1280.
2. Mieller AD. Human gene therapy comes of age. Nature. 1992;357:455–460.
3. Williamson B. Gene therapy. Nature. 1982;298:416–418.

4. Bennett J, Tanabe T, Sun D, et al. Photoreceptor cell rescue in retinal degeneration (rd) mice by in vivo gene therapy. Nat Med. 1996;2:649–654.

5. Kumar-Singh R, Farber DB. Encapsidated adenovirus minichromosome-mediated delivery of genes to the retina: application to the rescue of photoreceptor degeneration. Hum Mol Genet. 1998;7:1893–1900.

6. Takahashi M, Miyoshi H, Verma IM, et al. Rescue from photoreceptor degeneration in the rd mouse by human immunodeficiency virus vector-mediated gene transfer. J Virol. 1999;73:7812–7816.

7. Acland GM, Aguirre GD, Ray J, et al. Gene therapy restores vision in a canine model of childhood blindness. Nat Genet. 2001;28:92–95.

8. Mori K, Duh E, Gehlbach P, et al. Pigment epithelium-derived factor inhibits retinal and choroidal neovascularization. J Cell Physiol. 2001;188:253–263.

9. Gehlbach PL, Demetriades AM, Yamamoto S, et al. Periocular injection of an adenoviral vector encoding of pigment epithelium-derived factor inhibits choroidal neovascularization. Gene Ther. 2003;10:637–646.

10. Mori K, Gehlbach P, Ando A, et al. Regression of ocular neovascularization in response to increased expression of pigment epithelium-derived factor. Invest Ophthalmol Vis Sci. 2002;43:2428–2434.

11. Takita H, Yoneya S, Gehlbach PL, et al. Retinal neuroprotection against ischemic injury mediated by intraocular gene transfer of pigment epithelium-derived factor. Invest Ophthalmol Vis Sci. 2003;44:4497–4504.

12. Imai D, Yoneya S, Gehlbach PL, et al. Intraocular gene transfer of pigment epithelium-derived factor rescues photoreceptors from light-induced cell death. J Cell Physiol. 2005;202(2):570–578.

13. Ashery-Padan R. Somatic gene targeting in the developing and adult mouse retina. Methods. 2002;28:457–464.

14. Surace EM, Auricchio A. Adeno-associated viral vectors for retinal gene transfer. Prog Retin Eye Res. 2003;22:705–719.

15. Allikmets R, Shroyer NF, Singh N, et al. Mutation of the Stargardt disease gene (ABCR) in age-related macular degeneration. Science. 1997;277:1805–1807.

16. Weber BH, Vogt G, Pruett RC, et al. Mutations in the tissue inhibitor of metalloproteinases-3 (TIMP3) in patients with Sorsby's fundus dystrophy. Nat Genet. 1991;8:352–356.

17. Ali RR, Sarra GM, Stephens C, et al. Restoration of photoreceptor ultrastructure and function in retinal degeneration slow mice by gene therapy. Nat Genet. 2000;25:306–310.

18. Wivel NA, LeRoy W. Germ-line gene modification and disease prevention: some medical and ethical perspectives. Science. 1993;262:533–537.

19. Crystal RG. Transfer of genes to humans: early lessons and obstacles to success. Science. 1995;270:404–409.

20. Pleyer U, Ritter T. Gene therapy in immune-mediated disease of the eye. Prog Retin Eye Res. 2003;22:277–293.

21. Morsy MA, Alford EL, Bett A, et al. Efficient adenoviral-mediated ornithine transcarbamylase expression in deficient mouse and human hepatocytes. J Clin Invest. 1993;92:1580–1586.

22. Morsy MA, Mitani K, Clemens P, et al. Progress toward human gene therapy. JAMA. 1993;270:2338–2345.

23. Morsy MA, Zhao JZ, Warman AW, et al. Patient selection may affect gene therapy success. Dominant negative effects observed for ornithine trancarbamylase in mouse and human hepatocytes. J Clin Invest. 1996;97:826–832.

24. Muzzin P, Eisensmith RC, Copeland KC, et al. Correction of obesity and diabetes in genetically obese mice by leptin gene therapy. Proc Natl Acad Sci U S A. 1996;93:14804–14808.

25. Stratford-Perricaudet LS, Levrero M, Chasse J, et al. Evaluation of the transfer and expression in mice of an enzyme-encoding gene using a human adenovirus vector. Hum Gene Ther. 1990;1:241–256.

26. Mitani K, Graham FL, Caskey CT, et al. Rescue, propagation, and partial purification of a helper virus-dependent adenovirus vector. Proc Natl Acad Sci U S A. 1995;92:3854–3858.

27. Kumer-Singh R, Chamberlain JS. Encapsidated adenovirus minichromosomes allow delivery and expression of a 14 kb dystrophin cDNA to muscle cells. Hum Mol Genet. 1996;5:913–921.

28. Clemens PR, Kochanek S, Sunada Y, et al. In vivo muscle gene transfer of full-length dystrophin with an adenoviral vector that lacks all viral genes. Gene Ther. 1996;3:965–972.

29. Fisher KJ, Choi H, Burda J, et al. Recombinant adenovirus deleted of all viral genes for gene therapy of cystic fibrosis. Virology. 1996;217:11–22.

30. Lieber A, He CY, Kirillova I, et al. Recombinant adenoviruses with large deletions generated by Cre-mediated excision exhibit different biological properties compared with first-generation vectors in vitro and in vivo. J Virol. 1996;70:8944–8960.

31. Chaum E, Hatton MP. Gene therapy for genetic and acquired retinal disease. Surv Ophthalmol. 2002;47:449–469.

32. Campochiaro PA. Gene transfer for ocular neovascularization and macular edema. Gene Ther. 2012;2:121–126.

33. Flannery JG, Zolotukhin S, Vaquero MI, et al. Efficient photoreceptor-targeted gene expression in vivo by recombinant adeno-associated virus. Proc Natl Acad Sci U S A. 1997;94:6916–6921.

34. Miyoshi H, Takahashi M, Gage FH, et al. Stable and efficient gene transfer into the retina using an HIV-based lentiviral vector. Proc Natl Acad Sci U S A. 1997;94:10319–10323.

35. Olsson JE, Gordon JW, Pawlyk BS, et al. Transgenic mice with a rhodopsin mutation (Pro23His): a mouse model of autosomal dominant retinitis pigmentosa. Neuron. 1992;9:815–830.

36. Sarra GM, Stephes C, de Alwis M, et al. Gene replacement therapy in the retinal degeneration slow (rds) mouse: the effect on retinal degeneration following partial transduction of the retina. Hum Mol Genet. 2001;10:2353–2361.

37. Martin KR, Klein RL, Quigley HA. Gene delivery to the eye using adeno-associated viral vectors. Methods. 2002;28:267–275.

38. Auricchio A. Pseudotyped AAV vector for constitutive and regulated gene expression in the eye. Vision Res. 2003;43:913–918.

39. Beltran WA, Cideciyan AV, Lewin AS, et al. Gene therapy rescues photoreceptor blindness in dogs and paves the way for treating human X-linked retinitis pigmentosa. Proc Natl Acad Sci U S A. 2012;109(6):2132–2137.

40. Kavanaugh MP, Miller DG, Zhang W, et al. Cell-surface receptors for gibbon ape leukemia virus and amphotropic murine retrovirus are inducible sodium-dependent phosphate symporters. Proc Natl Acad Sci U S A. 1994;91:7071–7075.

41. Kozak SL, Siess DC, Kavanaugh MP, et al. The envelope glycoproteins of an amphotropic murine retrovirus binds specifically to the cellular receptor/phosphate transporter of susceptible species. J Virol. 1995;69:5110–5113.

42. Takahashi Saishin Y, Saishin Y, et al. Intraocular expression of endostatin reduces VEGF-induced retinal vascular permeability, neovascularization, and retinal detachment. FASEB J. 2003;17(8):896–898.

43. O'Reilly MS, Boehm T, Shing Y, et al. Endostatin: an endogenous inhibitor of angiogenesis and tumor growth. Cell. 1997;88(2):277–285.

44. Liang FQ, Dejneka NS, Cohen DR, et al. AAV-mediated delivery of ciliary neurotrophic factor prolongs photoreceptor survival in the rhodopsin knockout mouse. Mol Ther. 2001;3:241–248.

45. Bennett J, Duan D, Engelhardt JF, et al. Real-time, noninvasive in vivo assessment of adeno-associate virus-mediated retinal transduction. Invest Ophthalmol Vis Sci. 1997;38:2857–2863.

46. Faktorovich EG, Steinberg RH, Yasumura D, et al. Photoreceptor degeneration in inherited retinal dystrophy delayed by basic fibroblast growth factor. Nature. 1990;347:83–86.

47. Hahn P, Lindsten T, Ying G, et al. Proapoptotic Bcl-2 family members, Bax and Bak, are essential for developmental photoreceptor apoptosis. Invest Ophthalmol Vis Sci. 2003;44:3598–3605.

48. Jacobson SG, Cideciyan AV, Ratnakaram R, et al. Gene therapy for leber congenital amaurosis caused by RPE65 mutations: safety and efficacy in 15 children and adults followed up to 3 years. Arch Ophthalmol. 2012;130(1):9–24.

49. Garcia Valenzuela E, Sharma SC. Rescue of retinal ganglion cells from axotomy-induced apoptosis through TRK oncogene transfer. Neuroreport. 1998;9:165–170.

50. Lai CC, Wu WC, Chen SL, et al. Suppression of choroidal neovascularization by adeno-associated virus vector expressing angiostatin. Invest Ophthalmol Vis Sci. 2001;42:2401–2407.

51. Semkova I, Kreppel F, Welsandt G, et al. Autologous transplantation of genetically modified iris pigment epithelial cells: a promising concept for the treatment of age-related macular degeneration and other disorders of the eye. Proc Natl Acad Sci U S A. 2002;99:13090–13095.

52. The Macular Photocoagulation Study Group. Argon laser photocoagulation for neovascular maculopathy: five year results from randomized clinical trials. Arch Ophthalmol. 1991;109:1109–1114.

53. Klein R, Klein B. Vision disorders in diabetes. In: Group NDD, ed. Diabetes in America. Washington, DC: National Institutes of Health; 1995:293–330.

54. Rosenfeld PJ, Brown DM, Heier JS, et al. MARINA Study Group. Ranibizumab for neovascular age-related macular degeneration. N Engl J Med. 2006;355(Hirano 2003):1419–1431.

55. Brown DM, Kaiser PK, Michels M, et al. ANCHOR Study Group. Ranibizumab versus verteporfin for neovascular age-related macular degeneration. N Engl J Med. 2006;355(Hirano 2003):1432–1444.

56. Martin DF, Maguire MG, Ying GS, et al. Ranibizumab and bevacizumab for neovascular age-related macular degeneration. CATT Research Group. N Engl J Med. 2011;364:1897–1908.

57. Ezekowiyz RAB, Mulliken JB, Folkman J. Interferon alpha-2a therapy for life-threatening hemangioma of infancy. N Engl J Med. 1992;326:1456–1463.

58. Miller JW, Stinson W, Folkman J. Regression of experimental iris neovascularization with systemic alpha-interferon. Ophthalmology. 1993;100:9–14.

59. Aiello LP, Avery RL, Arrigg PG, et al. Vascular endothelial growth factor in ocular fluid of patients with diabetic retinopathy and other retinal disorders. N Engl J Med. 1994;331:1480–1487.

60. D'Amore PA. Mechanisms of retinal and choroidal neovascularization. Invest Ophthalmol Vis Sci. 1994;35:3974–3978.

61. Tobe T, Okamoto N, Vinores MA, et al. Evolution of neovascularization in mice with overexpression of vascular endothelial growth factor in photoreceptors. Invest Ophthalmol Vis Sci. 1998;39:180–188.

62. Aiello L, Pierce E, Foley H, et al. Inhibition of vascular endothelial growth factor suppresses retinal neovascularization in vivo. Proc Natl Acad Sci U S A. 1995;92:10457–10461.

63. Adamis AP, Shima DT, Tolentino MJ, et al. Inhibition of vascular endothelial growth factor prevents retinal ischemia associated iris neovascularization in non human primate. Arch Ophthalmol. 1996;114:66–71.

64. Seo M-S, kwak N, Ozaki H, et al. Dramatic inhibition of retinal and choroidal neovascularization by oral administration of a kinase inhibitor. Am J Pathol. 1999;154:1743–1753.

65. Fire A, Xu S, Montgomery MK, et al. Potent and specific genetic interference by double-strand RNA in *Caenorhabditis elegans*. Nature. 1998;391:806–811.

66. Hannon GJ. RNA interference. Nature. 2002;418:244–251.

67. Tolentino MJ, Brucker AJ, Fosnot J, et al. Intravitreal injection of vascular endothelial growth factor small interfering RNA inhibits growth and leakage in a nonhuman primate, laser induced model of choroidal neovascularization. Retina. 2004;24:132–138.

68. O'Reilly MS, Holmgren S, Shing Y, et al. Angiostatin: a novel angiogenesis inhibitor that mediates the suppression of metastases by a Lewis lung carcinoma. Cell. 1994;79:315–328.

69. Black WR, Agner RC. Tumor regression after endostatin therapy. Nature. 1998;391:450.

70. O'Reilly MS, Pirie-Sheherd S, Lane WS, et al. Anti-angiogenic activity of the cleaved conformation of the serpin antithrombin. Science. 1999;285:1926–1928.

71. Dawson DW, Volpert OV, Gillis P, et al. Pigment epithelium-derived factor: a potent inhibitor of angiogenesis. Science. 1999;285:245–248.

72. Tombran-Tink J, Johnson L. Neuronal differentiation of retinoblastoma cells induced by medium conditioned by human RPE cells. Invest Ophthalmol Vis Sci. 1989;30:1700–1709.

73. Rasmussen HS, Rasmussen CS, Durham RG, et al. Looking into anti-angiogenic gene therapies for disorders of the eye. Drug Discov Today. 2001;22:1171–1175.

74. Mori K, Gehlbach P, Yamamoto S, et al. AAV-mediated gene transfer of pigment epithelium derived factor inhibits choroidal neovascularization. Invest Ophthalmol Vis Sci. 2002;43:1994–2000.

25

NEW PHARMACOTHERAPIES FOR AGE-RELATED MACULAR DEGENERATION

SCOTT D. SCHOENBERGER • PAUL STERNBERG JR.

INTRODUCTION

The pathogenesis of age-related macular degeneration (AMD) is highly complex and incompletely understood. Its causes are multifactorial, with genetic predisposition and environmental factors likely playing a role. Numerous molecular and biochemical pathways have been suggested to be involved, leading to optimism for several potential therapies targeting these pathways. Perhaps the greatest success has been in the treatment of exudative AMD, with the emergence of several efficacious agents directed against vascular endothelial growth factor (VEGF). However, the only current therapy with documented benefit for dry AMD has been the use of nutritional supplements, as demonstrated in the Age-Related Eye Disease Study. A wide variety of therapies directed toward different pathways are being investigated in preclinical testing and human clinical trials for both forms of AMD.

Chronic inflammation, complement deposition, oxidative stress, angiogenesis, and visual cycle toxic by-products have been associated with the development and progression of AMD (1–5). In dry AMD, inflammatory cells, complement components, amyloid-β (Aβ), and oxidized lipids have been shown to localize within or near drusen (4–7). In addition, chronic inflammatory cells, complement components, and cytokines increase choroidal neovascularization (CNV) formation or are overexpressed in CNV (8,9). Laboratory in vitro studies and animal research have shown that these

pathways may be interconnected. Interferon-gamma (IFN-γ) is a proinflammatory cytokine that induces complement factor H (CFH) and promotes VEGF secretion (10,11). Aβ colocalizes with activation-specific fragments of complement C3 and activates the complement cascade (12). Oxidative stress generates reactive oxygen species (ROS) within lipofuscin, and this exposure leads to the deposition of complement components, microglia, and other inflammatory cells in the retina (3,13).

The above pathways have been targeted in animal studies and preclinical studies, and many are currently undergoing clinical testing in human patients with AMD.

INFLAMMATION

Chronic inflammation has been associated with multiple neurodegenerative disorders of aging (14), including AMD (4). Autoimmunity has been linked with AMD, as a majority of patients in one study had elevated serum retinal autoantibodies, as compared to 9% in controls (15). Serum C-reactive protein (CRP) levels have been shown to be elevated in some studies of patients with AMD (16). On a histologic level, several studies have linked AMD with inflammation. Inflammatory cells and proinflammatory cytokines have been demonstrated to contribute to both dry and exudative AMD. Macrophages and giant cells localize near drusen, at CNV, and at breaks in Bruch's membrane (8). Macrophages induce proliferation and migration of vascular endothelium, increasing CNV (17). Activated microglia, as part of the innate immune system, migrate within the retina, ingest debris, and produce cytokines (18). Inflammatory cytokines including tumor necrosis factor-alpha (TNF-α) and interleukin-1 (IL-1) have been shown to promote intercellular adhesion molecule-1 (ICAM-1) formation in the retinal pigment epithelium (RPE) and vascular endothelium, leading to a further increase in inflammatory cells, creating a self-perpetuating cycle of inflammation. IFN-γ is an important modulator of the immune system, up-regulating complement components and other cytokines, leading to increased leukocyte activation (11). IFN-γ transgenic mice developed inflammatory cell infiltration and photoreceptor loss (19). Thus, targeting chronic inflammation may be beneficial for both atrophic and exudative AMD.

Nonsteroidal Anti-Inflammatory Drugs

Nonsteroidal anti-inflammatory drugs (NSAIDs) are used systemically for their anti-inflammatory, analgesic, and antipyretic properties. They are used topically for inflammation, allergic conjunctivitis and keratitis, inhibition of miosis, and cystoid macular edema (20). Newer formulations have better penetration into the posterior segment of the eye. NSAIDs inhibit the cyclooxygenase (COX) pathway, including the COX-1 and COX-2 enzymes. COX-2 has been detected in the RPE and vascular endothelium within CNV (21). It is an inducible enzyme that produces prostaglandins that increase vascular permeability and modulate the expression of VEGF and its receptors (20).

Topical NSAIDs have been investigated in exudative AMD. Zweifel et al. (22) investigated topical bromfenac as an adjunct to intravitreal anti-VEGF therapy in patients with persistent subretinal or intraretinal fluid. They found no statistically significant benefit over 2 months. Chen et al. (23) similarly found no statistically significant benefit to the addition of topical nepafenac to intravitreal anti-VEGF agents in patients with persistently active exudative AMD. A prospective, randomized study found the addition of topical diclofenac to photodynamic therapy (PDT) to be no superior to PDT alone (24).

Intravitreal NSAIDs have been tested in animal models (25). Studies have shown intravitreal NSAIDs to have powerful anti-inflammatory effects in rabbit models (26). In rats, intravitreal ketorolac reduced laser-induced CNV leakage and vascular budding (25). Intravitreal NSAIDs have been evaluated more commonly in humans with diabetic macular edema and uveitis, but in one report of intravitreal diclofenac for various etiologies, increased visual acuity (VA) was noted in both patients with exudative AMD (27).

Corticosteroids

Corticosteroids have several anti-inflammatory effects: they induce lipocortin synthesis, which inhibits phospholipase A2 and arachadonic acid formation, leading to a decrease in prostaglandins and leukotrienes through the COX and lipo-oxygenase pathways (28); they inhibit the production of IL-1 and TNF-α (4) and down-regulate cytokine-induced expression of adhesion molecules, further inhibiting adhesion and migration of inflammatory cells (28); within the eye, they reduce vascular permeability, stabilize the blood–ocular barrier, and suppress VEGF expression (29).

Dexamethasone and triamcinolone have been studied in clinical settings. Intravitreal dexamethasone has been combined with anti-VEGF therapy and PDT. Intravitreal triamcinolone acetonide has been evaluated in combination with anti-VEGF and/or PDT, with mixed results (28). The addition of intravitreal dexamethasone or triamcinolone may decrease the anti-VEGF burden but have not demonstrated adequate efficacy as monotherapy compared to other agents (4).

The fluocinolone acetonide intravitreal implant is being investigated in patients with both dry and exudative AMD. It is involved in a randomized, double-masked, fellow eye controlled (sham-injected) phase II clinical trial designed to evaluate changes in geographic atrophy (GA) over 24 months in patients with bilateral GA (30). It is also involved in a phase II, randomized study investigating two doses of fluocinolone acetonide and its safety and efficacy over 36 months as an adjuvant agent in patients undergoing treatment with intravitreal ranibizumab for exudative AMD (31).

Immunomodulators

Methotrexate is a dihydrofolate reductase inhibitor and inhibits T-lymphocyte proliferation by reducing nucleotide formation (4). It inhibits cytokine production and decreases inflammation. In one report, two patients with exudative AMD who were unresponsive to anti-VEGF therapy were treated with intravitreal methotrexate (32). One patient had an improved VA and both patients had decreased subretinal fluid and perifoveal leakage 2 weeks after injection.

Infliximab is a chimeric (mouse/human) IgG1 monoclonal antibody to TNF-α. It neutralizes circulating TNF-α and prevents binding to its receptors, leading to cytokine and cellular inhibition (4). TNF-α is overexpressed in CNV (17), and TNF-α inhibitors significantly reduced laser-induced CNV after intravitreal injection in animal models (33). In three patients who were treatment naive or PDT resistant, intravenous infliximab for rheumatoid arthritis was noted to improve VA and cause CNV regression after several months (34). A pilot study of systemic immunosuppression for exudative AMD found no change in the frequency of anti-VEGF injections in patients receiving intravenous infliximab (35). Intravitreal infliximab has been studied in anti-VEGF nonresponders. In one study, three patients were given intravitreal infliximab, two of whom showed complete resolution of intraretinal fluid and the third had a temporary reduction of intraretinal fluid (36). Another four patients were treated with intravitreal infliximab, without a significant visual or anatomical benefit, but two developed severe intraocular inflammation (37).

Adalimumab is another antibody to TNF-α being investigated for AMD. It is fully humanized and less likely to cause human antichimeric antibodies than is infliximab. It is undergoing phase II studies to investigate electroretinogram (ERG) abnormalities, retinal thickness, VA, and adverse events after intravitreal administration for exudative AMD (38).

Daclizumab is a fully humanized IgG1 monoclonal antibody against the α chain of the IL-2 receptor (4). This results in decreased activation and proliferation of T lymphocytes and decreased IFN-γ expression in CD4 and CD8 cells. In one trial of systemic daclizumab for exudative AMD, there was a decrease in anti-VEGF injections from 0.73 to 0.42 per month after treatment with daclizumab for 6 months (35). The authors concluded that systemic immunosuppression may alter the course of exudative AMD but that further studies are needed.

MAMMALIAN TARGET OF RAPAMYCIN

Multiple molecular pathways exist that contribute to aging, including the mammalian target of rapamycin (mTOR) pathway. The mTOR protein is a serine/threonine protein kinase that processes signals and controls cell growth and proliferation (39). Reduced mTOR activity, through knocking out downstream protein signaling or with pathway inhibitors, has been observed in mice with extended life (40). The mTOR pathway has been implicated in different cancer types and resistance to chemotherapy (41).

As the RPE ages, mitochondrial function decreases and cells are more prone to oxidative damage (39). These early changes correlate with RPE hypertrophy and dedifferentiation and coincide with mTOR activation (42). The RPE cells contain mTOR complexes that are affected by various stimuli, and down-regulation of mTOR signaling may prolong cellular survival (39). As nutrient and growth factor signals affect the mTOR pathway, it may link environmental factors to cellular functions. mTOR inhibitors down-regulate markers of cellular senescence and may have a therapeutic effect in AMD, as they may slow down RPE aging.

The mTOR pathway also has a role in angiogenesis and is affected by inflammation and complement. IFN-γ plays an important role in intraocular inflammation, and promotes VEGF secretion from RPE cells via the mTOR pathway (10). Other angiogenic factors, including TNF-α, IL-1β, IL-6, IL-8, basic fibroblast growth factor (bFGF), and VEGF, depend on the mTOR pathway for cellular signaling (43).

mTOR Inhibitors

Sirolimus (rapamycin) is a macrolide antibiotic that inhibits T-lymphocyte activation and proliferation (44). It inhibits the mTOR pathway and has antiangiogenic properties. As it has dual effects against angiogenesis and inflammation,

it may be a therapeutic option for both exudative and dry AMD (10). Animal models of retinal and choroidal angiogenesis have been inhibited by sirolimus (44). It was effective in reducing VEGF from cultured RPE cells and was more effective in reducing endothelial cell sprouting than were VEGF inhibitors (45). In phase I studies in patients with diabetic macular edema, it was well tolerated and safe when administered intravitreally and subconjunctivally (46). It is being investigated in two phase I/II trials in patients with bilateral GA due to AMD. Patients will receive subconjunctival (47) or intravitreal (48) sirolimus in one eye every 2 months for 2 years, with the other eye as a control. Primary outcomes include change of GA and development of exudative AMD.

Palomid 529 is a small molecule drug that inhibits the mTOR pathway via dissociation of both target of rapamycin complexes, TORC1 and TORC2 (49). It inhibits tumor growth, angiogenesis, and vascular permeability in mutant glioma tumor cells and endothelial cells (50). As the mTOR pathway has several positive and negative feedback loops, dual TORC inhibitors may have a more effective and broad inhibition of angiogenesis than sirolimus. Phase I studies are under way to investigate safety and tolerability in patients with exudative AMD after intravitreal or subconjunctival administration (51).

COMPLEMENT

The complement system is part of the innate immune system but also has a role in adaptive immunity (5). It eliminates damaged, necrotic and apoptotic cells and facilitates the elimination of circulating immune complexes (52). This system is made of proteins that circulate normally and are activated by several triggers. Three pathways exist, and the final result is the generation of the membrane attack complex (MAC), a cell-killing protein.

The complement system is a highly regulated system but has the ability to damage host tissue (5). It may play a role in autoimmune disorders like asthma, systemic lupus erythematosus, multiple sclerosis (MS), inflammatory bowel disease, transplant rejection, and others (52). Complement-associated membranoproliferative glomerulonephritis type II is associated with deposits that resemble drusen. Complement is also thought to play a role in neurodegenerative disorders like Alzheimer's disease (AD). Deficiencies in complement factors predispose to infections and autoimmune diseases, and complement inhibitors may cause an increased risk of infection.

Complement Pathways

The complement system is shown in Figure 25.1, including the medications under investigation and their sites of action. The classical pathway requires an antigen–antibody complex and is the only pathway that is specific for a given antigen (5). It involves the components C1, C2, and C4 and is inhibited by C1 inhibitor (C1-INH). The alternative pathway is triggered

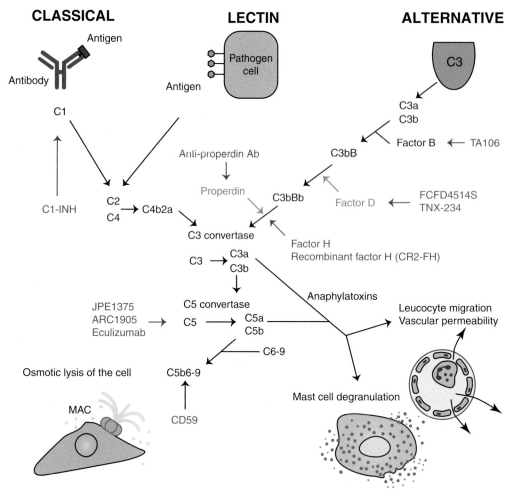

Figure 25.1 ■ A simplified schematic of the complement cascade. The sites of action of therapies being investigated are included.

by binding to a host cell or pathogen surface. C3b and the activated form of complement factor B (Bb) form the C3 convertase, and complement factor D is required. There is a spontaneous low-level activation of this pathway, and components of cigarette smoke can activate this pathway (53). CFH inhibits this pathway, and this is the main pathway thought to be involved in AMD (5). The lectin pathway is triggered by polysaccharides on microbial surfaces and requires C2 and C4.

All pathways form a C3 convertase, an enzyme that cleaves and activates C3 into C3a and C3b. C3b activates the C5 convertase, which cleaves C5 into C5a and C5b. C5b combines with C6-9, forming the terminal MAC, which causes lysis of cellular membranes and is deadly to cells and pathogens. C3a and C5a are anaphylatoxins that increase vascular permeability, cause degranulation of mast cells and neutrophils, induce cytokine release, and mediate leukocyte chemotaxis (54).

Complement and AMD

Several studies have shown that complement components may be deposited in drusen, including C3, C3a, C5a (55), and C5, the MAC (56), CFH, and complement receptor 1

(57,58). C1q and C3 have been shown to occur in CNV (9), and C3a and C5a increase VEGF production (55).

Genetic polymorphisms in complement encoding genes are associated with a predisposition for AMD. Complement factor B (CFB) and complement factor 2 genes have been associated with AMD, and genetic variations may be protective (59), as the production of the classical and alternative C3 convertases are diminished (60). Variations in the C3 gene are associated with AMD (61), as is the CFH gene; the most frequently reported factor implicated (62).

Complement Component 3

C3 is important for all three pathways, and animal and in vitro studies have demonstrated its importance in AMD. Subretinal injections of C3 in mice develop signs of AMD (63), while C3 knockout mice are protected from laser-induced CNV (64). C3a leads to increased VEGF production by RPE cells in vitro (55), and C3 has been demonstrated in surgically removed CNV (9). Plasma C3 levels appear to be elevated in patients with AMD (65).

POT-4/AL-78898A is a derivative of compstatin, a peptide inhibitor of C3 activation. Compstatin has been shown to decrease drusen formation in monkeys with early-onset macular degeneration (66). In phase I studies, POT-4 was demonstrated to be safe when injected intravitreally (67). AL-78898A is currently in a phase II randomized, double-blinded, crossover study in patients with exudative AMD designed to demonstrate a biologic effect after one intravitreal injection (68). Outcomes include time to escape to standard of care therapy, change in retinal thickness and VA.

Complement Component 5

Complement factor 5 is required for formation of the MAC. In humans, C5 is found in drusen (55), and serum levels of C5a are elevated in patients with AMD (69). C5a may increase RPE-mediated VEGF secretion (55). Mouse knockouts for the C5a receptor display reduced VEGF production and CNV formation in laser-induced models of CNV. There have not been clear associations between the C5 gene polymorphisms and AMD.

Eculizumab is a humanized monoclonal antibody against C5. It is given intravenously for paroxysmal nocturnal hemoglobinuria, another complement-mediated disorder (70). Chronic and systemic use increases the risk of *Neisseria meningitides* infection. Eculizumab is being tested in a phase II, randomized, placebo-controlled, double-masked study for dry AMD (71). After receiving a meningococcal vaccine, patients are randomized to eculizumab or placebo for 24 weeks. Patients are followed for 12 months after the initial infusion, and outcome measures include changes in the size of GA, drusen volume, and VA.

ARC1905 is an anti-C5 aptamer that blocks the cleavage of C5 into C5a and C5b, thus blocking further complement activation (52). Aptamers are nonimmunogenic, single-stranded oligonucleotides that display three-dimensional folding characteristics that allow inhibition of protein–protein interactions (72). A phase I study evaluating intravitreal ARC1905 in combination with intravitreal ranibizumab for exudative AMD has been completed (73). Results have not been released. Another phase I trial is ongoing to investigate safety and tolerability of intravitreal ARC1905 in the treatment of dry AMD with drusen and/or GA (74).

JPE1375 is a small molecule peptidomimetic antagonist against the C5 receptor. This compound exhibits high stability and receptor specificity. In mice, it has been demonstrated to have activity in an immune complex–mediated peritonitis model (75).

Complement Factor D

CFD is required for the activation of the alternative pathway C3 convertase. CFD knockout mice showed a significant reduction in photoreceptor damage after being exposed to constant light for several days (76). Genetic alterations in the CFD gene may (77) or may not be associated with AMD (78). There are conflicting data on whether or not systemic CFD is elevated in AMD patients (5,69,77). Nonetheless,

there still may be a therapeutic role for lowering CFD and inhibiting the alternative pathway C3 convertase.

FCFD4514S is a monoclonal antibody against CFD. A phase I study assessing the safety and tolerability, dosing, and pharmacokinetics of intravitreally delivered FCFD4514S is ongoing (79). A phase II, randomized, sham injection controlled study of safety, tolerability, and efficacy of intravitreal FCFD4514S in patients with GA is also ongoing (80). The main outcome measure is growth of GA at 12 months.

TNX-234 is a complement inhibitor that may be a therapeutic option for AMD. It is a humanized antibody against CFD (81).

Complement Factor B

CFB is a component of the alternative pathway C3 convertase (5). CFB has been localized in the neurosensory retina, in the RPE, in the choroid, and in drusen (59). In mice, its expression increases with age, and this was associated with increased C3 in the RPE and Bruch's membrane (82). Variations in the CFB gene are associated with AMD (59) and confer a protective effect through the reduction of alternative pathway C3 convertase. In vitro studies have shown a fourfold reduction in C3b binding affinity in certain variants, and this was associated with a reduction in C3 convertase formation (60).

TA106 is a Fab fragment of an anti-CFB antibody (52). Intraocular injections of anti–factor B antibodies appear to decrease light-induced photoreceptor loss (83). It is currently involved in preclinical testing.

Complement Factor H

CFH regulates the alternative pathway by promoting the breakdown of its C3 convertase. In vivo studies have shown that CFH is produced in the RPE and accumulates in drusen, RPE cells, choroid, and extracellular space (58). CFH knockout mice demonstrate increased autofluorescent material and C3 deposition in the retina (84). Subretinal injection of RNA directed against CFH showed increased MAC deposition and laser-induced CNV in mice (85). Genetic studies have revealed that polymorphisms in the CFH gene increase the development and progression of AMD. A substitution of tyrosine by histidine at the 402 position (Y402H) is the most reported polymorphism (62), but other variants also exist (86). High-risk CFH polymorphisms are additive with smoking (87) and may be associated with systemic complement activation (88).

Molecules resembling CFH or with a similar function represent a possible therapy for AMD. Animal models and in vitro studies have shown that RPE deterioration and CNV development are inhibited by CR2-fH, a recombinant protein consisting of CFH linked to a factor 2 targeting fragment that binds to activated complement products (89). Other recombinant CFH proteins have been developed (83,90) and may represent future therapies.

Other Therapies

CD59 is a natural membrane-bound inhibitor of MAC formation. In a murine model, subretinal delivery of an adenovirus vector expressing human CD59 can attenuate the formation of laser-induced CNV (91). Properdin stabilizes the C3 convertase and may also actively induce its formation on foreign surfaces (92). Antiproperdin antibodies have been developed that would destabilize the C3 convertase and may inhibit the complement system. C1-INH (SERPING1) is a protein that inhibits the classical pathway and has been shown to be associated with AMD (93). C1-INH has been used systemically in a complement disorder, hereditary angioneurotic edema, but has not been tested in AMD. Complement receptor type 1 has specificity for C3b and C4b (94). It inhibits the classical and alternative pathways. A form of the receptor has been developed, the soluble complement receptor type 1 (sCR1).

▮ AMYLOID

The extracellular accumulation of proteinaceous deposits has been implicated in several age-related conditions, including atherosclerosis, skin elastosis, AD (12), and AMD. Proteins include immunomodulators, inflammatory mediators, acute phase reactants, complement components, and immunoglobulins, highlighting a common chronic and localized inflammatory component in these disorders (95). One well-established protein in the brain is Aβ, a peptide that is produced by the cleavage of amyloid precursor protein (APP) by the β-site APP-cleaving enzyme and a presenilin complex (96). Aβ is a physiologic peptide that is synthesized but quickly degraded by peptidases such as neprilysin (97).

AD is the most common form of dementia and is the sixth leading cause of death in the United States (98). It is characterized by the extracellular deposition of amyloid plaques and neurofibrillary tangles. The accumulation and aggregation of Aβ form β-pleated sheets that form the insoluble amyloid plaques and cerebrovascular deposits in the brain of AD patients (99). Aβ is neurotoxic, as its accumulation leads to microglial and astrocyte activation and migration to the plaques (100). The microglia engulf Aβ and release cytokines, ultimately leading to neuronal apoptosis.

Amyloid Deposition in AMD

Studies have shown that Aβ is deposited in drusen (7,101). Dentchev et al. (101) found four of nine postmortem AMD human eyes to have Aβ-containing vesicles, as opposed to none in normal eyes. In postmortem eyes, the RPE was the source of APP, the precursor to Aβ (7). In mouse models for AD, RPE degeneration occurred with an accumulation of sub-RPE deposits (102). Injections of Aβ into the vitreous of rats have been shown to induce apoptosis of the outer and inner nuclear layers (103). With age, a diseased and thickened Bruch's membrane may impair clearance of Aβ into the choroid (99).

Aβ may also have a role in the progression of AMD. Dentchev et al. (101) showed that the highest quantity of Aβ-containing vesicles occurred at the borders of GA. Aβ was not present in the center of GA or within a disciform scar. Aβ is most prevalent in eyes with moderate-to-high amounts of drusen and may be associated with advanced AMD (12). Aβ may also have a role in exudative AMD. Cultured human RPE cells and mice disrupted for the neprilysin gene had an up-regulation of VEGF and a down-regulation of pigment epithelium–derived factor, an antiangiogenic protein (102). Furthermore, studies have shown that the high temperature requirement factor A1 (HTRA1) gene encodes a protein that is directly involved in the Aβ pathway, and it colocalizes with these deposits in the brain (104). Genetic polymorphisms in the HTRA1 gene have been linked with a higher risk of AMD (105).

Though AMD and AD share common features, the ultrastructural characteristics and localization of in the two are not the same (12). In AD, Aβ is deposited mostly around major retinal vessels in the inner retina, similar to that seen in amyloid angiopathy of the brain (99). While one prospective study identified an increased risk of developing AD in patients with advanced AMD (106), other studies have shown no significant association between AD and early AMD (107). Thus, there are clearly differences between the two, and medications targeting one may not necessarily be useful for the other.

Complement and Amyloid

Amyloid deposits have been shown to activate the complement system in both AD and AMD (108,109). In AD, Aβ directly and independently activate both the classical and alternative complement pathways through C3, C5, and MAC (108,110). CFH polymorphisms (Y402H) have also been shown to be overrepresented in AD in some studies (111), but not in others (112). Drusen may form, in part, due to activation of the complement system by Aβ. Aβ colocalizes with activation-specific fragments of C3 (12). A main activator of the alternative pathway, CFB, was shown to be indirectly up-regulated by Aβ in the presence of microglia and macrophages (111). C3b is inactivated by factors H and I, but factor I has been shown to be inhibited by the presence of Aβ, resulting in unregulated complement activation (109).

Amyloid-Based Therapies

Copaxone (glatiramer acetate) is approved for relapse prevention in MS. It is thought to modify the immune process that is responsible for MS, but its full mechanism is unknown. It is neuroprotective in mice models of AD, reducing amyloid plaques and prolonging neuronal survival (113,114). Landa et al. (113) investigated the use of Copaxone to reduce drusen number. Patients with intermediate dry

AMD were enrolled in a prospective, randomized, double-blinded, placebo-controlled trial. They received weekly subcutaneous Copaxone or placebo for 12 weeks. Four treated patients (eight eyes) showed a decrease in total drusen area, as compared to two control patients (four eyes) who displayed a slight increase. Another prospective study of patients with dry AMD received weekly subcutaneous Copaxone or sham injections for 12 weeks (114). Seven patients (14 eyes) were treated with Copaxone, and seven patients (12 eyes) received sham treatment. Copaxone-treated patients exhibited a disappearance/shrinkage of 19.2% of drusen, as opposed to 6.5% in the sham group (P = 0.13). No current clinical trials are registered investigating the use of Copaxone for AMD.

RN6G is an antibody to Aβ that targets the C-terminus of the Aβ peptides Aβ40 and Aβ42. In a mouse model of AMD, it improved the ERG response, reduced levels of Aβ and complement components in sub-RPE deposits, and preserved the RPE (115). A phase I, double-masked, placebo-controlled study was performed to evaluate its safety, tolerability, and dosing for dry AMD (116). Patients were randomized to an intravenous single dose of RN6G or placebo. Results have not been published. A second phase I double-masked study is under way to evaluate multiple doses of intravenous RN6G versus placebo (117).

GSK-933776 is a monoclonal antibody against Aβ that is involved in a phase II study designed to evaluate its effect on GA after intravenous administration (118). Patients are being recruited for this randomized, double-masked, placebo-controlled study, and estimated enrollment is 162. The primary outcome is the rate of change of GA over 12 and 18 months.

ANGIOGENESIS

Angiogenesis inhibitors have drastically changed the treatment and prognosis of exudative AMD. VEGF is a protein that regulates vasculogenesis and angiogenesis, is proinflammatory, and induces vascular permeability (1). Its expression is up-regulated by several growth factors, including fibroblast growth factor (FGF), platelet-derived growth factor (PDGF), insulin-like growth factor, and others. The VEGF gene family includes VEGF-A, -B, -C, -D, and placental growth factor (PlGF). VEGF-A appears to be the most associated with angiogenesis (1), while PlGF is the mostly expressed VEGF protein in endothelium (119). PDGF-β is another factor implicated in angiogenesis, as it stimulates pericytes, which support the endothelium (120).

Receptor tyrosine kinases (TKs) have been increasingly recognized as being important in the angiogenesis pathway. Three VEGF receptors exist with intrinsic TK activity (VEGFR-1, 2 and 3), and VEGFR-2 appears to be the primary mediator of angiogenesis and vasculogenesis (121). Other TK-based receptors may contribute to angiogenesis, including the PDGF receptor (CD140) and FGF receptors

α and β (122). Other receptor types have also been implicated in angiogenesis and targeted in studies; these include the nicotinic acetylcholine receptor (nAChR) (123), integrin α5β1 receptors (124), and sphingosine-1-phosphate (S1P) (125).

Bevasiranib

Bevasiranib is a small interfering RNA (siRNA) that acts by inducing breakdown of the VEGF messenger RNA (mRNA) (1). It was developed to match the protein-encoding nucleotide sequence of the mRNA to prevent translation into the protein. It does not target the VEGF protein itself. SiRNA directed against VEGF inhibited and regressed ocular neovascularization in mouse and primate models (126,127). After undergoing phase I and II studies, intravitreal bevasiranib was evaluated in a phase III study to assess its efficacy in exudative AMD after three loading doses of ranibizumab (128). Ranibizumab given every 4 weeks served as the control. Outcomes at 60 weeks showed that visual results were inferior to the ranibizumab arm. The study was terminated early, as the study was unlikely to meet its primary end point.

E10030

One mechanism of resistance to anti-VEGF therapy involves the ability of pericytes to protect endothelial cells from VEGF inhibition. PDGF-β stimulates pericytes and allows their integration into the vessel wall (120). Several lines of evidence support targeting PDGF and VEGF to enhance efficacy. Coinhibition of PDGF-β and VEGF-A is more effective in inhibiting mouse models of ocular neovascularization than anti-VEGF therapy alone (129). E10030 is an aptamer directed against PDGF-β that decreases pericyte density in CNV. Phase I studies confirmed safety, dosing, and tolerability (130). Twelve-week results of 22 patients treated with combined intravitreal E10030 and ranibizumab yielded an improvement of three lines in 59% and an 86% mean decrease in CNV size (131). E10030 is involved in a phase II clinical trial to assess safety and efficacy in exudative AMD (132). Patients are randomized to one of two doses of intravitreal E10030 or sham. All groups receive monthly ranibizumab. Outcomes include proportion of patients gaining 15 letters, change in VA, CNV area, and central subfield thickness and adverse events. Visual outcomes are measured at 12 weeks, and adverse events are monitored for 24 weeks.

Pazopanib

As part of angiogenesis, growth factors and pathways exist that signal through TK-based receptors (122). Two of three VEGF receptors (VEGFR-1 and VEGFR-2) are structurally related and possess TK activity. Other receptors possess TK activity and may contribute to angiogenesis, including PDGF receptors, FGF receptors α and β, and VEGFR-3.

Therapies targeting multiple TK receptors may allow for more potent suppression of angiogenesis than with VEGF inhibition alone (133).

Pazopanib is a small molecule inhibitor of multiple receptor TKs, including VEGF receptor-1, -2, and -3; PDGF receptors α and β; c-kit/CD117; FGF receptor-1, -2, and -3; and c-fms/CD115 (134). In vitro studies revealed that pazopanib inhibited VEGF expression by the RPE and choroidal endothelium (122). In laser-induced CNV in rats, topical pazopanib was found to statistically significantly decrease leakage and CNV size as compared to placebo. Pazopanib has undergone multiple phase I studies to date. It is currently involved in a phase IIb, dose-ranging study evaluating pazopanib eye drops versus intravitreal ranibizumab for exudative AMD (135). Five hundred and ten patients are enrolled, and outcomes include change in VA and number of intravitreal ranibizumab injections. Five pazopanib dosing regimens are being evaluated, and patients are able to receive ranibizumab injections as needed. Outcomes will be measured at 52 weeks.

TG100801

TG100572 is a molecule that inhibits multiple enzymes, including Src kinases and selected receptor TKs (136). Systemic TG100572 in a murine model of laser-induced CNV caused regression of the CNV, but systemic toxicity occurred. Topical administration of TG100801, a prodrug of TG100572, achieved a high retinal concentration, significantly suppressed laser-induced CNV, and reduced fluorescein leakage in mice. A phase II study of topically administered TG100801 was terminated early due to irreversible corneal toxicity (137).

Vatalanib

Vatalanib is a TK inhibitor that binds VEGFR-1, 2, 3, PDGF receptor-β, and c-kit (138). Vatalanib is an attractive option, as it has good oral bioavailability and can be given without intravitreal or intravenous injections. Mouse models of ischemic retinopathy have shown that it inhibits experimental retinal neovascularization (139). Orally administered vatalanib has been evaluated with PDT versus PDT alone in patients with subfoveal CNV due to AMD (140). The study was completed in 2007, but results were not published.

α5β1 Integrin Antagonists

Integrins are transmembrane receptors that have a large role in angiogenesis, and the α5β1 subtype is significantly up-regulated on tumor vessels (141), and expression is further increased by other growth factors. It is highly expressed in experimentally induced CNV (124) and promotes adhesion and proliferation of endothelial cells (142) and RPE (124).

JSM6427 is a small molecule inhibitor of α5β1 and has been shown to induce regression of murine models of CNV when given systemically (124). Further, it has been shown with intravitreal injection to provide dose-dependent inhibition of CNV in monkey and rabbit laser-induced and growth factor–induced models (141). JSM6427 has been investigated in a phase I study evaluating intravitreal administration in patients with exudative AMD (143). The study was completed in 2009, but results were not published.

Volociximab is a human IgG antibody to integrin α5β1 that has been shown to be a potent inhibitor in a cynomolgus model (144). A phase I clinical trial is under way to evaluate intravitreal volociximab in patients with subfoveal CNV (145).

Sonepcizumab

Sonepcizumab is an antibody to S1P (125). S1P is a lipid molecule on vascular endothelial cells that promotes their migration and survival. Receptors for S1P are up-regulated in ischemic retina, and deficiencies for these receptors demonstrate less neovascularization. Intraocular injections of sonepcizumab suppressed retinal neovascularization in murine models of oxygen-induced ischemic retinopathy. Furthermore, murine models of laser-induced CNV revealed that sonepcizumab reduced CNV area and fluorescein leakage. A phase I study has been completed (146) and a second is under way to evaluate its use in patients with persistent pigment epithelial detachments due to AMD or polypoidal choroidal vasculopathy (147). Patients are being recruited for a larger phase II study in exudative AMD (148).

ATG003

ATG003 is a topical eye drop formulation of mecamylamine, a nAChR antagonist toward one pathway that mediates angiogenesis (149). Nicotine has been shown to be proangiogenic, mediated through the nAChR (123). Antagonists toward this pathway suppress nicotine-induced retinal angiogenesis. Topical ATG003 (0.3% or 1.0%) was evaluated in a phase II randomized, placebo-controlled, double-masked study in exudative AMD (150). The study was terminated early. The primary outcome measure was proportion of patients losing fewer than 15 Early Treatment Diabetic Retinopathy Study (ETDRS) letters at 48 weeks compared to baseline, which was achieved in 88% in the 1% ATG003 group, 86% in the 0.3% ATG003 group, and 92% in placebo group ($P > 0.05$). ATG003 was completed in a second phase II study for exudative AMD, but results were not published (151).

Anti-VEGF Receptor Vaccine

Anti-VEGF receptor vaccine therapies represent an immune-related therapy for CNV. Inducing cytotoxic T lymphocyte responses to specific molecules expressed in vascular endothelium may decrease angiogenesis (152). Immunization with recombinant VEGFR2 protein has been shown to inhibit tumor growth and angiogenesis in mice (153).

In another study, mice immunized with the VEGFR2 peptide had a significantly lower size of laser-induced CNV as compared to controls (152). A phase I study to evaluate vaccination with the VEGFR peptide was started in 2008, but the status is currently unknown (154).

VISUAL CYCLE INHIBITORS

The initial steps of visual input include the absorption of light by a chromophore (2). Rhodopsin and the color opsins are photoreceptor proteins located in the outer segments that associate with the visual chromophore, 11-*cis*-retinal. When a photon of light is absorbed, 11-*cis*-retinal isomerizes to all-*trans*-retinal and a conformational change occurs in the rhodopsin and color opsin proteins, leading to a change in an outer segment cation channel. This hyperpolarizes the cell and transmits an electrical impulse that eventually reaches the brain. The visual cycle involves the regeneration of the chromophore.

The regeneration of the visual chromophore, 11-*cis*-retinal, is a complex sequence of steps that occurs in the photoreceptor, extracellular space, and the RPE (2). It can also be formed from dietary vitamin A. After the chromophore and rhodopsin or color opsins undergo conformational changes, all-*trans*-retinal is converted to all-*trans*-retinol. All-*trans*-retinol is then released into the extracellular space and is taken up by the RPE along with shed outer segments. Serum all-*trans*-retinol is also taken up by the RPE and is delivered by retinol-binding protein (RBP). The RPE-specific 65-kDa protein (RPE65), also known as isomerase, is the enzyme that generates 11-*cis*-retinol. 11-*cis*-retinol is then oxidized to 11-*cis*-retinal and transported back to the photoreceptor as a visual chromophore, or it is esterified and stored in the RPE.

There are several fundamental differences between rods and cones that have clinical implications (2). Rods detect single photons, are slower acting, and are very sensitive, whereas cones are much less sensitive, but respond several times faster. Rods require 11-*cis*-retinal from the RPE to regenerate rhodopsin. Cones use 11-*cis*-retinal but can also use 11-*cis*-retinol to regenerate opsins. For the above reasons, inhibition of the generation of 11-*cis*-retinal is expected to have a greater effect on rod function.

Lipofuscin

Lipofuscin is a heterogeneous aggregation of material that forms in the RPE in a number of retinal disorders, including AMD, Stargardt disease, and types of cone–rod dystrophy and retinitis pigmentosa (155). Lipofuscin builds up in the lysosomes of the RPE, which phagocytizes shed outer segments, and incomplete digestion of these retinaldehyde-rich segments result. The material is composed primarily of retinoid precursors and oxidatively damaged lipids (156). The main component is A2E, a complex of vitamin A aldehyde and ethanolamine in a 2:1 ratio (157) but also includes other bisretinoids (158). Lipofuscin is not present in mice when the visual chromophores are absent (159). A2E is cytotoxic. It has been shown to impair phospholipid degradation and lysosomal degradation (160), induce the release of pro-apoptotic proteins (161), destabilize cellular membranes (162), and cause DNA fragmentation (163). Blue light is within the excitation spectra of A2E and causes the generation of singlet oxygen, resulting in apoptosis and, ultimately, RPE cell death (164). The overlying photoreceptors are then lost.

Lipofuscin accumulates with age and in AMD (165). In AMD, phagocytosis and the metabolic load of the RPE is increased. As the RPE cells die, the metabolic demand of the remaining RPE cells increase, leading to a self-accelerating accumulation of lipofuscin and RPE cell death. This is especially evident in the macula, where the number of photoreceptors per RPE cell and the amount of lipofuscin is increased. Evidence suggests that areas rich in lipofuscin eventually lead to atrophy (166). This is evident in GA, where the atrophic area is hypoautofluorescent, but there is prominent hyperautofluorescence surrounding these areas in the junctional area adjacent to normal retina. New areas of atrophy may emerge from these areas of hyperautofluorescence.

The efficacy behind visual cycle inhibitors is in their ability to slow the synthesis of 11-*cis*-retinal, causing depletion of all-*trans*-retinal, the precursor to A2E (2). The visual cycle and the medications that inhibit it are shown in Figure 25.2. Lipofuscin accumulation is dependent, in part, on dietary vitamin A. Dietary retinol deficiency can reduce lipofuscin accumulation and autofluorescence (167). Visual cycle inhibitors have been found to have several effects in the human and animal eye. Inhibitors slow the rod recovery time after bleaching light (168) and reduce the levels of A2E in the RPE (169).

Isotretinoin

Isotretinoin (Accutane) is a systemic vitamin A derivative used in the treatment of severe acne. Also known as 13-*cis*-retinoic acid, it inhibits 11-*cis*-retinol dehydrogenase and decreases the regeneration of 11-*cis*-retinal in the RPE (169) and may also have an effect on the RPE65 enzyme (2). Animals treated with isotretinoin showed reduced lipofuscin and delayed rod recovery following exposure to bright light (169). Systemic toxicity occurred before photoreceptor death (168). In humans, isotretinoin therapy was linked with nyctalopia, daytime glare, abnormal dark adaptation, and abnormal ERG (170). Doses required to inhibit the visual cycle in humans are too high and carry significant systemic side effects.

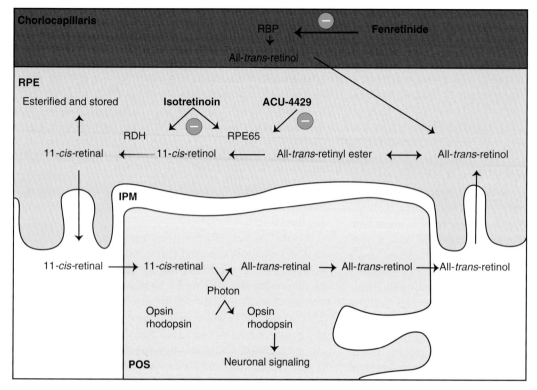

Figure 25.2 ■ A simplified diagram depicting the visual cycle and the regeneration of 11-*cis*-retinal. The sites of action of various therapies are included. RBP, retinol-binding protein; RPE, retinal pigment epithelium; RDH, retinol dehydrogenase; IPM, interphotoreceptor matrix.

Fenretinide

Fenretinide, also known as *N*-(4-hydroxyphenyl)retinamide, is a retinoid analog that has been used for systemic malignancies (2). It binds to RBP and competes with retinol (171). The binding of fenretinide–RBP prevents its association with transthyretin and leads to renal excretion of the complex (172). Treatment in mouse models of Stargardt disease slowed the accumulation of A2E and its precursors and led to delays in dark adaptation (155). In patients treated for systemic malignancy, there was a reversible and transient decrease in serum retinol and RBP, delayed dark adaptation, and reduced scotopic ERG (173,174).

Fenretinide was tested in a 24-month, double-masked, placebo-controlled, prospective phase II study involving 246 patients with GA (175). Patients received daily fenretinide (100 or 300 mg) or placebo. A reduction of RBP of 60% (achieved in 43% of those treated with 300 mg) experienced a lesion growth of 30%, as compared to 50% in the placebo group. In those who experienced less lesion growth, vision loss was six letters as compared to 11 in the placebo group. Rates of CNV were lower in the fenretinide groups (13%–14%) versus placebo (22%).

ACU-4429

ACU-4429 is a nonretinoid molecule that inhibits RPE65, slows the visual cycle in the rods, and decreases the accumulation of A2E. Phase I studies have been completed

(158). Adverse effects were not uncommon, as 50% experienced a dose dependent but transient and reversible visual change (dyschromatopsia, nyctalopia, blurred vision, or photophobia), but none of the adverse effects were serious. Mildly abnormal dark adaptation did occur, but cone responses were unchanged. A placebo-controlled phase II study is ongoing (176). Estimated enrollment is 84 patients, and patients are given one of several doses daily for 90 days. The primary outcome measure is safety, and serum drug levels are being checked.

■ OXIDATIVE STRESS

ROS include free radicals, hydrogen peroxide, and singlet oxygen (1,3). Free radicals contain one or more unpaired electrons, and hydrogen peroxide and singlet oxygen are unstable molecules. All of these compounds damage carbohydrates, membrane lipids, proteins, and nucleic acids. ROS are increased in the setting of irradiation, aging, inflammation, high oxygen tension, air pollutants, cigarette smoke, and reperfusion injury (177). The body has several ways of protecting from ROS-induced damage, including compartmentalization of the ROS, antioxidant enzymes, antioxidant vitamins, and others.

The retina is prone to oxidative damage (178). There are high levels of irradiation exposure, large amounts of oxygen consumption, and photosensitive chemical buildup (3).

The photoreceptor outer segments are rich in polyunsaturated fatty acids, which are easily oxidized (179), and phagocytosis by the RPE generates ROS (180). Lipofuscin is derived from photoreceptor outer segments and is more concentrated in the posterior pole (181). It is a photosensitizer, leading to oxidative damage, and impairs the RPE lysosomal functions, further leading to buildup of cellular debris. Blue light generates ROS within lipofuscin (182). The above mechanisms are more prominent with age and in the macula (183).

Animal models have confirmed the role of oxidative stress in retinal disease. Blue light exposure damages photoreceptors, causes cellular proliferation, and RPE loss in monkey retinas, resembling atrophic AMD (184). Mutated superoxide dismutase predisposes to light-induced retinal damage in mice (185). Oxidative stress has been linked with complement activation. CFH, an alternative pathway inhibitor, is down-regulated by peroxide treatment of cells (186). In vitro studies showed that photoactivation of bisretinoid-laden RPE activated the alternative pathway and led to complement deposition (13). Blue light exposure in rats has led to the deposition of complement components, microglia, and inflammatory cells in the retina (187).

In humans, oxidative damage and excessive light have been linked to the progression and severity of AMD (188). Excessive light has been linked to photoreceptor damage through the generation of ROS and lipid peroxidation of retinal tissues (189). Oxidized lipids have been demonstrated in drusen (6). The ability of the RPE to protect from light-induced damage declines with age (190).

Iron

Iron has a role in oxidative stress. In addition to AMD, it has been implicated in other age-related conditions including AD and Parkinson's disease (191), and iron chelation may help the treatment of these disorders (192). Iron, in its ferrous state (Fe^{2+}), reacts with hydrogen peroxide to generate ROS that damage cellular proteins, lipids, and nucleic acids (193). Light irradiation causes iron release from ferritin, generating Fe^{2+} (188). Rats treated with deferoxamine, an iron chelator, may be protected against photic injury (194). Iron has several other roles in the eye. It is a component of the RPE65 enzyme, a cofactor for generation of photoreceptor outer segments and a cofactor for an enzyme necessary for steps in phototransduction (193). Iron may contribute to the loss of photoreceptors seen in subretinal hemorrhages (195). In animal models, iron chelation may help prevent this degeneration (Youssef TA et al. *IOVS* 2002;43:ARVO E-Abstract 3000). Hereditary disorders of iron overload exhibit retinal degeneration (196). Iron levels have been found to be increased in the RPE and photoreceptors of AMD patients, as compared to age-matched controls (197). Iron may also activate the complement cascade (198).

NtBHA

NtBHA is an antioxidant that has been shown to have protective effects against iron-induced mitochondrial damage (199). In cultured RPE cells, it can delay mitochondrial loss, reduce oxidizing substances and oxidative stress, increase the antioxidant glutathione, and decrease iron accumulation and its storage protein ferritin (200). It may restore some mitochondrial function in iron-overloaded RPE cells.

TEMPOL and OT-551

TEMPOL (4-hydroxy-2,2,6,6-tetramethylpiperidine-*N*-oxyl) is an antioxidant that may be protective in disorders involving ROS, such as ischemic stroke, cardiac reperfusion injury, and Parkinson's disease (201). TEMPOL and its derivative, TEMPOL-H, have superoxide dismutase and ferroxidase-like activity (188). TEMPOL also has anti-inflammatory activity (202). TEMPOL-H is able to penetrate into posterior segment of the eye and may quench singlet oxygen. TEMPOL and TEMPOL-H protect against retinal ganglion cell damage in iron-loaded optic nerve crush models in vivo (203). In vitro studies have shown that TEMPOL-H suppresses short wavelength light-induced oxidative cell damage in lipofuscin-laden RPE cells, and it reduces A2E photooxidation (204). OT-551 is a hydroxylamine antioxidant that is converted by esterases to TEMPOL-H (188,202). Systemically administered OT-551 in rats protects photoreceptors from light-induced damage (188). It improved ERG amplitudes and outer nuclear layer thickness, and lowered oxidative end products in rats after intensive light exposure, as compared to controls. Similarly, systemic OT-551 preserved more RPE cell nuclei as compared to controls after oxidative stress (202).

OT-551 was evaluated in ten patients with bilateral GA, with one eye receiving topical OT-551 0.45% and the other as a control (178). At the 2-year end point, results were promising, as treated eyes had a significantly lower decrease in VA, and the proportion of patients losing ≥5, 10, and 15 letters was lower in the treated eyes. Scotoma size, retinal sensitivity, and change in drusen area did not differ significantly. OT-551 was evaluated in a larger phase II study for patients with GA (Sternberg et al. IOVS 2010;51:ARVO E-Abstract 6416). In a randomized, double-masked, placebo-controlled study, it was given topically for 24 months at one of two doses (0.3% and 0.45%). Forty-four of the 137 patients finished the 24 month end point at the time of study termination. The increase in size of GA from baseline to month 18 was not statistically different between the treated and placebo groups. The change in VA and percentage of subjects losing ≥15 letters at month 18 was also not different. Thus, although topically administered OT-551 was safe and well tolerated, it did not slow GA progression or maintain VA.

5-HT1A agonists

AL-8309A is a potent serotonin 5-HT1A agonist, a class of compounds that have been found to be protective in animal models of CNS ischemia and traumatic brain injury (205). This compound also provides structural and functional protection against blue light–induced retinal damage in rats, as topical pretreatment decreased microglial and T-lymphocyte activation and migration into the retina (187). The deposition of alternative complement components was nearly completely inhibited. Up-regulation of antioxidant enzymes and other antiapoptotic proteins occurred. The HCl salt of this compound, AL-8309B, is being evaluated in the treatment of GA in a phase III study (206). Five hundred and fifty patients were randomized to topically administered AL-8309B at doses of 1.75% or 1.0% or the vehicle given twice daily. Patients are treated for 24 months, and the outcome measures include VA and growth of the GA.

◼ OTHER PATHWAYS

RNA-144101

Toll-like receptors (TLRs) are a family of membrane receptors that are expressed in ocular tissues and, when activated, induce the secretion of proinflammatory cytokines and angiogenic factors (207). The presence of TLR3 in CNV membranes was evaluated by Maloney et al. (208). Immunostaining on eight AMD patients and four controls without CNV revealed that TLR3 was found in all CNV membranes and was expressed in the RPE but was not seen in the posterior pole of three of the four controls. TLR3 may also contribute to GA, as this pathway triggers caspase-3–mediated apoptosis of the RPE (209). SiRNAs have been developed that suppress angiogenesis through the TLR3 pathway (210). RNA-144101 is a siRNA targeted against TLR3. A phase I study is under way to evaluate its safety, tolerability, and dosing when administered intravitreally in patients with GA (211).

Vasodilators

Studies have suggested that impaired choroidal perfusion may play a role in AMD. Some have hypothesized that the accumulation of hydrophobic lipids in Bruch's membrane decreases perfusion, resulting in deposition of protein and lipids and decreasing the permeability of nutrients and waste products (212). The choriocapillaris may be maintained by factors secreted by the RPE, and the diffusion of these factors may be limited by a thickened Bruch's membrane. Regulation of choroidal blood flow may be abnormal in patients with CNV, as pericytes within the CNV may exhibit altered contraction capabilities (213).

In a recent study of dry AMD, there was an association between increased drusen extent and decreased choroidal blood flow (214). Color Doppler (215) and indocyanine green angiography (216) studies revealed perfusion defects in aged

and AMD eyes. Piguet et al. (217) found that prolonged choroidal filling was associated with vision loss. In eyes with prolonged choroidal filling, 38% lost two lines at 2 years, as compared to 14% of eyes with normal choroidal filling. Chen et al. (218) found that patients with and without abnormal choroidal perfusion were identical in VA and fundus appearance. It is unknown if choroidal filling defects are the primary cause or secondary to the disease process in AMD and that hypofluorescence may be due to abnormal staining or permeability of Bruch's membrane, not choroidal ischemia (212).

Prostaglandin E1 (PGE1) is used for limb ischemia by enhancing blood flow (219). It has been noted that patients receiving PGE1 infusions for peripheral arterial disease reported spontaneous improvements in vision. One study revealed improvements in visual function and foveal sensitivity in patients with AMD receiving intravenous PGE1 for 3 to 5 weeks (220). Another study found that 6-month therapy with PGE1 showed a mild improvement of vision relative to controls in 11 patients. A phase III study of PGE1 (Alprostadil) for dry AMD revealed no difference between PGE1 and control groups at 3 months, but this study was terminated early (221).

Trimetazidine (TMZ) is an anti-ischemic agent used in Europe for angina pectoris, VA and visual field loss due to presumed vascular causes, vertigo and tinnitus (222). Ischemic retinal injury is mediated in part by the excitatory neurotransmitter glutamate, a potent neurotoxin (223). In animal models, TMZ can decrease damage from retinal ischemic injury (224) and inhibit the buildup of glutamate (223). TMZ was evaluated for patients at high risk of advanced AMD in a phase III, prospective, double-blinded, randomized, placebo-controlled trial (222). Seven hundred and twelve patients completed the 3 years of follow-up. Thirty-three percent of patients in both treatment groups (TMZ and placebo) developed CNV. The incidence of GA nonsignificantly favored the TMZ group.

SUMMARY

In summary, several different pathways, including chronic inflammation, complement deposition, oxidative stress, angiogenesis, and visual cycle toxic by-products, have been associated with the development and progression of AMD. Several therapies are being investigated in ongoing clinical trials, and additional therapies are in preclinical testing, and new, unrecognized pathways may also become apparent. We are likely going to see new medications become available for both dry and exudative AMD in the near future.

REFERENCES

1. Zampros I, Praidou A, Brazitikos P, et al. Antivascular endothelial growth factor agents for neovascular age-related macular degeneration. J Ophthalmol. 2012; 319728:2012.

2. Travis GH, Golczak M, Moise AR, et al. Diseases caused by defects in the visual cycle: retinoids as potential therapeutic agents. Annu Rev Pharmacol Toxicol. 2007;47:469–512.

3. Beatty S, Koh HH, Phil M, et al. The role of oxidative stress in the pathogenesis of age-related macular degeneration. Surv Ophthalmol. 2000;45:115–134.

4. Wang Y, Wang VM, Chan CC. The role of anti-inflammatory agents in age-related macular degeneration (AMD) treatment. Eye (Lond). 2011;25:127–139.

5. Khandhadia S, Cipriani V, Yates JRW, et al. Age-related macular degeneration and the complement system. Immunobiology. 2012;217:127–146.

6. Crabb JW, Miyagi M, Gu X, et al. Drusen proteome analysis: an approach to the etiology of age-related macular degeneration. Proc Natl Acad Sci U S A. 2002; 99:14682–14687.

7. Johnson LV, Leitner WP, Rivest AJ, et al. The Alzheimer's Aβ-peptide is deposited at sites of complement activation in pathologic deposits associated with aging and age-related macular degeneration. Proc Natl Acad Sci U S A. 2002;99:11830–11835.

8. Dastgheib K, Green WR. Granulomatous reaction to Bruch's membrane in age-related macular degeneration. Arch Ophthalmol. 1994;112:813–818.

9. Baudouin C, Peyman GA, Fredj-Reygrobellet D, et al. Immunohistological study of subretinal membranes in age-related macular degeneration. Jpn J Ophthalmol. 1992;36:443–451.

10. Liu B, Faia L, Hu M, et al. Pro-angiogenic effect of IFNγ is dependent on the PI3K/mTOR/translational pathway in human retinal pigmented epithelial cells. Mol Vis. 2010;16:184–193.

11. Kim YH, He S, Kase S, et al. Regulated secretion of complement factor H by RPE and its role in RPE migration. Graefes Arch Clin Exp Ophthalmol. 2009;247:651–659.

12. Anderson DH, Talaga KC, Rivest AJ, et al. Characterization of β amyloid assemblies in drusen: the deposits associated with aging and age-related macular degeneration. Exp Eye Res. 2004;78:243–256.

13. Zhou J, Kim SR, Westlund BS, et al. Complement activation by bisretinoid constituents of RPE lipofuscin. Invest Ophthalmol Vis Sci. 2009;50:1392–1399.

14. McGeer PL, McGeer EG. Inflammation and the degenerative diseases of aging. Ann N Y Acad Sci. 2004;1035:104–116.

15. Morohoshi K, Goodwin AM, Ohbayashi M, et al. Autoimmunity in retinal degeneration: autoimmune retinopathy and age-related macular degeneration. J Autoimmun. 2009;33:247–254.

16. Seddon JM, Gensler G, Milton RC, et al. Association between C-reactive protein and age-related macular degeneration. JAMA. 2004;291:704–710.

17. Oh H, Takagi H, Takagi C, et al. The potential angiogenic role of macrophages in the formation of choroidal neovascular membranes. Invest Ophthalmol Vis Sci. 1999;40:1891–1898.

18. Gupta N, Brown KE, Milam AH. Activated microglia in human retinitis pigmentosa, late-onset retinal degeneration, and age-related macular degeneration. Exp Eye Res. 2003;76:463–471.

19. Geiger K, Howes E, Gallina M, et al. Transgenic mice expressing IFN-gamma in the retina develop inflammation of the eye and photoreceptor loss. Invest Ophthalmol Vis Sci. 1994;35:2667–2681.

20. Kim SJ, Flach AJ, Jampol LM. Nonsteroidal anti-inflammatory drugs in ophthalmology. Surv Ophthalmol. 2010;55:108–133.

21. Maloney SC, Fernandes BF, Castiglione E, et al. Expression of cyclooxygenase-2 in choroidal neovascular membranes from age-related macular degeneration patients. Retina. 2009;29:176–180.

22. Zweifel SA, Engelbert M, Khan S, et al. Retrospective review of the efficacy of topical bromfenac (0.09%) as an adjunctive therapy for patients with neovascular age-related macular degeneration. Retina. 2009;29:1527–15231.

23. Chen E, Benz MS, Fish RH, et al. Use of nepafenac (Nevanac®) in combination with intravitreal anti-VEGF agents in the treatment of recalcitrant exudative macular degeneration requiring monthly injections. Clin Ophthalmol. 2010;4:1249–1252.

24. Boyer DS, Beer PM, Joffe L, et al. Effect of adjunctive diclofenac with verteporfin therapy to treat choroidal neovascularization due to age-related macular degeneration: phase II study. Retina. 2007;27:693–700.

25. Kim SJ, Toma HS. Inhibition of choroidal neovascularization by intravitreal ketorolac. Arch Ophthalmol. 2010;128:596–600.

26. Baranano DE, Kim SJ, Edelhauser HF, et al. Efficacy and pharmacokinetics of intravitreal non-steroidal anti-inflammatory drugs for intraocular inflammation. Br J Ophthalmol. 2009;93:1387–1390.

27. Soheilian M, Karimi S, Ramezani A, et al. Pilot study of intravitreal injection of diclofenac for treatment of macular edema of various etiologies. Retina. 2010;30:509–515.

28. Jermak CM, Dellacroce JT, Heffez J, et al. Triamcinolone acetonide in ocular therapeutics. Surv Ophthalmol. 2007;52:503–522.

29. Wang YS, Friedrichs U, Eichler W, et al. Inhibitor effects of triamcinolone acetonide on bFGF-induced migration and tube formation in choroidal microvascular endothelial cells. Graefes Arch Clin Exp Ophthalmol. 2002;240:42–48.

30. Fluocinolone acetonide intravitreal inserts in geographic atrophy. Available at: http://clinicaltrials.gov/ct2/show/NCT00695318. Accessed January 17, 2012.

31. The MAP study: fluocinolone acetonide (FA)/Medidur (TM) for age related macular degeneration (AMD) pilot. Available at: http://clinicaltrials.gov/ct2/show/NCT00605423. Accessed January 17, 2012.

32. Kurup SK, Gee C, Greven CM. Intravitreal methotrexate in therapeutically resistant exudative age-related macular degeneration. Acta Ophthalmol. 2010; 88:e145–e146.

33. Lichtlen P, Lam TT, Nork TM, et al. Relative contribution of VEGF and TNF-alpha in the cynomolgus laser-induced CNV model: comparing the efficacy of bevacizumab, adalimumab and ESBA105. Invest Ophthalmol Vis Sci. 2010; 51:4738–4745.

34. Theodossiadis PG, Liarakos VS, Sfikakis PP, et al. Intravitreal administration of the anti-tumor necrosis factor agent infliximab for neovascular age-related macular degeneration. Am J Ophthalmol. 2009;147:825–830.

35. Nussenblatt RB, Byrnes G, Sen N, et al. A randomized pilot study of systemic immunosuppression in the treatment of age-related macular degeneration with choroidal neovascularization. Retina. 2010;30:1579–1587.

36. Giganti M, Beer PM, Lemanski N, et al. Adverse events after intravitreal infliximab (Remicade). Retina. 2010;30:71–80.

37. Arias L, Caminal JM, Badia MB, et al. Intravitreal infliximab in patients with macular degeneration who are nonresponders to antivascular endothelial growth factor therapy. Retina. 2010;30:1601–1608.

38. Intravitreal adalimumab in patients with choroidal neovascularization secondary to age-related macular degeneration. Available at: http://clinicaltrials.gov/ct2/show/NCT01136252. Accessed January 17, 2012.

39. Chen Y, Wang J, Cai J, et al. Altered mTOR signaling in senescent retinal pigment epithelium. Invest Ophthalmol Vis Sci. 2010;51:5314–5319.

40. Harrison DE, Strong R, Sharp ZD, et al. Rapamycin fed late in life extends life span in genetically heterogeneous mice. Nature. 2009;460:392–395.

41. Ghayad SE, Cohen PA. Inhibitors of the PI3K/Akt/mTOR pathway: new hope for breast cancer patients. Recent Pat Anticancer Drug Discov. 2010;5:29–57.

42. Zhao C, Vollrath D. mTOR pathway activation in age-related retinal disease. Aging. 2011;3:346–347.

43. Lee DF, Hung MC. All roads lead to mTOR: integrating inflammation and tumor angiogenesis. Cell Cycle. 2007;6:3011–3014.

44. Dejneka NS, Kuroki AM, Fosnot J, et al. Systemic rapamycin inhibits retinal and choroidal neovascularization in mice. Mol Vis. 2004;10:964–972.

45. Stahl A, Paschek L, Martin G, et al. Rapamycin reduces VEGF expression in retinal pigment epithelium (RPE) and inhibits RPE-induced sprouting angiogenesis in vitro. FEBS Lett. 2008;582:3097–3102.

46. Dugel PU, Blumenkranz MS, Haller JA, et al. A randomized, dose-escalation study of subconjunctival and intravitreal injections of sirolimus in patients with diabetic macular edema. Ophthalmology. 2012;119:124–131.

47. Sirolimus to treat geographic atrophy associated with age-related macular degeneration. Available at: http://clinicaltrials.gov/ct2/show/NCT00766649. Accessed January 21, 2012.

48. Sirolimus for advanced age-related macular degeneration. Available at: http://clinicaltrials.gov/ct2/show/NCT01445548. Accessed January 21, 2012.

49. Palomid 529 in patients with neovascular age-related macular degeneration. Available at: http://clinicaltrials.gov/ct2/show/NCT01271270. Accessed January 21, 2012.

50. Qi X, Hopkins B, Perruzzi C, et al. Palomid 529, a novel small-molecule drug, is a TORC1/TORC2 inhibitor that reduces tumor growth, tumor angiogenesis, and vascular permeability. Cancer Res. 2008;68:9551–9557.

51. Phase I study of Palomid 529 a dual TORC1/2 inhibitor of the PI3K/Akt/mTOR pathway for advanced neovascular age-related macular degeneration (P52901). Available at: http://clinicaltrials.gov/ct2/show/NCT01033721. Accessed January 21, 2012.

52. Gehrs KM, Jackson JR, Brown EN, et al. Complement, age-related macular degeneration and a vision for the future. Arch Ophthalmol. 2010;128:349–358.

53. Kew RR, Ghebrehiwet B, Janoff A. Cigarette smoke can activate the alternative pathway of complement in vitro by modifying the third component of complement. J Clin Invest. 1985;75:1000–1007.

54. Markiewski MM, Lambris JD. The role of complement in inflammatory diseases from behind the scenes into the spotlight. Am J Pathol. 2007;171:715–727.

55. Nozaki M, Raisler BJ, Sakurai E, et al. Drusen complement components C3a and C5a promote choroidal neovascularization. Proc Natl Acad Sci U S A. 2006;103:2328–2333.

56. Johnson LV, Ozaki S, Staples MK, et al. A potential role for immune complex pathogenesis in drusen formation. Exp Eye Res. 2000;70:441–449.

57. Johnson LV, Leitner WP, Staples MK, et al. Complement activation and inflammatory processes in drusen formation and age-related macular degeneration. Exp Eye Res. 2001;73:887–896.

58. Hageman GS, Anderson DH, Johnson LV, et al. A common haplotype in the complement regulatory gene factor H (HF1/CFH) predisposes individuals to age-related macular degeneration. Proc Natl Acad Sci. 2005;102:7227–7232.

59. Gold B. Variation in factor B (BF) and complement component 2 (C2) genes is associated with age-related macular degeneration. Nat Genet. 2006;38:458–462.

60. Montes T, Tortajada A, Morgan BP, et al. Functional basis of protection against age-related macular degeneration conferred by a common polymorphism in complement factor B. Proc Natl Acad Sci. 2009;106:4366–4371.

61. Thakkinstian A, McKay GJ, McEvoy M, et al. Systematic review and meta-analysis of the association between complement component 3 and age-related macular degeneration: a HuGE review and meta-analysis. Am J Epidemiol. 2011;173:1365–1379.

62. Thakkinstian A, Han P, McEvoy M, et al. Systematic review and meta-analysis of the association between complement factor H Y402H polymorphisms and age-related macular degeneration. Hum Mol Genet. 2006;15:2784–2790.

63. Cashman SM, Desai A, Ramo K, et al. Expression of complement component 3 (c3) from an adenovirus leads to pathology in the murine retina. Invest Ophthalmol Vis Sci. 2011;52:3436–3445.

64. Bora PS, Sohn JH, Cruz JM, et al. Role of complement and complement membrane attack complex in laser-induced choroidal neovascularization. J Immunol. 2005;174:491–497.

65. Sivaprasad S, Adewoyin T, Bailey TA, et al. Estimation of systemic complement C3 activity in age-related macular degeneration. Arch Ophthalmol. 2007;125:515–519.

66. Chi ZL, Yoshida T, Lambris JD, et al. Suppression of drusen formation by compstatin, a peptide inhibitor of complement C3 activation, on cynomolgus monkey with early-onset macular degeneration. Adv Exp Med Biol. 2010;703:127–135.

67. Potentia: a clearer vision of the future. Available at: http://www.potentiapharma.com. Accessed January 7, 2012.

68. Evaluation of AL-78898A in exudative age-related macular degeneration (AMD). Available at: http://clinicaltrials.gov/ct2/show/NCT01157065. Accessed January 7, 2012.

69. Reynolds R, Hartnett ME, Atkinson JP, et al. Plasma complement components and activation fragments: associations with age-related macular degeneration genotypes and phenotypes. Invest Ophthalmol Vis Sci. 2009;50:5818–5827.

70. Parker C. Eculizumab for paroxysmal nocturnal haemoglobinuria. Lancet. 2009;373:759–767.

71. Complement inhibition with eculizumab for the treatment of non-exudative macular degeneration (AMD) (COMPLETE). Available at: http://clinicaltrials.gov/ct2/show/NCT00935883. Accessed January 7, 2012.

72. Mayer G, Jenne A. Aptamers in research and drug development. BioDrugs. 2004;18:351–359.

73. ARC1905 (Anti-C5 Aptamer) given either in combination therapy with Lucentis® 0.5 mg/eye in subjects with neovascular age-related macular degeneration. Available at: http://clinicaltrials.gov/ct2/show/NCT00709527. Accessed January 7, 2012.

74. A study of ARC1905 (anti-C5 aptamer) in subjects with dry age-related macular degeneration. Available at: http://clinicaltrials.gov/ct2/show/NCT00950638. Accessed January 7, 2012.

75. Schnatbaum K, Locardi E, Scharn D, et al. Peptidomimetic C5a receptor antagonists with hydrophobic substitutions at the C-terminus: increased receptor specificity and in vivo activity. Bioorg Med Chem Lett. 2006;16:5088–5092.

76. Rohrer B, Guo Y, Kunchithapautham K, et al. Eliminating complement factor D reduces photoreceptor susceptibility to light-induced damage. Invest Ophthalmol Vis Sci. 2007;48:5282–5289.

77. Stanton CM, Yates JR, den Hollander AI, et al. Complement factor D in age-related macular degeneration. Invest Ophthalmol Vis Sci. 2011;52:8828–8834.

78. Zeng J, Chen Y, Tong Z, et al. Lack of association of CFD polymorphisms with advanced age-related macular degeneration. Mol Vis. 2010;16:2273–2278.

79. A study of the safety, tolerability, pharmacokinetics, and immunogenicity of intravitreal injections of FCFD4514S in patients with geographic atrophy. Available at: http://clinicaltrials.gov/ct2/show/NCT00973011. Accessed January 2, 2012.

80. A study of safety, tolerability, and evidence of activity of FCFD4514S administered monthly or every other month to patients with geographic atrophy. Available at: http://clinicaltrials.gov/ct2/show/NCT01229215. Accessed January 7, 2012.

81. Ricklin D, Lambris JD. Complement-targeted therapeutics. Nat Biotechnol. 2007;25:1265–1275.

82. Chen M, Muckersie E, Robertson M, et al. Up-regulation of complement factor B in retinal pigment epithelial cells is accompanied by complement activation in the aged retina. Exp Eye Res. 2008;87:543–550.

83. Tailgen therapeutics: targeting complement. Controlling inflammation. Available at: http://www.ophthalmologysummit.com/presentations/Taligen.pdf. Accessed January 11, 2012.

84. Coffey PJ, Gias C, McDermott CJ, et al. Complement factor H deficiency in aged mice causes retinal abnormalities and visual dysfunction. Proc Natl Acad Sci U S A. 2007;104:16651–16656.

85. Lyzogubov VV, Tytarenko RG, Jha P, et al. Role of ocular complement factor H in a murine model of choroidal neovascularization. Am J Pathol. 2010;177:1870–1880.

86. Klein RJ, Zeiss C, Chew EY, et al. Complement factor H polymorphism in age-related macular degeneration. Science. 2005;308:385–389.

87. Deangelis MM, Ji F, Kim IK, et al. Cigarette smoking, CFH, APOE ELOVL4 and risk of neovascular age-related macular degeneration. Arch Ophthalmol. 2007;125:49–54.

88. Scholl HP, Charbel Issa P, Walier M, et al. Systemic complement activation in age-related macular degeneration. PLoS One. 2008;3:e2593.

89. Rohrer B, Long Q, Coughlin B, et al. A targeted inhibitor of the complement alternative pathway reduces RPE injury and angiogenesis in models of age-related macular degeneration. Adv Exp Med Biol. 2010;703:137–149.

90. Schmidt CQ, Slingsby FC, Richards A, et al. Production of biologically active complement factor H in therapeutically useful quantities. Protein Expr Purif. 2011;76:254–263.

91. Cashman SM, Ramo K, Kumar-Singh R. A non membrane-targeted human soluble CD59 attenuates choroidal neovascularization in a model of age related macular degeneration. PLoS One. 2011;6:e19078.

92. Hourcade DE. The role of properdin in the assembly of the alternative pathway C3 convertases of complement. J Biol Chem. 2006;281:2128–2132.

93. Mullins RF, Faidley EA, Daggett HT, et al. Localization of complement 1 inhibitor (C1INH/SERPING1) in human eyes with age-related macular degeneration. Exp Eye Res. 2009;89:767–773.

94. Swift AJ, Collins TS, Bugelski P, et al. Soluble human complement receptor type 1 inhibits complement-mediated host defense. Clin Diagn Lab Immunol. 1994;1:585–589.

95. Anderson DH, Mullins RF, Hageman GS, et al. A role for local inflammation in the formation of drusen in the aging eye. Am J Ophthalmol. 2002;134:411–431.

96. Vassar R, Bennett BD, Babu-Khan S, et al. Beta-secretase cleavage of Alzheimer's amyloid precursor protein by the transmembrane aspartic protease BACE. Science. 1999;286:735–741.

97. Iwata N, Tsubuki S, Takaki Y, et al. Metabolic regulation of brain Aβ by neprilysin. Science. 2001;292:1550–1552.

98. Alzheimer's disease & dementia guide. Available at: http://www.alz.org/alzheimers_disease_what_is_alzheimers.asp. Accessed December 17, 2011.

99. Ohno-Matsui K. Parallel findings in age-related macular degeneration and Alzheimer's disease. Prog Retin Eye Res. 2011;30:217–238.

100. Wyss-Coray T, Mucke L. Inflammation in neurodegenerative disease—a double edged sword. Neuron. 2002;35:419–432.

101. Dentchev T, Milam AH, Lee VM, et al. Amyloid-β is found in drusen from some age-related macular degeneration retinas, but not in drusen from normal retinas. Mol Vis. 2003;9:184–190.

102. Yoshida T, Ohno-Matsui K, Ichinose S, et al. The potential role amyloid β in the pathogenesis of age-related macular degeneration. J Clin Invest. 2005;115:2793–2800.

103. Walsh DT, Montero RM, Bresciani LG, et al. Amyloid-beta peptide is toxic to neurons in vivo via indirect mechanisms. Neurobiol Dis. 2002;10:20–27.

104. Grau S, Baldi A, Bussani R, et al. Implications of the serine protease HtrA1 in amyloid precursor protein processing. Proc Natl Acad Sci. 2005;102:6021–6026.

105. Tong Y, Liao J, Zhang Y, et al. LOC387715/HTRA1 gene polymorphisms and susceptibility to age-related macular degeneration: a HuGE review and meta-analysis. Mol Vis. 2010;16:1958–1981.

106. Klaver CC, Ott A, Hofman A, et al. Is age-related maculopathy associated with Alzheimer's disease? The Rotterdam Study. Am J Epidemiol. 1999;150:963–968.

107. Baker ML, Wang JJ, Rogers S, et al. Early age-related macular degeneration, cognitive function, and dementia: the Cardiovascular Health Study. Arch Ophthalmol. 2009;127:667–673.

108. Bradt BM, Kolb WP, Cooper NR. Complement-dependent proinflammatory properties of the Alzheimer's disease beta-peptide. J Exp Med. 1998;188:431–438.

109. Wang J, Ohno-Matsui K, Yoshida T, et al. Altered function of factor I caused by amyloid β: implication for pathogenesis of age-related macular degeneration from drusen. J Immunol. 2008;181:712–720.

110. Webster S, Lue LF, Brachova L, et al. Molecular and cellular characterization of the membrane attack complex, C5b-9, In Alzheimer's disease. Neurobiol Aging. 1997;18:415–421.

111. Wang J, Ohno-Matsui K, Yoshida T, et al. Amyloid-β up-regulates complement factor B in retinal pigment epithelial cells through cytokines released from recruited macrophages/microglia: another mechanism of complement activation in age-related macular degeneration. J Cell Physiol. 2009;220:119–128.

112. Hamilton G, Proitsi P, Williams J, et al. Complement factor H Y402H polymorphism is not associated with late-onset Alzheimer's disease. Neuromolecular Med. 2007;9:331–334.

113. Landa G, Butovsky O, Shoshani J, et al. Weekly vaccination with Copaxone (glatiramer acetate) as a potential therapy for dry age-related macular degeneration. Curr Eye Res. 2008;33:1011–1013.

114. Landa G, Rosen RB, Patel A, et al. Qualitative spectral OCT/SLO analysis of drusen change in dry age-related macular degeneration patients treated with Copaxone. J Ocul Pharmacol Ther. 2011;27:77–82.

115. Ding JD, Johnson LV, Hermann R, et al. Anti-amyloid therapy protects against retinal pigment epithelium damage and vision loss in a model of age-related macular degeneration. Proc Natl Acad Sci U S A. 2011;108:E279–E287.

116. Safety and tolerability study of RN6G in patients with dry, age-related macular degeneration. Available at: http://clinicaltrials.gov/ct2/show/NCT00877032. Accessed December 17, 2011.

117. Safety and tolerability study of RN6G in subjects with advanced dry, age-related macular degeneration including geographic atrophy. Available at: http://clinicaltrials.gov/ct2/show/NCT01003691. Accessed December 17, 2011.

118. Clinical study to investigate safety and efficacy of GSK933776 in adult patients with geographic atrophy secondary to age-related macular degeneration. Available at: http://clinicaltrials.gov/ct2/show/NCT01342926. Accessed January 28, 2012.

119. Yonekura H, Sakurai S, Liu X, et al. Placenta growth factor and vascular endothelial growth factor B and C expression in microvascular endothelial cells and pericytes. Implication in autocrine and paracrine regulation of angiogenesis. J Biol Chem. 1999;274:35172–35178.

120. Bergers G, Hanahan D. Modes of resistance to anti-angiogenic therapy. Nat Rev Cancer. 2008;8:592–603.

121. Ferrara N, Gerber HP, LeCouter J. The biology of VEGF and its receptors. Nat Med. 2003;9:669–676.

122. Yafai Y, Yang XM, Niemeyer M, et al. Anti-angiogenic effects of the receptor tyrosine kinase inhibitor, pazopanib, on choroidal neovascularization in rats. Eur J Pharmacol. 2011;666:12–18.

123. Dom AM, Buckley AW, Brown KC, et al. The α7-nicotinic acetylcholine receptor and MMP-2/-9 pathway mediate the proangiogenic effect of nicotine in human retinal endothelial cells. Invest Ophthalmol Vis Sci. 2011;52:4428–4438.

124. Umeda N, Kachi S, Akiyama H, et al. Suppression and regression of choroidal neovascularization by systemic administration of an α5β1 integrin antagonist. Mol Pharmacol. 2006;69:1820–1828.

125. Xie B, Shen J, Dong A, et al. Blockade of sphingosine-1-phosphate reduces macrophage influx and retinal and choroidal neovascularization. J Cell Physiol. 2009;218:192–198.

126. Reich SJ, Fosnot J, Kuroki A, et al. Small interfering RNA (siRNA) targeting VEGF effectively inhibits ocular neovascularization in a mouse model. Mol Vis. 2003;9:210–216.

127. Tolentino MJ, Brucker AJ, Fosnot J, et al. Intravitreal injection of vascular endothelial growth factor small interfering RNA inhibits growth and leakage in a nonhuman primate, laser-induced model of choroidal neovascularization. Retina. 2004;24:132–138.

128. Safety & efficacy study evaluating the combination of bevasiranib & Lucentis therapy in wet AMD (COBALT). Available at: http://clinicaltrials.gov/ct2/show/NCT00499590. Accessed January 24, 2012.

129. Jo N, Mailhos C, Ju M, et al. Inhibition of platelet-derived growth factor B signaling enhances the efficacy of anti-vascular endothelial growth factor therapy in multiple models of ocular neovascularization. Am J Pathol. 2006;168:2036–2053.

130. A phase 1, safety, tolerability and pharmacokinetic profile of intravitreous injections of E10030 (anti-PDGF pegylated aptamer) in subjects with neovascular age-related macular degeneration. Available at: http://clinicaltrials.gov/ct2/show/NCT00569140. Accessed January 24, 2012.

131. Inhibiting VEGF and PDGF to treat AMD. Available at: http://www.revophth.com/content/d/retinal_insider/c/29979/. Accessed January 28, 2012.

132. A safety and efficacy study of E10030 (anti-PDGF pegylated aptamer plus Lucentis for neovascular age-related macular degeneration. Available at: http://clinicaltrials.gov/ct2/show/NCT01089517. Accessed January 24, 2012.

133. Bergers G, Song S, Meyer-Morse N, et al. Benefits of targeting both pericytes and endothelial cells in the tumor vasculature with kinase inhibitors. J Clin Invest. 2003;111:1287–1295.

134. Kumar R, Knick VB, Rudolph SK, et al. Pharmacokinetic-pharmacodynamic correlation from mouse to human with pazopanib, a multikinase angiogenesis inhibitor with potent antitumor and antiangiogenic activity. Mol Cancer Ther. 2007;6:2012–2021.

135. Dose ranging study of pazopanib to treat neovascular age-related macular degeneration. Available at: http://clinicaltrials.gov/ct2/show/NCT01134055. Accessed January 24, 2012.

136. Doukas J, Mahesh S, Umeda N, et al. Topical administration of a multitargeted kinase inhibitor suppresses choroidal neovascularization and retinal edema. J Cell Physiol. 2008;216:29–37.

137. Ho AC, Regillo CD, eds. Age-related macular degeneration: diagnosis and treatment. New York: Springer; 2011.

138. Gerstner ER, Sorensen AG, Jain RK, et al. Anti-vascular endothelial growth factor therapy for malignant glioma. Curr Neurol Neurosci Rep. 2009;9:254–262.

139. Maier P, Unsoeld AS, Junker B, et al. Intravitreal injection of specific receptor tyrosine kinase inhibitor PTK787/ZK222 584 improves ischemia-induced retinopathy in mice. Graefes Arch Clin Exp Ophthalmol. 2005;243:593–600.

140. Safety and efficacy of oral PTK787 in patients with subfoveal choroidal neovascularization secondary to age-related macular degeneration (AMD) (ADVANCE). Available at: http://clinicaltrials.gov/ct2/show/NCT00138632. Accessed January 28, 2012.

141. Zahn G, Vossmeyer D, Stragies R, et al. Preclinical evaluation of the novel small-molecule integrin α-5-β-1 inhibitor JSM6427 in monkey and rabbit models of choroidal neovascularization. Arch Ophthalmol. 2009;127:1329–1335.

142. Wilson SH, Ljubimov AV, Morla AO, et al. Fibronectin fragments promote human retinal endothelial cell adhesion and proliferation and ERK activation through alpha5beta1 integrin and PI 3-kinase. Invest Ophthalmol Vis Sci. 2003;44:1704–1715.

143. A phase 1 safety study of single and repeated doses of JSM6427 (intravitreal injection) to treat AMD. Available at: http://clinicaltrials.gov/ct2/show/NCT00536016. Accessed January 28, 2012.

144. Ramakrishnan V, Bhaskar V, Law DA, et al. Preclinical evaluation of an anti-α5β1 integrin antibody as a novel anti-angiogenic agent. J Exp Ther Oncol. 2006;5:273–286.

145. A phase 1 ascending and parallel group trial to establish the safety, tolerability and pharmacokinetics profile of volociximab (alpha 5 beta 1 integrin antagonist) in subjects with neovascular age-related macular degeneration. Available at: http://clinicaltrials.gov/ct2/show/NCT00782093. Accessed January 28, 2012.

146. Safety study of iSONEP (sonepcizumab/LT1009) to treat neovascular age-related macular degeneration. Available at: http://clinicaltrials.gov/ct2/show/NCT00767949. Accessed January 28, 2012.

147. iSONEP to treat persistent pigment epithelial detachment (PED) in subjects with exudative age-related macular degeneration (AMD) or polypoidal choroidal vasculopathy (PCV). Available at: http://clinicaltrials.gov/ct2/show/NCT01334255. Accessed January 28, 2012.

148. Efficacy and safety study of iSONEP with and without Lucentis/Avastin to treat age-related macular degeneration (AMD) (Nexus). Available at: http://clinicaltrials.gov/ct2/show/NCT01414153. Accessed January 28, 2012.

149. Ni Z, Hui P. Emerging pharmacologic therapies for wet age-related macular degeneration. Ophthalmologica. 2009;223:401–410.

150. Safety and efficacy of ATG003 in patients with wet age-related macular degeneration (AMD). Available at: http://clinicaltrials.gov/ct2/show/NCT00414206. Accessed January 28, 2012.

151. Safety and efficacy of ATG003 in patients with AMD receiving anti-VEGF. Available at: http://clinicaltrials.gov/ct2/show/NCT00607750. Accessed January 28, 2012.

152. Mochimaru M, Nagai N, Hasegawa G, et al. Suppression of choroidal neovascularization by dendritic cell vaccination targeting VEGFR2. Invest Ophthalmol Vis Sci. 2007;48:4795–4801.

153. Li Y, Wang MN, Li H, et al. Active immunization against the VEGF receptor flk1 inhibits tumor angiogenesis and metastasis. J Exp Med. 2002;195:1575–1584.

154. Anti-VEGFR vaccine therapy in treating patients with neovascular maculopathy. Available at: http://clinicaltrials.gov/ct2/show/NCT00791570. Accessed January 28, 2012.

155. Radu RA, Han Y, Bui TV, et al. Reductions in serum vitamin A arrest accumulation of toxic retinal fluorophores: a potential therapy for treatment of lipofuscin-based retinal diseases. Invest Ophthalmol Vis Sci. 2005;46:4393–4401.

156. Feeney-Burns L, Eldred GE. The fate of the phagosome: conversion to "age pigment" and impact on human retinal pigment epithelium. Trans Ophthalmol Soc U K. 1984;103:416.

157. Sakai N, Decatur J, Nakanishi K, et al. Ocular age pigment A2E: an unprecedented pyridinium bisretinoid. J Am Chem Soc. 1996;118:1559–1560.

158. Kubota R, Boman NL, David R, et al. Safety and effect on rod function of ACU-4429, a novel small-molecule visual cycle modulator. Retina. 2012;32:183–188.

159. Katz ML, Redmond TM. Effect of RPE65 knockout on accumulation of lipofuscin fluorophores in the retinal pigment epithelium. Invest Ophthalmol Vis Sci. 2001;42:3023–3030.

160. Finnemann SC, Leung LW, Rodriguez-Boulan E. The lipofuscin component A2E selectively inhibits phagolysosomal degradation of photoreceptor phospholipid by the retinal pigment epithelium. Proc Natl Acad Sci U S A. 2002;99:3842–3847.

161. Sparrow JR, Cai B. Blue light-induced apoptosis of A2E-containing RPE: involvement of caspase-3 and protection by Bcl-2. Invest Ophthalmol Vis Sci. 2001;42:1356–1362.

162. De S, Sakmar TP. Interaction of A2E with model membranes. Implications to the pathogenesis of age-related macular degeneration. J Gen Physiol. 2002;120:147–157.

163. Sparrow JR, Vollmer-Snarr HR, Zhou J, et al. A2E-epoxides damage DNA in retinal pigment epithelial cells. Vitamin E and other antioxidants inhibit A2E-epoxide formation. J Biol Chem. 2003;278:18207–18213.

164. Sparrow JR, Zhou J, Ben-Shabat S, et al. Involvement of oxidative mechanisms in blue light induced damage to A2E-laden RPE. Invest Ophthalmol Vis Sci. 2002;43:1222–1227.

165. Dorey CK, Wu G, Ebenstein D, et al. Cell loss in the aging retina: relationship to lipofuscin accumulation and macular degeneration. Invest Ophthalmol Vis Sci. 1989;30:1691–1699.

166. Holz FG, Bellman C, Staudt S, et al. Fundus autofluorescence and development of geographic atrophy in age-related macular degeneration. Invest Ophthalmol Vis Sci. 2001;42:1051–1056.

167. Katz ML, Norberg M. Influence of dietary vitamin A on autofluorescence of leupeptin induced inclusions in the retinal pigment epithelium. Exp Eye Res. 1992;54:239–246.

168. Sieving PA, Chaudhry P, Kondo M, et al. Inhibition of the visual cycle in vivo by 13-*cis* retinoic acid protects from light damage and provides a mechanism for night blindness in isotretinoin therapy. Proc Natl Acad Sci U S A. 2001;98:1835–1840.

169. Radu RA, Mata NL, Nusinowitz S, et al. Treatment with isotretinoin inhibits lipofuscin accumulation in a mouse model of recessive Stargardt's macular degeneration. Proc Natl Acad Sci U S A. 2003;100:4742–4747.

170. Weleber RG, Denman ST, Hanifin JM, et al. Abnormal retinal function associated with isotretinoin therapy for acne. Arch Ophthalmol. 1986;104:831–837.

171. Berni R, Formelli F. In vitro interaction of fenretinide with plasma retinol-binding protein and its functional consequences. FEBS Lett. 1992;308:43–45.

172. Noy N, Xu ZJ. Interactions of retinol with binding proteins: implications for the mechanism for uptake by cells. Biochemistry. 1990;29:3878–3883.

173. Kaiser-Kupfer MI, Peck GL, Caruso RC, et al. Abnormal retinal function associated with fenretinide, a synthetic retinoid. Arch Ophthalmol. 1986;104:69–70.

174. Torrisi R, Parodi S, Fontana V, et al. Factors affecting plasma retinol decline during long-term administration of the synthetic retinoid fenretinide in breast cancer patients. Cancer Epidemiol Biomarkers Prev. 1994;3:507–510.

175. Phase 2b data suggest ReVision's oral fenretinide (RT-101) slows lesion growth, preserves vision and reduces incidence of neovascularization in geographic atrophy patients. Available at: http://www.pipelinereview.com/index.php/2010101837764/Other-Disease-Areas/Phase-2b-Data-Suggest-ReVisions-Oral-Fenretinide-RT-101-Slows-Lesion-Growth-Preserves-Vision-and-Reduces-Incidence-of-Neovascularization-in-Geographic-Atrophy-Patients.html. Accessed December 29, 2011.

176. Study of the safety, tolerability, pharmacokinetics and pharmacodynamics of ACU-4429 in subjects with geographic atrophy. Available at: http://clinicaltrials.gov/ct2/show/NCT01002950. Accessed December 29, 2011.

177. Machlin LJ, Bendich A. Free radical tissue damage: protective role of antioxidant nutrients. FASEB J. 1987;1:441–445.

178. Wong WT, Kam W, Cunningham D, et al. Treatment of geographic atrophy by the topical administration of OT-551: results of a phase II clinical trial. Invest Ophthalmol Vis Sci. 2010;51:6131–6139.

179. Bazan NG. The metabolism of omega-3 polyunsaturated fatty acids in the eye: the possible role of docosahexaenoic acid and docosanoids in retinal physiology and ocular pathology. Prog Clin Biol Res. 1989;312:95–112.

180. Tate DJ Jr, Miceli MV, Newsome DA. Phagocytosis and H2O2 induce catalase and metallothionein gene expression in human retinal pigment epithelial cells. Invest Ophthalmol Vis Sci. 1995;36:1271–1279.

181. Kennedy CJ, Rakoczy PE, Constable IJ. Lipofuscin of the retinal pigment epithelium: a review. Eye (Lond). 1995;9:262–274.

182. Rozanowska M, Jarvis-Evans J, Korytowski W, et al. Blue light-induced reactivity of retinal age pigment. In vitro generation of oxygen-reactive species. J Biol Chem. 1995;270:18825–18830.

183. De La Paz M, Anderson RE. Region and age-dependent variation in susceptibility of the human retina to lipid peroxidation. Invest Ophthalmol Vis Sci. 1992;33:3497–3499.

184. Ham WT Jr, Ruffolo JJ Jr, Mueller HA, et al. Histologic analysis of photochemical lesions produced in rhesus retina by short-wave-length light. Invest Ophthalmol Vis Sci. 1978;17:1029–1035.

185. Mittag TW, Bayer AU, La VM. Light-induced retinal damage in mice carrying a mutated SOD 1 gene. Exp Eye Res. 1999;69:677–683.

186. Wu Z, Lauer TW, Sick A, et al. Oxidative stress modulates complement factor H expression in retinal pigmented epithelial cells by acetylation of FOXO3. J Biol Chem. 2007;282:22414–22425.

187. Collier RJ, Wang Y, Smith SS, et al. Complement deposition and microglial activation in the outer retina in light-induced retinopathy: inhibition by a 5-HT1A agonist. Invest Ophthalmol Vis Sci. 2011;52:8108–8116.

188. Tanito M, Li F, Elliott MH, et al. Protective effect of TEMPOL derivatives against light-induced retinal damage in rats. Invest Ophthalmol Vis Sci. 2007;48:1900–1905.

189. Wiegand RD, Giusto NM, Rapp LM, et al. Evidence for rod outer segment lipid peroxidation following constant illumination of the rat retina. Invest Ophthalmol Vis Sci. 1983;24:1433–1435.

190. Liang FQ, Godley BF. Oxidative stress-induced mitochondrial DNA damage in human retinal pigment epithelial cells: a possible mechanism for RPE aging and age-related macular degeneration. Exp Eye Res. 2003;76:397–403.

191. Perry G, Sayre LM, Atwood CS, et al. The role of iron and copper in the aetiology of neurodegenerative disorders: therapeutic implications. CNS Drugs. 2002;16:339–352.

192. Zheng H, Weiner LM, Bar-Am O, et al. Design, synthesis, and evaluation of novel bifunctional iron-chelators as potential agents for neuroprotection in Alzheimer's, Parkinson's, and other neurodegenerative diseases. Bioorg Med Chem. 2005;13:773–783.

193. Dunaief JL. Iron induced oxidative damage as a potential factor in age-related macular degeneration: The Cogan lecture. Invest Ophthalmol Vis Sci. 2006;47:4660–4664.

194. Li ZL, Lam S, Tso MO. Desferrioxamine ameliorates retinal photic injury in albino rats. Curr Eye Res. 1994;10:133–144.

195. Glatt H, Machemer R. Experimental subretinal hemorrhage in rabbits. Am J Ophthalmol. 1982;94:762–773.

196. Dunaief JL, Richa C, Franks EP, et al. Macular degeneration in a patient with aceruloplasminemia, a disease associated with retinal iron overload. Ophthalmology. 2005;112:1062–1065.

197. Hahn P, Milam AH, Dunaief JL. Maculas affected by age-related macular degeneration contain increased chelatable iron in the retinal pigment epithelium and Bruch's membrane. Arch Ophthalmol. 2003;121:1099–1105.

198. Vogi W, Nolte R, Brunahl D. Binding of iron to the 5th component of human complement directs oxygen radical-mediated conversion to specific sites and causes nonenzymatic activation. Complement Inflamm. 1991;8:313–319

199. Atamna H, Robinson C, Ingersoll R, et al. N-t-butyl hydroxylamine is an antioxidant that reverses age-related changes in mitochondria in vivo and in vitro. FASEB J. 2001;15:2196–2204.

200. Voloboueva LA, Killilea DW, Atamna H, et al. *N-tert*-butyl hydroxylamine, a mitochondrial antioxidant, protects human retinal pigment epithelial cells from iron overload: relevance to macular degeneration. FASEB J. 2007;21:4077–4086.

201. Liang Q, Smith AD, Pan S, et al. Neuroprotective effects of TEMPOL in central and peripheral nervous system models of Parkinson's disease. Biochem Pharmacol. 2005;70:1371–1381.

202. Tanito M, Li F, Anderson RE. Protection of retinal pigment epithelium by OT-551 and its metabolite TEMPOL-H against light-induced damage in rats. Exp Eye Res. 2010;91:111–114.

203. Thaler S, Fiedorowicz M, Rejdak R, et al. Neuroprotective effects of tempol on retinal ganglion cells in a partial optic nerve crush rat model with and without iron load. Exp Eye Res. 2010;90:254–260.

204. Zhou J, Jang YP, Chang S, et al. OT-674 suppresses photooxidative processes initiated by an RPE lipofuscin fluorophore. Photochem Photobiol. 2008;84:75–80.

205. Mauler F, Horvath E. Neuroprotective efficacy of repinotan HCl, a 5-HT1A receptor agonist, in animal models of stroke and traumatic brain injury. J Cereb Blood Flow Metab. 2005;25:451–459.

206. Geographic atrophy treatment evaluation (GATE). Available at: http://clinicaltrials.gov/ct2/show/NCT00890097. Accessed January 21, 2012.

207. Cho Y, Wang JJ, Chew EY, et al. Toll-like receptor polymorphisms and age-related macular degeneration: replication in three case–control samples. Invest Ophthalmol Vis Sci. 2009;50:5614–5618.

208. Maloney SC, Antecka E, Orellana ME, et al. Choroidal neovascular membranes express toll-like receptor 3. Ophthalmic Res. 2010;44:237–241.

209. Kleinman ME, Kaneko H, Cho WG, et al. Short-interfering RNAs induce retinal degeneration via TLR3 and IRF3. Mol Ther. 2012;20:101–108.

210. Kleinman ME, Yamada K, Takeda A, et al. Sequence- and target-independent angiogenesis suppression by siRNA via TLR3. Nature. 2008;452:591–597.

211. A phase I open label dose escalation trial of RNA-144101 in the treatment of geographic atrophy. Available at: http://clinicaltrials.gov/ct2/show/NCT01093170. Accessed January 28, 2012.

212. Staurenghi G, Bottoni F, Lonati C, et al. Drusen and "choroidal filling defects": a cross-sectional survey. Ophthalmologica. 1992;205:178–186.

213. Pournaras CJ, Logean E, Riva CE, et al. Regulation of subfoveal choroidal blood flow in age-related macular degeneration. Invest Ophthalmol Vis Sci. 2006;47:1581–1586.

214. Berenberg TL, Metelitsina TI, Madow B, et al. The association between drusen extent and foveolar choroidal blood flow in age-related macular degeneration. Retina. 2012;32:25–31.

215. Ciulla TA, Harris A, Chung HS, et al. Color Doppler imaging discloses reduced ocular blood flow velocities in non-exudative age-related macular degeneration. Am J Ophthalmol. 1999;128:75–80.

216. Ciulla TA, Harris A, Chung HS, et al. Choroidal perfusion perturbations in non-neovascular age-related macular degeneration. Br J Ophthalmol. 2002;86:209–213.

217. Piguet B, Palmvang IB, Chisholm IH, et al. Evolution of age-related macular degeneration with choroidal perfusion abnormality. Am J Ophthalmol. 1992;113:657–663.

218. Chen JC, Fitzke FW, Pauleikhoff D, et al. Functional loss in age-related Bruch's membrane change with choroidal perfusion defect. Invest Ophthalmol Vis Sci. 1992;33:334–340.

219. Ladewig MS, Ladewig K, Güner M, et al. Prostaglandin E1 infusion therapy in age-related macular degeneration. Prostaglandins Leukot Essent Fatty Acids. 2005;72:251–256.

220. Heidrich JP, Harnisch J, Ranft J. PGE1 in senile macular degeneration. A pilot study. Klin Monatsbl Augenheilkd. 1989;194:282–284.

221. Alprostadil in maculopathy study (AIMS). Available at: http://clinicaltrials.gov/ct2/show/NCT00619229. Accessed January 28, 2012.

222. Cohen SY, Bourgeois H, Corbe C, et al. Randomized clinical trial France DMLA2: effect of Trimetazidine on exudative and nonexudative age-related macular degeneration. Retina. 2012;32(4):834–843.

223. Payet O, D'Aldin C, Maurin L, et al. Anti-excitotoxic activity of trimetazidine in the retina. J Ocul Pharmacol Ther. 2004;20:85–92.

224. Mohand-Said S, Jacquet A, Lucien A, et al. Protective effect of trimetazidine in a model of ischemia-reperfusion in the rat retina. Ophthalmic Res. 2002;34:300–305.

26

ARTIFICIAL VISION, RETINAL IMPLANTS, AND IMPLANTABLE TELESCOPE

NANCY KUNJUKUNJU

Vision results from light transmission. Light is converted to electrical impulses that are then relayed to the brain. After traveling through the cornea and lens, light reaches the retina and the optic nerve and is converted to electrical energy. This energy is conducted intracranially through the lateral geniculate nucleus to the primary visual cortex in the occipital lobe. The information is subsequently transmitted to higher cortical areas of the brain, thus making the optic nerve and retina vital components of the pathway of light transmission.

According to a recent report by the World Health Organization, 285 million people are visually impaired worldwide, 39 million are blind, and 246 million have low vision (October 2011 Fact sheet WHO). Blindness, the inevitable result of irreparable damage to the visual pathway, is often a result of injury to either the neural retina or the optic nerve. Retinitis pigmentosa (RP) is a leading cause of inherited visual blindness, while age-related macular degeneration (AMD) is a leading cause of degenerative visual loss in the elderly.

Research is currently under way to offer patients suffering from visually debilitating diseases viable prosthetic options for visual rehabilitation. Approaches to visual rehabilitation involve electrical microstimulation of the visual cortex, the lateral geniculate nucleus, the optic nerve, and the retina to generate the impression of light or phosphenes. Beginning in the early 1900s, experiments in cortical stimulation were performed in attempt to assist the blind. For example, in 1929,

the German neurosurgeon Foerster observed that electrical stimulation of the cortex enabled his subject to detect a spot of light. This phenomenon of electrically induced light perception was defined as a phosphene (1).

In 1974, an electrode was used in a blind patient to stimulate the visual cortex to generate light perception (2). Experiments conducted by Dobelle et al. and Normann et al. (3–6) utilized either implanted surface electrodes or intracortical microelectrodes to excite the visual cortex. Over 50 electrodes were implanted over the occipital pole, and although some form of visual perception was obtained in the experiment, it was difficult to control the number of phosphenes induced by each electrode and the interaction between phosphenes. Furthermore, electrical stimulation was seen to cause an increase in the incidence of epileptic activity and to cause meningeal pain induced by high currents and large electrodes.

A contemporary form of the intracortical prosthesis, the Utah electrode array, consists of multiple silicon spikes. In testing of the array, the silicon tissue reaction ranges from none to gliosis and buildup of fibrotic tissue between the array and meninges (7). Recently, research was conducted to determine the feasibility of implanting a neural prosthesis in the lateral geniculate nucleus of the thalamus, which relays visual information from the retina to the visual cortex (8). Initial research demonstrated that electrical stimulation of the lateral geniculate body can generate neural responses in the visual pathway: electrical stimuli delivered to the thalamus engendered responses similar to those of when images are presented to the eye. Further research is currently under way.

Cortical prosthesis may bypass diseased visual pathway neurons rostral to the primary cortex and allow for visual restoration regardless of the insult to the eye. However, the organization of the visual field is more complex at the level of the primary cortex than at the level of the optic nerve or retina and may result in limited spatial resolution. Intracranial surgery also runs the risk of central nervous system (CNS) infection, epilepsy, and disturbance of blood flow to the optic nerve. Surgical complications carry significant morbidity and mortality risks for the patient.

Given the potential dangers of approaching artificial vision from the cortical approach, other groups have chosen to pursue an ocular prosthesis from within an eye possessing remaining viable tissue. Previous reports show that in spite of the level of vision loss in patients with RP, viable cells in the eye are able to transmit information with 30% of ganglion cells and 80% of inner nuclear layer cells that remain histologically intact after the death of photoreceptors (9). Investigations are ongoing in regard to a viable ocular prosthesis at the levels of suprachoroidal, subretinal, and epiretinal space by utilizing the preexisting signal processing network. This requires that sufficient bipolar cells or ganglion cells remain to elicit a response to electrical stimulation. In cortical prosthesis experiments, an array of electrodes is used to deliver an electrical current to the retina, thus stimulating functional retinal neurons to send signals to the visual cortex to be perceived as phosphenes (Fig. 26.1). In contrast to cortical electrodes, the use of preexisting signal processing network is expected to have higher visual resolution.

Sakaguchi and Tano et al. (10) investigated suprachoroidal transretinal stimulation in which an electrode was inserted into the suprachoroidal space to elicit electrical evoked potential (EEP). In the subretinal approach, explored by Chow et al. (11–13) and Zrenner et al. (14), lost photoreceptor function was replaced by a subretinal microphotodiode array (MPDA) that activated the remaining functioning retinal network. In the epiretinal approach, investigated by Eckmiller et al. (15), Humayun et al. (16,17), Rizzo et al. (18,19), and Walter et al. (20,21), devices stimulated the ganglion cells from the vitreous side of the retina.

SUPRACHOROIDAL–TRANSRETINAL STIMULATION

A new approach in artificial retina stimulation considers suprachoroidal–transretinal stimulation (STS) to elicit phosphenes. In 2010, STS implantation was shown to be safe and functional in two patients with advanced RP (22). This method involves insertion of a retinal prosthesis in the sclera pocket and placement of a reference electrode in the vitreous cavity. The device consists of a secondary coil that receives signals from an external coil and a decoder that generates pulses, which are then delivered to individual electrodes. The internal device was implanted under the skin of the temporal portion of the skull, and a 49-electrode array was implanted in the sclera pocket of one eye (Figs. 26.2 and 26.3).

Functional testing using head scanning revealed that the detection and discrimination of objects was possible with a small number of active electrodes. The resolution of the image with STS prosthesis may be lower because the electrodes

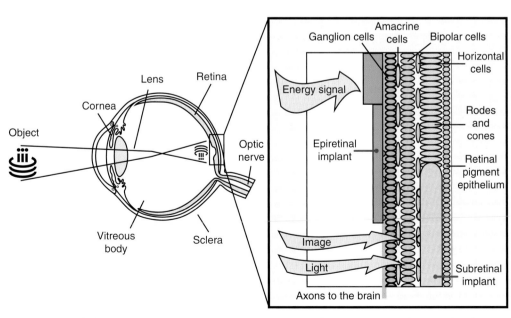

Figure 26.1 ■ Light is transmitted through the anterior segment of the eye to reach the posterior elements and reaches the electrodes at either the subretinal or epiretinal layer.

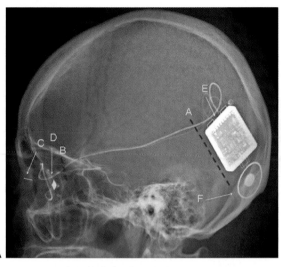
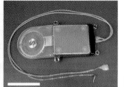

Figure 26.2 ■ Diagram of retinal prosthesis system. **A.** Lateral view of the skull XP of Pt 1 after implantation surgery. *A*, Position of skin incision to insert and anchor the device. *B*, Position of skin incision to fix the cable to the bone of the lateral orbital wall. *C*, Return electrode. *D*, Stimulating electrode. *E*, Decoder. *F*, Secondary coil. **B.** The implanted devices, cable, and electrodes. *Scale bar, 3 cm.* (Reprinted with permission from Fujikado T, Kamei M, Sakaguchi H. Testing of semichronically implanted retinal prosthesis by suprachoroidal-transretinal stimulation in patients with retinitis pigmentosa. Invest Ophthalmol Vis Sci. 2011;52(7):4726. Copyright 2011. The Association for Research in Vision and Ophthalmology, Inc.)

are farther from the retina than they would be when utilizing either the subretinal or epiretinal approach. In addition, there is a potential need for greater stimulation thresholds, and a demand for increased power given the added distance. It is considered safer, however, as the electrodes do not touch the retina and are stably fixed in the sclera pocket.

SUBRETINAL IMPLANTS

In 1956, a retinal prosthesis was described in which a light-sensitive selenium cell was placed behind the retina of a blind patient, allowing the patient to discern a moment of light perception (23). Subsequently, microchips containing light-sensitive MPDAs were implanted between the neural retina and the retinal pigment epithelium. Access to the subretinal space is gained through internal or external mechanisms. It is achieved externally by a process in which the sclera is dissected down to the choroid, the choroid is excised, and the implant is placed in the desired location under the retina. Internal access is accomplished by a vitrectomy and retinotomy (24). A combination of the two methods may also be employed: fluid is used to detach the retina internally, and a choroidal incision is made externally. MPDAs are used to replace degenerated photoreceptors by rendering the transmitted light into small currents proportional to the light stimulus. Essentially, there is direct replacement of lost photoreceptor function.

In the case of hereditary retinal degenerations, the remaining intact neural tissue may be used to transmit and process image information. Subretinal implants require

less current for stimulation because they are placed anatomically closer to the surviving bipolar cells, and they do not need adhesives or mechanical fixation. Inserting the microchip under transparent retina allows the microchip to sense light while simultaneously generating a signal through use of an array. Additionally, there is no need for either external cameras or processing units. It was considered that subretinal implantation may affect neurotrophic factors and enable a level of neuroprotection to the remaining viable tissue. Electroretinograms were assessed, which led to later suggestions that subretinal stimulation may preserve photoreceptors (25).

A consortium of universities in Germany developed and tested subretinally implanted MPDAs and used the device to transform visual scenes into electrical stimuli (26). Experimenting with in vitro and animal studies, they created a compatible and biostable implant. In addition, they employed a transchoroidal surgical technique for feasibility of implantation. Functionally, their subretinal implant moved in conjunction with the eye. There are two aspects to the implant: the MPDA with 1,500 elements that senses light using a photodiode, amplifies the signal, and connects the signal to the respective microelectrode (Fig. 26.4) and the additional electrode array of 16 electrodes for light-independent direct stimulation (Fig. 26.5).

A pilot study was undertaken in order to provide evidence that subretinally planted multielectrode arrays may restore visual function in patients affected by a retinal dystrophy. This study concluded that visual perception may be restored enough to provide patients with a degree of localization and recognition of objects; moreover, the potential to acquire

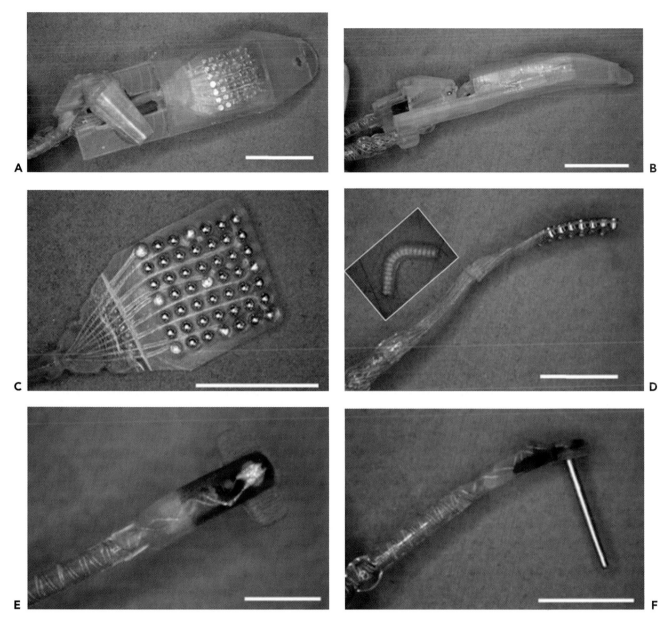

Figure 26.3 ■ Photograph of 49-channel stimulating electrode (**A–D**) and return electrode (**A,B,E,F**). Top (**A**) and side (**B**) views of stimulating and return electrode protected by protective silicone cover. Top (**C**) and side (**D**) views of 49-channel stimulating electrode. The diameter of each electrode is 0.5 mm, and the center-to-center electrode distance is 0.7 mm. The *inset* in (**D**) shows the protective cover that reinforced the junction between the electrode array and the cable. Top (**E**) and side (**F**) views of return electrode. The diameter of return electrode is 0.5 mm. Scale bars in (**A–F**), 5 mm. (Reprinted with permission from, Fujikado T, Kamei M, Sakaguchi H. Testing of semichronically implanted retinal prosthesis by suprachoroidal-transretinal stimulation in patients with retinitis pigmentosa. Invest Ophthalmol Vis Sci. 2011;52(7):4726. Copyright 2011. The Association for Research in Vision and Ophthalmology, Inc.)

enough vision to affect daily living (27). Further work is being performed to increase the level of spatial resolution.

In 2004, Chow et al. (28) reported on a pilot study in which an artificial silicon retina microchip was implanted in the subretinal space. The chip was composed of approximately 5,000 independent functioning electrodes and was powered entirely by incoming light. Their microchip was well tolerated; successful implantation was seen in six patients over 1 to 1.5 years with some degree of visual function improvement. As with other subretinal devices, visual improvement may result from the neuroprotective effect of

the subretinal implant on photoreceptors (28). Rizzo and Wyatt produced a subretinal stimulator chip that receives information from a camera mounted on a pair of glasses. The subretinal implant decodes the information from the camera and stimulates ganglion cells accordingly.

There are certain limitations to the subretinal prosthesis, which include a more complex implant procedure and the potential for subretinal damage from thermal energy. There have been reports of histologic changes to the surrounding retina such as a decrease in the cellular density of the inner retina and a presence of macrophages at the implantation site (29,30). Additionally, an external power source is needed to achieve adequate power levels for signal amplification (31,32). Subretinal implants are subject to corrosion over time, which may change the surface characteristic of the implant and disintegrate the electrode (24). Furthermore, there is currently no method available to noninvasively determine the viability of the remaining retinal cells needed for the implant to work successfully (33). Damage to the remaining cells could mean that the transmitted information is nonspecific. For this reason, direct stimulation of the ganglion cells by an epiretinal implant may be preferred.

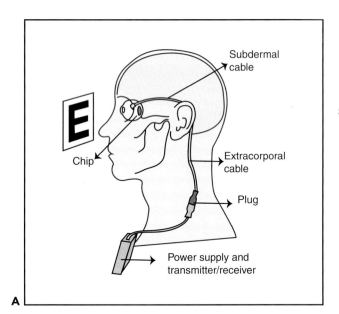

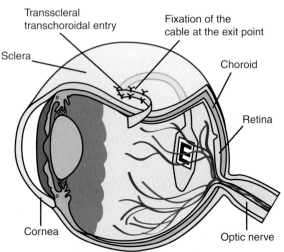

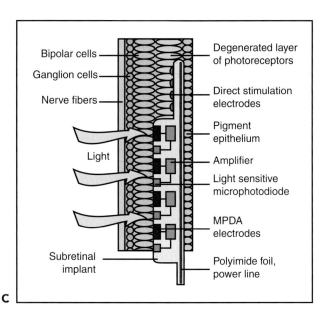

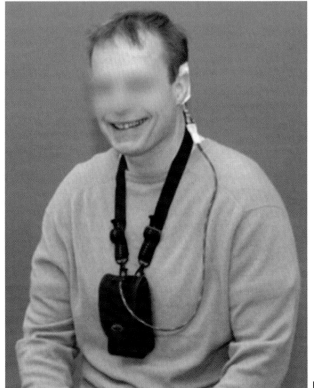

Figure 26.4 ■ Implant position in the body **A.** The cable from the implanted chip in the eye leads under the temporal muscle to the exit behind the ear and connects with a wirelessly operated control unit. **B.** Position of the implant under the transplanted retina. **C.** MPDA photodiodes, amplifiers, and electrodes in relation to retinal neurons and pigment epithelium. **D.** Patient with wireless control unit attached to a neckband.

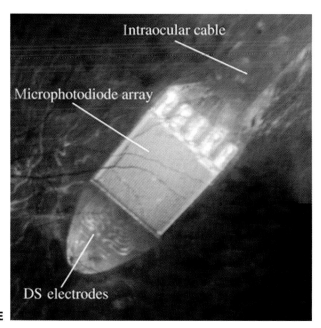

E

Figure 26.4 ■ *(Continued)* **E.** Photograph of the subretinal tip at the posterior eye pole through a patient pupil. (**A**, **B**, **C** modified from; **D**, **E**. Reprinted from, Zrenner E, Bartz-Schmidt KU, Benav H, et al. Subretinal electronic chips allow blind patients to read letters and combine them to words. Proc Biol Sci. 2011;278:1489–1497.)

EPIRETINAL IMPLANTS

The epiretinal prosthesis is composed of extraocular and intraocular components. In contrast to subretinal electrodes, which rely on information transmitted posteriorly through the cornea and lens, the epiretinal implant requires a supplementary optical system. Moreover, there is no light-sensitive element, so additional processing is necessary to prepare the visual information. The optical system consists of a camera built into a pair of glasses, a battery source, and a small processing unit. The camera captures and digitizes information from the environment. The images are then transmitted electronically to the remaining surviving inner retinal neurons. These images are preprocessed and modified in such a way that they are easily transmitted from the retinal implant to the optic nerve and subsequently to the brain. Essentially, information is transmitted from an external device to an internal receiver and microelectrode array (34).

One of the greatest difficulties the epiretinal implant faces is the affixation of the structure to the retinal surface. A functional, chronic prosthesis was implanted for the first time by Humayun (35). A blind test subject was able to see phosphenes upon stimulating an electrode array. The patient could detect light, discern motion, and recognize simple shapes. In late 2011, interim results from Second Sight's visual prosthesis were published, in which the Argus II retinal prosthesis system was evaluated. An electronic stimulator and antenna was sutured onto the sclera using an encircling silicon band. Following pars plana vitrectomy, electrode array and cable were introduced into the eye and tacked to the epiretinal surface. The camera first captured video before sending it to the processor, where it was converted to an electronic signal sent to the transmitter coil in the glasses. The antenna and receiver coil wirelessly received the data and sent the information to the electrode array where electrical stimulation pulses were emitted. The microelectrode induced cellular responses in the retina that traveled to the optic nerve and brain producing visual precepts. There was a 10% incidence of presumed endophthalmitis, which was treated medically, and two retina detachments, one of which may have been due to blunt trauma. The most common reported adverse event was conjunctival dehiscence over the extraocular implant. Subjects in the study had better ability in terms of object localization and motion discrimination. The best recorded visual acuity obtained in Second Sight's visual prosthesis study was 20/1,260 (36). The Argus II retinal prosthesis was approved for sale in Europe.

Epiretinal implants may also nonspecifically stimulate the bipolar cells and ganglion cells of the inner retinal layer (37). Learning retinal implants, which are employed by Intelligent Medical Implants (IMI), use an epiretinal stimulator that is fixed onto the retina by a sclera tack. Using a wireless control, information is received through a camera mounted on eyeglasses. The information is modulated through an encoder; the settings on the encoder are calibrated in an iterative process until visual perception matches picture information (38,39).

A completely intraocular retinal prosthesis (Fig. 26.6) is under investigation by the Epiret 3 study group. The system is comprised of a computer system, a transmitter, and a transmitter coil. The receiver is implanted similarly to that of an intraocular lens within the sulcus but with a wired connection to the epiretinal array that is anchored to the retina with retinal tacks (40).

There are pros and cons to the epiretinal approach. Advantages include the vitreous serving as a sink for the heat generated to prevent further retinal compromise. The implantable portion of the device has little microelectronics, and the extraocular portion of the device allows for easy upgrades. Disadvantages include the prolonged adhesion to the inner retina using retinal tacks, the possibility of retinal detachment and endophthalmitis, the large amount of current needed to reach the bipolar cells, and the close proximity of the current to the target cells.

OPTIC NERVE PROSTHESIS

Epiretinal and subretinal implants rely heavily on preexisting processing retinal neural cells, as such direct stimulation of the optic nerve may be more effective in circumstances when the retinal network is heavily damaged. Sakaguchi et al. (41) determined that transvitreous electrical stimulation of the optic nerve would elicit EEP in albino rabbits. In Belgium, a group of researchers implanted a spiral cuff

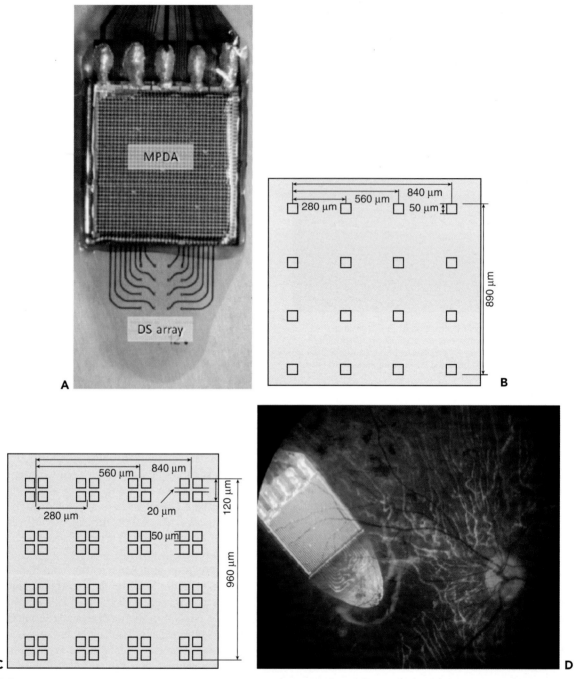

Figure 26.5 ■ Implanted device and DS electrode arrays. **A.** Prototype of the implant with the MPDA on the polyimide substrate containing gold leads as conductive paths for the DS array and the MPDA. The 16 TiN electrodes of the DS array are visible at the inferior part of the implant. **B.** Layout of first-generation DS array. Electrodes are rectangular with dimensions of 50 × 50 μm with a grid spacing of 280 μm. **C.** Layout of second-generation DS array. Four TiN elements are grouped to form a single electrode. Those elements are separated by 20 μm from each other creating a compound electrode that covers an area of 120 × 120 μm. **D.** Fundus photo of participant 10 showing the chip implanted subretinally. Note the retinal vessels passing over the chip. (Reprinted with permission from, Wilke R, Gabel VP, Sachs H. Spatial resolution and perception of patterns mediated by a subretinal 16-electrode array in patients blinded by hereditary retinal dystrophies. Invest Ophthalmol Vis Sci. 2011;52(8):5995–6003. Published on June 21, 2011 as Manuscript iovs.10-6946.)

electrode with four electrodes around the optic nerve of a blind RP patient. By altering the pulse width, intensity, frequency, and current of the stimulus, the patient perceived phosphenes at the corresponding locations (10,42). A Japanese group tested electrical stimulation with the optic nerve with wire-type electrodes and reported on their efficacy and safety in acute and long-term animal studies (43). This group then examined and reported on artificial vision by direct optic nerve electrode (AV-DONE) implantation in a blind patient with RP. Phacoemulsification was performed prior to implantation. The device was comprised of three 0.05-mm-diameter wire electrodes. A silicone tube

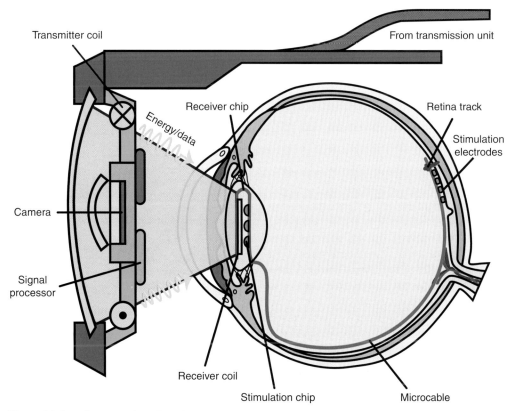

Figure 26.6 ■ Concept of the EPIRET3 system. A transmitter coil sends data and energy to the receiver unit of the implant, which is located in the posterior chamber of the eye. The receiver unit is connected with the stimulator unit carrying an array of 25 3D IrOx electrodes by a flexible microcable. The stimulator is placed safely onto the retinal surface and fixed with retinal tacks. (Reprinted with permission from, Roessler G, Laube T, Brockmann C. Implantation and explanation of a wireless epiretinal retina implant device: observations during the EPIRET3 prospective clinical trial. Invest Ophthalmol Vis Sci. 2009;50(6):3003–3008. Copyright Association for Research in Vision and Ophthalmology.)

containing Parylene-coated platinum wires (each 0.05 mm) encircled the globe and sutured at the four scleral quadrants with a 5-0 suture. A standard pars plana vitrectomy was performed with confirmed posterior vitreous detachment. The wire bundle was then inserted into the vitreous through the sclerotomy at 3.5 mm from the limbus. Three wire tips were inserted into the optic nerve using vitreoretinal forceps. The tips were inserted into the disc at a 1- to 2-mm depth away from the vessels. Another wire was left in the vitreous cavity as a reference electrode. The external wires were covered with Tenon's capsule and conjunctival tissue. At the time of electrical stimulation, a peritomy was performed and the wires were connected to the outside stimulator. The wires were functionally stable for 12 months. Phosphenes and visual sensations were elicited by electrical stimulation through each electrode. The threshold for phosphene perception was elicited by pulses of 0.25 ms duration per phase and a pulse frequency of 320 Hz. The phosphenes ranged in size from a match head to an apple; they were round, oval, or linear in shape; primarily yellow in color; and focally distributed. There were no complications during the follow-up period, and the wires were stable for a 6-month period. The trial was limited by the absence of a transcutaneous

transmission system to draw a complete and accurate phosphene map; nonetheless, it was successful in showing that localized phosphene perceptions were elicited by stimulating the optic nerve in a patient with advanced RP (44).

Although the AV-DONE system is limited by the need for an active nerve fiber and cannot treat blindness resulting from late-stage glaucoma or optic neuropathy, it does not have the same heavy reliance on residual functioning retinal nerve fibers as other retinal implants.

The AV-DONE system utilizes three linear-shaped electrodes implanted after vitrectomy. Recently, researchers studied a new device for optic nerve stimulation with a seven-wire stimulation electrode (45). The device was successfully implanted in a rabbit model. AV-DONE system is being developed in collaboration with NIDEK Co., Ltd.

IMPLANTABLE MINIATURE TELESCOPE

Implanted in one eye, the Implantable Miniature Telescope (IMT) provides a magnified image onto a healthy portion of the retina. The nonimplanted eye serves as a basis for peripheral vision. The device is implanted into patients 75 years or older with stable bilateral central scotomas resulting from AMD and a visually significant cataract. Prior to implantation, patients undergo training with an external telescope with a low vision specialist to determine whether they benefit from an implanted telescope. Postoperatively, patients must undergo a visual training program.

The prosthesis (IMT; VisionCare Ophthalmic Technologies, Saratoga, CA) was developed to reduce visual impairment caused by end-stage AMD. The prosthesis is a fixed-focus telescopic system integrated in a carrier with two rigid continuous haptics. The device enlarges the objects in the central visual field and reduces the peripheral field accordingly. A 20- to 24-degree forward field of view is projected onto 55 degrees of retina. The central visual field is enlarged 2.2 to 3 times that of the image normally projected onto the retina. Eyeglasses are given after surgery to enhance the focus of near and distance vision. After 1 year in the multicentered study, 67% of implanted eyes achieved a three-line or more improvement in best-corrected distance visual acuity, versus 13% of fellow eye controls. Mean quality of life was assessed in association with implantation of the lens and was considered to be increased significantly postimplantation (46).

The IMT is a large device, and implantation can lead to extensive endothelial cell loss. Endothelial cell density, associated with postsurgical edema, was reduced 20% at 3 months and 25% at 1 year. There were two cases of corneal decompensation after 1 year (46). The device is FDA approved, and the base cost is suggested to be $14,389; however, "substantial human gain from device implantation contributes to making the intervention cost-effective by conventional standards" (47).

REFERENCES

1. Rizzo J, Tombran-Tink J, Colin J. Visual prosthesis and ophthalmic devices: new hope in sight. Totowa, NJ: Humana Press; 2007:160.

2. Brindley GS, Lewin WS. The sensations produced by electrical stimulation of the visual cortex. J Physiol. 1968;196:479–493.

3. Dobelle WH, Mladejovsky MG. Phosphenes produced by electrical stimulation of human occipital cortex, and their application to the development of a prosthesis for the bind. J Physiol. 1974;243:553–576.

4. Dobelle WH. Artificial vision for the blind by connecting a television camera to the visual cortex. ASAIO J. 2000;46:3–9.

5. Normann RA, Warren DJ, Ammermuller J, et al. High-resolution spatio-temporal mapping of the visual pathways using micro-electrode arrays. Vision Res. 2001;41:1261–1275.

6. Schmidt EM, Bak MJ, Hambrecht FT, et al. Feasibility of a visual prosthesis for the blind based on intracortical microstimulation of the visual cortex. Brain. 1996;119:507–522.

7. Normann RA, Maynard EM, Roushe PJ, et al. A neural interface for a cortical vision prosthesis. Vision Res. 1999;39(15):2577–2587.

8. Pantesos F, Sanchez-Jimenez A, Diaz-de Cerio E, et al. Consistent phosphenes generated by electrical microstimulation of the visual thalamus. An experimental approach for the thalamic visual neuroprosthesis. Front Neurosci. 2011;5(84):1–12.

9. Santos A, Humayun MS, de Jaun E Jr, et al. Preservation of the inner retina in retinitis pigmentosa. A morphometric analysis. Arch Ophthalmol. 1997;115:511–515.

10. Sakaguchi H, Fujikado T, Fang X, et al. Transretinal electrical stimulation with a suprachoroidal multichannel electrode in rabbit eyes. Jpn J Ophthalmol. 2004;48:256–261.

11. Chow AY, Chow VY. Subretinal stimulation of the rabbit retina. Neurosci Lett. 1997;225:13–16.

12. Peachey NS, Chow AY. Subretinal implantation of semiconductor-based photodiodes: progress and challenges. J Rehabil Res Dev. 1999;36:371–376.

13. Schwahn HN, Gekeler F, Kohler K et al. Studies on the feasibility of a subretinal visual prosthesis: data for the Yucatan micropig and rabbit. Graefes Arch Clin Exp Ophthalmol. 2001;239:961–967.

14. Zrenner E, Miliczek KD, Gabel VP, et al. The development of subretinal microphotodiodes for replacement of degenerated photoreceptors. Ophthalmic Res. 1997;29:269–280.

15. Eckmiller R. Learning retina implants with epiretinal contacts. Ophthalmic Res. 1997;29:281–289.

16. Humayun MS, de Juan E Jr, Dagnelie G, et al. Visual perception elicited by electrical stimulation of retina in blind humans. Arch Ophthalmol. 1996;114:40–46.

17. Humayun MS, de Juan E Jr, et al. Pattern electrical stimulation of the human retina. Vision Res. 1999;39:2569–2576.

18. Grumet AE, Wyatt JL Jr, Rizzo JF III. Multi-electrode stimulation and recording in the isolated retina. J Neurosci Methods. 2000;101:31–42.

19. Rizzo JF III, Wyatt J, Humayun M, et al. Retinal prosthesis: an encouraging first decade with major challenges ahead. Ophthalmology. 2001;108:13–14.

20. Walter P, Szurman P, Vobig M, et al. Successful long-term implantation of electrically inactive epiretinal microelectrode arrays in rabbits. Retina. 1999;19:546–552.

21. Walter P, Heimann K. Evoked cortical potentials after electrical stimulation of the inner retina in rabbits. Graefes Arch Clin Exp Ophthalmol. 2000;238:315–318.

22. Fujikado T, Kamei M, Sakaguchi H, et al. Testing of a semichronically implanted retinal prosthesis by suprachoroidal-transretinal stimulation in patients with retinitis pigmentosa. Invest Ophthalmol Vis Sci. 2011;52(7):4726–4733.

23. Tassiker GE. US patent 2,760,483. 1956.

24. Sachs HG, Gabel VP. Retinal replacement—the development of microelectric retinal prostheses-experience with subretinal implants and new aspects. Graefes Arch Clin Exp Ophthalmol. 2004;242:717–723.

25. Pardue MT, Phillips MJ, Yin H, et al. Neuroprotective effect of subretinal implants in the RCS Rat. Invest Ophthalmol Vis Sci. 2005;46:674–682.

26. Wilke R, Gabel VP, Helmut S, et al. Spatial resolution and perception of patterns mediated by a subretinal 16-electrode array in patients blinded by hereditary retinal dystrophies. Invest Ophthalmol Vis Sci. 2011;52:8:5995–6003.

27. Zrenner E, Bartz-Schmidt KU, Benav H. Subretinal electronic chips allow blind patients to read letters and combine them to words. Proc Biol Sci. 2011;278:1489–1497.

28. Chow AY, Chow VY, Packo KH, et al. The artificial silicon retina microchip for the treatment of vision loss from retinitis pigmentosa. Arch Ophthalmol. 2004;122:460–469.

29. Zrenner E, Stett A. Can subretinal microphotodiode arrays successfully replace degenerated photoreceptors. Vision Res. 1999;39:2555–2567.

30. Pardue Mt, Stubbs EB Jr, Perlman J, et al. Immunohistochemical studies of the retina following long-term implantation with subretinal microphotodiode arrays. Exp Eye Res. 2001;73:333–343.

31. Maynard EM. Visual prostheses. Annu Rev Biomed Eng. 2001;3;145–168.

32. Chow AY, Peachey NS. The subretinal microphotodiode array retinal prosthesis. [comment]. Ophthalmic Res. 1998;30(3):195–198.

33. Lowenstein JL, Montezuma SR, Rizzo JF. Outer retinal degeneration. Arch Ophthalmol. 2004;122:587–596.

34. Awdeh RM, Lakhanpal RR, Weiland JD, et al. Artificial vision, visual prosthesis, and retinal implants. Age related macular degeneration: a comprehensive textbook. Philadelphia, PA: Lippincott Williams & Wilkins; 2006.

35. Humayun MS, Weiland JD, Fuji GY, et al. Visual perception in a blind patient with a chronic microelectronic retinal prosthesis. Vision Res. 2003;43:2573–2581.

36. Humayun MS, Dorn JD, Cruz LD, et al. Interim results from the International Trial of Second Sight's Visual Prosthesis. Ophthalmology. 2012;119(4):779–788. January 11, 2012. [Epub ahead of print]

37. Fried SL, Lasker AC, Eddington DK, et al. Two different parts of the ganglion cell axon are activated by epi-retinal stimulation. Invest Ophthalmol Vis Sci. 2008;49:E-abstract 3034.

38. Keserue M, Feucht M, Post N, et al. Clinical study on chronic electrical stimulation of the human retina with an epiretinal electrode array. Fluorescein angiography and OCT findings. Invest Ophthalmol Vis Sci. 2008;49:E-abstract 1785.

39. Richard G, Keserue M, Feucht M, et al. Visual perception after long term implantation of a retinal implant. Invest Ophthalmol Vis Sci. 2008;49:E-abstract 1786.

40. Walter P, Mokwa W, Messner A. Epiret-Epiret 3 wireless intraocular retina implant system: design of the Epiret 3 prospective clinical trial and overview. Invest Ophthalmol Vis Sci. 2008;49:e-abstract 3023.

41. Sakaguchi H, Fujikado T, Kanda H, et al. Electrical stimulation with a needle-type electrode inserted into the optic nerve in rabbit eyes. Jpn J Ophthalmol. 2004;48:552–557.

42. Veraart C, Wanet-Defalque MC, Gerard B, et al. Pattern recognition with the optic nerve visual prosthesis. Artif Organs. 2003;27:996–1004.

43. Fang X, Sakaguchi H, Fujikado T, et al. Electrophysiological and histological studies of chronically implanted intrapapillary electrodes in rabbit eyes. Graefes Arch Clin Exp Ophthalmol. 2006;244:364–375.

44. Sakaguchi H, Kamei M, Ozawa M, et al. Artificial vision by direct optic nerve electrode (AV-DONE) implantation in a blind patient with retinitis pigmentosa. J Artif Organs. 2009;12:206–209.

45. Sakaguchi H, Kamei M, Nishida K, et al. Implantation of a newly developed direct optic nerve electrode device for artificial vision in rabbits. J Artif Organs. 2012;15(3):295–300.

46. Hudson HL, Lane SS, Heier JS, et al. Implantable miniature telescope for the treatment of visual acuity loss resulting from end-stage age-related macular degeneration: 1-year Results. Ophthalmology. 2006;113(11):1987–2001.

47. Brown GC, Brown MM, Lieske HB, et al. Comparative effectiveness and cost-effectiveness of the implantable miniature telescope. Ophthalmology. 2011;118:1834–1843.

27

RETINAL TRANSPLANTATION

ANTONIO LÓPEZ BOLAÑOS

The possibility of rebuilding a damaged retina has been the aim of multiple researchers. Because of improved technology and the molecular biology, it is now possible to manage many diseases that were previously untreatable. However, retinal degenerations, such as retinitis pigmentosa and age-related macular degeneration (AMD), among others, continue to be devastating causes of progressive vision loss and blindness. These diseases primarily affect the photoreceptors or the retinal pigment epithelium (RPE). There are currently no effective treatments available to prevent the loss of photoreceptors in most of these disorders.

A variety of approaches to preserve or restore vision are under investigation. Treatment strategies for retinal degeneration are aimed at either preventing photoreceptor loss or restoring vision by replacing the lost photoreceptors and/or the RPE. Retinal transplantation is based on the hypothesis that the degenerated retina can be repaired by introducing normal RPE and photoreceptor cells that may develop appropriate connections with the still functional part of the host retina.

Retinal transplantation was first performed in 1946 by Tansley (1), who demonstrated features of retinal differentiation in embryonic ocular tissue transplanted into the brains of young rats. In 1959, Royo and Quay (2) reported the first intraocular retinal transplantation procedure and demonstrated that fetal mice retina could survive in the anterior chamber of the maternal parent. In 1980, del Cerro et al. (3) transplanted full-thickness strips of retina into the anterior chamber of a mouse and demonstrated survival of both allografts and xenografts. Turner and Blair (4) transplanted neonatal rat retina into the subretinal space via a transscleral approach and demonstrated survival and differentiation of the graft into retinal layers.

Dissociated retinal microaggregates and retinal cell suspensions were subsequently tried by a numerous investigators (5–7). These preparations were easily manipulated and introduced into the subretinal space with a minimal amount of trauma. After transplantation, however, microaggregate suspensions are often organized into rudimentarily differentiated rosettes rather than well-organized layers (8,9).

Several sources of cells have been tested for their ability to replace photoreceptors. Fetal or embryonic retinal progenitors can be grown in vitro (10) and used for transplantation. Neurospheres can be grown from the adult pigmented ciliary epithelium, and these cells can also be transplanted to the retina (11). Neural stem cells derived from the hippocampus show a remarkable ability to integrate into the retinal layers and form morphologically normal-appearing retinal neurons (12). The best evidence for functional photoreceptors comes from the study of MacLaren et al. (13), in which freshly dissociated, postmitotic rod photoreceptors were transplanted to the subretinal space; however, the number of cells cannot be increased in vitro due to their postmitotic state.

Embryonic stem cells (ESCs) might also be a source for replacement of photoreceptors. Their indefinite self-renewal and pluripotency make them an ideal source (13). Lamb et al. in 2009 transplanted human ESC–derived photoreceptors. After transplantation of the cells into the subretinal space of a mice model of Leber's congenital amaurosis, the cells differentiated into functional photoreceptors and restored light responses to the animals. These results demonstrate that ESCs can, in principle, be used for photoreceptor replacement therapies.

In principle, successful transplantation requires graft survival and integration with the host. Graft survival depends on a number of factors, both immunologic and nonimmunologic. Immune privilege in the eye is the result of (a) the blood–ocular barrier, which minimizes contact of allografts with the cells and molecules of the immune system, thus blunting the immune response to alloantigens; (b) deficient lymphatic drainage of the eye; (c) an unusual distribution and functional properties of bone marrow–derived antigen-presenting cells; and (d) an ocular microenvironment rich in soluble or cell membrane–associated immunomodulatory factors.

Synapse formation between retinal grafts and the host retina is much more complex (14).

The prospective transplant interconnections with the host retina need to be improved and enhanced, which is expected to occur in future experiments outlined below. Retinal interneurons in the transplant may interfere with the synaptic connectivity of transplant photoreceptors with the host retina. Connectivity could be supported by factors that reduce glial reactivity and trauma to the retina because the formation of glial scars is another barrier to integration. Treatment with trophic factors or gene delivery into donor cells also needs to be explored. This requires carefully controlled experiments to account for the normal up-regulation of trophic factors that are seen after injury (15).

Retinal transplantation and approaches to develop retinal prostheses are presently the only potential treatments once photoreceptors are lost. Growth factor and gene therapy can only work to delay retinal diseases, not replace lost photoreceptors. In the future, one can conceive of stimulating stem cells in the adult eye to regenerate the lost photoreceptors or the bioengineering of a retina from stem cells (15).

RETINAL PIGMENT EPITHELIAL TRANSPLANT

Aging pathophysiology of the RPE and Bruch's membrane

Retinal pigment epithelial dysfunction is believed to be the main cause of many debilitating retinal diseases of which AMD is the most common. In this disease, the retinal pigment epithelial dysfunction leads to photoreceptor damage causing severe vision loss. The RPE and Bruch's membrane (BM) suffer cumulative damage over lifetime, which is thought to induce AMD in susceptible individuals.

There is a continuous "physiologic" increase in lipofuscin within the RPE cells, evident between 20 and 70 years of age. The concentration is higher in the posterior pole. In AMD, lipofuscin accumulates in the lysosomes of RPE and is associated with several adverse effects on RPE function and survival (16). In the aging human eye, apoptosis of RPE cells was found to be four times higher in the macular center than in the rest of the retina (17). Lipofuscin is also known to be a photoinducible generator of reactive oxygen species. RPE phagocytosis of photoreceptor outer segments is associated with oxidative stress, and H_2O_2 is probably the reactive oxygen intermediate involved (18).

The RPE seems to play an important role in sustaining the microenvironment and protecting it from various noxious insults. In vivo protection of photoreceptors from light damage by pigment epithelium derived growth factor (PEDF) has been reported by Cao et al. (19). PEDF also inhibits retinal and choroidal neovascularization (CNV) (20). It has been suggested that RPE cells may control the growth of new vessels from the choroid because of the membrane protein Fas ligand, which is highly expressed on the RPE (21).

The RPE maintains retinal function as the metabolic gatekeeper between photoreceptors and the choriocapillaris. The RPE and BM suffer cumulative damage over lifetime. BM plays a crucial role in the pathogenesis of AMD. It is believed that BM forms a physical barrier against the invasion of new vessels into the retina (22). With its strategic location between the retina and the choroidal circulation, BM is involved in the exchange of numerous biomolecules, oxygen, nutrients, and waste products between the RPE and choriocapillaris. It plays a crucial role in cell-to-cell communication, cellular differentiation, proliferation, migration, and tissue remodeling (23).

BM thickness greatly varies among individuals and has been shown to double in size throughout life, from an average 2 μm in the first decade of life to 4.7 μm 80 years later. This thickening is caused by the deposition of waste products of the RPE, such as oxidized lipids and proteins. Over time, granular, membranous, filamentous, and vesicular material accumulates into the different layers of BM (24–27). This accumulation eventually leads to the formation of focal or diffuse sub-RPE deposits in BM, best known as drusen. The accumulation of biomolecules in BM causes changes in hydrostatic pressure and permeability, resulting in hypoxia and lack of nutrient exchange. This leads to the release of cytokines and growth factors, including vascular endothelial growth factor (VEGF), from the RPE cells (28).

RPE Transplantation

RPE transplantation is conceptually easier because the RPE is only a monolayer of cells between the systemic circulation and the photoreceptors. It works by being next to the outer segments of the photoreceptors, separated by a narrow extracellular space, uniquely enriched with specialized proteins. Although all of the functional roles of the RPE have not been elucidated yet, most of the major ones have. We know that without an RPE layer, the photoreceptors as well as the choriocapillaris degenerate. Transplanted RPE corrects this defect and prevents the photoreceptor cells from degenerating.

In the past 20 years, a huge amount of research has been conducted in the area of transplantation of RPE. This technique aims to restore the subretinal anatomy and reestablish the critical interaction between the RPE and the photoreceptor, which is fundamental to sight.

The success of RPE transplantation depends largely on the origin of introduced RPE cells: *autologous* transplants taken from the patient's own eye and *allogenic* transplants using foreign cells. Two different transplantation techniques are currently used in clinical studies: the RPE-suspension technique and the RPE–choroid sheet technique. Both allogenic and autologous transplants have advantages and disadvantages. The RPE-cell suspension, providing limited amounts of cells on a partially defective basal lamina, can easily be delivered subretinally through small retinotomies, which can be sealed with a gas bubble; the words "transplantation" and "risk of rejection" are often spoken in the same breath. Today, autologous RPE is used in clinical studies because homologous transplants make necessary long-term combined immunosuppressive therapies, and these are not well tolerated by elderly patients (28,29). On the other hand, the translocation of a full-thickness RPE–choroidal sheet, providing a regular cell sheet of polarized RPE on its own basal lamina, carries a high risk for intra- and postoperative complications.

A new potential alternative is a human embryonic stem cell (hES)–derived RPE. The *pluripotentiality* is part of the promise and the problem of hES transplantation. The question is: How can a specific type of cell needed for transplantation be created from a cell that has not decided which part of the body it will become? To create transplantable RPE cells, the scientists moved the hES cells from medium to medium and from culture to culture. The most crucial step in cell development did not require any intervention; however, the hES cells spontaneously differentiated into RPE cells using a default path of neural induction (30). Stem cells are full of the theoretical power of possibility. In short, human epithelial stem cell–derived RPE transplantation may be more feasible than other applications of hES technology.

Falkner-Radler et al. evaluated the outcome after two types of RPE transplantation techniques in patients with advanced exudative AMD. They were assigned to RPE–choroid sheet transplantation or RPE-cell suspension transplantation. They conclude that the anatomical and functional outcome after both RPE transplantation techniques was comparable, and the functional outcome was comparable between both groups. Transplantation of RPE–choroid sheet provides an organized cell layer over its own basal lamina, whereas transplantation of RPE-cell suspension has the disadvantage that a limited amount of cells is distributed over a damaged basal lamina with an uncertain fate. This implies that uneventful transplantation of RPE–choroid sheet, being a better cell source than RPE-cell suspension, may offer a greater chance of regaining normal retinal structures and thus visual function (31,32).

RPE transplantation technique

Despite the introduction of anti-VEGF treatment resulting in significant improvement of vision in patients with neovascular AMD, the treatment for advanced AMD such as geographic atrophy and/or nonresponders is still controversial. A possible alternative is the autologous translocation of the choroid and RPE.

Peyman et al. (33) first suggested translocation of peripheral choroid and RPE. Others later demonstrated the clinical feasibility of the new technique (34–36). Preoperative examinations are basic to determine which patient is the best candidate, even when the criteria are not yet well established. A key point is patients with early visual loss, perhaps within 6 months of presentation. Other investigations included fundal photography with fundus fluorescein angiography (FFA) and optical coherence tomography (OCT). If it is possible, it is better to perform visual function tests using a microperimeter to assess fixation patterns and retinal sensitivity.

The surgical procedure began with phacoemulsification and implantation of an intraocular lens. After the induction of a posterior vitreous detachment by active suction, a complete 23-gauge vitrectomy was performed, taking care to make an excellent shaving of the vitreous base in order to reduce the possibility of retinal incarceration at the sclerotomy site during surgery and the risk of vitreous base contraction with secondary retinal detachment during the postoperative period.

Two retinotomies are made. In the first retinotomy, we dissect and remove the damaged subfoveal membrane with forceps, hemostasis of the membrane bed is achieved by elevating the infusion bottle, and the blood is aspirated through the retinotomy with an aspirating cannula. In the second retinotomy, we remove gently a block of retina, RPE cells, BM, and choroid in a different region of the eye, preferably in the uppers quadrants. To accomplish this, previously diode laser is applied in the superior midperiphery outside the vascular arcade (Fig. 27.1A). After demarcation of a rectangular excision area of 6 to 8 disk diameters, the graft is subsequently cut out as a full-thickness RPE choroid graft after peeling off the overlying neurosensory retina.

The graft is gripped on the choroidal surface with an aspirating cannula and then slid through the original retinotomy into the subfoveal space (Fig. 27.1B). The patch is held with forceps, and the graft is gently pulled to the subfoveal area (Fig. 27.1C). A perfluorocarbon bubble is used to hold the graft to ensure correct unfolding and a subfoveal position (Fig. 27.1D). Retinopexy laser is not applied to the macular retinotomy, and the eye is filled with silicone oil or C3F8.

In another technique, the surgeon creates a retinal detachment of temporal retina by injecting a balanced salt solution into the subretinal space through a 42-gauge subretinal cannula; this retinal detachment includes the macula and involves repeated fluid air exchanges (Fig. 27.2A and B). A 180-degree temporal retinotomy is performed with curved scissors, as close as possible to the ora serrate (Fig. 27.2C and D). The retina is folded on itself exposing the subretinal space, facilitating to remove the RPE damage

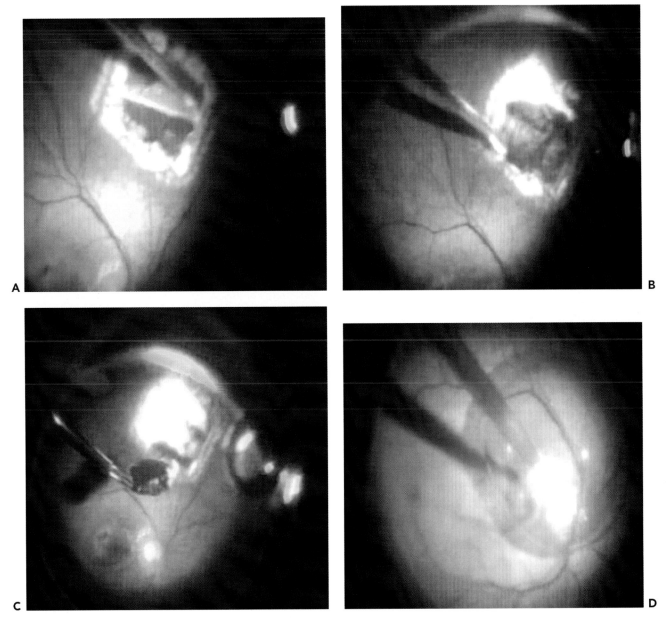

Figure 27.1 ■ Surgical technique of RPE–choroid transplantation. **A.** Delimitation with laser at the site which the graft is taking. **B.** The graft is gripped on the choroidal surface with an aspirating cannula. **C.** The patch is held with forceps, and the graft is gently pulled to the subfoveal area. **D.** A perfluorocarbon bubble is used to hold the graft to ensure correct unfolding and a subfoveal position.

and the CNV. The bleeding from the choroidal feeder vessels of the CNV is stopped with gentle pressure or diathermy. A full-thickness patch of choroid, choriocapillaris, BM, and RPE is isolated from the midperiphery. First the graft is delineated with three intense crowns of diode laser. After demarcation of a rectangular excision area helped by the use of diathermy, the graft is subsequently cut out as a full-thickness RPE choroid graft after peeling off the overlying neurosensory retina. When the patch is fully cut to 360 degrees, choroidal bleeding was controlled by diathermy or intraocular pressure elevation (Fig. 27.2E). The graft is gently pulled to the subfoveal area. During this maneuver, the patch is held with forceps at its anterior edge, in order to prevent damaging it with extensive manipulation. In order to assure adequate adhesion between the patch and the posterior pole, the temporal retina is flipped over its original position, and the perfluorocarbon liquid (PFCL) is injected into the preretinal space to reattach the retina. Peripheral laser endophotocoagulation is performed at the edge of the retinotomy being careful to avoid the pigment epithelium. The eye is filled with silicone oil. This technique facilitates the manipulation and implantation of the graft, less cell loss of RPE, and better centering. However, intraoperative and postoperative complications are more likely. Proliferative vitreoretinopathy is the most frequent complication, affecting visual outcome irremediably.

Anatomical and Functional Outcome

Following autologous RPE–choroid graft transplant, the graft has a brown appearance. Unfortunately, the graft can fold over (Fig. 27.3) or become a fibrotic patch. Sometimes an irregular accumulation of hyperpigmentation at the margins, near the graft or on the graft, can be seen.

Angiographic patterns in patients with revascularization of the graft (Fig. 27.4) may be observed if the large choroidal vessels of the graft are visible. The revascularization pattern of the grafts suggests connection of the choroidal channels of the transplant with those of the underlying recipient choroid. There are different revascularization patterns. Most patients will have revascularization of the graft as early as 3 weeks after translocation.

If the graft is not rejected, the OCT imaging shows an intact outer nuclear layer, an external limiting membrane, and a junction between photoreceptor inner and outer segments, indicating the presence of intact photoreceptors (Figs. 27.5 and 27.6). In the rejected graft, a photoreceptor layer cannot be identified. A late postoperative complication is the development of classic or occult CNV.

In regard of the functional outcome, the visual acuity must be carefully assessed before and after surgery. Relevant studies in which visual acuities were evaluated

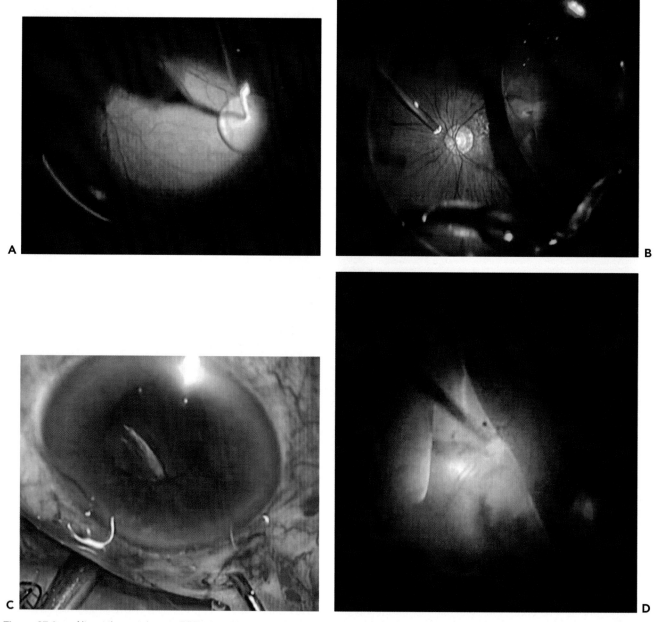

Figure 27.2 ■ Alternative autologous RPE–choroid transplantation technique. **A.** After vitrectomy, we perform a controlled retinal detachment with BSS in the temporal sector. **B.** Exchange liquid air to increase the macular detachment. **C.** A 180-degree temporal retinotomy is performed as close as possible to the ora serrata. **D.** The temporal retina is overlying the nasal retina and the graft is taking.

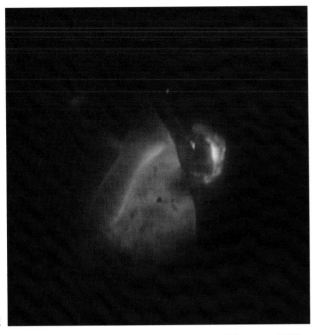

E

Figure 27.2 ■ (*Continued*) **E.** When the patch is fully cut to 360°, choroidal bleeding was controlled by diathermy or intraocular pressure elevation.

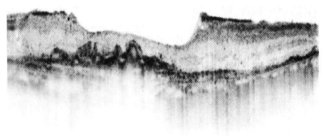

Figure 27.4 ■ Optic coherent tomography shows the RPE–choroid complex folded and the presence of an epiretinal membrane after 3 months to perform a surgical procedure.

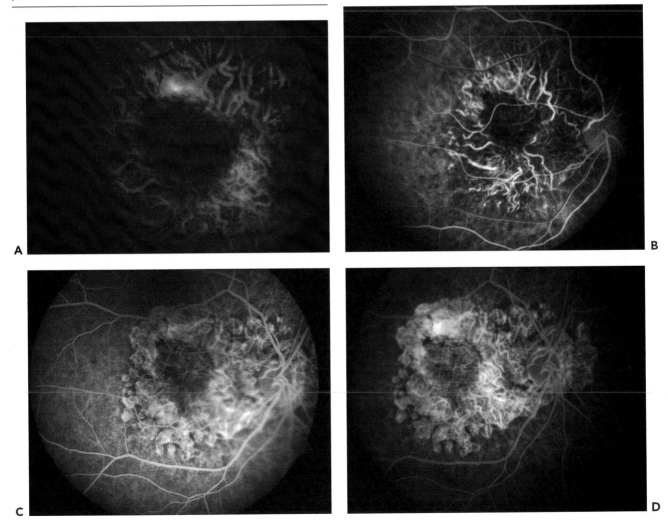

A
B
C
D

Figure 27.3 ■ **A.** Follow-up of a patient presenting after autologous translocation of the RPE and choroid in geographic atrophy. **B–D.** The graft showed good vascularization.

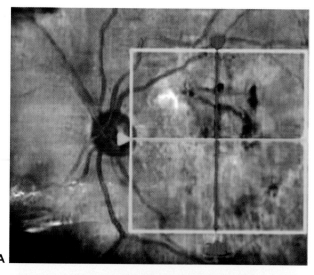

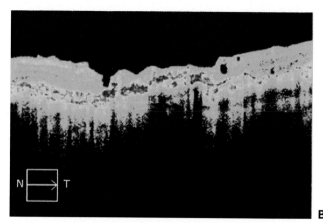

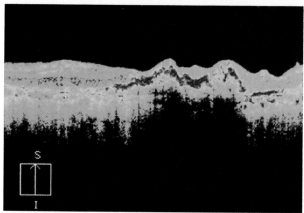

Figure 27.5 ■ Autologous RPE–choroid transplantation OCT of the left eye. **A.** The picture shows the folding complex placed in the macula. **B, C.** OCT shows integration of the graft to the original choroid.

are summarized in Table 27.1. There is a disparity in the improvement of visual acuity between research studies. One factor for the variability in outcomes may be variability in the degree and type of disease, including CNV, geographic atrophy, and/or nonresponders. Moreover, the type of graft is another factor to consider. If it is allogenic,

this is accompanied by the risk of immunosuppression. Another possible explanation for the visual loss after RPE–choroid patch transplant is an inadequate positioning of the graft. Even though a functioning and intact RPE cell layer is transplanted, patients with initial extrafoveal fixation may have no benefit from the patch. Thus,

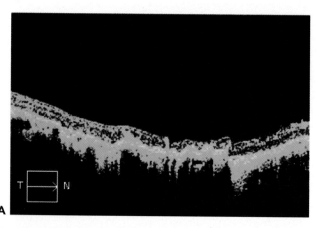

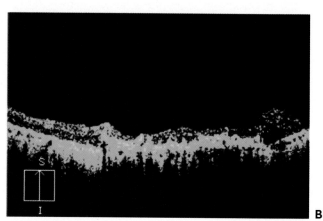

Figure 27.6 ■ OCT imaging **(A)** and **(B)** 12 months after autologous RPE–choroid transplant. This patient has improvement in visual acuity from 5/200 to 20/200.

Table 27.1 SUMMARY OF RETINAL TRANSPLANTATION STUDIES

Article	Type of transplantation	Disease	Patients included	Improvement/ stabilization of vision acuity	Worsening of visual acuity	Complications
Tezel et al. (37), 2006	RPE allogenic cells. Human cadaver	AMD	12	33%	67%	Ocular hypertension. Immune suppression complications. Died
Cereda et al. (38), 2010	Autologous RPE–choroid graft	AMD	13	92%	8%	RD
Van Meurs et al. (39), 2004	Autologous RPE cells	AMD	8	75%	25%	PVR
Caramoy et al. (40), 2009	Autologous RPE–choroid graft	AMD	10	30%	70%	EM, PVR, RD, patch not vascularized
Maaijwee et al. (41), 2007	Autologous RPE–choroid graft	AMD	83	24%	76%	Inadequate positioning or incomplete flattening of the graft, RD, PVR, EM
MacLaren et al (42), 2007	Autologous RPE–choroid graft	AMD	12	20%	80%	PVR, RD, macular pucker, vitreous hemorrhage, and patch were renewed

RD, retinal detachment; PVR, proliferative vitreoretinopathy; EM, epiretinal membrane.

preoperative microperimetry and spectral domain OCT is essential to select patients with central fixation and intact photoreceptor.

On the other hand, the neurosensory retina of a patient with geographic atrophy is more adherent to the choroid compared to exudative AMD. Separating the macula intraoperatively from the choroid may damage the outer retina irreversibly; even a macular hole can be formed. Another cause of failure to improve visual acuity is nonperfusion of the graft.

Finally, it is worthwhile to mention that surgical skill is an important variable. During the surgery, complications may occur, such as trauma of the subfoveal choroid with bleeding, tearing of the retinotomy with bleeding, a peripheral retinal tear, a retinal detachment, failure of the subfoveal release of the graft, and an inadequate positioning or incomplete flattening of the graft, which was partly folded or wrinkled underneath the fovea. An important postoperative complication is proliferative vitreoretinopathy with a high risk of retinal detachment. The excision of peripheral full-thickness retina and choroid generates inflammation, which probably stimulates proliferative vitreoretinopathy. Recurrent CNV membrane, rhegmatogenous retinal detachment, postoperative hemorrhages, acute glaucoma, and retinal puckering/cellophane maculopathy (Fig. 27.3) are other causes of poor prognosis.

Future perspectives

Transplantation of RPE–choroid sheet provides an organized cell layer over its own basal lamina. This strategy of retinal transplantation may offer a greater chance of regaining normal retinal structures and thus visual function. Transplantation of RPE offers an alternative approach in advanced AMD and is also suitable for geographic AMD and other degenerative retinal diseases. However, the functional results with RPE transplantation techniques do not approach the levels of outcome seen with anti-VEGF treatment. Although complications after transplantation of RPE are common, refinement of surgical technique to allow for an adequate graft size, improvement of the quality of RPE and BM, and combination therapies might be future options to improve outcome after transplantation of RPE. Refined indications for treatment, such as duration of vision loss, may be a significant predictor of the functional outcome after RPE–choroid sheet transplantation and macular translocation. Microperimetry and other functional studies may be important parameters in the assessment of retinal function. These may help better determine which candidates are most likely to benefit.

REFERENCES

1. Tansley K. The development of the rat eye in graft. J Exp Biol. 1946;22:221–223.
2. Royo PE, Quay WB. Retinal transplantation from fetal to maternal mammalian eye. Growth. 1959;23:313–336.
3. del Cerro M, Gash DM, Rao GN, et al. Intraocular retinal transplants. Invest Ophthalmol Vis Sci. 1985;26:1182–1185.
4. Turner JE, Blair JR. Newborn rat retinal cells transplanted into a retinal lesion site in adult host eyes. Brain Res. 1986;26:91–104.
5. Gouras P, Du J, Gelanze M, et al. Transplantation of photoreceptors labeled with tritiated thymidine into RCS rats. Invest Ophthalmol Vis Sci. 1991;32:1704–1707.
6. Du J, Gouras P, Kjeldbye H, et al. Monitoring photoreceptor transplants with nuclear and cytoplasmic markers. Exp Neurol. 1992;115:79–86.
7. Lazar E, del Cerro M. A new procedure for multiple intraretinal transplantation in mammalian eyes. J Neurosci Methods. 1992;43:157–169.
8. Juliusson B, Bergstrom A, van Veen T, et al. Cellular organization in retinal transplants using cell suspensions or fragments of embryonic retinal tissue. Cell Transplant. 1993;2:411–418.
9. Gouras P, Algvere P. Retinal cell transplantation in the macula: new techniques. Vision Res. 1996;36:4121–4125.
10. Anchan RM, Reh TA, Angello J, et al. EGF and TGF-alpha stimulate retinal neuroepithelial cell proliferation in vitro. Neuron. 1991;6:923–936.
11. Coles BL, Angenieux B, Inoue T, et al. Facile isolation and the characterization of human retinal stem cells. Proc Natl Acad Sci U S A. 2004;101:15772–15777.
12. Banin E, Obolensky A, Idelson M, et al. Retinal incorporation and differentiation of neural precursors derived from human embryonic stem cells. Stem Cells. 2006;24:246–257.
13. MacLaren RE, Pearson RA, MacNeil A, et al. Retinal repair by transplantation of photoreceptor precursors. Nature. 2006;444:203–207.
14. Streilein JW. Immunoregulatory mechanisms of the eye. Prog Retin Eye Res. 1999;18:357–370.
15. Lamba DA, Gust J, Reh TA. Transplantation of human embryonic stem cell-derived photoreceptors restores some visual function in crx-deficient mice. Cell Stem Cell. 2009;4:73–79.
16. Delori FG, Goger DG, Dorey K. Age-related accumulation and spatial distribution of lipofuscin in RPE of normal subjects. Invest Ophthalmol Vis Sci. 2001;42:1855–1866.
17. Del Priore L, Newark NJ, Tezel TH, et al. The retinal pigment epithelium undergoes age-related apoptosis in human eyes. The Retina Society, USA, 33rd Annual Meeting, 2000; Coral Gables, FL.
18. Beatty S, Koh H-H, Phil M, et al. The role of oxidative stress in the pathogenesis of age-related macular degeneration. Surv Ophthalmol. 2000;454:115–134.
19. Cao W, Tombran-Tink J, Elias R, et al. In vivo protection of photoreceptors from light damage by pigment epithelium-derived factor. Invest Ophthalmol Vis Sci. 2001;42:1646–1652.
20. Mori K, Duh E, Gehlbach P, et al. Pigment epithelium-derived growth factor inhibits retinal and choroidal neovascularization. J Cell Physiol. 2001;188:253–263.
21. Kaplan HJ, Leibole MA, Tezel T, et al. Fas ligand (CD95 ligand) controls angiogenesis beneath the retina. Nat Med. 1999;5:292–297.
22. Chong NH, Keonin J, Luthert PJ, et al. Decreased thickness and integrity of the macular elastic layer of Bruch's membrane correspond to the distribution of lesions associated with age-related macular degeneration. Am J Pathol. 2005;166:241–251.
23. Booij JC, Baas DC, Beisekeeva J, et al. The dynamic nature of Bruch's membrane. Prog Retin Eye Res. 2010;29:1–18.
24. Okubo A, Rosa RH Jr, Bunce CV, et al. The relationships of age changes in retinal pigment epithelium and Bruch's membrane. Invest Ophthalmol Vis Sci. 1999;40:443–449.
25. van der Schaft TL, Mooy CM, de Bruijn WC, et al. Histologic features of the early stages of age-related macular degeneration. A statistical analysis. Ophthalmology. 1992;99:278–286.
26. Ramrattan RS, van der Schaft TL, Mooy CM, et al. Morphometric analysis of Bruch's membrane, the choriocapillaris, and the choroid in aging. Invest Ophthalmol Vis Sci. 1994;35:2857–2864.
27. Huang JD, Presley JB, Chimento MF, et al. Age-related changes in human macular Bruch's membrane as seen by quick-freeze/deep-etch. Exp Eye Res. 2007;85:202–218.
28. Moore DJ, Hussain AA, Marshall J. Age-related variation in the hydraulic conductivity of Bruch's membrane. Invest Ophthalmol Vis Sci. 1995;36:1290–1297.
29. Algvere PV, Gouras P, et al. Long-term outcome of RPE allografts in non-immunosuppressed patients with AMD. Eur J Ophthalmol. 1999;9:3:217–230.

30. Zhang X, Bok1 D. Transplantation of retinal pigment epithelial cells and immune response in the subretinal space. Invest Ophthalmol Vis Sci. 1998;39:1021–1027.

31. Lund RD, Wang S, et al. Human embryonic stem cell-derived cells rescue visual function in dystrophic RCS rats. Cloning Stem Cells. 2006;8:3:189–199.

32. Falkner-Radler CI, Krebs I, Glittenberg C, et al. Human Retinal Pigment Epithelium (RPE) transplantation. Outcome after autologous RPE-choroid sheet and RPE cell-suspension in a randomised clinical study. Br J Ophthalmol. 2011;95(3):431.

33. Peyman GA, Blinder KJ, Paris CJ, et al. A technique for retinal pigment epithelium transplantation for age-related macular degeneration secondary to extensive subfoveal scarring. Ophthalmic Surg. 1991;22:102.

34. van Meurs JC, ter Averst E, Croxen R, et al. Comparison of the growth potential of retinal pigment epithelial cells obtained during vitrectomy in patients with age-related macular degeneration or complex retinal detachment. Graefes Arch Clin Exp Ophthalmol. 2004;242:442–443.

35. Stanga PE, Kychenthal A, Fitzke FW, et al. Retinal pigment epithelium translocation after choroidal neovascular membrane removal in age-related macular degeneration. Ophthalmology. 2002;109:1492–1498.

36. Stanga PE, Kychenthal A, Fitzke FW, et al. Functional assessment of the native retinal pigment epithelium after the surgical excision of subfoveal choroidal neovascular membranes type II: preliminary results. Int Ophthalmol. 2001;23:309–316.

37. Tezel TH, Del Priore LV, Berger AS, et al. Adult retinal pigment epithelial transplantation in exudative age-related macular degeneration. Am J Ophthalmol. 2007;143:584–595.

38. Cereda MG, Parolini B, Elisa Bellesini E, et al. Surgery for CNV and autologous choroidal RPE patch transplantation: exposing the submacular space. Graefes Arch Clin Exp Ophthalmol. 2010;248:37–47.

39. van Meurs JC, ter Averst E, Hofland LJ, et al. Autologous peripheral retinal pigment epithelium translocation in patients with subfoveal neovascular membranes. Br J Ophthalmol. 2004;88:110–113.

40. Caramoy A, Liakopoulos S, Menrath E, et al. Autologous translocation of choroid and retinal pigment epithelium in geographic atrophy: long term functional and anatomical outcome. Br J Ophthalmol. 2010;94(8):1040–1044.

41. Maaijwee K, Heimann H, Missotten T, et al. Retinal pigment epithelium and choroid translocation in patients with exudative age-related macular degeneration: long-term results. Graefes Arch Clin Exp Ophthalmol. 2007;245: 1681–1689.

42. MacLaren RE, Uppal GS, Balaggan KS, et al. Autologous transplantation of the retinal pigment epithelium and choroid in the treatment of neovascular age-related macular degeneration. Ophthalmology. 2007;114:561–570.

INDEX

Note: Page numbers followed by "f" indicate figures; those followed by "t" indicate tabular material.